Psychology
for Nurses

Devinder Rana and Dominic Upton

PEARSON
Education

Harlow, England • London • New York • Boston • San Francisco • Toronto • Sydney • Singapore • Hong Kong
Tokyo • Seoul • Taipei • New Delhi • Cape Town • Madrid • Mexico City • Amsterdam • Munich • Paris • Milan

Pearson Education Limited
Edinburgh Gate
Harlow
Essex CM20 2JE
England

and Associated Companies throughout the world

Visit us on the World Wide Web at:
www.pearsoned.co.uk

First published 2009

ISBN: 978-0-13-200107-6

British Library Cataloguing-in-Publication Data
A catalogue record for this book is available from the British Library

Library of Congress Cataloging-in-Publication Data
A catalog record for this book is available from the Library of Congress

10 9 8 7 6 5 4 3 2 1
12 11 10 09 08

Typeset in 10/12.5pt Sabon by 30
Printed and bound by Graficas Estella, Navarro, Spain

The publisher's policy is to use paper manufactured from sustainable forests.

Brief Contents

Contents

Supporting resources

Visit **www.pearsoned.co.uk/rana** to find valuable online resources

Companion Website for students

- Extensive links to valuable resources on the web
- Self-assessment questions to check your understanding

For instructors

- PowerPoint slides that can be downloaded and used for presentations

Also: The Companion Website provides the following features:

- Search tool to help locate specific items of content
- E-mail results and profile tools to send results of quizzes to instructors
- Online help and support to assist with website usage and troubleshooting

For more information please contact your local Pearson Education sales representative or visit **www.pearsoned.co.uk/rana**

Guided Tour

Case study

Colin Butt is a 60-year-old builder who is currently working in his own business but is looking forward to retiring shortly. He has worked continuously since he started his apprenticeship when he was 15 years old, and he is very proud of his achievements. He is still married to Nicki, the woman he met when he was 16 years old. He has two grown-up children and three grandchildren he adores. He loves to play football in the back garden with his grandchildren but is finding himself getting breathless frequently and thus not being able to enjoy playing with them as much as he would like. His grandson – Billie – worships his grandfather. However, Colin has noticed that Billie has started acting like him, plays 'smoking cigarettes', is refusing to eat anything other than chips and certainly isn't eating his portions of fruit and vegetables every day. Colin has had Type II diabetes for a number of years but it has recently become more poorly controlled. He drinks alcohol and eats typical 'builder's meals': a traditional fry-up in the morning, a sandwich or a pie at lunchtime with a couple of pints and a large evening meal with his family later. Colin likes a couple of pints at lunchtime as he thinks it is good to get together with his colleagues but his major drinking is at the weekend when he goes out with his friends and his wife down the local club. Here, Colin can drink nearly 15 pints during an evening while he enjoys the relaxing and social environment in the pub. Colin has smoked cigarettes since he was a teenager. He used to smoke heavily but has recently cut down to about 15 cigarettes a day. He suffers from early peripheral vascular disease and has a mild degree of lower limb neuropathy. He has been attending the clinic for routine care and monitoring. In order to prevent development of the more negative consequences of his condition it is essential for Colin to stop smoking and improve his diet.

Colin knows that he has to stop smoking but he has been doing it for over 40 years and feels he cannot stop. He is also aware that this behaviour and his diet are poor and are adversely affecting his health. However, he does not think he can change either of these. He sees you in the clinic and you realise that his health is severely compromised by his behaviour and he must change it or suffer serious consequences. How would you go about this?

Why is this relevant to nursing practice?

Over 30 years ago, Belloc and Breslow (1972) reported the impact on mortality of seven different behaviours (so-called **behavioural immunogens**, those behaviours that can protect health):

- sleeping seven or eight hours a night;
- not smoking;
- consuming no more than two alcoholic drinks per day;
- getting regular exercise;
- not eating between meals;
- eating breakfast;
- being no more than 10 per cent overweight.

This study followed up over 7000 healthy adults for over 15 years. The results of the study indicated that there were benefits of completing these types of behaviour and that these benefits were cumulative. The more an individual engaged in the behaviours, the more likely they were to live to an older age (Figure 12.1). At the 15-year follow-up, fewer than 4 per cent of those who were engaged in all seven types of activities had died, compared with 7–13 per cent of those who performed fewer that four of these activities. Also of note

Case studies. Provide a range of scenarios across all branches of nursing, and demonstrate the role of psychology in nursing practice.

Definitions of health

There are a number of different definitions of health, which may vary from group to group and from individual to individual. At its most basic, a strong, fit swimmer may consider themselves unhealthy when they cannot swim 100 m in less than a minute, but some would consider this an exceptional performance. Others may consider healthy to be about going to the gym regularly, or eating a healthy breakfast (some may define this as the traditional 'British fry-up' whereas others would consider it muesli). Hence, there is no real agreement about what health is and how it should be defined. Obviously this has consequences in terms of measuring health and finding out whether the people we see are, indeed, healthy or not from our perspective (as a health care professional) and from theirs.

Think about this

Which one of these would you consider healthy: a happy new-age traveller who lives on the road and smokes 20 roll-up cigarettes a day; a person in a wheelchair who is an active member of the local basketball club; a rugby player who plays regularly but weighs 20 stone (125 kg) and drinks excessively at the weekend? How would you characterise the health of all these people? What does this mean for the definition of health? How will this influence your practice?

When you try to explore these definitions you realise that it is extremely difficult, but if you attempt to classify some of these descriptions you find that there is a form of consensus. For example, if you have words such as 'not being ill' or 'not having a cold' then these can be classified as a *negative* definition (i.e. something is missing). Alternatively, you may have definitions that are *positive* (i.e. something is there), for example being 'fit and well' or being described as 'being full of beans' or 'full of energy'. The definitions provided in this field can thus be broadly defined into three different groups: negative definitions, positive definitions and the rest (rather that a rag-bag of ideas) and each of these explanations will be explored in turn.

Negative definitions

Health can be defined as the *absence of something*. There are two main ways of seeing health negatively; the first equates it with the absence of disease or bodily **abnormality**. The second is the absence of illness. Obviously, it is important to note the difference between disease and illness (Wikman *et al.*, 2005): disease is the biological concomitant of ill-health and is diagnosed by the physician (the change in white blood cells, the presence of a bacterium or anatomical or physiological change) whereas illness is the subjective feeling of ill-health (for example, being in pain or discomfort).

Negative definitions of health refer to health as the absence of disease or illness. According to this definition people are healthy as long as they show no signs of bodily abnormality. If a person is not suffering any symptoms – they are not sneezing, coughing or aching for example and if they feel 'fit and well' – then they can be defined as healthy.

Think about this. Questions throughout the text encourage self-reflection and self-awareness in relation to practice.

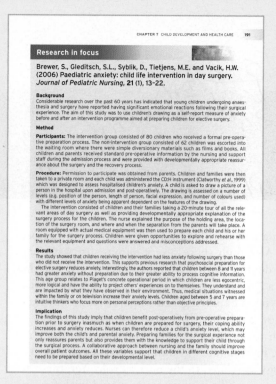

Research in focus

Brewer, S., Gleditsch, S.L., Syblik, D., Tietjens, M.E. and Vacik, H.W. (2006) Paediatric anxiety: child life intervention in day surgery. *Journal of Pediatric Nursing*, **21** (1), 13–22.

Background
Considerable research over the past 60 years has indicated that young children undergoing anaesthesia and surgery have reported having significant emotional reactions following their surgical experience. The aim of this study was to use children's drawing as a self-report measure of anxiety before and after an intervention programme aimed at preparing children for elective surgery.

Method
Participants: The intervention group consisted of 80 children who received a formal pre-operative preparation process. The non-intervention group consisted of 62 children was escorted into the waiting room where there were simple diversionary materials such as films and books. All children and parents received standard pre-operative information by the nursing and support staff during the admission process and were provided with developmentally appropriate reassurance about the surgery and the recovery process.

Procedure: Permission to participate was obtained from parents. Children and families were then taken to a private room and each child was administered the CD:H instrument (Clatworthy *et al*, 1999) which was designed to assess hospitalised children's anxiety. A child is asked to draw a picture of a person in the hospital upon admission and post-operatively. The drawing is assessed on a number of levels (e.g. position of the person, length of person, facial expression, and number of colours used) with different levels of anxiety being apparent dependent on the features of the drawing.

The intervention consisted of children and their families taking a 20-minute tour of all the relevant areas of day surgery as well as providing developmentally appropriate explanation of the surgery process for the children. The nurse explained the purpose of the holding area, the location of the surgery room, and where and when the separation from the parents will take place. A room equipped with actual medical equipment was then used to prepare each child and his or her family for the surgery process. Children were given opportunities to explore and rehearse with the relevant equipment and questions were answered and misconceptions addressed.

Results
The study showed that children receiving the intervention had less anxiety following surgery than those who did not receive the intervention. This supports previous research that psychosocial preparation for elective surgery reduces anxiety. Interestingly, the authors reported that children between 8 and 11 years had greater anxiety without preparation due to their greater ability to process cognitive information. This age group relates to Piaget's concrete operational period in which children are less egocentric, more logical and have the ability to project others' experiences on to themselves. They understand and are impacted by what they have observed in their environment. Thus, medical situations witnessed within the family or on television increase their anxiety levels. Children aged between 5 and 7 years are intuitive thinkers who focus more on personal perceptions rather than objective principles.

Implication
The findings of this study imply that children benefit post-operatively from pre-operative preparation prior to surgery inasmuch as when children are prepared for surgery, their coping ability increases and anxiety reduces. Nurses can therefore reduce a child's anxiety level, which may improve both the child's and parental anxiety. Preparing families for the surgical experience not only reassures parents but also provides them with the knowledge to support their child through the surgical process. A collaborative approach between nursing and the family should improve overall patient outcomes. All these variables support that children in different cognitive stages need to be prepared based on their developmental level.

Research in focus. These give examples of recent research in psychology, and show the relevance of this research to nursing practice.

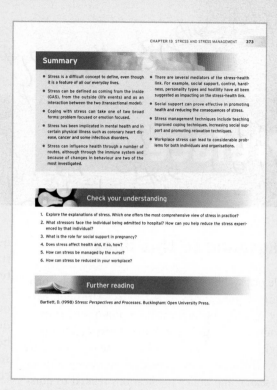

Summary

- Stress is a difficult concept to define, even though it is a feature of all our everyday lives.

- Stress can be defined as coming from the inside (GAS), from the outside (life events) and as an interaction between the two (transactional model).

- Coping with stress can take one of two broad forms: problem focused or emotion focused.

- Stress has been implicated in mental health and in certain physical illness such as coronary heart disease, cancer and some infectious disorders.

- Stress can influence health through a number of routes, although through the immune system and because of changes in behaviour are two of the most investigated.

- There are several mediators of the stress-health link. For example, social support, control, hardiness, personality types and hostility have all been suggested as impacting on the stress-health link.

- Social support can prove effective in promoting health and reducing the consequences of stress.

- Stress management techniques include teaching improved coping techniques, increasing social support and promoting relaxation techniques.

- Workplace stress can lead to considerable problems for both individuals and organisations.

Check your understanding

1. Explore the explanations of stress. Which one offers the most comprehensive view of stress in practice?

2. What stressors face the individual being admitted to hospital? How can you help reduce the stress experienced by that individual?

3. What is the role for social support in pregnancy?

4. Does stress affect health and, if so, how?

5. How can stress be managed by the nurse?

6. How can stress be reduced in your workplace?

Further reading

Bartlett, D. (1998) *Stress: Perspectives and Processes*. Buckingham: Open University Press.

Check your understanding. Questions at the end of each chapter test your knowledge, and act as a revision tool.

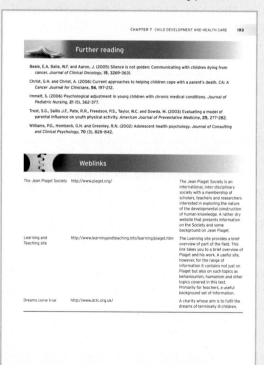

Further reading

Beale, E.A, Baile, W.F. and Aaron, J. (2005) Silence is not golden: Communicating with children dying from cancer. *Journal of Clinical Oncology*, **15**, 3269–3631.

Christ, G.H. and Christ, A. (2006) Current approaches to helping children cope with a parent's death. *CA: A Cancer Journal for Clinicians*, **56**, 197–212.

Immelt, S. (2006) Psychological adjustment in young children with chronic medical conditions. *Journal of Pediatric Nursing*, **21** (5), 362–377.

Trost, S.G., Sallis J.F., Pate, R.R., Freedson, P.S., Taylor, W.C. and Dowda, M. (2003) Evaluating a model of parental influence on youth physical activity. *American Journal of Preventative Medicine*, **25**, 277–282.

Williams, P.G., Hombeck, G.N. and Greenley, R.N. (2002) Adolescent health psychology. *Journal of Consulting and Clinical Psychology*, **70** (3), 828–842.

Weblinks

The Jean Piaget Society	http://www.piaget.org/	The Jean Piaget Society is an international, inter-disciplinary society with a membership of scholars, teachers and researchers interested in exploring the nature of the developmental construction of human knowledge. A rather dry website that presents information on the Society and some background on Jean Piaget.
Learning and Teaching site	http://www.learningandteaching.info/learning/piaget.htm	The Learning site provides a brief overview of part of the field. This link takes you to a brief overview of Piaget and his work. A useful site, however, for the range of information it contains not just on Piaget but also on such topics as behaviourism, humanism and other topics covered in this text. Primarily for teachers, a useful background set of information.
Dreams come true	http://www.dctc.org.uk/	A charity whose aim is to fulfil the dreams of terminally ill children.

Further reading and Weblinks. These will point the way forward for continued and more in-depth study.

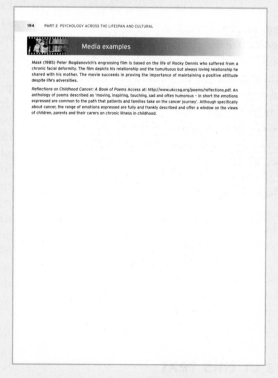

Media examples

Mask (1985) Peter Bogdanovich's engrossing film is based on the life of Rocky Dennis who suffered from a chronic facial deformity. The film depicts his relationship and the tumultuous but always loving relationship he shared with his mother. The movie succeeds in proving the importance of maintaining a positive attitude despite life's adversities.

Reflections on Childhood Cancer: A Book of Poems Access at: http://www.ukccsg.org/poems/reflections.pdf. An anthology of poems described as 'moving, inspiring, touching, sad and often humorous – in short the emotions expressed are common to the path that patients and families take on the cancer journey'. Although specifically about cancer, the range of emotions expressed are fully and frankly described and offer a window on the views of children, parents and their carers on chronic illness in childhood.

Media examples: Illuminate topics in psychology in books, films and plays.

Preface

Background to this book

The role of psychology in nursing practice has become ever more significant in recent years. Although psychology has always had a role in nursing education and practice (although it was not always called psychology), in recent years this has come ever more to the fore. This has led to an increase in the number of texts, research and policy publications related to nursing, health care and psychology. This substantial body of literature has formed the backdrop to this book. We have read many (or perhaps, in reality, *some*) of these publications – from the classic texts of yesteryear (i.e. anything before 2000!) and those more recent. However, we are not claiming that we have read all of these publications – an impossible task. Nonetheless, we have read, for the preparation of this text, hundreds of such papers and we hope that this academic rigour comes through.

More important than simply the number of publications, however, was the interpretation and presentation of these. We wanted to write a psychology textbook that would be academic in tone and presentation and would be useful and relevant to student nurses from all backgrounds and with a range of professional aspirations. In this way we wanted to be inclusive and demonstrate the importance of psychology in both the nursing role and in health care in general. We are both passionate about psychology and communicating its relevance and effectiveness in nursing practice. We hope that this comes through.

Aims of this text

The aims of the text were, therefore, to be inclusive and to demonstrate the value of psychology in nursing and health care from a European perspective. Although there are a number of American texts dealing with psychology, there are few that have a European perspective. There are, of course, other texts exploring health psychology but these do not explicitly link psychological aspects of health to the nursing role. Furthermore, there are some, more limited in number, texts exploring psychology as related to the nursing role. Yet, these are not as comprehensive as many would wish for, and may omit some key aspects of psychology that have a direct bearing and relevance to health care. We have tried, therefore, to cover all the psychological aspects and concepts that have a direct role in health care.

This has proved a contentious decision and there are competing perspectives on what the limits of psychology are. So, for example, there is some debate about social class and health – should this be included in a psychology textbook? What about the sociological definitions of health? Or the physiological components of pain and stress? We have included these issues, along with other material that some may argue is not the true province of psychology. We did not aim to be restrictive and narrow in our definition – we want to be inclusive and therefore our definition of psychology is broad, including the social and biological arms of the subject. We apologise if this upsets the purists but we think the relevance and importance of psychology deserve this inclusivity.

This book has been approached with two aims in mind. Firstly, for the student nurse to become familiar with how the role of psychology and health psychology can be applied to nursing and health care practice. Secondly, for the student nurse to be able to apply theories and ideas to both their own placement practice and student nurse portfolios. This has been included in particular sections of the book, and reflection and self-awareness are emphasised – a core theme throughout nurse portfolios and clinical placements. Reflection, self-awareness, communication and care plan construction are also included in various chapters. There are also sections dedicated to cycles of reflection, and what is involved in reflection. All of these should be useful for a nurse as they form a necessary part of the student nurse training and learning experience – along with being a key component of life-long learning.

Psychology has many perspectives that enable the nurse student to appreciate the individuality and diversity of patients. This is important in the construction and delivery of individualised care plans as stated throughout nursing courses and, of course, the Nursing and Midwifery Code of Conduct. Material presented in this text includes specific material dedicated to explaining how this can be successfully achieved in practice.

Creating a Patient Led NHS – Delivering the NHS Improvement Plan (DoH, 2005a) is a Government health paper that highlights the importance of patient-centredness, including patient choice and needs that should be addressed within any interaction with a patient. Hopefully, this book builds on the vision of such government statements and encourages the reader to appreciate the input psychology can have with such emerging visions of the future. There are, of course, many other policy developments that highlight the importance of a patient-centred NHS, ill-health prevention and promoting health and well-being (e.g. *Our Health, Our Care, Our Say: A New Direction for Community Services*, 2006); *Independence, Well-being and Choice. Our Vision for the Future of Social Care for Adults in England*, 2005) in which psychology has a key role to play.

Structure of this book

We thought long and hard about the structure of this book and it has evolved over its writing to the present state. At the outset, we knew the content, we knew how we wanted to present the material, we knew the order of the material we thought we knew the structure. So what was our problem? The difficulty was in the individual chapters: how could

we differentiate the material, indeed should we differentiate it? Ultimately, the final chapter structure we settled on was as follows:

Part 1 Basic principles

This first part outlines the underlying approaches to explaining behaviour from different schools of thought in psychology. So, for example, the approaches to explaining behaviour from a behavioural and cognitive perspective are presented. Within this chapter we also explore the social psychological concepts that may be important in nursing and health care. However, another basic principle is also introduced in this part: that of health, what it is, how it is defined and how it can be measured. The chapters in this part therefore include:

1. The meaning and measurement of health
2. The principles of behaviourist psychology
3. Patient-centred nursing
4. Anxiety and psychodynamic principles
5. Cognitive psychology
6. Social psychology

Thus, we hope that this part has set the scene for the rest of the text – both from a psychological and a health care perspective.

Part 2 Psychology across the lifespan and cultures

In this part the use of psychology when nursing individuals from different cultures and age groups will be explored. Hence, the first chapter explores how psychological explanations of child development can be applied to health and illness and ultimately how it can be used to further the nursing role. The subsequent chapters explore how the social factors in adulthood (for example social class and gender) and culture can impact on health. The final chapters deal with the elderly and then loss, death and dying. Death and dying come to us all and it is not necessarily when we are old – death can come to children, teenagers and young adults. However, we have put it at the end of the part as a full stop: it is the end of life.

The chapters in this part were:

7. Child development and health care
8. The impact of social group on health

9. Cultural awareness and transcultural issues
10. Working with older adults
11. Patient loss, bereavement and terminal illness

Part 3 Health psychology

This part explores health psychological concepts and how they can be applied to nursing. For example, the concept of stress is outlined – how it is defined and its consequences on health status, followed by how psychology can be used in nursing to reduce stress both by the nurse and for the nurse. Similarly, there are chapters on social cognition models – loved by health psychologists – and how they can be applied to the practical role of the nurse. There are also chapters on the psychological approaches to, and management of, pain, adherence to treatment and how it can be improved, the psychological consequences of entering hospital and how behaviours risky to an individual's health can be both explained and modified by psychological techniques. Hence, the chapters in this part include:

12. Risky behaviours: smoking, alcohol, diet and exercise
13. Stress and stress management
14. The psychology of pain
15. Psychological models in health and health care
16. Exploring patient adherence to medical information and lifestyle change
17. Communication and counselling skills
18. Being admitted to hospital

Part 4 Practical applications

This is the final part and consists of just two chapters. It draws on the information presented in all the previous chapters to demonstrate how they can be applied to particular illnesses and treatments. The shortness of this part should not hide its importance – the models relevance of the research material cited in other parts is highlighted and related to the practice of nursing and health care. These chapters, we hope, bring together the complete text. The final chapters are:

19. Applying psychology to specific conditions: part I
20. Applying psychology to specific conditions: part II

Is this book for you?

This book is geared towards those nursing students during their undergraduate studies, but it works equally well for those on postgraduate courses that require an additional psychological component. Students on any nursing branch will find the text useful, as will those on midwifery programmes. We also hope that practising nurses and other health care professionals will find some value in this text and it can act as a useful reference text.

Features of this book

We have tried to use a variety of pedagogical devices throughout this book with the intent of focusing the reader, reiterating the relevance of key points, and acting as a revision device. At the outset of the chapters we have tried to orientate the reader and demonstrate the relevance of the topic by starting all chapters with a case study followed by a clear exposition of why the topic is relevant to nursing practice. We have also included inserts throughout the individual chapters in order to demonstrate key points and promote learning. For example, all chapters include 'Think about this' boxes which ask the reader to consider a specific issue related to an individual topic under discussion. Obviously you can do this by yourself, or with a colleague in order to increase your learning. There are also 'Research in focus' boxes. These highlight a research report that has been completed in a certain area and the relevance of this academic research to nursing practice.

Finally, we have also included a series of sources of further information at the end of each chapter. For example:

- **Future reading:** We have included a number of items that will provide additional information – some of these are in journals and some are full texts.
- **Media examples:** We have also presented some media examples that we hope will illuminate a particular topic in an entertaining (and often) humorous manner. Some are books, others films and some plays or poems.
- **Web resources:** These weblinks can be accessed with minimum of fuss and immediately so we

hope you can gather up-to-date information as soon as you have completed the reading of the chapter. Unfortunately, a caveat: we checked all of these weblinks when writing and just before publishing. However, some of these can become dated rather quickly and the exact address may change – apologies, but this is beyond our control. We have set up a web page for these weblinks and we hope that they will remain more up to date.

- **Summary points**: At the end of each chapter we present a summary of the chapter in a series of bullet points. We hope that these will match the learning outcomes presented at the outset of the chapter.
- **Check your understanding**: In order to assess your awareness of the topic we have also produced a series of questions for you to discuss and debate with your colleagues. You can also use these questions as revision materials.

Throughout the text, links will be made to contemporary literature and studies drawn from the professions' research base in order to exemplify points will be outlined. This is an important point that we should stress: the clinical examples we have provided have come from events we are familiar with. We have selected them because they provide clear examples of how research and evidence-based material can be applied to the nursing role. However, these clinical examples can also be applied to other professions and the underlying values and principles explored will be relevant to all health professionals. For some cases it may appear as if the cases have been created to include every single disastrous event that could possibly occur, and to a certain extent this is true. However, each of the cases has some basis in reality. We have come across cases that have made our hearts bleed and have challenged every sinew of our professional practice. We have had to tone down some of these cases so they do not appear too unrealistic and imaginative. We hope that these examples and the text in general will help improve the psychological care that these patients and clients deserve.

There is a full glossary at the end of the book which includes the definitions of various words and phrases that either may not be immediately familiar or are technical in nature.

Supplementary material

There is a website to accompany the text, the details of which are presented at the end of this section. This book and its accompanying materials are not a substitute for your lectures and seminars but it should form part of your learning experience – make the most of all the resources available to you.

Acknowledgements

This project has been a major undertaking for both of us and has involved the reading and reviewing of a considerable number of research and review papers published in psychological, nursing and health care journals, texts and websites for both researcher and practitioner. This reading has helped us identify some of the key issues facing nursing from both practice and research. We obviously thank the researchers, clinicians and policy makers for all this work and the contributions they have made to the current knowledge base.

On a more personal level, several key colleagues have acted as informal reviewers for each of our chapters: they have provided honest and robust reviews of our work for which we are truly thankful (although sometimes we felt the bruises!). They have spotted errors and inconsistencies that were inevitable during the first draft – we hope that we have ironed them all out during this final, published, version. However, if any errors remain we accept, of course, ultimate responsibility. We also thank those who acted as formal reviewers for their thorough feedback. Furthermore, the comments from our student reviewers were constructive and valuable and we thank them for their unique insight.

Many thanks also to the team at Pearson Education for helping us through this project: Kate Brewin for her support throughout the project, and the constant nagging, constructive comments and encouragement from the rottweiler that was Peter Hooper. We also thank those in the production of the project – the designers and production editors for enhancing the text with some excellent features, which we hope has provided guidance, direction and added value for all readers.

We must offer thanks and acknowledge those that have provided the support both at work and at home. First, thanks to our friends and colleagues at the University of Worcester and Birmingham City University for their help, advice, friendship and practical guidance. Obviously, we would also like to thank our many students. Some were excellent students – we learnt from you. Some were terrible and made us think and made us work harder. Some were there begrudgingly but we hope at the end of the sessions, you appreciated the value and experience of psychology and the role it has to your professional practice.

Finally, we would also like to thank our family for bringing us sustenance and calming us down during our manic periods when we could think of nothing else other than 'the book'. So special thanks to Penney (Ken), Francesca, Rosanna and Gabriel. Also thanks to Balbir and Jass for being there and a special thank you to Kashmira Singh Rana (deceased) who was and always will be an inspiration to me, who sadly passed away during this project.

Aknowledgements

We are grateful to the following for permission to reproduce copyright material:

Table 1.1 from *Health and Illness: the Lay Perspective*, Calnan, M., London: Tavistock Publications (1987); Table 3.1 from Reynolds, W., Scott, P. and Austin, W., Nursing, empathy and perception of the moral, *Journal of Advanced Nursing*, Blackwell Publishing Ltd.; Figure 3.2 from J. Prochaska and C. Diclemente (1986) Towards a comprehensive model of change, in *Treating addictive behaviours: Processes of change*, Miller, W. and Heather, N. (eds), Copyright © 1986 Plenum Press, New York, with kind permission of Springer Science and Business Media; Figure 5.1 from Morris, Charles G.; Maisto, Albert A., *Understanding Psychology*, 6th Edition, © 2003, p. 203. Reprinted by permission of Pearson Education, Inc., Upper Saddle River, NJ; Table 5.1 from Delp, C. and Jones, J. (1996) Communicating information to patients: the use of cartoon illustrations to improve comprehension of instructions, *Academic Emergency Medicine*, 3, 264–70, Blackwell Publishing; un-numbered table, p. 118 © Stokes, 2000. *Challenging Behaviour in Dementia*. Reproduced with kind permission; Table 6.1 from Tuckman, B.W. (1965) Developmental sequences in small groups in *Psychological Bulletin*, 63 (6) 384–99, APA, reprinted and adapted with permission; Figure 6.2 from Joseph Luft, *Of Human Interaction* (1969), Mayfield Publishing Company, reproduced with permission of The McGraw-Hill Companies; Figure 6.3 from *Learning by Doing: A Guide to Teaching and Learning Methods*, Further Education Unit, (Gibbs, G. 1988); Table 6.4 from Aggressive incidents on a psychiatric intensive care unit, *Nursing Standard*, 14 (35), 33–36 (Saverimuttu, A. and Lowe, T. 2000); Table 6.5 from Hogg, M.A. and Vaughan, G. (2002) *Social Psychology*, 3rd Edition, Harlow: Pearson Prentice Hall; Figure 7.1 Reprinted from *Journal of Pediatric Nursing*, Vol. 21 (2), McCarthy, A.M. and Kleiber, C., A conceptual model of factors influencing children's responses to a painful procedure when parents are distraction coaches, pp. 88–98, Copyright 2006, with permission from Elsevier; Figure 7.2 from Holmbeck, G.N. and Shapera, W.E. (1999) Research methods with adolescents in *Handbook of Research Methods in Clinical Psychology*, 2nd Edition. New York: Wiley, (Kendall, P.C., Butcher, J.N. and Holbeck, G.N. [Eds]); Figures 8.1, 8.2, 8.3 and 8.5, Tables 9.1 and 10.1 Source: National Statistics website: www.statistics.gov.uk Crown copyright material is reproduced with the permission of the Controller Office of Public Sector Information (OPSI); un-numbered table, p. 272 from Schaie, K. Warner; Willis, Sherry L., *Adult Development And Aging*, 5th Edition, © 2002, Pgs. 16–17. Reprinted by permission of Pearson Education, Inc., Upper Saddle River, NJ; Table 11.2 from *Bereavement Studies of Grief in Adult Life*, Parkes, C.M., London: Tavistock Publications (1986); Figure 12.1 Reprinted from *Preventative Medicine*, Vol. 1 (3), Belloc, N.B. and Breslow, L. Relationship of physical health status and health practices, pp. 409–421, Copyright 1972, with permission from Elsevier; Table 13.1 Reprinted from *Journal of Psychosomatic Research*, Vol. 11 (2), Holmes, T.H. and Rahe, R.H., The social readjustment rating scale, pp. 213–218, Copyright 1967, with permission from Elsevier; Table 13.2 from The hassle assessment scale for students in college: measuring the frequency and unpleasantness of and dwelling on stress events in *Journal of American College Health*, 48 (2), 75–83, Heldref Publications, (Sarafino, E.P. and Ewing, M. 1999); Table 13.3 from Folkman, S. and

Lazarus, R.S., Coping as a mediator of emotion in *Journal of Personality and Social Psychology*, **54** (3), 466–475 (1988), APA, reprinted and adapted with permission; Figure 14.1 from The McGill pain questionnaire: major properties and scoring methods in *Pain*, 1 (Melzack, R. 1975); Figure 14.2 Wong-Baker FACES pain rating scale from Hockenberry, M.J., Wilson, D., Winkelstein, M.L. *Wong's Essentials of Pediatric Nursing*, ed. 7, St. Louis, 2005, p. 1259. Used with permission. Copyright, Mosby; Figure 14.3 Neurological transmission of pain stimuli from http://www.wildirismedicaleducation.com/courses/127/index_nceu.html; Figure 14.4 from *Health Psychology: Biopsychosocial Interactions* 5th Edition, John Wiley & Sons, Inc. (Sarafino, E.P. 2005); Figure 15.1 from *Sexual Behaviour in Britain*, London: Penguin, (Wellings, K. et al. 1994); Figures 15.2, 15.6, 15.7 and 19.2 from Ogden, J. (2004) *Health Psychology: A Textbook*, 3rd Edition, Open University Press. Reproduced with the kind permission of the Open University Press Publishing Company; Figures 15.4 and 15.5 from Stroebe, W. (2000) *Social Psychology and Health*, 2nd Edition, Open University Press. Reproduced with the kind permission of the Open University Press Publishing Company; Table 16.1 from Patient-centered communication: do patients really prefer it? in *Journal of General Internal Medicine*, **19** (11), 1069–1079, Blackwell Publishing (Swenson, S.L., Buell, S., Zettler, P., White, M., Ruston, D.C., and Lo, B. 2004) With kind permission from Springer Science and Business Media; figure on p. 469 from Egan. *The Skilled Helper*, 5th Edition. © 1994 Wadsworth, a part of Cengage Learning, Inc. Reproduced by permission. www.cengage.com/permissions; figure on p. 472 reproduced by permission of SAGE Publications, London, Los Angeles, New Delhi and Singapore, from Heron, J., *Helping the client: A creative practical guide* 5th Edition, Copyright (© John Heron, 1975, 2001); Figure 19.1 from Cancer Research UK, http://info.cancerresearchuk.org/cancerstats/types/breast/survival/, (accessed November 2007); Figure 20.1 from Andersen, B.L., Kiecolt-Glaser, J.K. and Glaser, R., A biobehavioural model of cancer stress and disease course, *American Psychologist*, **49** (5) 389–404, 1994, APA, reprinted with permission.

Photographs (key: b-bottom; c-centre; l-left; r-right; t-top): **Advertising Archives:** 189, 319; **Alamy Images:** Alaska Stock LLC 84; Allstar Picture Library 45; Allstar Pictures 264; Bubbles Photolibrary 278; Christopher Baines 464r; Geoffrey Kidd 443t; Mary Evans Picture Library 83; Peter Banos 448; Phototake Inc. 41; Picture Partners 211tr; Profimedia International 211tl; Watergate Creative 118; **Corbis:** Adrianna Williams/Zefa 238; Comstock 134, 143; Dan McGowan/Illustration Works 335bl; Dmitri Baltermants/Collection 383; Douglas Pearson 346; Heide Benser/Zefa 463tl; Laura Dwight 172; Ralph A Clevenger 14; Reuters 310; **Getty Images:** 176, 337; **Kobal Collection Ltd:** MGM 214; **PA Photos:** 509; **Photo Edit Inc:** 252, 270, 390; **Rex Features:** ABC/Everett 31; **Science Photo Library Ltd:** 381; Christian Darkin 335br; Doug Goodman 170; **Shout Pictures:** John Callan 231; **University of Wales, Bangor:** University of Wales, Bangor 335t.

Research in focus, p. 293 reprinted with the permission of Scribner, an imprint of Simon & Schuster Adult Publishing Group, from *On Death and Dying*, Elisabeth Kubler-Ross. Copyright © 1969 by Elisabeth Kubler-Ross; copyright renewed ©1997 by Elisabeth Kubler-Ross. All rights reserved. Reproduced also by permission of Taylor & Francis Books UK; ABCDEs of Delivering Bad News, p. 300 from Beyond breaking bad news: how to help patients who suffer in *Western Journal of Medicine* 171 (4), 260–263, (Rabow, M.W. and McPhee, S.J. 1999), adapted and reproduced with permission from the BMJ Publishing Group; The Twelve Steps of Alcoholics Anonymous (p.330). The Twelve Steps are reprinted with permission of Alcoholics Anonymous World Services, Inc. (A.A.W.S.) Permission to reprint the Twelve Steps does not mean that A.A.W.S. has reviewed or approved the contents of this publication, or that A.A.W.S. necessarily agrees with the views expressed herein. A.A. is a program of recovery from alcoholism only – use of the Twelve Steps in connection with programs and activities which are patterned after A.A., but which address other problems, or in any other non-A.A. context, does not imply otherwise; Dialogue page 398 from *Pain Management: A Handbook of Psychological Treatment Approaches*, Elmsford, NY: Pergamon Press, (Holzman, A.D. and Turk, D.C. (eds) 1986); Typical Distraction Techniques for Children, p. 396 from Incorporating psychological approaches into routine paediatric venepuncture in *Archives of Disease in Childhood*, 2003, Vol. **88**, 931–937, (Duff, A.J.A. 2003), reproduced with permission from the BMJ Publishing Group; The Threatening Medical Situations Inventory, p. 501 reprinted from *Personality and Individual Differences*, Vol. **21** (1), van Zuuren, F.J., de Groot, K.I., Mulder, N.L. and Muris, P., Coping with medical threat: an evaluation of the threatening medical situations inventory (T.M.S.I.), pp. 21–31, Copyright 1996, with permission from Elsevier.

In some instances we have been unable to trace the owners of copyright material, and we would appreciate any information that would enable us to do so.

Part 1
Basic principles

Part 1

Basic principles

Chapter 1

The meaning and measurement of health

Learning outcomes

When you have read through this chapter you should understand:

- How health has been defined by professionals and by the general public.
- How the definition of health differs among different groups of society.
- Why the definition of health is important to the practising nurse.
- The development and importance of the biopsychosocial model of health and illness.
- The role of illness behaviours in seeking out health care.
- How health can be measured.
- How the different measurement techniques can be used by the nurse in developing and assessing interventions.

Case study

Margaret Bruce is a 60-year-old woman who lives in a one-bedroom flat on the 21st floor of a tower block in a 'poor' area of her home town. Her block of flats was built several decades ago and is now suffering from the passage of time – it is both damp and vandalised, being covered with graffiti with the lift regularly out of order or being defaced by some of the local youths. There are very few shops or amenities nearby, other than a single corner shop at which Mrs Bruce has worked for a number of years, part time as a shelf stacker and check-out operator. She works from 10.00am until 3.00pm so she can look after her grandchildren when they come home from school. She enjoys the work and likes the flexibility and the social interaction that it offers. Other than this she rarely goes out, although she does play bingo once a week at the local centre. However, her primary pleasure is her grandchildren – Mrs Bruce enjoys spending time with her grandchildren, who bring joy and pleasure into her life.

The shop is regularly subjected to vandalism and has installed additional security lights and shutters to deal with the almost constant harassment from local teenagers. The owner has threatened to close down the shop if there are too many incidents of further vandalism. The local youths tend to 'run riot' – for example there are many joyriders – during the night-time and because of this the older residents tend not to go out of their homes at night. The locals claim it is because they are bored and have nothing to do – there is no community centre in the locality – and unemployment rates are above average.

Mrs Bruce lives alone and has done for the previous 15 years when she split from her last partner. She has one daughter, a lone parent, who lives in a nearby block of flats with her two children, Steve and Chloe. Mrs Bruce helps to look after her grandchildren, enabling her daughter to work part time and also to have an occasional break from childcare.

Once a month she attends her GP surgery for her blood pressure to be checked by the community nurse. She has high blood pressure which is exacerbated by Mrs Bruce smoking and being obese. She also has diabetes mellitus which is also being exacerbated by her behaviours. The GP surgery is near her grandchildren's school so it is convenient. It is also in the centre of town so the appointment is also an opportunity for her do to some shopping in the main shops.

Mrs Bruce has been a patient at the GP practice for a number of years and has developed a friendly and comfortable relationship with the nurse who takes her blood pressure. Over the recent months, however, the nurse has noticed that Mrs Bruce appears somewhat fraught and anxious – the conversation is no longer going well but is rather stilted and Mrs Bruce appears distant. The nurse has also recently noticed that Mrs Bruce has begun to smell and is wearing a number of layers of clothes, which is inappropriate given the weather. When this was mentioned to Mrs Bruce she became defensive and said she was tired – mainly because of a lack of sleep due to the pressures of looking after her grandchildren and holding down her job. As time progresses, the smell becomes more obvious until the nurse feels obliged to question further and become more direct. At this point Mrs Bruce finally breaks down and reveals that she had been very worried about her health for some months – she is tired, anxious and has no energy and asks the nurse if she can show her what the problem is: 'I have no one else to turn to and need some advice on whether this is important or not'.

Mrs Bruce unbuttons her blouse and removes layers of bandages and padding from her breast, finally revealing what is obviously a fungating tumour. The wound is deep, with a purulent, offensive discharge.

Why is this relevant to nursing practice?

There are a number of reasons why this is important to your practice. Why didn't Mrs Bruce tell the nurse about the problem when it first started? She has a good rapport with the nurse and had been seeing her for a number of years. If people get ill and have strange and serious symptoms surely they will report it to the health care services? We have a free NHS service that has access for all.

If we look at the case study there may be a number of important factors in this case. For example, Mrs Bruce may be scared that she will be given a diagnosis of cancer since she may believe that this is always fatal and she couldn't deal with it. Alternatively, she may also be concerned about letting her daughter and grandchildren down: worrying that treatment might involve hospitalisation. In addition, a stay in hospital would mean that she could not care for the grandchildren, and hence her daughter would have to start caring for them full time, which would mean that she would lose her job as well. The grandchildren are the love of Mrs Bruce's life and she fears that if she is not able to help out with their care in the short term then her daughter will be forced to give up work. This would, obviously, have negative consequences as she will lose her carer role with her grandchildren, which could result in her losing contact with them – something that she fears beyond everything else. She also believes that cancer treatment is serious and long term. This would mean that she would lose her job, which would have knock-on effects for her both financially and socially.

This case example highlights the important concepts of illness behaviour and perceptions of illness. The way that Mrs Bruce has perceived her symptoms is not the same way as everyone would perceive it. Some people, for example, would go to the GP at the first sign of anything amiss. Hence the same 'illness' or 'symptom' may be experienced differently by different people and has different meanings for them. Consequently, different people behave in different ways when they perceive their illness (Kasl and Cobb, 1966).

Furthermore (as we can see from Mrs Bruce), the patient's perception of symptoms may not correlate with the seriousness of the condition (as we, as health care professionals, may define it). Patients' perceptions of illness or disease severity often have a cultural component, and the manner in which the individual is meant to respond is then culturally determined. This culture is not simply restricted to the differences among different countries but also includes the differences between different groups in society – the way a woman defines her health may differ from a man. The way somebody in the working class defines their health may differ from somebody in the higher social classes.

There are a number of factors that may influence a patient's perception of their illness – for example their previous experience and knowledge of that condition (hence our perception as health care professionals will always differ from that of the lay public). We also know from our own experience that symptoms do not always result in consultation with a health care professional. When people experience unusual, abnormal or persistent symptoms, they may turn to a number of resources available to them. On the one hand, they may use the local pharmacy or an alternative therapist, or they may turn to what is known as the '**lay referral system**'. This involves consulting family and friends for advice about their condition. More importantly, it is through the lay referral system that the patient learns how they are *meant to respond* to the symptoms in a way that is normatively acceptable.

Seeking professional help may be further delayed as a result of fear, ignorance of the condition and embarrassment. The way in which patients describe their symptoms varies widely and is also affected by cultural and demographic factors. Many people who experience symptoms choose to wait to see whether they develop further before seeking professional advice (Wikman *et al.*, 2005).

Perspectives on health

Knowledge of health and illness grew rapidly during the eighteenth and nineteenth centuries with the development of new techniques and equipment. Scientists began to learn how the body functioned and, just as importantly, how it went wrong. At this stage they realised that micro-organisms caused certain diseases and therefore rejected the humoral theories of the past. These advancements led to the conceptualisation of health and illness according to a particular approach: the **biomedical** model.

The biomedical model suggested that the causes of illness were outside the control of the individual: all physical disorders can be explained by disturbances in physiological processes, which result from injury, biochemical imbalance, bacterial or viral infections and so on. Hence, there was a need for a biomedical treatment (e.g. vaccination, surgery, medication) administered by a trained medical professional. Psychology had very little role in either health or illness and no relationship was postulated between the mind and physical illness (so-called '**Cartesian dualism**'). This perspective on health and illness held sway for a number of years and still represents the dominant view in medicine today.

However, during the twentieth century there was a challenge to the biomedical model and the realisation that a simple biomedical explanation for all illnesses is not sufficient (Engel, 1977, 1980). For example, it was noted that lifestyle could impact on health and that certain stresses could cause illness. In light of this a new perspective was promoted: the **biopsychosocial** model of health and illness. This new model proposed that biological, psychological and social factors were all important. Specifically, all three factors affect health and are affected by the person's health.

An important development for the patient from the biomedical to the biopsychosocial model is that in the former the individual is seen as a passive recipient of treatment. They have 'caught' or developed the illness or injury and hence they are not responsible for their illness: they are merely regarded as 'victims' of external forces. Consequently, the patient is no longer responsible for their health and their treatment. The treatment is something that is 'done to them' by the trained medical profession.

In contrast to this, the biopsychosocial model considers illness to be a result of a number of factors and hence the individual is no longer simply seen as a passive individual: the person can contribute to their health and to their ill-health. This has consequences when we come to explore who has responsibility for treatment. The person is no longer a passive victim but takes an active role in their treatment: they are responsible for taking their medication (for example) and, more importantly, for changing their beliefs and behaviours.

If we explore what causes illness from a biopsychosocial perspective then it is not simply a case of looking for a biological causative agent or physiological or genetic marker, we have to look additionally at both social and psychological factors.

Bio	Psycho	Social
Viruses	Behaviour	Class
Bacteria	Beliefs	Gender
Genetics	Stress	Ethnicity

Biological factors are, perhaps, more apparent and include such factors as the genetic make-up of the individual along with anatomy and physiology and chemical balance. Illness is caused by involuntary physical changes caused by such factors as chemical imbalance, bacteria, viruses and genetic predisposition.

Psychological factors include such variables as lifestyle (e.g. smoking, drinking) and personality. It also includes such variables as cognition – thinking and interpreting – and beliefs. For example, if you believe that smoking is not bad for you and looks cool, then you are more likely to smoke than if you held more negative thoughts about the behaviour. Emotional factors are also important in determining whether we seek out medical or some other form of health care assistance. Motivational factors are another factor under the psychological variable: if we are motivated when we start an exercise programme we are more likely to keep up with the programme.

Social factors are both broad and deep. All of us live in a social world – we all have relationships with others, whether these be our family, our friends or our work colleagues. Children may start smoking if their peer group encourages it because it may make them feel more grown up. These may be referred to as social **norms** of behaviour (whether it is OK to smoke or thought 'cool' to drink to excess), social values on health (e.g. as we have seen with Mrs Bruce whether her peer group considers health to be the primary factor) and the pressures to change behaviour (expectations from parents or friends). But as we will see in Chapter 8 there is a range of other social influences on health – our social class, our sex and ethnic group for example.

Think about this

Consider a person who comes to you after suffering a myocardial infarction/heart attack. What biological, psychological and social factors could be implicated? Is any one of the factors alone sufficient?

Now consider how you would treat them: what intervention would you suggest? How would you employ psychological and social variables?

Definitions of health

There are a number of different definitions of health, which may vary from group to group and from individual to individual. At its most basic, a strong, fit swimmer may consider themselves unhealthy when they cannot swim 100 m in less than a minute, but some would consider this an exceptional performance. Others may consider themselves healthy if they can 'get through the day'. Others may consider healthy to be about going to the gym regularly, or eating a healthy breakfast (some may define this as the traditional 'British fry-up' whereas others would consider it muesli). Hence, there is no real agreement about what health is and how it should be defined. Obviously this has consequences in terms of measuring health and finding out whether the people we see are, indeed, healthy or not from our perspective (as a health care professional) and from theirs.

Think about this

Which one of these would you consider healthy: a happy new-age traveller who lives on the road and smokes 20 roll-up cigarettes a day; a person in a wheelchair who is an active member of the local basketball club; a rugby player who plays regularly but weighs 20 stone (125 kg) and drinks excessively at the weekend? How would you characterise the health of all these people? What does this mean for the definition of health? How will this influence your practice?

When you try to explore these definitions you realise that it is extremely difficult, but if you attempt to classify some of these descriptions you find that there is a form of consensus. For example, if you have words such as 'not being ill' or 'not having a cold' then these can be classified as a *negative* definition (i.e. something is missing). Alternatively, you may have definitions that are *positive* (i.e. something is there), for example being 'fit and well' or being described as 'being full of beans' or 'full of energy'. The definitions provided by experts in this field can thus be broadly defined into three different groups: negative definitions, positive definitions and the rest (rather that a rag-bag of ideas) and each of these explanations will be explored in turn.

Negative definitions

Health can be defined as the *absence of something*. There are two main ways of seeing health negatively; the first equates it with the absence of disease or bodily **abnormality**. The second is the absence of illness. Obviously, it is important to note the difference between disease and illness (Wikman *et al.*, 2005): disease is the biological concomitant of ill-health and is diagnosed by the physician (the change in white blood cells, the presence of a bacterium or anatomical or physiological change) whereas illness is the subjective feeling of ill-health (for example, being in pain or discomfort).

Negative definitions of health refer to health as the absence of disease or illness. According to this definition people are healthy as long as they show no signs of bodily abnormality. If a person is not suffering any symptoms – they are not sneezing, coughing or aching for example and if they feel 'fit and well' – then they can be defined as healthy.

There are a number of problems with this form of definition. Firstly, the notion of 'abnormality' or **pathology** implies that certain universal 'norms' exist against which an individual can be assessed when making the judgement whether a person is healthy or not: but do these exist (MacIntyre, 1986)? More importantly, this means that anyone who is 'abnormal' is unhealthy. Thus, a person in a wheelchair is unhealthy, as is someone who is HIV-positive or who has early signs of cancer. Finally, what about cultural differences? In some cultures vivid expression of emotions is considered normal, whereas in other cultures this would be considered a sign of 'mental illness'.

Think about this

An 18-year-old is sent to see you by his parents since they think he has been using drugs. His blood tests show a high white blood cell count and he has a persistent dry cough. However, he puts this cough down to a long party the other night. Do you think this man is ill? Why? Or why not?

The other negative definition is health as the absence of illness. According to this definition so long as someone does not experience anxiety, pain or distress, they are healthy. They can have some disease, but still be healthy. Thus somebody in a wheelchair would be healthy, as would a person with cancer or with heart disease if they did not feel anxiety, pain or distress. The problem with this definition is one of **'relativism'**. That is, this definition is all relative: what one person says is healthy may not be the same as another person. Since this is the case, then how would you measure health?

Positive definitions

Positive definitions refer to those in which health is defined as something that is achieved or gained. The most famous (or infamous?) definition of health is that provided by the **WHO** (World Health Organization) and this interpretation is a positive definition. It is the one that is cited most frequently in textbooks and by most health care professionals – in fact by the time you finish your course you will probably be able to cite it like a mantra. The WHO definition (1946) of health states that:

> Health is a state of complete physical, mental and social well-being and not merely the absence of disease or infirmity.

It was first conceptualised just after the Second World War and emphasises that peace and health are inseparable. It made something clear from the outset: disease and infirmity cannot be isolated from subjective experience and that any definition of health must include a social and psychological dimension.

The definition sets a high standard: does anybody actually achieve this high status? Indeed, it appears as if it is such an idealised state that nobody would be described as healthy. Because the concept of health is still unclear and represents an unreachable ideal state, Svedberg *et al.* (2004) argue that is it important to concretise the definition so that the concept of health can be used as a realistic goal in nursing care (Lindsey, 1996; Pender, 1996;

Simmons, 1989). However, the definition does provide something that countries and local communities should aspire to and so it can be extremely useful as a guide and prompter for development. However, others have argued that the definition provided is merely a definition of happiness rather than health (Saracci, 1997) and that this has important consequences in the allocation of resources for 'proper' health care. However, the WHO definition has remained as it was first conceptualised in 1946 and, as mentioned, has become the byword for health in health care practice in the twenty-first century (Blaxter, 1995).

Other definitions

Finally, there are a number of other definitions of health that have been provided. For example, some (Parsons, 1951b) have suggested that health can be defined as 'The state of optimum capacity of an individual for the effective performance of the roles and tasks for which (s)he has been socialised'. This definition suggests that each of us have a role in life (for example, mother, father, son, lecturer, student, doctor, nurse and so on) and if we can perform these roles we are healthy, but if we can't then we are unhealthy. This is related to the more contemporary concept of 'sickness' which is related to the social role a person with illness or sickness takes or is given in society (Yeandle and Macmillan, 2003). Obviously, a problem with this is that on some occasions you will be able to do some of them (or be forced to do some of them) such as being a parent, but will not be able to do others (i.e. go to work). In this example, are you healthy or not?

Seedhouse (1986) suggests 'Health is a commodity. That is something – albeit an amorphous thing – which can be supplied. Equally it is something that can be lost'. He suggested that we can buy health (for example health insurance), and lose health (in an accident) – it was just another commodity that we all have access to. There are problems with this definition – is health clearly definable and measurable? Can we really 'buy' and 'sell' health like we can with various goods? Secondly, it also suggests that health is something we are born with and something that is removed – the health care practitioner simply has to be a technician to restore health.

Health can also be defined as a reserve of strength or energy. For example, we talk about the ability to 'fight off a cold' (i.e. physical strength) or the ability to 'cope with illness' (i.e. mental strength). Thus the reserve can either be mental – an attitude or outlook on life – or physical – the ability to resist a disease or illness. Finally, Dubos (1959) suggests that health is the human capacity to adapt to new situations. These forms of definition do have some merit from a common-sense perspective. However, how can we define these personal strengths and abilities? How can they be measured?

Seedhouse (1986) also defines health in terms of factors that help people to achieve their maximum personal potential – these *foundations for achievement*. Some of these foundations are unique, whereas others are common to all. Common foundations include the basic necessities of life such as food, water and shelter, as well as other factors such as access to information and the ability to make sense of this. Unique foundations vary considerably – they will differ between an elderly person and a young child, for example. However, this is also a rather vague definition – the notion of 'personal potential' remains rather mystical and undefined.

These definitions are, however, rather theoretical and unlikely to be of use in day-to-day practice. It is rare that any patient/client comes in and says 'I am not feeling in a complete state of complete physical, mental and social well-being today – please can you do something about it.' Hence, we should really ask the general public what they consider health to be.

So what happens when you ask the general public what they consider health to be? The majority of studies have been from a **social anthropological** perspective. For example, Herzlich (1973) reported that her participants classified health into one of three categories: 'health in a vacuum' (i.e. the absence of illness); 'the reserve of health' (i.e. physical strength); and '**equilibrium**' – a state rarely achieved that is characterised by happiness, relaxation and getting on with others.

Later, Blaxter (1990) asked over 9000 individuals what it meant to be healthy. A range of responses as received that indicated health was seen in terms of a reserve, a healthy life filled with health behaviours, physical fitness, having energy and vitality, social relationships with others, being able to function effectively and an expression of psychosocial well-being. In contrast, others saw it simply as not being ill. Thus, these studies have indicated what we already know: defining health is problematic and definitions vary from individual to individual. However, are there any group differences that may lead to problems?

Another study provides some evidence for group differences. Calnan (1987) examined health and illness within a British context. He asked respondents to select the explanation for what is healthy and what is not healthy. The definition of 'being healthy' provided by Calnan's respondents is provided in Table 1.1. The table suggests that social class can have an impact on the definition of health. Hence, the working class may define health from a different perspective from the middle classes – the latter defining it in terms of being active and energetic whereas those in the working class tend to define it in terms of 'getting through the day'. Since many health care professionals may be drawn from the middle classes, there could be a serious communication breakdown.

Svedberg *et al.* (2004) report on a study on the definitions of health in people with a mental health problem. The results indicated that autonomy and dignity were important to health. An important aspect of this was the ability to do things according to one's individual wishes, being able to

Table 1.1
Explanations for health provided by Calnan (1987)

Type of explanation	Upper/middle social class	Working class (number of respondents)
Getting through the day	8	15
Being active/energetic	14	4
Never being ill	0	10
Feeling fit	7	2
Feeling strong	6	0
State of mind	5	0
Being able to cope with life's stresses	5	0
Plenty of exercise	4	0
Not overweight	4	0

Think about this

A patient from a working class background comes to see you and states that they are healthy since they are keeping their job down (they work as a labourer). However, they report that they have limited energy when they get home, are overweight and don't get any exercise. What would you conclude?

manage daily routines, and not be dependent on others. Furthermore, health was associated with meaning in life – seeing the positive things and experiencing happiness from one's family and interests (Hwu *et al.*, 2002). This adds to the evidence from other studies that indicates that chronic illness – either physical or mental – may have an impact on the individual's definitions of health (e.g. Hedelin and Strandmark, 2001; McMullen O'Brien, 1998; Pavis *et al.*, 1998).

What about being ill? When people are asked to suggest what makes them ill two broad responses are provided. At the one end illnesses are caused by forces outside the individual (**exogenous**) rather than within the individual (**endogenous**). The exogenous beliefs often emphasise the environment, stress, germs and debilitating work factors. On the other hand, endogenous beliefs emphasise inborn disposition, heredity and genetics defects. Studies have generally indicated that exogenous factors are the ones that people blame for ill-health rather than the endogenous factors (Blaxter, 1983), although with increasing technological advance and health literacy there may be a change in this pattern.

Exploring the examples provided and the evidence produced it is probably best to consider health and illness as a continuum rather than as distinct entities. Hence, there are degrees of illness/wellness ranging from death at one end to optimal wellness at the other (see Figure 1.1). Antonovsky (1987, p. 3) suggests that 'we are all terminal cases. And we all are, so long as there is breath of life in us, in some measure healthy'. This neatly side-steps the issue of what health is and isn't: if you are alive then you are healthy but there are simply different graduations of this. The role of the health care practitioner is to enable all to be as near the 'optimal wellness' end of the continuum as possible.

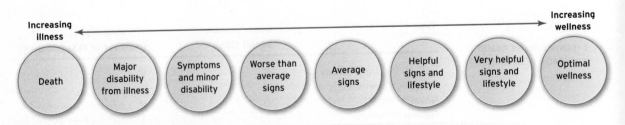

Figure 1.1 Degress of illness/wellness.

Source: Sarafino (2005), p. 3.

Research into practice

But what does this all mean for you as the nurse? What do all these various definitions of health mean for the health care professional? Does it have relevance or is it merely an academic exercise? Ogden *et al.* (2001) suggest that the differing models of health can have an impact on consultation patterns. Their study, which, although exploring the GP consultation, is relevant to the nurse, sought to explore the models of health of general practitioners and their patients.

Over 470 patients and 64 of their GPs responded to a questionnaire on what being healthy meant to them, along with a demographic questionnaire detailing their sex, age, ethnicity and social class. Although there were a number of similarities (for example, sleep, energy and sex drive) there were also a number of differences. GPs placed significantly more importance upon mood and exercise than their patients as markers of health. However, the patients considered a number of markers such as appetite, complexion, heartbeat, a desire to eat sweet things, the colour of their urine, the regularity of their bowels and so on as more important markers of their health.

So what does this mean for practice? It indicates that patients have much more varied models of health – GPs tended to focus on the emphasis of 'healthy minds and bodies', which, although considerably more diverse than previous biomedical models was not as broad as the patients model of health. Ogden *et al.* (2001) suggest that patients and doctors have '... different ways of conceptualising health, the very essence of any consultation. Such a difference between GPs and patients could potentially result in difficulties in reaching a shared understanding within the consultation with GPs and patients speaking a fundamentally different language'. They further conclude that 'consultations may involve two parties who speak not only from different perspectives and educational backgrounds, but also interpret the language they use in different ways'.

Think about this

How does this relate to the nurse consultation? How does this suggest you change your practice when talking to patients about their health?

Health in the community

When you ask people how they rate their own health an interesting picture is obtained. Blaxter (1990) in a national survey found that 71 per cent of participants defined their health as at least 'good'. This did not mean that all those that rated their health as good were without disability or objective signs of illness, or that those rating their health as 'poor' had a disability or objective signs of ill-health. For example, many disabled people rated their health as excellent, whereas 10 per cent of men and 7 per cent of women in the top category of objectively measured health (i.e. measures of disease – that diagnosed by medical practitioners), described their health as either 'fair' or 'poor'. In contrast, 40 per cent of those with objectively measured health problems described their health as 'good' or 'excellent'.

In a more recent survey the General Household Survey (2002) 59 per cent of those asked rated their health as 'good' and 27 per cent as 'fairly good' with only 14 per cent rating their health as 'not good'. In contrast, the proportion of individuals rating themselves as having a long-standing illness was 34 per cent. Hence, there must be individuals with a chronic illness who rate their health as good. Interestingly, the same survey suggested that 16 per cent of those asked reported an acute illness in the previous fortnight. This figure seems to relate to those rating their health as 'not good' (although it is of course possible that those with acute illness rated their health as excellent and those without an acute illness rated their health as poor!).

A number of studies have indicated, however, that people who are 'ill' (or properly have some symptoms) rarely report the illness to their health care practitioner (Bentzen *et al.*, 1989; Morris *et al.*, 2003; Scambler *et al.*, 1981). Although it is obvious that many of these symptoms may be 'trivial' and minor, there are some studies that have indicated that serious symptoms may be missed: people do not always report their symptoms to their GP or health care practitioner. This is the '**clinical iceberg**' (Hannay, 1977): there is a large unmet need since many people are in pain or discomfort which could be treated if they accessed appropriate services.

If all of these people did attempt to access the service, however, then the service would be swamped. But the question is, why do people attend health

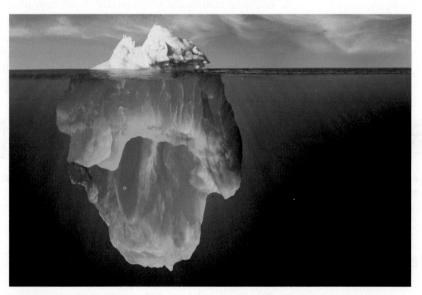

© Ralph A. Clevenger/CORBIS

Think about this

The evidence suggests that people who have symptoms of ill-health do not consult their health care practitioner. Where do these ill people go? What impact does this have on the practice of the nurse and how can they go out and help those people who need medical assistance but do not currently access it?

care services? And, just as importantly, why do they not attend health care services? This type of behaviour is known as 'illness behaviour'.

At its most basic a number of studies have indicated that sociodemographic characteristics differ between users and non-users of medical services (e.g. Stoller, 2003). For example, women consult more than men, children and the elderly more frequently than young adults. Social class (less in the working class), ethnicity (less in ethnic minority groups) and marital status (less in those married) are all factors that have appeared related to utilisation. However, on top of this information we must ask why people do not seek out health care.

But where do people go when they are ill? We have seen that most people do not go to the GP when they are ill, but they seek health care assistance from others. The most frequent resource drawn on is the family as a source of social support and information (see Chapter 8 on social support). If we are ill then we will consult our families first for their advice and interpretation. This helps to guide us as to what is considered appropriate. If, on the basis of this, the symptoms are not thought to be particularly serious then it is likely that there will be no medical consultation. However, there could be other forms of consultation – for example at the local pharmacy or with friends, or (increasingly) through information gathered on the Internet.

The most important piece of information that must be remembered is that people do not simply respond to the mere presence of disease, nor to the presence of some symptoms. It depends on how they and others around them respond to the symptoms. But what about Mrs Bruce? We can note from the case study that she did not consult her GP as soon as the symptom became immediately apparent – there were a number of factors that were relevant. Mechanic (1978) has suggested ten key variables (although acknowledged that these were only the start of the list) that may be relevant to consulting a health care provider. These are listed in Table 1.2, with how they relate to Mrs Bruce.

Think about this

Consider the case of Mrs Bruce: which factors were the most important for her in deciding whether to go and seek out assistance for her symptoms? Was it simply the medical factors? What implications does this have for your practice?

Although the Mechanic study was an important element in our understanding of health-seeking behaviour there are other factors that may be relevant. One of these can be considered the lay referral system, which we have already touched upon. It is notable that not all people go to the GP when they are ill, so where do they go? One of those places is their family or friend (e.g. Biddle et al., 2004; Schoenberg et al., 2003). If a person goes along and says they have a particular symptom and the response is 'Nothing serious – I had that last year and it got better within a week' then the person is less likely to go than if the response was 'Urgghh, that is disgusting, I would seek help for that straight away!' Thus, it is likely that married people or those living within a strong family are more likely to access this lay system at the outset and go on the recommendations of the family.

Variables	Relationship to Mrs Bruce
Visibility and recognisability of symptoms	She could see the symptoms, but did she recognise them as such?
Personal estimate of seriousness of symptoms	Did she consider the symptoms to be important?
Extent to which symptoms disrupt personal life	Since she managed to keep up with her job and social activities the symptoms were obviously not disruptive
Frequency of appearance of signs and symptoms	The signs and symptoms were continuous but she managed to avoid them until they became too apparent
Tolerance threshold	Mrs Bruce obviously has a high threshold and other competing factors
Available information	Did she have any information on the potential symptoms?
Basic needs that lead to denial	There were more important factors in her life and hence she denied that the symptoms were serious
Competing needs	Her family and her work life were more important to her than the symptoms
Competing interpretations of symptoms	She may have interpreted them as minor
Availability of treatment resources	This did not appear to be a problem

Table 1.2
Key variables relevant to consulting a health care provider

Another factor in accessing health care has been described as the 'cost–benefit' models of health. Most health care practitioners (and it was the belief of the founding figures of the NHS) believe that if a rational person has a symptom or is ill then they will immediately seek help. Obviously this is not the case with all symptoms, as we have seen. One of the key reasons for this is that 'good health' (however defined) is not always the priority for the individual since it might (as in Mrs Bruce's case) disrupt work, social functioning and other activities that are *perceived* as more important than accessing health care for herself. Thus the value of health varies in accordance with the perception of the benefits versus the costs of its accomplishment. There are a number of models representing attempts to bring together various factors relating to the cost–benefit analysis of health and these are more fully outlined in Chapter 15.

Finally, ease of access to health care has implications for usage. The **inverse care law** (Tudor, 1971) has been suggested as operating in Britain: that is, the provision of health care is inversely related to the need for it. Although this is more fully explored in Chapter 8 it is also worth considering here – certainly it has been shown that as the distance between home and general practice increases, the likelihood of consultation decreases: this is particularly true for elderly or disabled people who, it may be argued, may need the service more (Whitehead, 1992).

Measurement of health

Defining health is a problem, but how do we measure it? We have to be able to measure it so we can see whether our interventions and practice actually improve health. If we are supposed to be health care professionals then we need to be able to demonstrate that we are being effective. In consequence, this section seeks to explain the terms mortality and morbidity and their usefulness in measuring health and then on the basis of this describe the various ways of measuring health including measures of mortality (e.g. crude death rates, standardised mortality rates) and morbidity. Obviously all of this will be related to your practice. Look at the case study of Mrs Bruce – how could you measure health in her case? You could, for example, explore whether she is 'ill' (i.e. feels that she is in pain or in discomfort), or whether she has a disease (i.e. some bacterial or physiological problem) or we could see whether she has reported her illness to a GP or other health care worker, or we could see whether she has taken any time from her work or other usual activities. All of these putative measures of health have been used in studies exploring health and health values in the community or in the country. Indeed, as there are many ways of defining health, there are, similarly, many ways of measuring it. At its most basic the two main ways in which health has been measured are:

- Mortality rates: That is, how many people have died of a particular cause or in a specific region or area.
- Morbidity rates: That is, whether a person has an illness, or whether there are higher rates of illness within a particular region or area.

However, each of these has individual sub-components of health measurement and each of these will be explored in turn: firstly the mortality measures of health.

Life expectancy

The life expectancy of an individual can also be used as a measure of health. It allows us to explore how healthy a particular area, region, historical period (see Table 1.3) or group is. Life expectancy provides a useful age-standardised measure of mortality. Since the middle of the nineteenth century the expectation of life at birth for both women and men has almost doubled. Neither men nor women born in England and Wales in 1841 had an average life expectancy from birth much beyond 40, although those who survived to the age of 15 could expect another 45 years of life. However, by 1998 the life expectancy at birth of women in Great Britain had almost reached 80, and men nearly 75 years. It is important to note when the life expectancy is derived from. When you are born your life expectancy is lower than it is at 60, 70 or 80 years of age. This isn't anything to worry about as it just means you have reached that age and hence when working out the average it is bound to be higher.

		1841	1901	1931	1961	1981	1986	1991	1997	1998
Table 1.3 Life expectancy at birth by gender	Males	41.0	45.7	58.1	67.8	70.9	72.0	73.2	74.6	74.9
	Females	43.0	49.6	62.1	73.7	76.8	77.7	78.8	79.6	79.8

Crude death rates

One way of measuring health is to simply count the number of people who die in a particular area, or in a particular month or are from a particular group. In this way it is possible to compare these rates from group to group (e.g. between men and women) or from area to area (e.g. between Cardiff and London) or from period to period (e.g. from the nineteenth century to the present day). That area, group or time period with the highest death rate is, obviously, the unhealthiest. Since death rates have been collected from the mid-nineteenth century to the present day it is possible to investigate a number of important factors.

To start with, the figure was just totalled – the *crude death rate*. It is then possible to use this to provide an overview of the death rate over the years (since we also know the population of the country at the time), then we can provide a simple overview of say X per 1000 (the death rate in 2004). Data can then be collected and analysed at the simple level and we can compare area, group or historically (see Table 1.4).

There are problems with this approach, however – the death rate in Eastbourne may be quite high, whereas in Birmingham it may be lower. This is not because Eastbourne is a particularly unhealthy place to live but that it is the place where people go to retire and hence it is bound to have a higher death rate. Crude death rates ignore the fact that many different factors impact upon the death rate (for example, an individual's sex, age or their previous health) and because of these problems they are not often used any more when sensitive statistics are required.

To deal with the age-related problems, often age-specific death rates are calculated using, in particular, the stillbirth rate (the number of stillbirths for every 1000 births registered) and the infant mortality rate (the number of deaths in infants under 1 year of age for every 1000 live births). The other measure of mortality is expectation of life at birth, or the average length of life.

Standardised mortality rate

The standardised mortality rate (SMR) compares the mortality rate for the whole population with that of a particular region or group (the so-called *index population*) and expresses this as a ratio. Thus, the observed death rate is divided by the expected rate (derived from the index population) and then multiplied by 100.

Year	Men		Women	
	Deaths (thousands)	**Death rate (per 1000 population)**	**Deaths (thousands)**	**Death rate (per 1000 population)**
1976	300.1	12.5	298.5	11.8
1981	289.0	12.0	288.9	11.3
1986	287.9	11.8	293.3	11.4
1991	277.6	11.2	292.5	11.2
1996	268.7	10.4	291.5	11.0
2001	252.4	9.9	277.9	10.4
2004	245.2	9.4	269.0	9.9

Table 1.4
Deaths

SMRs are calculated in order to be able to make comparisons of death rates from a single cause (e.g. heart attacks, breast cancer) between geographical areas or different groups (according to sex, class, ethnicity and so on). The SMR for deaths from a particular disease is calculated by expressing the actual number of deaths in the group of interest in the index area as a ratio of the expected number of deaths from the standard population data. In most analyses a value of 100 equals the average mortality. Any value greater than 100 indicates above-average mortality and less than 100 equates to a mortality better than average. For example, if we look at Figure 1.2 we can see the SMR for coronary heart disease (CHD) in selected areas of London. For some the SMR is above 100 (e.g. Bethnal Green South – there are above-average rates of CHD), whereas in others the SMR is below 100 and therefore below average (e.g. Millwall).

Although SMRs are used frequently and presented as evidence of the health of a country or area, they have a major problem as a measure of health:

Just because you are alive does not mean you are healthy!

SMRs and crude death rates measure death, but just because a person is alive does not necessarily mean that they are healthy. There is more to health than simply not being dead. They tell us nothing about the health of the person when they were alive – they do not tell us about the possible pain, discomfort and disability that the individual was in before their death.

Hence, what we have to do is to measure health according to morbidity or sickness. There are a variety of ways in which this can be measured – some of these focus on illness, whereas others focus on disease (as we have previously outlined the difference can be important).

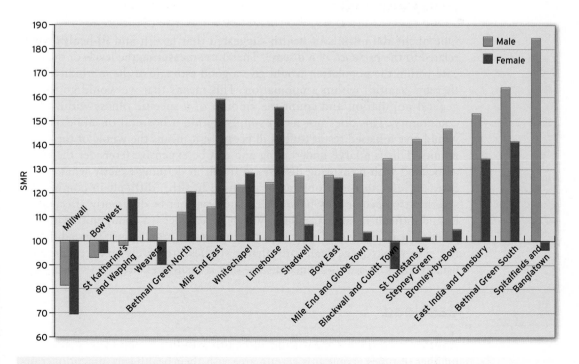

Figure 1.2 SMR for CHD in selected wards in London, 2000–2004.

© London Borough of Tower Hamlets

Morbidity statistics

Since we can't assume that just because somebody is alive then they are healthy, we have to explore how we can measure health in terms of morbidity, or ill-health. This is a more difficult task than creating mortality statistics. As we have seen there is still some confusion when we examine death statistics, as on many occasions the cause of death is either inaccurate or confused. An issue with mortality statistics is that although they we can be relatively accurate when recording death, we are somewhat uncertain about the cause of death. Although death certificates are always produced often doctors have to make a subjective judgement about the cause of death. Nonetheless, death rates from specific causes are often calculated but caution must be taken when attempting to interpret these figures given the difficulties in trying to determine the cause of death.

This problem may be exaggerated in the living since the diagnosis and recording of objective ill-health may not be easily achieved. Of course, valuable statistical data can be gleaned from hospital records, from consultations and from records detailing the causes of absence from work (although see later for the problems inherent in this approach). However, the data achieved from epidemiologists have two key features: the **incidence** (i.e. the number of new cases occurring in a specified period) and **prevalence** (i.e. the number of people who have the disease or illness at a specified time). Knowing these figures, plus the total number of people at risk, it is possible to calculate the incidence rate and the prevalence rates (usually per 10 000 or per 100 000 population) for a specific disease or illness.

Prevalence rates

One of the definitions of health suggested that health and ill-health were related to the presence of a disease. Therefore, measuring the levels of the disease within the population would give a good estimate of the morbidity (and thereby 'health') within a population. This means that we would go to the general population and count the amount of a specific illness within that community. This does not mean simply within a hospital or clinic as this would give a biased result (full of ill people!), it means the whole of the community. This is a large undertaking and can be expensive (consider the costs associated with measuring disease), difficult in defining exactly what is the disease (refer to the problems of defining health), difficult in comparing severity (two people may have the same disease but be differently affected by it) and difficult in comparability. (Which is healthier – a community with ten cases of heart disease or another with ten cases of bronchitis?) These difficulties mean that large-scale prevalence studies are rarely undertaken and usually focus on a well-defined disease that is easily measured.

Caseload

Another method for measuring ill-health would be simply to count the number of times people in a certain area visit their health care practitioner or attend a local hospital. This is easy information to collect and could be relatively easy to compare between areas, shouldn't it? It should be useful because it provides an indication of health status and illness – it is a subjective measure of how people perceive their own health.

However, there are a number of assumptions that underlie this method for measuring health and these could cause problems. First, this measure of health assumes that when people are ill they visit the doctor. Hence it also reflects illness behaviour. As we have noted earlier in this chapter there are a number of reasons why some people attend their GP and some do not. It is not simply a consequence of their illness or the symptoms that they are suffering. It also reflects health demand. Just as some people will not seek out health care when they have symptoms, there are some individuals who will demand health care irrespective of whether they need it or not. Some individuals may go to private practitioners, or alternative/complementary therapists, or just ask their friends and family for advice rather than having to go through the hassle of getting an appointment at the local GP surgery. It also assumes that the health services are available – if there is no service available, then there is no caseload figure: does this mean that the area is healthy? Finally, some people cannot afford to take time off work when they are ill, so they do not go to the doctor. Hence a very confusing picture can be obtained which reflects ability to go to the doctor rather than the need to go.

All of these issues mean that caseload cannot be used as a measure of health for the population.

Sickness absence rates

In this method we assume that the health of a community can be assessed by measuring how much time people take off from work and then divide this by the actual working population. Since these figures are recorded, as are the number of days worked, we can work out the sickness absence rate (number of days off sick divided by the number of days worked). We can then compare two or more populations (or communities). Although this information is collected routinely, there are several problems. Sickness absence rates can be affected by a number of factors. Firstly, they can be affected by illness behaviour: some people are more likely than others to seek absence from work than others. Secondly, some jobs require different levels of registration for sickness. For example, if a person has to have a 'sick-note' in order to get paid for a day off, then they are probably less likely to have some time off work because of the problems associated with accessing the health services. With some jobs, the person will not get paid (e.g. a labourer, brick layer or agency workers) if they do not turn up for work. Hence, these individuals are less likely to have a day off work and less likely to go to the doctors. Finally, and the most serious problem, is that sickness absence rates cannot deal with those who are not in paid employment. For example, it cannot account for some housewives, students, the elderly and disabled who may not be paid employed. Bizarrely, these are believed to have higher sickness rates than other members of the population.

Self-report measures

A number of methods have been employed which can be classified as self-report measures – the major one being **quality of life**, which we will explore in more detail later. The overall self-report method, however, is to ask the informant about their acute or chronic sickness within a given period. The classic example of this is given by the questions used in the General Household Survey (ONS, 2006). This survey asks a series of questions about an individual and their family's life. In particular the health section requests information on a number of measures of health status. For example:

ADULT HEALTH

Over the last twelve months would you say your health has on the whole been good, fairly good, or not good?

Good 1

Fairly Good 2

Not Good 3

2. Do you have any long-standing illness, disability or infirmity? By long-standing, I mean anything that has troubled you over a period of time or that is likely to affect you over a period of time?

Yes 1

No 2

3. Now I'd like you to think about the 2 weeks ending yesterday. During those 2 weeks, did you have to cut down on any of the things you usually do (about the house/at work or in your free time) because of some other illness or injury?

Yes 1

No 2

4. How many days was this in all during these 2 weeks, including Saturdays and Sundays?

5. During the 2 weeks ending yesterday, apart from any visit to a hospital, did you talk to a doctor for any reason at all, either in person or by telephone?

Yes 1

No 2

Although these are all relatively simple questions given the range of questions asked in the survey and the large size of the sample the General Household Survey provides extremely valuable information. Furthermore, although asking people to simply rate their health as 'good', 'fair' or 'poor' seems a rather simplistic measure, it can be used as a predictor of subsequent mortality.

Although self-report measures are extremely useful and simple, there are some drawbacks. Firstly, as with all self-reporting, they depend to a large extent on the individual responding. For example, there may be a gender bias to respond positively or certain stoical individuals will rate their health as 'good' whereas others may exaggerate their poor health. Secondly, this measure of health relies on the perception of health rather than any objective measure. Hence, it depends on how the individual has perceived their health and any symptoms – again it is a problem of relativism. Furthermore, this can be extended to ask people about their level of function: what they can and cannot do, or their quality of life.

Measures of functioning

The self-report measures we mentioned above are simply crude measures of whether a person thinks they have an illness or not. The measures of functioning ask a person what they can and cannot do and hence can be considered more comprehensive. These are termed subjective health measures because they rely on the respondent's view of their own health.

The same diseases may cause differential effects on the level of functioning. Therefore, ask the respondent how they perform with their illness. One such measure is the 'activities of daily living' (ADL), which rates individuals on how much they can and cannot do (e.g. climbing stairs). Self-report measures ask the individual about their health/illness. For example, the Nottingham health profile classifies an individual's health status into such groupings as pain, physical mobility and energy.

A popular health profile is the SF-36 (Short-Form – 36 items) which was developed from large-scale studies in the United States. It contains 36 items that produce eight individual dimensions:

- physical functioning;
- social functioning;
- role limitation due to physical problems;
- role limitation due to emotional problems;
- general mental health;
- energy/vitality;
- bodily pain;
- general health perceptions.

The authors argue that the SF-36 only takes 5–10 minutes to complete so it is useful in both clinical practice and in research studies. However, there are shorter forms: the SF-12 and SF-6 (guess how many questions they include!). This measure of functioning can also be classified as a quality of life (QoL) measure, which are currently being employed in health care in a range of settings.

When various measures of health are compared a range difference in health status is found. Policy and public health interventions often use different measures of health interchangeably. However, Wikman *et al.* (2005) found that this was not possible. Indeed, they found a difference between 'illness', 'disease' and 'sickness absence'. Not surprisingly, they found that most people had some sort of illness or health complaint, but fewer were registered with a disease and even fewer had taken sick leave (i.e. caseload). Consequently, there are two consequences that can be drawn from this. Firstly, there is a need to consider a range of measures when devising interventions and measuring their success. Secondly, the lack of overlap between the different measures means that they represent a different form of realities. Of course one other way of exploring health is to measure its impact on the individual's quality of life.

Quality of life

Quality of life measures are also mainly self-report measures and it is argued that since illness affects quality of life, then simply assess quality of life. Although there is no general consensus on the definition of QoL, the WHO defines it as 'a broad ranging concept affected in a complex way by the person's physical health, psychological state, level of independence, social relationships and their relationship to the salient features in the environment' (WHOQoL Group, 1993). Obviously this has implications in the way that QoL is operationalised. We have already seen that the SF-36 characterises it as a series of terms. Fallowfield (1990), in contrast, defined the four main dimensions of quality of life as psychological (mood, emotional distress, adjustment to illness), social (relationships, social and leisure activities), occupational (paid and unpaid work) and physical (mobility, pain, sleep and appetite).

There are many measures of QoL – some are generic and some are specific for individual illnesses (see Bowling, 2004). Early measures used to attempt to classify QoL as a function of the objective concomitants of the illness whereas more modern-day measures have explored the subjective components of the disorder (what it stops you from doing). Hence they try to combine the physical functioning impairment along with the psychological well-being.

Although there are a number of different QoL measures and there is a lack of agreement about which are 'best', it is generally agreed that they are useful and offer a tacit way of exploring the benefits of medical intervention.

Using quality of life in the clinical setting

Higginson and Carr (2001) describe the way in which QoL indicators can be used in the clinical setting. Although they contend that QoL measures have found a use in the research arena they are less well used in the clinical setting despite the fact that 'Florence Nightingale was one of the first clinicians to insist on measuring the outcomes of routine care to evaluate treatment' (p. 1297). They suggest that they can be used, potentially, in eight different areas of clinical practice (see Table 1.5) – five immediately in the clinical encounter (see table) and the remaining three (contribute to training, reviewing care and improving care in the future) are more long term.

Think about this

Think about the case study of Mrs Bruce. What measure of health would you use for her when she first arrives in clinic and then again when she reveals her tumour? How could you use quality of life measures with her?

Table 1.5 Five areas of clinical practice	Area	
	Prioritise problems	The QoL measure will explore a range of issues and enable the patient and nurse to identify which problems are most important together.
	Facilitate communication	The QoL measure should provide clear information on the range of problems experienced by the patient. It should therefore aid communication by providing more information in a more concise fashion. It may, therefore, also have the added benefit of speeding the encounter.
	Screen for potential problems	Some patients may have problems that can be overlooked and the QoL measure may highlight some of these issues that may have been overlooked (particularly social and psychological problems).
	Identify preferences	The QoL assessment may help identify the patient's preferred outcome or treatment goal. Obviously if these are unknown at the time of the clinical encounter then there is a likelihood that the treatment will not meet expectations and that the adherence to treatment will not be as strong as preferred.
	Monitor changes or response to treatment	Change is usually monitored in a clinical fashion by reporting to 'clinical indicators'. However, these may not be of most importance to the patient – the change or improvement in QoL may be of key concern.

Research in focus

McCarthy, M.C., Ruiz, E., Gale, B.J., Karam, C. and Moore, N. (2004) The meaning of health: perspectives of Anglo and Latino older women. *Health Care for Women International*, **25**, 950–969.

Background

There are increasing numbers of older adults and, as the population ages, it becomes more diverse in terms of ethnicity, gender and social class. Furthermore, as the population ages there are associated chronic diseases and disabilities and these can result in functional limitations. Although this is appreciated by the health care system and appropriate interventions are being developed and implemented, there is a lack of knowledge on the sociocultural influences and descriptors of health. It was argued by the authors that most health care planners are from a white middle-class background and this ethnocentrism leads to barrier in the development of health care services. This study aimed to describe sociocultural influences on the definitions of health.

Method

This was a qualitative study undertaken in the United States. A series of focus group interviews were undertaken with older Anglo and older Latino women (a series of 29 participants) aged between 51 and 85 years of age. The primary theme of the groups was the description and meaning of functional health in everyday life. Each focus group lasted two hours and tapes of the

▶

groups were transcribed. The tapes were analysed through a qualitative technique known as the 'dimensional analysis' approach which aims to answer the question, 'What is involved here?'

Results

There were clear differences between the Anglo and the Latino groups. The Anglo groups were more individualistic in their description, describing health in terms of 'not being sick, not feeling bad, being able to do the things I need to do'. In contrast the Latino groups rarely described their health in terms of well-being or the absence of disease. Instead they consistently appeared to perceive health as part of the self: health was part of life and the business of living.

Implications

Findings from this study highlight the different conceptualisation of health in different cultures. Although it was an American study this result can also be applied to the developments in the United Kingdom. As the authors suggest: 'understanding the meaning given to the concept of health can only enhance our ability to provide culturally competent care to people of different racial/ethnic, age, socioeconomic and gender groups' (p. 966).

Think about this

How would you measure health in the following examples?

- Children attending the local school in comparison with other children in the locality.
- A homeless person who comes in an alcoholic state.
- An educated professor who complains of chest pain.
- An old man with dementia.
- How effective a new tablet was in improving a person's epilepsy.

Conclusion

There are a range of definitions of health – it is not merely whether you are ill or not. It is important to appreciate how individuals differ in their definition of health since this can impact on their reporting behaviour and their subsequent reactions to ill-health. Not surprisingly, there are also a number of methods of measuring health, from the standardised mortality rates (SMRs) through to self-report quality of life measures. These are useful in different situations, from the clinic through to the community.

Summary

- There are a variety of definitions of health.

- Positive definitions stress the importance of achieving or gaining something.

- Negative definitions define health as the absence of illness or disease.

- The most frequently cited definition of health is that from the World Health Organization.

- The way that an individual defines their health can impact upon their use of the health service and the benefit they derive from it.

- There are a number of different measurements of health.

- The most frequently used measure of population health is the standardised mortality rate (SMR), although it has to be remembered that just because a person is alive does not mean that they are healthy!

- Self-report measurement of health is possible but is influenced by the way individuals and groups view their own health. It is a very subjective measure.

- Measuring the caseload of individual hospitals and general practitioners is not very useful since these vary according to the provision of service and the factors that influence the use of services.

- Similarly, measuring sickness absence rate is not very useful since a person may still go to work even though they are ill, or take time off even if they are not. This may be influenced by the type of job they have.

- Quality of life indicators are now widely used in the measurement of health and they can be used for both clinical and research purposes.

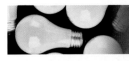

Check your understanding

1. Discuss the concept of health: which definition is of the most use to the nurse?

2. Why is the WHO definition of health useful for the general population?

3. What problems can differing health definitions of the nurse and patient present for the practising nurse?

4. How can health be best assessed in the clinic, and in the community?

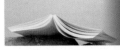

Further reading

Aggleton, P. (1990) *Health*. London: Routledge.

Calnan, M. (1987) *Health and Illness – The Lay Perspective*. London: Tavistock.

Wikman, A., Marklund, S. and Alexanderson, K. (2005) Illness, disease, and sickness absence: an empirical test of difference between concepts of ill health. *Journal of Epidemiology and Community Health*, **59**, 450–454.

Weblinks

World Health Organization	http://www.who.int/about/definition/en/	Offers the key definition of health and provides additional information on health statistics across the globe
World Health Organization	http://www.who.int/en/	WHO home page where considerable information can be accessed
Wellcome library	http://library.wellcome.ac.uk/	The history of medicine library funded and hosted by Wellcome
SF-36	http://www.sf-36.org/	The home page of the SF-36 and the other SF measures of quality of life. Provides considerable information on the measurement technique and its development

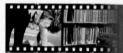

Media example

Whose life is it anyway? A serious road accident forces the protagonist (Richard Dreyfuss in the 1981 film) to contemplate a future in which they will remain constantly dependent on those around them. Left with only the use of a sharp mind, wit and indomitable spirit, the play/film raises issues concerning quality of life and euthanasia.

Chapter 2

The principles of behaviourist psychology

Learning outcomes

When you have read through this chapter you should understand

- How previous learning and associations can explain current behaviour.
- How the principles of behaviourism can help nurses shape behaviour.
- How behaviour modification techniques can be applied in practice.
- How patients and nurses learn through observation.
- How patient's medical fears, anxiety and phobias can be addressed by the nurse.
- How behavioural therapy can be adapted and applied to the patient.
- How self-efficacy is central to the patient's health and well-being.

Case study

Samuel McNube has come to the accident and emergency department with his 7-year-old, Buba. Buba has cuts to both of his arms and legs after falling on broken glass in the garden. The consultant examines Buba and instructs the nurse to bandage both his arms, which have deep lacerations, as well as administer the prescribed injection to prevent any infection.

As soon as the consultant mentions the word 'injection', Buba becomes agitated and repeatedly shouts, 'no' and 'I want to go home'. The nurse realises that administering the injection is not going to be easy. Samuel suggests to the nurse that he will hold his son while the nurse carries out the procedure. The nurse decides not to administer the injection immediately but instead decides to sit with Buba, talk to him and calm him down. After asking Buba and his father a few questions, the nurse concludes that Buba has had this reaction to injections since the age of 4. According to Buba, injections are painful and all adults, especially nurses, seem to pretend that they are not. He even maintains that he does not like people in hospitals because they all seem to cause pain to children.

The nurse first talks to Buba about nurses and how they are there to get children better. She then asks Buba to hold out his arm while she scrapes her nail lightly against his hand. The nurse then informs him that the injection will result in the level of pain that the scratch evoked. Buba still looks unconvinced, so the nurse brings in two dolls; one dressed as a nurse and one dressed as a superhero. Buba plays with the superhero doll until the nurse informs him that the superhero doll cannot play as he is not feeling well. Both Buba and the nurse agree that the superhero doll needs an injection so that he can play again. Buba holds the superhero doll while the nurse pretends that the doll dressed up as the nurse administers an injection. The nurse emphasises to Buba how well the superhero doll is and how nice the nurse was to the superhero doll. She then provides a gold reward sticker for the superhero doll.

Samuel asks his son if he would like to get better like the superhero doll, to which Buba pulls out his arm and nods a yes. The nurse administers the injection, throughout which Buba is calm and unchallenging. The nurse praises Buba for how calm he has been while having his injection. Buba smiles and sits patiently while having his arm bandaged. The nurse then gives Buba a gold star sticker for being a good patient.

Why is this relevant to nursing practice?

The opening case study exemplifies how behaviourist principles can be applied in practice. The nurse noted Buba's negative reaction to the word 'injection', which resulted in the nurse addressing his adverse reaction before administering the injection. Behaviourist psychologists postulate that behaviour is a product of previous learning. For example, behaviourism would explain Buba's reaction towards injections as being negative and arising from previous experiences.

The two strands of behaviourism that will help the reader identify associations and prior learning are classical conditioning and operant conditioning. By being familiar with such principles, the nurse will be able to answer such questions as: Why is the patient fearful? Why do cancer patients feel sick even when not having chemotherapy? Why has the patient taken a dislike to the nurse without even talking to her? And as shown in the case study above, why are so many people, irrespective of age, fearful of injections? All of these questions can be comfortably addressed with the basic principles of classical and operant conditioning, which will be examined further in this chapter.

The nurse in the case study above used dolls to explain to Buba that injections do not hurt. This is another example of behaviourism, which is referred to as social learning theory. According to this perspective, learning takes place through observation rather than actually participating in the learning process. Social learning theory highlights areas such as modelling which are important to consider when attempting to change old or learn new behaviour. In the case study above, dolls were used because of the age of the patient. Modelling can be applied to other age groups, which this chapter will consider.

The case study above portrayed the shaping of Buba's behaviour from disliking injections to not having an extreme dislike. The nurse first ensured that Buba was taught a new association which replaced injections and pain. This chapter will look at how behavioural techniques can be applied to change the patient's behaviour. The chapter will also focus on particular techniques such as behaviour modification, which focus solely on the behaviour change of patients, and are based on behaviourist principles. This will also be useful for nurses working with patients who may need to modify their current behaviour but are finding it difficult. Hence, such principles are useful to take into consideration when promoting the health and well-being of the patient.

During the consultation the nurse praises Buba; this is later reinforced when the nurse provides Buba with a yellow reward sticker. Praise is just one example of reinforcement and is a useful technique for the nurse to become familiar with. The aim of this technique is to increase the probability of a behavioural response by pairing it with either a pleasant or unpleasant outcome (punishment). Thus reinforcement is a useful tool which will enable the nurse to shape or modify behaviour. There are many examples of reinforcement in the media. The most recent of these is 'Supernanny', which exemplifies how reinforcement and associated principles can help parents discipline unruly children.

There are many therapies and specialised techniques that have built on the work of behaviourist principles. **Token economies**, behaviour modification and therapies used to treat phobias are just a few techniques that a nurse will find useful to be familiar with when thinking about shaping patient behaviour.

'Supernanny'
The nanny who has famously applied the basic principles within behaviourism to disciplining children. The 'naughty step' and the 'reward chart' feature as part of the discipline programme.

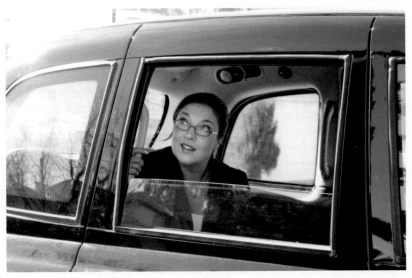

Rex Features/ABC/Everett

What is behaviouristic psychology and how does it explain patient behaviour?

Behaviourists maintain that only behaviour that is observable can be studied (Eysenck, 2002). In turn behaviour that is not observable, such as attitudes, thinking and memory, cannot be studied but only inferred. This is in complete contrast to the cognitive psychology perspective (Chapter 5) which believes that there are many factors that need to be considered between the stimulus and response relationship. For example, when a person feels cold they will put on a jumper. According to cognitive psychologists, it is not as simple as putting on a jumper. Instead your previous experiences with the cold weather and seeing others around you with jumpers entails thinking and memory processes that result in a person putting a jumper on.

Think about this

Think about the everyday tasks a nurse performs. Do these tasks involve thinking, problem-solving and the use of other mental states, or are all these tasks as simple as responding to the environment? The answer to this question will make it evident that mental processes are involved in most of the tasks that are new or those that pose new scenarios. At the same time responding to several patients and observing their reactions has to the same stimuli, i.e. an injection, will result in the nurse concluding they have similar reactions. For example, patients will either be highly fearful, slightly fearful or show no fear at all.

According to early behaviourist theories, learning and behaviour are the result of **conditioning**. Below we explore two early strands within behaviourist psychology, referred to as classical and operant conditioning.

Classical conditioning

Ivan Pavlov (1849–1936) is the famous physiologist who explained learning by the principle of **classical conditioning.** Pavlov's initial interest was studying dogs and their digestive system from a physiological perspective. During his observations he became intrigued with the dogs and their salivating patterns, which would occur when the dogs would see the laboratory assistants in white coats without food. This began Pavlov's exploration of the process of classical conditioning and responses that occur in relation to the environment.

Pavlov firstly noted that the dogs would salivate when food was presented to them. Pavlov referred to the food as the **unconditional stimulus** and the response of salivation as the **unconditional response**. An unconditional response refers to a response that is reflexive and does not require any learning; hence it is unconditional. For example, feeling tired and sleeping is an example of a reflex that is not learned but one we are born with.

Pavlov then began to refer to the learning process within classical conditioning. He manipulated this by pairing the unconditional stimulus (food) with a neutral stimulus (something that does not result in salivation, e.g. a bell). Every time the food was presented with the neutral stimulus, the dog had the obvious response of salivation (unconditional response). This was repeated several times.

The aim of the learning process was to see if the dog's behaviour had been conditioned. Over time the dog began to associate the bell with food and would salivate upon hearing it even when there was no food present. Hence, salivation became a **conditioned response** to the bell, now a **conditioned stimulus.** See Figure 2.1 for each of these stages.

Classical conditioning in practice and breaking the association

There are many contexts in which the patient's current behaviour can be explained by classical conditioning. Finding out about previous associations as an explanation for the patient's current behaviour can enable a nurse to help the patient more effectively. This was illustrated in the case study above as the nurse acknowledged that Buba's anxiety resulted from a prior experience and that he associated injections with pain and distress.

Current patient behaviour can also be explained by the associations the patient could have made with previous treatments within the hospital. One example that has been widely researched has been that of cancer patients undergoing chemotherapy treatment. Research has shown that up to 25 per cent of chemotherapy patients tend to experience anticipatory nausea and vomiting prior to treatment (Morrow *et al.*, 1998). This is explained as a conditioned response to the hospital in general, where the act of vomiting is initially associated with chemotherapy treatment and then becomes associated with the hospital or ward itself (Aapro *et al.*, 2005). Classical conditioning has been documented by other researchers as being a plausible

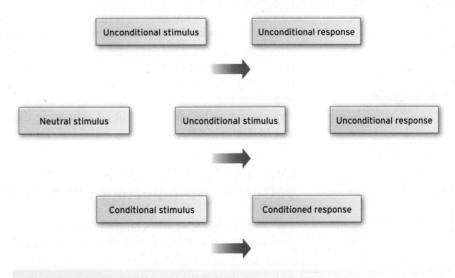

Figure 2.1 Classical conditioning association.

explanation for anticipatory nausea and vomiting among cancer chemotherapy patients (Stockhorst *et al.*, 2000).

Anticipatory nausea and vomiting is more likely to occur with patients who experienced nausea and vomiting during their initial chemotherapy sessions, thus resulting in an association between the chemotherapy and feeling nausea and/or actual vomiting. This can further extend to the patient feeling nausea and vomiting when attending the same hospital for another matter, as a trigger within the hospital, e.g. the smell, may become associated with chemotherapy and feeling sick. According to behaviourist psychologists this is referred to as stimulus **generalisation** where the conditioned stimulus (chemotherapy) is paired with a similar stimulus (treatment within the hospital) which will evoke the same conditioned response (nausea and vomiting). For example, in one experimental study, it was shown that a novel beverage could become a conditioned stimulus to nausea when paired with several chemotherapy treatments (Bovbjerg *et al.*, 1992).

So what can nurses do to ensure that associations by the patient are not made or, if such associations are inevitable, how they can be lessened in their effect? According to behaviourist psychologists what can be learned can also be unlearned. Pavlov explored the possibility of being able to unlearn associations that had been conditioned through experimentation. Presenting food to the dogs several times without the bell resulted in the dogs not salivating when the bell was presented alone. Pavlov referred to this as **extinction.**

Researchers have found that there a number of steps that a nurse can take to ensure that the chemotherapy patient will not suffer from the effects of anticipatory vomiting and nausea. According to Rhodes and McDaniel (2001) pre-chemotherapy preparation and patient education in the palliative care setting are essential to preventing distress and anticipatory symptoms from vomiting and nausea. Managing the symptoms of nausea and vomiting or avoiding such symptoms during the initial stages of treatment is important (i.e. Aapro *et al.*, 2005), as this will assist in preventing associations between chemotherapy, nausea and vomiting.

Introducing **progressive muscle relaxation** has been found to reduce the effects of anticipatory vomiting and nausea when carried out pre-chemotherapy and during the initial session (refer to Chapter 13 for progressive muscular relaxation). Arakawa (1997) documented the beneficial effects of progressive muscle relaxation in 60 Japanese patients receiving chemotherapy and found that it reduced nausea and vomiting. Other methods that have been found to reduce the effects of chemotherapy include **guided imagery** (Scott *et al.*, 1986) and music therapy (Frank, 1985) which can be practised alone by the patient and also have the added benefit of enhancing the feeling of control (Rhodes and McDaniel, 2001).

Learned associations for smoking and dietary patterns: the importance of environmental cues

The principles of classical conditioning can also in part explain why patients may find it difficult to change their current health behaviours when advised to do so. A nurse who acknowledges possible triggering factors and then addresses these with the patient will increase the chances of a care plan being put together that is individualised and hence more effective in facilitating behaviour change. Studies have shown that nicotine craving tends to occur on presentation of smoking-related stimuli, e.g. drinking in a pub (Payne *et al.*, 1990) which results in an increased desire for a cigarette. This has been referred to as **cue reactivity.**

Cue reactivity in a health care setting is where a classically conditioned response to an environmental cue coincides with drug administration (Ferguson and Miller, 2001). This can result in associations being made even in relation to medical drugs and side-effects, resulting in poor compliance (see Chapter 16). Cue reactivity can also stem from the internal state of an individual. For example, research has extensively documented the link between alcohol uptake and moods. Litt *et al.* (1990) concluded from their study testing alcoholics that exposure to alcohol cues had no effect on desire for alcohol while subjects were in a relaxed, neutral mood state. Instead, the desire for alcohol was elicited when there was a negative mood states, irrespective of whether alcoholic beverages were present or not. However, other researchers have not found a link between negative mood states and an increase in alcohol consumption among alcoholics (Jansma *et al.*, 2000).

Studies looking at individuals who have attempted to stop smoking have identified factors such as not being aware of triggers, not having an alternative means of handling pressure and having a bad or pressurised day, as being common reasons for relapse (Wilkinson *et al.*, 2004). All of these are examples of associations that the smoker has made with environmental and emotional factors. A nurse who can identify these factors and provide alternative solutions or ways of dealing with potential triggers will result in the patient being less likely to relapse as they will be prepared when faced with triggering factors.

Providing patients with relaxation techniques to use when faced with stress or a pressurised day is one way of managing the triggering factor and, in turn, breaking down the association between stress and smoking. Another frequent factor that is associated with smokers who find it difficult to abstain from smoking is the association between stopping smoking and an increase in weight. Croghan and Johnson (2005) recommend keeping a diary that documents dietary changes as one way of attributing control and breaking the association between weight increase and stopping smoking. Addressing potential triggers is an important consideration in any effective behaviour change intervention.

Operant conditioning

Researchers within operant conditioning explore how a response becomes more or less likely to occur, depending on its consequences. Skinner (1956) is the renowned psychologist who dedicated much of his career to the exploration of **operant conditioning** principles, which built on the work of Edward Thorndike (1898).

Skinner showed how likely a behaviour is to occur depending on its consequences by his famous experiment where he placed rats within a Perspex box (Skinner box) with a lever and a mechanical food dispenser fitted to one side. Once placed inside the box the rats were free to play and explore their environment. While exploring the environment, the rats would accidentally learn that when the lever was depressed a pellet of food would be dispensed. This resulted in the rats continually depressing the lever, as there would be a reward of food. The food in turn acted as a **reinforcer**, which encouraged the rats to depress the lever (target response) yet again. The reverse was also found to this association where the rats depressed the lever and were given a mild electric shock instead of food. The mild shock (consequence of behaviour) resulted in the rats avoiding the lever. The principles of operant conditioning are useful for nursing practice, as they will enable the nurse to understand what is required in order to to enhance or reduce particular reactions/interactions by the patient.

Think about this

How did the nurse in the opening case study encourage Buba's positive reaction towards needles?

Reinforcement is responsible for increasing behaviour

One of the concepts from Skinner's exploration of operant conditioning has been that of **reinforcement**. Reinforcement has been defined as 'the process by which a stimulus or event strengthens or increases the probability of the response that it follows' (Wade and Tavris, 2003, p. 241). There are two types of reinforcement: negative and positive. They both enhance behaviour or the response of the individual, but in different ways. **Positive reinforcement** is where a pleasant consequence makes a response more likely to occur again. Positive reinforcement could be seen in Skinner's experiment where response behaviour (pressing a lever) was reinforced by a pleasant consequence (food).

On the other hand **negative reinforcement** involves the removal, delay or decrease in intensity of an unpleasant stimulus, which results in the response becoming stronger or more likely to occur. For example, in the opening case study Buba, prior to meeting the nurse, may have become distressed and cried each time he saw an injection. Buba's father would take the child away each time he was distressed. Hence, each time Buba increased the likelihood of avoiding injections by crying and in turn his father reinforced this behaviour by taking him away. Another example of negative reinforcement is where an individual may have taken a medication that resulted in a severe side effect. After this they increased the likehood of avoiding that particular medication because of the unpleasant consequences.

Think about this

Is it possible for nurses and patients to negatively reinforce each other's behaviour?

Nurses reinforcing patient behaviour

There are numerous interactions that take place between the nurse and the patient which impact on the patient's behaviour. Part of this process involves shaping the patient's behaviour through reinforcement; however this may prove counterproductive to the patient's wellbeing. Baltes and Skinner (1983) showed how nurses can unintentionally reinforce the dependency behaviours of the patient with the **instrumental passivity hypothesis**. According to this hypothesis, hospitals and nursing homes reinforce the dependent behaviours of older people by supporting and encouraging them. The hypothesis draws upon the basic principles within operant conditioning.

According to Baltes, independent behaviours (e.g. a patient attempting to walk to the toilet, or to get up in bed by themselves) tend to get punished (**positive punisher**) or ignored (**negative punisher**). On the other hand, dependent behaviours tend to be reinforced by nurses and health care staff, for example by giving patients more attention (positive reinforcement) or ending their disapproval of independence-seeking behaviours when patients no longer display them (negative reinforcement). Because patients associate dependency behaviours with social rewards and independent behaviours with social punishment, this results in an increase of dependency behaviours.

Faulkner (2002) highlights two main reasons why nurses can be responsible for dependency patient behaviours. Firstly, nursing staff have a high workload, which enhances the probability of the nurse prioritising dependent patients because of their high need of nursing care. Secondly, nurses may shape dependency behaviour as a means to reduce accidents. For example, rather than encouraging a patient to walk alone in the ward for 10 minutes a day, the nurse may hold the patient so that they will not fall, hence increasing dependency. Faulkner (2002) suggests that in line with the *National Service Framework for Older People* (Department of Health, 2001b), which highlights the importance of promoting patient independence and speeding up discharges, nurses should be aware of the possible reinforcement of dependency behaviour. This will in turn make it possible to alleviate such reinforcement of behaviour by being aware of how it can occur. Faulkner (2002) goes as far as to suggest that the principles of operant conditioning can be 'both friend and foe to those delivering patient care' (p. 21).

Although much of the research in relation to the instrumental passivity hypothesis was carried out among elderly patient, the basic principles apply much the same to other patients who are to some degree reliant on the nurse and/or other health care professionals. For example, in the opening case study the nurse had taken time away from the administration of the injection and investigated why Buba was distressed. By doing this, the nurse decreased the patient's distress and encouraged him to be calm and less reliant on his father. This all transpired because the nurse took time away to investigate how the distressing behaviour came to be associated with the administration of the injection.

Reinforcement and avoidance behaviour of the patient

The principles of reinforcement can provide a useful framework when caring for patients with depression or anxiety related disorders. An awareness of the principles of reinforcement will aid the nurse in her understanding of the patient and enable her to implement more effective intervention strategies. According to Rogers *et al.* (2002) an individual who has depression or an anxiety related disorder would strive to avoid situations that evoke anxiety or unpleasant feelings. The avoidance of anxiety or unpleasant feelings will tend to reinforce the avoidance behaviour. This is an example of negative reinforcement.

The nurse will need to raise the patient's awareness as to the long-term implications of avoidance. One of the key points to highlight is that avoiding anxious situations is a short-lived strategy and will not be beneficial for their depression over a longer period of time. For example, a patient who has been diagnosed with severe depression may feel that their anxiety is increased when in a situation consisting of many people and new faces. As a result, the patient will avoid this feeling by not venturing out of the home and even possibly not attending health appointments. The avoidance behaviour will result in the patient sitting at home and not interacting with many people. Hence the individual is more likely to exacerbate their depression because of their overall passive role.

Martell *et al.* (2001) developed a behavioural strategy which can help depressed patients, known as **behavioural activation**. This principle emphasises and makes workable reinforced avoidance behaviours which patients need to encompass. Understanding behavioural activation will enable the nurse to help patients to gradually stop participating within avoidance behaviour and instead begin to focus on strategies that will enable them to get better over the long term. This is achieved by raising the patient's awareness of the implications and consequences of their current behaviour and, in turn, reinforcing behaviour that does not involve avoidance of anxiety-related situations.

Below are some treatment approaches that can help not only patients with a mental health illness but also patients like Buba, who may fear particular medical interventions. The strategies themselves are applicable and popular among those who receive treatment for phobias. These all fall under the general behavioural activation treatment approach.

Overcoming medical and other phobias

Many of the approaches have been based on the principles of conditioning and operant conditioning. **Phobia** is defined as 'anxiety that has turned into a powerful fear by avoidance' (Anxiety Care, 2007). This clearly applies to many patients who access health care, as figures suggest that as many as one person in ten is affected by a phobia at some time in their life. Medical phobias concerning hospitals, dentists, injections and blood are the most common (Anxiety Care, 2007).

Exposure-based therapies can be defined as 'facing something that has been avoided because it provokes anxiety' (Hawton *et al.*, 1989). Curran *et al.* (2006) maintain that for exposure-based therapies to be effective, the therapy needs to be graded (taking one step at a time), repeated (patients who carry out exposure tasks as homework are more successful at beating their phobia; Marks, 1987) and prolonged so that it becomes habitual just like the habitual reaction that characterises the phobia. It does not necessitate that the nurse needs to be well read around the area of exposure-based therapies and breaking up previous learned associations. Instead a nurse who is familiar with the underlying principles can incorporate these into practice. In the case study above, the nurse incorporated the graded component of exposure therapy. Rather than administering the injection immediately, she took a step-by-step approach. To begin with, she spoke about injections. She then demonstrated the administration of the injection using the dolls and finally administered the injection to Buba. The case study exemplifies how principles of exposure therapy can be applied within contexts where there is limited time and within interactions where the nurse will see the patient only once.

Exposure-based therapies are based on the principle of **desensitisation**. This refers to the process in which patients are gradually exposed to their phobia and, in turn, a deconditioning process takes place. Any type of desensitisation will involve a personal plan being drawn up that mirrors the steps of gradual exposure according to the patient's needs. For example, fear of hospital can be common.

The first step within desensitisation would be to find out what the patient is afraid of within the hospital. Many of the fears will be related to previous experiences, e.g. bad news or panic within the hospital setting as a result of an earlier visit. It will then be necessary to build gradual steps, such as being present within the waiting room. At the same time the new experience of the hospital will need to be associated with being calm. One example could be asking the patient to listen to relaxing music. Keeping a diary is another way to find out which situation will evoke high anxiety. This approach will be limited to patients who will have frequent contact with the hospital environment.

Positive reinforcement and social reinforcers

Positive reinforcement or **social reinforcers** can be used to strengthen the associations and new learning that the patient makes. In the opening case study, the nurse used praise as a way of strengthening the association Buba made with having an injection and feeling calm. Praise also acknowledges the patient's efforts and increases the likelihood of the behaviour occurring again. However, positive reinforcers such as praise need to be given immediately and consistently (Hand, 2006) for them to have an effect on behaviour. In addition to this, praise should be used sparingly as it can begin to be taken for granted. Consequently, the patient may show a decrease in behaviour when praise has not been given, as it then becomes expected.

There are many benefits of praise and reward apart from the obvious encouragement of desired behaviour. For example, praise and reward have been found to help children cope positively. It has also been found to play an important part within the emergence of **self-efficacy**, which lowers the anticipatory anxiety that can be experienced within the accident and emergency setting (Bentley, 2004). The opening case study is a prime example of how Buba's behaviour was praised. This not only decreased his anxiety during that particular interaction but will also have a beneficial effect during his future interactions with health care professionals. However, research has found that staff may not fully appreciate the importance of such strategies (Bentley, 2002).

Other examples of positive reinforcement that encourage the same behaviour to be repeated are non-verbal communications such as smiling and nodding. These are referred to as social reinforcers (Hinchliff, 2004). Non-verbal social reinforcers also encourage the patient to carry on with their desired behaviour without feeling patronised as well as not falling into the trap of taking praise for granted. This can be seen in the case study above where praise was only used once when the injection was administered by the nurse. Before the administration of the injection, social reinforcers such as smiling and head nodding were used within the interaction.

Negative reinforcement and not providing rewards

In relation to negative reinforcement where behaviour is motivated by the avoidance of states that cause anxiety or unpleasantness, the actual concept can explain certain types of challenging behaviour. For example, children who have temper tantrums will have this behaviour further reinforced every time the parent gives in and begins to pay attention to the child. Not reinforcing such behaviour, i.e. not paying attention, will result in the behaviour ceasing (Hand, 2006).

To an extent, Buba's father has negatively reinforced Buba's behaviour by holding on to him. Even though a link does exist between ignoring behaviour and not providing reinforcements such as attention, they have no place within a clinical area (Hinchliff, 2004) where every patient needs to be attended to. However, familiarity with this particular association can help a nurse to understand why patients may display certain kinds of behaviour. Harbourne and Solly (1996) go as far as to state that instead nurses should be trained to reduce both **negative affect** and their own reactions to patients with challenging behaviour while at the same time still attending to them. By nurses being familiar with why challenging behaviour is occurring, they can address the causative origins of the challenging behaviour.

In the case study above, the nurse still attended to Buba but focused on why Buba was distressed, so that care could be more effective. On the other hand, Buba's father attended to his son when he was distressed.

Think about this

Think about the television programmes that look at children and challenging behaviour, e.g. 'Supernanny'. How do the principles of operant conditioning and in particular positive and negative reinforcement explain their current behaviour? How are these principles manipulated to shape behaviour that is desired from the child?

Biofeedback

Biofeedback is an intervention that is based wholly on the principles of operant as well as classical conditioning. The focus of biofeedback sessions is for the patient to learn through reinforcement and challenge patterns of their abnormal behaviour (Mills, 2005); this works on the same principle as a treadmill machine that gives instant feedback on heart rate, etc. (see picture). Biofeedback has been used in the management of several health conditions, including functional bowel and bladder control and severe migraine. Electronic sensors are placed on the patient, who is then taught methods of control or relaxation while at the same time being able to visually see the improvements that are being made. For example, normalising bowel frequency is the aim of feedback sessions for this particular group (Norton and Chelvanayagam, 2004).

The principle of operant conditioning operates within biofeedback by demonstrating to the patient that practising exercises or relaxation techniques is beneficial to the management of particular states of ill health. This is continually reinforced by the visual feedback system which is central to the biofeedback method. This method is usually provided by specialist practitioners and nurses who are trained in its administration.

Human beings prefer to have instant rather than long-term positive results, as these enhance motivation. Biofeedback is effective because of the immediate feedback that is provided to the individual. A close example that is based on the biofeedback method is that of the pedometer, which calculates the number of steps as the individual walks or runs; this can contribute to weight management. This is in contrast to an approach where the individual may be calculating their walking sessions and being weighed after a week or a month.

Different versions of the biofeedback method can also be seen within health practice. For example, children who have problems in controlling their bladder can be given an enuresis alarm, which has been found to have a success rate of 70 per cent (Houts *et al.*, 1994). There are two types of alarm

Treadmill: an example of biofeedback where there is immediate visual feedback on the person's behaviour.

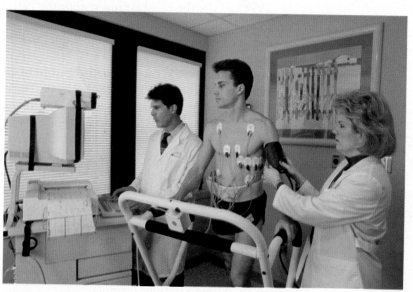

PHOTOTAKE Inc./Alamy

available: the bed or pad buzzer alarm and the body or mini alarm (Rogers, 1998). The mat is placed under the bed sheet on which the child sleeps and every time the child begins to wet the bed, the sensor triggers the alarm which wakes the child (Rogers, 2002).

The alarm method works on the basis of the child associating the release of urine with having to get up to go to the toilet. This is reinforced by the alarm as well as the support of family and practitioners around the child. Nurses should ensure that issues such as the disruption to sleep and how to handle this are taken into consideration if the method is to work.

Token economy system

The token economy system is another method of behaviour modification based on the principles of positive and negative reinforcement. The principle works by making the individual aware that when they carry out a desired behaviour they will be given a token (reinforcement), which can later be exchanged for material goods or other privileges. If it is not possible to provide tokens for material goods, a scoring board can be used instead. The token economy system has been highly recommended in psychiatric units where it has been found to be highly effective (Lin *et al.*, 2006).

The token economy works in line with positive reinforcement whereby you are rewarded or recognised for desired behaviour; behaviour that is not desired is not rewarded. The opening case study documented how the nurse gave patient Buba a gold reward sticker after he displayed calmness when having the injection administered. This exemplifies how the token economy can be applied to patients.

Social learning theory

Social learning theory originated from the work of Albert Bandura (1965, 1991) and is the third strand within the behaviourist approach. According to social learning theory learning can take place through observation and does not necessarily need the individual to be actively involved in the learning process.

Bandura (1965) exemplified the role of observation in learning in his famous study involving the 'Bobo Doll'. During the study, children sat and watched a film in which an adult behaved aggressively towards an inflated doll which bounced back every time it was hit. After the children had watched the film they were taken to a playroom which had the same Bobo Doll placed in the centre. The children were left to play, throughout which they were observed. It was found that the children within the experimental group who had viewed the film were also aggressive during their play activities with the Bobo Doll. The control group who had not watched the film were not aggressive towards the Bobo Doll. Bandura concluded that the principles of operant conditioning could not explain the learning that had taken place, as there was no reinforcement of behaviour. This led Bandura to explain the learning that had occurred solely from observation; this is also referred to as **vicarious learning**.

A nurse can use social learning theory to explore how individuals learn from observation and base their behaviour on 'models' (individuals) that are around them. This will enable the nurse to firstly be aware that patients can learn from people around them and, secondly, that they themselves may be seen as a role model. Ost and Hughdahl (1985) found that 12 per cent of adult dental phobics can trace their dental fear back to a vicarious experience in the past, which demonstrates how individuals from a young age learn from vicarious learning.

Many initiatives have manipulated observational learning, especially for a child who may have a particular fear that becomes a barrier to the care that they are receiving. For example, films can be used to reduce anxiety, since children model their behaviour on characters seen in a film. Do (2004) provides one example in which children were instructed to sit through a film where a child role model successfully endures a medical procedure that is similar to the one the patient is due to undergo. The film had many advantageous features such as demonstrating positive coping skills, deep breathing and relaxation. Do concluded from his study that children did learn and incorporate some of these behaviours during their treatment.

Studies have found that children who observe a modelling film have significant reductions in disruptive behaviour when compared to children who do not observe such a film (Allan and Strokes, 1989). The opening case study also demonstrates role modelling which can be applied to a context where showing a film is not viable. The nurse in the case study used the principles of vicarious observational learning when using the dolls to demonstrate the administration of the injection. This demonstrates how the basic principles of observational learning can be incorporated into an interaction where there is no time or access to video equipment.

Role modelling and learning both for the patient and the student nurse

Looking up to role models and observing behaviour that is then emulated is equally applicable to adult patients as well as student nurses. Rosenthal and Zimmerman (1987) suggest that much of our learning occurs through observation, watching other people and analysing what happens to them. Others suggest that within nurse training, role modelling can be the most important part of early nurse education, with Driggers *et al.* stating that:

> often I learnt by watching and copying the third year student nurse or staff nurse with whom I was working. Much of my nursing socialisation and behaviour was learnt not within the school of nursing but by observing others in practice. (Driggers *et al.*, 1993, cited in Charters, 2000, p. 27)

Bandura describes four phases to the process of social learning:

- attentional phase;
- retentional phase;
- reproduction phase;
- motivational phase.

Think about this

Think back to your last placement. If you have not had a placement yet, think back to a manual handlings or skills class. From whom did you learn and how? The chances are that you learnt from someone who has more experience as a nurse than you and who is someone you aspire to in terms of gaining eventual registration as a nurse. This shows how nurses as learners tend to base their professional conduct according to those who are experienced in practice. Behaviourists would explain this as learning through vicarious learning from a role model who is an experienced registered nurse.

The attentional phase involves the initial observation of the role model. This stage also contributes to variables that result in the learner being more likely to place the individual before them as a role model. Bastable (1997) suggests that role models who are perceived to have high status and competence are more likely to be observed and gain the attention of the learner. Campbell *et al.* (1994) further state that people are more likely to learn from role models who are organised, popular, encouraging and outgoing. Patients who are within the hospital setting will also place nurses and other health care staff as role models and will observe the nurse and how they conduct themselves. For example, emotional responses are influenced and learnt by role modelling (Quinn, 2001). When encouraging independence and assertiveness to a patient, the nurse should also be **congruent** (see Chapter 6) in mirroring these within their own behaviour.

The next phase is the retention phase in which information will be stored and rehearsed (see Chapter 5). The reproductive phase will involve the learner rehearsing the information either mentally or in actual interaction. The nurse at this stage should be aware that reinforcement will be needed so that positive behaviour is further encouraged. The motivational phase will determine how a patient can be motivated to practise such behaviour, which will depend on the reinforcement that is provided by nurses and family members.

Applying the above four phrases is simplistic within the relationship of the student nurse and their mentor. At the same time these phases can also be reinforced to patients who may make an effort to include observed behaviour into practice. For example, a nurse may show a patient how to relax while having a medical intervention administered to them. Although relaxation and how to handle anxiety will have been demonstrated, the patient will have to be further encouraged once they begin to carry out the observed behaviour. In the opening case study the nurse showed Buba as well as his father how to handle anxiety when faced with an injection. She further reinforced this to Buba with the help of the dolls. This was further strengthened with the nurse stating how calm the doll was after having the injection, as well as praising Buba for his calmness during the procedure.

There can be inherent problems when learning through observation from role models which nurses should be aware of. The most obvious one is that of 'good' and 'bad' role models. Calley (1990) has suggested that this can be a problem for a learner who cannot discriminate between good and bad role models. For these learners, they will mimic the behaviour of the role model irrespective of whether they are good or bad. At times, as a nurse on a busy ward, certain aspects of the daily routine may be overlooked. The nurse her-

Think about this

Think about children as well as adolescents and how the media and famous, successful people influence them. Victoria Beckham famously went on stage with a 'false' lip piercing. After that there were concerns in how many young girls would emulate the piercing. The famous pop star had to declare immediately that the piercing was false. More recently, Victoria has hit the headlines again, this time related to 'size zero' which influenced many others around her to lose weight. However, it is not only children or adolescents who are influenced by role models. Take, for example, magazines and the fashion trends and lifestyles that they publish and how many readers they influence. The long-standing fashion magazine *Vogue* is one example that shows high fashion trends, which influence many readers.

Victoria Beckham – how many readers will be influenced by this famous role model?

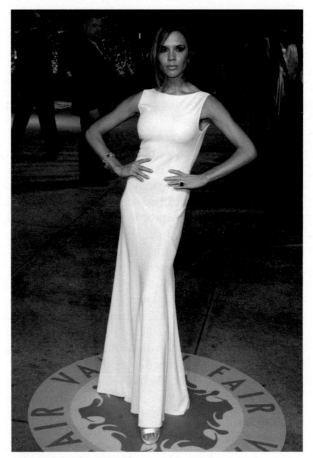

Allstar Picture Library/Alamy

self may not even be aware of this. As soon as this becomes obvious, it is important for the nurse to explain her mistake to any student nurse who could be observing.

However, studies have found that learners such as first-year nursing students can discriminate between good and bad practices (Davies, 1993). At the same time classic research reminds nurses of the high professional standards that have to be maintained within clinical work at all times because of the large influence of the nurse's behaviour on other potential learners (Melia,

1987). Research reminds us of what makes an effective model. Characteristics similar to that of a learner, such as age or the same or aspiring profession, provide one example of an effective model (Do, 2004). A model is also more likely to be effective if the learners look up to the model or hold the model in high regards (Bandura, 1977).

Learning may also be hindered by high-achieving, outstanding role models, who have the effect of dampening the learner's motivation (Lockwood and Kunda, 1999) as well as their self-esteem (refer to Chapter 6). A student nurse should be aware that nurses who have had more clinical experience will in turn be more competent within the ward area. Acknowledging this will prevent any potential problems arising. Good practice for more experienced nurses, will be to state to the assigned student nurses that they have a lot to learn and are not expected to be competent in every aspect of care during their initial learning. This kind of reassurance will not only decrease the possible negative implications of observing role models but will equally make the role model more effective in how they can understand the learner.

Self-efficacy

Self-efficacy is an overarching concept in social learning theory which can be defined as 'the conviction that one can successfully execute behaviour to produce a specified outcome which is one of the central features which distinguish one person from another' (Bandura, 1977) or from a lay person's perspective, having control within one's life. The goal of social learning theory is to build on self-efficacy or an individual's perception of capabilities for performance (Bandura, 1977). Understanding the concept of self-efficacy is important for nurses, as it considers how an individual can have control within a situation. This is becoming a central concept within health care as it interlinks with the area of patient empowerment (see Chapter 3) and self-management (Fleming *et al.*, 2003). For example, in the opening case study, patient Buba had more control over his anxious feelings when faced with the administration of an injection. There is a direct link between patients (or individuals in general) who feel that they have control within an environment, i.e. where they will be able to control and predict threatening events, and how vulnerable he or she will be to anxiety or stress in response to traumatic experiences (Bandura, 1977).

First, the nurse needs to make an assessment of the patient's self-efficacy in relation to the particular health condition; this can be carried out by asking a few questions. For example, Larner (2005) looked at assessing self-efficacy for patients with a newly acquired disability. Larner found many questions useful when measuring self-efficacy, such as asking the patient how difficult they consider a particular rehabilitation activity to be, or how confident he or she is in their ability to perform certain activities or movements. Resnick and Jenkins (2000) recommend the use of a percentage scale when assessing self-efficacy, with 0 being not confident, 50 partly confident and 100 as fully confident.

Questions from a general questionnaire can also be used to assess the patient's general self-efficacy and motivation on a day-to-day basis. The following questionnaire is originally from Bosscher and Smit (1998) but was adapted by Fleming *et al.* (2003) to include three additional questions (questions 13 to 15) for use within a psychiatric setting.

15-point questionnaire to assess self-efficacy adapted by Fleming *et al* (2003). Partly originated from Bosscher and Smit (1998).

1. If something looks too complicated, I will not even try it.
2. I avoid trying to learn new things when they look difficult.
3. When trying to learn something new I soon give up if I am not successful.
4. When I make plans I am certain I can make them work.
5. If I can't do a job first time, I keep on trying until I can.
6. When I have something unpleasant to do I stick to it until I have finished.
7. When I decide to do something I go right to work on it.
8. Failure just makes me try harder.
9. When I set important goals for myself I rarely achieve them.
10. I do not seem capable of dealing with most problems that come up in my life.
11. When unexpected problems occur, I don't handle them very well.
12. I feel insecure about my ability to do things.
13. I am a self-reliant person.
14. I am able to reduce my own anxiety levels easily.
15. I am in control of my own mood and feelings.

Each question can be answered 'strongly disagree', 'disagree', 'neither', 'agree' or 'strongly agree'. A score of 0 to 4 is attached to each answer, graded depending on whether it is a negative or a positive question. For negative questions (1, 2, 3, 9, 10, 11, 12) strongly disagree = 4, disagree = 3, neither = 2, agree = 1 and strongly agree = 0. For positive questions (4, 5, 6, 7, 8, 13, 14 and 15) strongly disagree = 0, disagree = 1, neither = 2, agree = 3 and strongly agree = 4. Hence for both positively and negatively framed questions an improvement in self-efficacy results in a higher score.

There are many strategies that the nurse can incorporate which enhance self-efficacy. For example, Litt *et al.* (1995) highlighted the importance of letting patients know that they are managing well. This will not only improve self-efficacy but also helps them to cope much better. Having prior experience of a situation also enhances self-efficacy. This was demonstrated by Lee (2001) who looked at violence in A&E and the role of staff training and self-efficacy (see Research in focus box below).

This study exemplifies how self-efficacy can be enhanced through experience. The study concluded that self-efficacy is much lower for those patients who have had a new diagnosis or a particular ill state of health which they are not familiar with. Within such contexts, patient self-efficacy will be dramatically low compared with patients who have had a diagnosis for a longer period, as they will be more familiar with the diagnosis, already built up coping responses and be able to better predict their health on a day-to-day basis. One of the four components that Bandura refers to which contribute to self-efficacy is that of performance accomplishment, where individuals experience mastery over their environment (see Chapter 6).

Research in focus

Lee, F. (2001) Violence in A&E: the role of training and self-efficacy. *Nursing Standard*, 15, 46, 33-38.

Aim
To determine the amount of violence experienced by A&E staff during a three month period and to explore the effect of aggression management training and exposure to violence on their self-efficacy in dealing with aggressive patients.

Method
A small-scale questionnaire survey was undertaken of 130 staff.

Results
Seventy-six (58%) members of staff responded. The findings suggested that verbal and physical violence were a common occurrence. The type and amount of aggression management training were variable. Greater self-efficacy in managing aggressive behaviour was observed in higher grades of staff and in staff who had experienced higher levels of verbal aggression.

Conclusion
Violence against nurses was widely reported. Their aggression management training did not appear to equip them with the skills required to manage this behaviour.

Think about this

Think back to the last time you achieved a high grade in an assignment or exam or had excellent feedback for a placement portfolio. How did you feel? In control? Keen to take on the next hurdle?

Each of your answers would have resulted in your thinking back to a time when your self-efficacy was high. How could high self-efficacy be achieved for a patient who feels that they have no control in their life since they have been ill or in hospital?

Managing chronic pain over a long-term period is another example of where self-efficacy has a central role to play. Oliver and Ryan (2004) suggest that successful pain management is determined by the improvement of self-efficacy. The researchers advocate the following skills which will enhance the self-efficacy of a patient experiencing chronic pain.

● Cognitive and social skills: understand the reason for such behaviour.
● Psychomotor skills: learn how to engage in relaxation techniques.
● Self-regulatory skills: to incorporate the principles of self-management into a daily routine.

Another attribute that Bandura outlines as contributing to self-efficacy is that of vicarious experience/learning which refers to the process of learning through the observation of a role model. For example, a nurse (role model) could exemplify to the patient (learner) effective coping strategies during times of stress from which the patient could then learn and practice.

According to Walker (2001), the enhancement of self-efficacy is dependent on the 'role in informing interventions designed to help people to gain new and relevant skills, have the confidence to use them, believe they can do them and that they will work' (p. 95). Underlying this is the incorporation of modelling, teaching skills to patients and consistent encouragement and praise, which will enhance the self-efficacy of the patient by building on the previously-mentioned principles of behaviourism. The nurse can take these into account when information-giving and attempting to build the patient's self-efficacy. Browes (2006) found that education and information were vital components in the enhancements of self-efficacy within the area of sexual health.

The beneficial effects of incorporating self-efficacy within a care plan is that patients with high self-efficacy on the whole tend to report less intense pain, increased perception of control, less emotional distress and higher activity levels (Anderson *et al.*, 1995). Self-efficacy has also been seen to play an important role within expert patient programmes, where there is emphasis on the patient or carer to carry out care routines that a nurse would normally do. The nurse can play a key role by ensuring that there is emotional support such as listening, counselling and promoting self-confidence and self-efficacy as well as practical help which encourages independence (Kirk and Glendinning, 2002). Self-efficacy features within many health models (see Chapter 15) as well as forming the main premise of stress and control research (Chapter 13), locus of control (Chapter 13) and self-esteem (Chapter 6). Each of these share the commonality of gaining control and mastery over one's environment as well as being able to accomplish set tasks. Understandably, self-efficacy as a construct has a vital role to play in patient management and behaviour modification programmes.

Conclusion

Behaviourist principles and theories can help a nurse better understand a patient's behaviour. If this behaviour becomes challenging or becomes distressful to the patient, it begins to act as a barrier to the care being provided or as a barrier to enhancing the well-being of the patient. Principles within behaviourism and associated behaviour modification therapies can help the nurse to direct the patient's behaviour in a beneficial way.

Even though behavioural therapies require a specialist practitioner or nurse, the principles of behaviourism can still be applied to patients, especially those who are highly anxious, have negative experiences of the hospital setting or have low self-efficacy. Such principles will be highly beneficial in moving the patient forward within the proposed care plan, while at the same time promoting independence and empowerment and the encouragement of the expert patient.

Summary

- Classical conditioning is the first strand within behaviourism which was put forward by Ivan Pavlov (1849–1936). According to this perspective learning occurs as a result of associations that are made between stimuli and responses that become conditioned.

- Generalisation can occur in patients who pair their conditioned response, e.g. feeling nausea or vomiting, with the original stimulus, e.g. treatment, and other associated stimulus, e.g. smell of the hospital. Extinction of a response occurs when the original stimuli is presented without the conditioned stimulus several times.

- Operant conditioning is the second strand within behaviourism, which was put forward by Skinner (1956). This strand postulates that learning and the occurrence of behaviour is dependent on its consequences.

- Reinforcement is the process by which a stimulus or event strengthens or increases the probability of the response that it follows. Positive reinforcement, e.g. praise, is a reinforcer that strengthens behaviour. Negative reinforcement is where avoidance of unpleasantness results in an avoidance behaviour.

- Instrumental passivity hypothesis looks at dependency behaviour that is reinforced by health care staff.

- Behavioural activation is a strategy where avoidance behaviours are addressed and, in turn, behaviour that helps an individual not to avoid situations is reinforced. Exposure-based therapies also address situations that are avoided because they evoke anxiety. Desensitisation refers to the process of gradual exposure to what the patient may fear.

- Biofeedback is an intervention that provides immediate feedback on behaviour, hence strengthening the behaviour through reinforcement. A token economy system is where the individual is rewarded by tokens each time the individual carries out desired behaviour.

- Social learning theory is the third strand of behaviourism, which was put forward by Bandura (1965, 1991). This strand emphasises that learning can take place without the learner being active in the process. This was exemplified with the famous Bobo doll study, which concluded that observation alone is enough for learning to take place. This is also known as vicarious learning.

- Self-efficacy is the confidence that one can carry out a desired behaviour. This concept features within most of the health belief models and plays a central role when looking at behaviour modification such as lifestyle or behaviour change.

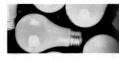 ## Check your understanding

1. Name the three strands within behaviourism and describe how each of these explains learning.

2. Positive and negative reinforcement both increase behaviour, but how do they differ?

3. Chemotherapy patients may, after a few sessions, begin to feel physically sick and experience vomiting. How can classical conditioning be applied to these patients and what can nurses do to prevent this or minimise the association of being sick and attending chemotherapy sessions?

4. Name three interventions that are based on operant and/or classical conditioning which can help patients feel less anxious and help them to face, rather than avoid, anxious situations.

5. Define vicarious learning and explain how both patients and nurses can learn from this.

6. Define self-efficacy and justify addressing this concept within patient care.

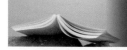

Further reading

Aapro, M.S., Molassiotis, A. and Olver, I. (2005) Anticipatory nausea and vomiting. *Support Care Cancer*, **13**, 117-121.

Charters, A. (2000) Encouraging student centred learning in a clinical environment: role modelling as a teaching method. *Emergency Nurse*, **7** (10), 25-29.

Curran, R.P. and Gournay, K. (2002) Depression: nature, assessment and treatment using behavioural activation (part 1). *Mental Health Practice*, **5** (10), 32-37.

Curran, J., Machin, C. and Gournay, K. (2006) Cognitive behavioural therapy for patients with anxiety and depression. *Nursing Standard*, **21** (7), 44-52.

Mills, P. (2005) Establishing a biofeedback (behavioural therapy) service. *Gastrointestinal Nursing*, **3** (3), 35-39.

Rogers, J. (2002) Managing daytime and night-time enuresis in children. *Nursing Standard*, **16** (32), 45-52.

Weblinks

Athabasa University Centre for Psychology	http://psych.athabascau.ca/html/prtut/reinpair.htm	Basic principles of positive and negative reinforcement are explored in depth
Encyclopedia of Psychology	http://www.psychology.org/links/ Paradigms_and_Theories/Behavior_Analysis/	This site provides a substantial collection of links to behaviourism and its founding principles
Social Anxiety Facts for Health Organisation	http://www.socialanxiety.factsforhealth.org/ treatment/behavior.asp	A site dedicated to therapies to help those with anxiety problems which are based on the principles of behaviourism. Behaviour therapy is given extensive coverage
The Behavioural Model of Abnormal Psychology Site	http://www.simplypsychology.pwp.blueyonder.co.uk/ behaviour-therapy.html	A look at therapies and interventions which have been covered within this chapter, ranging from systematic desensitisation to the token economy system
National Cancer Institute: Cancer Web	http://cancerweb.ncl.ac.uk/cancernet/304466.html	A look at nausea and vomiting in chemotherapy patients which are in part explained by the principles within behaviourism

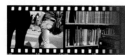

Media example

Supernanny A look at behaviouristic principles in practice among parents and their children.

Chapter 3

Patient-centred nursing

Learning outcomes

When you have read through this chapter you should understand:

- The definition of empathy and how it can be measured and applied within the nurse–patient relationship.

- What unconditional positive regard is and how the nurse can apply this to the nurse–patient relationship.

- How the terms congruence and incongruence can be distinguished and how the recognition of the two terms can benefit the nurse when understanding their patient.

- How Abraham Maslow's five-stage hierarchy of needs model can be applied to patients, when attempting to change their behaviour.

- How Prochaska and DiClemente's stage change model can help a nurse when motivating a patient to change their behaviour.

- What empowerment is and how the nurse can empower their patients.

- What the role of a patient advocate entails.

Case study

After one miscarriage, Rejoice has had a healthy baby boy. Her husband, family and friends are overjoyed by the new arrival. Several months after the birth of her baby, Rejoice is still feeling 'low'. Her GP has prescribed Rejoice a course of anti-depressants. She has decided not to take these.

Over a seven-month period, Rejoice's symptoms of depression become worse. The GP is concerned for the well-being of Rejoice and her baby. She has persistently rejected medication and counselling. The GP has invited the community nurse to become involved with the care of Rejoice and her baby.

The community nurse, Ragpal, visits Rejoice. During their first meeting, Rejoice is adamant that she does not need any help and is not feeling down. After the first meeting, the community nurse concludes that the patient is 'putting on a brave face' and will not acknowledge her feelings of depression. During the next meeting, the community nurse talks to Rejoice. The nurse makes a concerted effort to understand how Rejoice perceives her new role as a mother. After the second meeting, the community nurse feels that she is making progress, as Rejoice has begun to talk about her feelings.

During the next meeting, Rejoice begins to open up about her feelings. She has a healthy baby boy but is not happy. In addition to this, Rejoice says she is finding it difficult to meet the everyday demands that her child requires from her.

The community nurse has found that Rejoice opens up more about her feelings when the nurse explicitly states that she will not judge her in any way. During the forthcoming visits, Rejoice begins to acknowledge that 'feeling down' is common among first-time mothers. In addition to this, Rejoice has begun to use successful coping strategies when feeling under pressure. Rejoice has now begun enjoying being a mother.

The community nurse now starts to concentrate on Rejoice's self-esteem, which is very low. It becomes apparent that Rejoice had always enjoyed working, but had to stop because of health problems in her final trimester. Although Rejoice has now realised that she loves being a mother, she does miss the interaction she used to have at work with colleagues. In addition to this, her husband works away from home during the week, which has further limited contact with people of her own age. To overcome this, the community nurse and Rejoice have discussed 'tea mornings' with other mothers, as well as looking into short adult courses, to begin building up the confidence that Rejoice has lost.

Three years later Rejoice no longer feels 'low'. She now works part-time and leaves her son at the local crèche. She also discussed with her husband the importance of coming home mid-week so that they could spend more time together. Rejoice has now begun to feel better in herself, as well as gaining more confidence on a day-to-day-basis. Most importantly, she is now enjoying being a mother and is three months pregnant with her second child. When Rejoice looks back, she can never forget Ragpal, the community nurse who helped her. Today, Rejoice keeps a diary, where she reflects on her feelings, as well as setting goals for the future.

The case of Rejoice highlights many thinking points for a nurse. Should a nurse deal with the 'here and now' or should a wider focus be taken, including factors that led up to the present state of health? Are there psychological factors that can influence the individual's health? How can you help a patient who feels helpless? How can a nurse motivate a patient who has no confidence? This chapter will answer these questions and help the nurse gain confidence when caring for patients in similar situations to Rejoice.

Why is this relevant to nursing practice?

This case study is relevant to nursing practice as there will be patients who will need that 'extra' help on issues other than their medical diagnosis or problem. It highlights 'other issues' that the community nurse may have to address, such as confidence, **self-esteem** and motivation. **Humanistic psychology** is a perspective within psychology that aims to understand the individual as fully as possible, including factors such as those mentioned above, before treating their symptoms.

The basic principles within humanistic psychology can be applied when addressing such issues. For example, the community nurse used principles from **person-centred** counselling, which stem from the work of Dr Carl Rogers (1902–1987). Rogers was a famous American psychologist and therapist, who pioneered person-centred counselling in the 1930s and 1940s. According to him, the patient is 'the most important' and 'knows best' when attempting to make any change (Mearns and Thorne, 2005). Rogers highlighted **three core conditions** as central to person-centred counselling, these being **empathy**, **unconditional positive regard** and **congruence**, which are important for any therapeutic relationship. The community nurse in the opening case study used all three, which facilitated in her helping Rejoice more effectively.

Empathy can be defined as:

> a continuing process whereby the counsellor lays aside her own way of experiencing and perceiving reality, preferring to sense and respond to the experiences and perceptions of her client. Sensing may be intense and enduring with the counsellor actually experiencing her client's thoughts and feelings as powerfully as if they had originated in herself. (Mearns and Thorne, 2005, p. 41)

The community nurse used the skill of empathy when attempting to understand how Rejoice understood the world around her. Empathy will be explored in this chapter, as nurses are required to use empathy within the nurse–patient relationship when attempting to understand their patient's perception of their current state of health and their interpretation of the world around them.

The second core component within person-centred counselling that the community nurse used was *unconditional positive regard*. This can be defined as:

> a label given to the fundamental attitude of the person-centred counsellor towards her client. The counsellor who holds this attitude provides care for the individual irrespective of what beliefs and values the individual (patient) may hold. The attitude manifests itself in the counsellor's consistent acceptance of and enduring warmth towards her client. (Mearns and Thorne, 2005, p. 64)

The community nurse used the skill of unconditional positive regard, as the care that was offered was not influenced by any negative characteristics or expectations of depression, such as Rejoice's not being able to do anything. The community nurse expressed this verbally to the patient by reassuring Rejoice that she did not see her as a 'bad mother' or an individual who had 'given up'. Throughout practice it will be important to provide care for a patient without being influenced by their previous medical or other history, to ensure that the patient feels fully accepted.

The third component that Carl Rogers highlights is *congruence*. Congruence can be defined as:

> the state of being of the counsellor when her outward responses to her client consistently match the inner feelings and sensations, which she has in relation to the client. (Mearns and Thorne, 2005, p. 84)

For example, a nurse who states that they want to help the patient will mirror this in their behaviour when listening to the patient. By recognising congruence, a nurse can understand the thoughts and feelings of their patients more effectively.

The community nurse recognised the lack of congruency that Rejoice demonstrated during their first interaction. This was seen when Rejoice stated that 'she was fine' but her case notes suggested that she was depressed. Her stated feelings did not match her actual feeling, which is the opposite of congruence, referred to as **incongruence**. Within the case study, Rejoice had higher expectations of herself, which did not mirror her present resources or environment. As a result, there was a decrease in self-esteem and feeling low, which resulted in low motivation. This had a negative effect on the patient who needed to make changes within her lifestyle or follow instructions to manage her illness. Self-esteem will be explored in Chapter 4.

Motivation will be explored with reference to Abraham Maslow's (1943) **five-stage hierarchy of needs model**, which can be seen in Figure 3.1. According to this model, basic needs need to be met before an individual can achieve **self-actualisation** (SA), the peak need level. Self-actualisation can be defined as 'the need to find fulfilment and realise one's potential' (Watkinson and Scott, 2004). Clearly in the case of Rejoice many of her basic needs, such as belonging (feeling part of a group, e.g. a work team), love needs (having friends, family and loved ones around) and esteem needs (feeling a

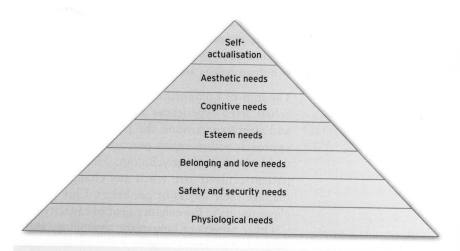

Figure 3.1 Maslow's five-stage hierarchy of needs model.

Source: A.H. Maslow (1943) A Theory of Human Motivation, *Psychological Review*, **50**(4), 370-96 © 1943 by the American Psychological Association.

sense of achievement and accomplishing important goals), were not being met since she had left work and given birth. This could have explained her lack of motivation. In the case study, the community nurse highlighted that Rejoice's basic needs that were not being met. Rejoice was no longer part of the workforce, her husband was away a lot and she did not feel capable as a mother. Addressing these needs enabled Rejoice to overcome her depression. This model is important for nurses when they care for patients who could be feeling 'low' or may not have the motivation to initiate any change in their present behaviour. Maslow's five-stage hierarchy of needs model will enable the nurse to address basic needs before the patient's behavioural change is explored. This model will be explored in greater depth further on in the chapter.

Many of the principles mentioned above are embedded within 'patient-centred care', which is the main framework that promotes holistic care within nursing. The above concepts are important to consider both from a theoretical standpoint as well as an understanding of how these principles can be applied in practice.

Humanistic psychology

Humanistic psychology emerged during the 1950s, in reaction to both the behaviourist and psychodynamic schools within psychology. Behaviourism (discussed in full detail within Chapter 2) is the first force psychodynamic (discussed in full detail within Chapter 4) is the second force and the humanistic school of psychology is the **third force** in psychology. The humanistic perspective strives to highlight a more holistic vision of both psychology and the understanding of the person.

This has been exemplified by the five main principles that underpin humanistic psychology, as put forward by James Bugental (1964):

- human beings cannot be reduced to components;
- human beings have in them a uniquely human context;
- human consciousness includes an awareness of oneself in the context of other people;
- human beings have choices and responsibilities;
- human beings are intentional; they seek meaning, value and creativity.

The aim of humanistic psychology is to understand 'the person' and the actual 'lived experiences' of the individual as well as planning therapy, care and treatment around the patient. The person-centred, or client-centred, approach within health practice is based on the basic theoretical principles within humanistic psychology. This approach highlights the importance of patient-centred care when any change is needed for the patient to better manage their illness or get better. Clay (2002) states that 'centring on the client results in the enhancement of capacity for self-direction'.

Other aspects of humanistic psychology include **empowerment**, which can be defined as having control and confidence over one's life and when interacting with others, and **advocacy**, where an individual such as a nurse may act as an advocate for the patient in voicing their concerns and needs on their behalf. The community nurse empowered Rejoice by working on smaller goals, so that she could gain more confidence. The nurse also acted as Rejoice's advocate by making links with social support networks, such at the 'tea mornings with new mothers'. Empowerment and advocacy are two areas that are important to look at, especially when working with patients who are depressed, feeling low or have no confidence to make any changes by themselves.

Think about this

Before reading the following sections, think about the humanistic strands that have been mentioned in the above section, such as empathy, holistic care and patient-centredness. How can these promote better understanding of the patient?

Principles of person-centred counselling

There are many roles that the nurse is expected to fill when caring for a patient. The most important role is to attend to the medical needs of the patient. However, there will be patients who have other 'non-medical' issues, which may be impacting on their well-being and therefore need to be addressed. The community nurse dealt with issues 'other' than depression itself. The following section will explore the main principles that the community nurse used when helping Rejoice.

The patient resource

Carl Rogers emphasised the client/patient being the most important resource when attempting to help them. This is illustrated in his famous quote:

> it is the client who knows what hurts, what direction to go, what problems are crucial, what experiences have been deeply buried. It began to occur to me that unless I had a need to demonstrate my own cleverness and learning, I would do better to rely upon the client for the direction of movement in the process. (Rogers, 1961, pp. 11–12)

Rogers highlighted the importance of three core conditions as being central to understanding the client:

- genuine and congruent;
- offering unconditional positive regard and total acceptance; and
- feel and communicate a deep empathetic understanding, which facilitate patient-centredness.

The community nurse in the case study above relied on Rejoice's perspective and insight when helping her to put together an effective plan. For example, Rejoice highlighted issues such as not working and having reduced adult contact as a big difference in her life as a new mother. The community nurse used this information as a base before thinking about strategies that could help Rejoice, rather than just providing advice.

Empathy

What is empathy?

Kunyk and Olson (2001) analysed and reviewed nursing literature between 1992 and 2000 and revealed five views or definitions of empathy. These are: empathy as a human trait, empathy as a professional state, empathy as a communication process, empathy as caring and empathy as a special relationship.

The first view of empathy as a *human trait* focuses on empathy being a basic, natural response that cannot be taught, although it can be identified, reinforced and refined (Kunyk and Olson, 2001). Many personal attributes can be called upon to enhance empathy. Experience, creativity, maturity and self-awareness (Kunyk and Olson, 2001) are all seen as such attributes. In the opening case study, the community nurse used self-awareness when looking back at how she communicated with Rejoice during her first meeting. She then used this as a base from which to plan her working goals for the second meeting. As a training nurse, with little if any experience working with patients, using self-awareness when interacting with the patient will be wholly beneficial (refer to Chapter 4).

Think about this

What questions would the community nurse have asked herself, when reflecting back and raising awareness of the extent to which she used empathy with Rejoice during her first visit?

One way of raising awareness as to the extent of empathy used within the nurse–patient relationship is to fill in an empathy scale (Table 3.1). This will not only help a nurse raise awareness of the extent to which empathy is being used in their practice, but will also be useful to those who are new to practising the skill of empathy within a professional capacity.

The scale contains 12 items that describe behaviours or attitudes of a counsellor (e.g. a nurse) during verbal interaction with his/her client or patient. Read each statement and decide the degree to which you perceive the person that you are rating (e.g. yourself, your nurse helper or an associate) as like or unlike the statement when applied to a recent relationship. There are positive as well as negative empathy statements in the grid.

The scale raises awareness as to what extent empathy has been used within the helping relationship.

The second view of empathy, outlined by Kunyk and Olson (2001), refers to empathy as a *professional state*. The main emphasis here is for the nurse to remain objective and to keep at 'arms length' from the emotional and personal experiences of the patient. The community nurse in the opening case study used open questions (refer to Chapter 17), which enabled the nurse to understand Rejoice, without the patient becoming dependent on her and allowing emotional detachment to be maintained.

The third view of empathy refers to it as a *communication process*. This *tends* to embrace the overall communication process that occurs when a nurse uses empathy. The communication process of empathy can be broken down into three phases:

	Always 100%	Nearly always 90%	Frequently 75%	Quite often 50%	Occasionally 25%	Seldom 10%	Never 0%
1. Attempts to explore and clarify feelings							
2. Leads, directs and diverts							
3. Responds to feelings							
4. Ignores verbal and non-verbal communication							
5. Explores personal meanings of feelings							
6. Judgemental and opinionated							
7. Responds to feelings and meaning							
8. Interrupts and seems in a hurry							
9. Provides the client with direction							
10. Fails to focus on solutions/does not answer direct questions/lacks genuineness							
11. Appropriate voice tone, sound relaxed							
12. Inappropriate voice tone sounds curt							

Source: Reynolds, W. et al., Journal of Advanced Nursing, **32** (1), 235-242.

Table 3.1 The empathy scale

- Phase One – nurse perceives the patient's emotions and situation;
- Phase Two – nurse expresses understanding;
- Phase Three – the patient perceives the understanding of the nurse.

By acknowledging the above phases when communicating and attempting to understand a patient, the outcome should be a more accurate perception of the patient and in turn the patient feeling understood. The actual process will be further endorsed by counselling skills, such as paraphrasing, summarising and open questioning, which are explored in Chapter 7.

Another important perspective of empathy is *caring*. From this perspective, the patient being understood is not considered an outcome of the empathetic process. Instead, the outcome of the empathetic process is a nursing intervention that meets the physical needs of the patient *and* alleviates emotional suffering.

Empathy can be divided into four phases which enable the nurse to meet the physical needs of the patient and alleviate their emotional suffering (Sutherland, 1993):

- Phase One – identification; whereby the nurse becomes engrossed in the experiences and situation of the patient and loses their own self in the process. For example, the nurse will not use his or her own experiences and will attentively listen to the patient.
- Phase Two – introjection; which involves the nurse emotionally feeling what the patient is feeling and reflecting on the meaning that the experience has for the patient.
- Phase Three – intervention; a nursing action is taken on behalf of the patient and is based on the scrutiny that has been carried out by the nurse when listening and thinking about what the patient has said and is feeling.
- Phase Four – response phase; involves having the physical needs of the patient met or their emotional suffering alleviated.

The model above shows that empathy alone is not adequate when caring for a patient, as there are many other basic needs of the patient that need to be met. This has been made evident by researchers who have distinguished between counsellors who do not have to attend to basic physical needs and nurses who have to meet the basic needs of the patient. Hudson (1993) highlights the relationship between empathy and the physical needs of the patient. He suggests that empathy is valuable, but only after the patient's basic needs have been met.

Finally, empathy is also considered to be a *special caring relationship* between the patient and the nurse with a focus on friendship, which is in contrast to the view of empathy as a professional state and objectivity being paramount. This conceptualisation stems from the work of Raudonis (1993), who explored the patient's perspective on the nature, meaning and impact of empathetic relationships with hospice nurses. According to the hospice patients in Raudonis's study, an empathetic relationship develops through a process of reciprocal sharing. Friendship emerged frequently in responses and was defined as an intense, deep and meaningful relationship. Also, the nurse's willingness to spend time getting to know a patient as an individual and the patient's reciprocal sharing were critical in the development of the empathetic relationship. According to this perspective, such a relationship is fundamental in providing the foundation for patients and nurses to work together to fulfil the patient's goals.

Think about this

Look back at the opening case study: which conceptualisations of empathy would have been useful for the community nurse to use when helping Rejoice?

Empathy in communication

Much of the literature that explores empathy tends to focus on the relationship between the counsellor and the client. The literature that does look at empathy within the context of nurse and patient interaction tends to be mixed. On one hand, literature tends to question the concept of empathy within the nurse–patient relationship. For example, Morse *et al.* (1992) argue that empathy is not possible within acute and medical settings because high workload does not give a nurse the time to spend 30 minutes or longer listening to one patient. However, the majority of literature that looks at empathy in relation to the nursing context highlights its usefulness, even though such barriers exist.

Carver and Hughes (1990) state that:

> The sterility of a mechanical (high technology) environment makes the caring, comforting functions of professionals critically important, yet difficult to achieve. Technical competence is necessary, but must be combined with interpersonal skills such as empathy, warmth and respect; before the patient feels health professionals care. (p. 15)

Empathy acts as a crucial element in a supportive interpersonal climate between nurse and patient. This view was accepted as early as the 1960s, for example, Kalman (1967) stated that:

> Relationship therapy refers to a prolonged relationship between a nurse therapist and a patient, during which the patient can feel accepted as a person of worth, and feels free to express himself without fear of rejection or censure. (p. 226)

Many studies have cited empathy as being the primary ingredient within any helping relationship (e.g. MacKay *et al.* 1990). For example, the beneficial outcome of the use of empathy has also been found within the context of helping children with learning disabilities. Seigal (1972) found improvement among children with learning disabilities in both verbal and behavioural spheres, which were related to time in play therapy, and the therapist's levels of empathy, warmth and genuineness.

Despite the mixture of evidence, empathy remains crucial to effective interpersonal processes and essential at the onset of a relationship (e.g. Barker *et al.*, 1998; MacKay *et al.* 1990).

Think about this

With the help of the various definitions of empathy, think about the different aspects of empathy that can be used when time is limited. Do patients with differing states of ill-health require different levels of empathy?

Sympathy and empathy – what is the difference?

Sympathy can be defined as 'an expression of the caregiver's own sorrow at another's plight' (Morse *et al.*, 2006). Sympathy is characterised by using 'I' statements and expressions from the practitioner to the patient. For example, in the opening case study, the community nurse would be using sympathy if she had made verbal statements such as, 'I'm sorry that you are feeling down' or 'I feel for you that it is a difficult time for you'. If Rejoice had cried and the nurse held her hand, this would have been another example of sympathy, via the non-verbal channel.

This differs from empathy, as when expressing sympathy the listener (nurse) becomes emotionally involved by sharing their own sorrow and pain. This could result in the nurse feeling emotional, as well as the possibility of the patient becoming overly dependent on the nurse to find answers for them. In contrast, empathy removes the listener (nurse) from becoming emotionally involved and keeps the listener at an emotional distance whilst attempting to understand what the speaker (patient) is feeling. For example, the community nurse would be using empathy if she used statements such as, 'you are telling me that you are feeling down' or 'from what you have told me, it seems that you are having a difficult time at the moment'.

As the process of sympathy encompasses emotional involvement, this can be a barrier to the nurse attempting to be objective about the patient. This can be seen in the following definition of sympathy, where sympathy has been defined as 'a means to share another's emotions such as sorrow or anguish, becoming emotionally involved which distorts clear and measured thinking' (*Health and Age*, 2006).

Another concern highlighted in relation to the use of sympathy is that of encouraging the patient to become more dependent on the nurse, as well as an increase in negative and helpless thinking. Take the following case study as an example:

Case study

Mike is a mental health nurse who is taking care of Tigbimawe, a 27-year-old male who has bipolar depression. The patient's wife died several months ago in a car accident. Mike has helped the patient by using his own experience of coping with his mother's death. Tigbimawe requests to see Mike and no other nurse. Mike has become frustrated, as he finds that Tigbimawe has made no progress in helping himself to get better.

The above case study exemplifies how sympathy when used inappropriately can result in the patient becoming overly dependent and helpless. It would have been more appropriate for Mike to leave out his personal experience of coping with death when helping Tigbimawe. Instead, the use of empathy would have been more advantageous for the patient. Sympathy could have still been used but in a different manner and not throughout the whole interaction. For example, the nurse could have stated that, 'I feel for you', rather than 'I know how you feel'.

The use of sympathy within the nurse–patient relationship is not forbidden when used appropriately alongside empathy. This can be seen in the following example of a patient experiencing alopecia for the first time:

Nobody has much sympathy for my feelings about my hair, which makes me feel misunderstood. 'What's more important?' the purveyors of optimism try to convince me 'your hair or your life?' I don't need convincing: of *course* my life, of course. But they have missed the point. Cook (1981)

Sympathy can also help when a patient is 'putting on a brave face' and is in constant neglect of their true feelings. The actual act of sympathy by a nurse can aid a patient to move from 'putting on a brave face' to feeling that it is fine to feel that way at the present moment.

Think about this

What are the advantages and disadvantages of using sympathy? What particular context or states of health warrant the nurse to use sympathy when helping a patient?

Unconditional positive regard

The second component Carl Rogers highlighted as being necessary for any change within a client or patient is *unconditional positive regard*, which can be defined as not judging a patient within the nurse–patient relationship, irrespective of their illness, lifestyle or previous lifestyle/medical history.

In order to display unconditional positive regard, the nurse needs to talk to the patient without any conditions and judgements placed on the patient. In turn, it will then be possible for the patient to feel accepted and worthy. These are necessary conditions in order for the patient to initiate change and to move out of their present mindset. Rogers refers to moving on as **self-growth.**

According to Rogers, as a result of initiating unconditional positive regard into the relationship, the patient will be able to draw upon their own resources when moving forward and growing. It is important for this to be delivered by a nurse who is congruent at all times. For example, if a nurse listens to a patient and does not make any judgement about them but, at the same time, takes a dislike to the patient, the nurse will be incongruent. This could manifest itself via the verbal or non-verbal channel.

Unconditional positive regard should be incorporated at the onset of a relationship between the nurse and patient, especially within interactions where the nurse may not agree with the patient's perspective. When a patient is unconditionally provided care and warmth and is accepted for who they are during their present state, the change that the nurse is encouraging is more likely. In the opening case study, the community nurse showed unconditional positive regard for Rejoice. This was demonstrated by the community nurse not making any judgements when referring to Rejoice and her negative mindset. As a result, Rejoice felt accepted and felt self-worth, which resulted in her initiating and actually participating in change within her life.

The converse of unconditional regard is that of conditional regard, which family members and friends may hold towards an individual. For example, Rejoice may have had comments from family members such as, 'what do you have to be ungrateful about, you finally have a lovely child', or 'what about those women who cannot have children?', which tend to be judgemental statements. Also, Rejoice may have felt that her husband or close family had high expectation of her being a good mother, which she had to live up to. A nurse who practises unconditional positive regard is someone who does not express a judgement towards the patient and does not have any expectations of the patient.

Genuineness and congruence

The third and final component that Rogers advocates to bring about change in a person is **genuineness** and congruency. Genuineness can be defined as the basic ability to be aware of inner experiences and to allow the quality of that inner experience to be apparent in relationships. Hence, genuineness excludes playing a role or putting up a façade.

In order for empathy and unconditional positive regard to be successful in bringing about change to a patient, the patient has to perceive them as genuine feelings. In turn, the patient is more likely to feel accepted and feel that the nurse is there 'for them' and 'accepts their present state'. A nurse needs to be aware that being genuine is expressed by two channels: verbal and non-verbal communication. **Self-awareness** of one's own behaviour and interaction is paramount. There may be times when a nurse may not, despite their efforts, be able to feel a genuine concern or find it extremely difficult because of beliefs that may clash. As a result, the nurse should use self-awareness to monitor how they are coming across to the patient and the implications on the nurse–patient relationship.

If a patient does not perceive a nurse as genuine, they may 'close up' and be less likely to change their current mindset. For example, in the opening case study, the nurse stated that she understood that is was a difficult time for Rejoice. This was mirrored by her non-verbal communication, which was expressed by her sympathetic facial expressions. However, had the community nurse not believed in what she had said, her non-verbal communication may not have been sympathetic and in turn the patient could have received mixed messages. If a nurse finds it difficult to be genuine for a valid reason, it is important for the nurse to excuse themselves from the patient (if possible) and speak to a senior staff nurse about their feelings as soon as possible.

The contradiction between verbal and non-verbal behaviour is referred to as being *incongruent*. This occurs when what the individual states is not what they actually feel. It is important for a nurse to ensure that they are congruent at all times, in order to appear genuine when empathising with their patient. Mirroring verbal statements via the non-verbal channel, i.e. expression of the face and body language, is referred to as being *congruent*.

The awareness of congruency and incongruence can also be valuable when the nurse is attempting to understand the patient. Incongruence between what a patient states and what they actually feel may be a sign of anxiety. This is a cue for the nurse to use empathy and unconditional positive regard when communicating with the patient and facilitating a patient's understanding of their current state. In the opening case study, the community nurse noted during her first meeting that when she asked Rejoice how she felt, her reply was that she was fine and nothing was wrong with her.

For the community nurse it was clear that there was incongruency between the patient stating that she was fine and her actual medical notes, which made it clear that Rejoice had severe postnatal depression. The first aim for the community nurse was to work with Rejoice, so that she could understand and receive help about her current mindset. The second aim was to ensure that Rejoice became congruent in the way that she felt and how she acknowledged her feelings. This acted as a base which on progressive change could be made, from her current mindset of being helpless to that of being more positive and proactive.

Think about this

Those who have issues with alcohol or drug misuse, tend to be taken care of by a multi-disciplinary team. However, they will only get better once they acknowledge that their current habit and aspects of their current lifestyle could be a trigger to their participation in risky behaviour. A patient who is being taken care of but is incongruent in terms of acknowledging their own risky behaviour or that they have a problem, is usually a patient who will relapse or will not be able to cease their risky behaviour.

Empathy, congruence and unconditional positive regard all contribute to a more patient-centred consultation with the patient. Theoretical aspects of patient centredness are given in Chapter 16 and how to achieve patient-centredness is explored within Chapter 17.

Motivation

Abraham Maslow's hierarchy of needs

Abraham Maslow (1908-1970) is one of the founding pioneers of humanistic psychology. His most famous contribution is the **five-stage hierarchy of needs model**, which explores how human beings can be motivated and reach eventual self-actualisation, the best that one can achieve (as introduced in the beginning of the chapter).

Maslow proposed the idea that growth needs – higher-order needs of a human being such as aesthetic, cognitive and self-actualisation needs – cannot be met unless the basic needs of a human being have been satisfied. These basic needs are referred to as **deficiency needs**, such as physiological, esteem, love and belonging, and security and safety needs. Maslow outlined these needs within his model, which are presented in order from the most basic needs to the eventual need of self-actualisation (Figure 3.1).

Physiological needs

Physiological needs are the first level of Maslow's hierarchy of needs, and encompass the most basic physical needs of a human being: e.g. sleep, oxygen, water and vitamins.

Think about this

The cravings of a pregnant woman could be her body telling her about possible vitamin deficiencies. Even though Rejoice had her baby several months ago, she could be lacking in particular vitamins or minerals, which could be contributing to her negative state of mind.

Safety and security needs

When the physiological needs are largely taken care of, the second level comes to the forefront: **safety and security needs**. This level includes needs such as protection, security and freedom from anxiety.

In the case study, the community nurse explored why Rejoice was not able to manage her symptoms of depression. It was evident that not working was causing Rejoice enormous anxiety. Anxiety regarding financial circumstances and having the comfortable life that she had become accustomed to before the birth of her baby may have been the result of Rejoice's unemployment.

Belongingness and love needs

When the physiological and safety needs levels have been met, the level of **belongingness and love needs** comes to the forefront. Within this level needs such as having friends, family, children, a partner, as well as the need to belong to a community, come into play. Failure to satisfy these needs can lead to feelings of isolation and loneliness.

Rejoice was feeling lonely, as she did not have contact with her work friends or regular contract with her husband who was working away from home during the weekdays. The community nurse explored this level well and found some workable ideas, so that Rejoice would not feel lonely.

Esteem needs

Once the previous levels have been adequately met, the **esteem needs** level comes into play, where the need for self- and social esteem is important. Maslow distinguished between the two levels of esteem. Lower (social) self-esteem stems from the need to be recognised by others, have attention, status and dignity. The higher level (self) esteem needs consist of the need for self-respect, which includes feelings such as confidence, competence, achievement, mastery, independence and freedom. Satisfaction of these needs moves the individual to a higher order of functioning and make the individual a more effective person. When self-esteem needs are not met, the result can be low self-worth, helplessness, depression, incompetence and inferiority.

The community nurse explored the issue of self-esteem, as it was apparent that Rejoice had low self-esteem in relation to her confidence as a mother. This was further heightened as Rejoice missed the recognition and confidence she used to gain at work. It is important for a nurse to take this particular level into consideration as, more often than not, there will be patients who are not fit and healthy, who will have low self-esteem as they will feel that they themselves are not in control of their state of health.

Maslow refers to these four needs as *deficit needs* or *D-needs*. If you don't have all of the needs, you feel deficient. These levels can be seen during the initial stages of infant development. For example, a newborn baby will tend to be focused on wanting a feed or having their nappy changed (physiological). This soon changes to wanting to be safe and secure (safety needs), which is indicative of a child crying when their parental figure is not with them (see Chapter 7). Affection and esteem needs come soon after, and this all happens within a couple of years.

Think about this

What have you most needed or required during a spell of flu? Sleep? Food? Liquids? Attention? All of these are regressive states, which take individuals back to their basic deficit needs levels. Do you think that patients will regress to any of these states? When the deficit needs are regularly met, the individual is an effective person both mentally and physically.

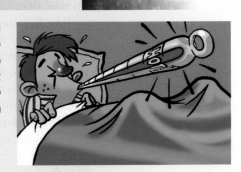

During stressful situations, e.g. not feeling well, it is possible for an individual to regress to these basic needs. For example, Rejoice had post-natal depression, which resulted in her reassessing her role in society (esteem), as well as wanting more contact with her husband and friends (affection and love). There is also a possibility of fixation at any level of the four deficit needs during early childhood development, if states such as loss, hunger, neglect or abuse occurred. (See links with Chapter 4.)

Growth needs

When all of the deficit needs are regularly satisfied, the **growth needs** come into existence. Needs such as **cognitive needs**, which stem from the need for understanding and knowledge, are growth needs. Nurses provide information to patients at all times, both when it is necessary and when the patient requires information or clarification on their state of health/medical procedure/treatment or medication. Patients who do not understand a medical procedure or treatment tend not to be satisfied with the medical practitioner and are less likely to adhere to a nurse's advice. (Refer to Chapters 5 and 16 for more detail.) Hence, the patient needs to be well informed in relation to their proposed care plan.

Alongside the cognitive needs are the needs that come under the umbrella level of **aesthetic needs**, which include needs for order and beauty. Satisfaction of these needs moves the individual to a higher state of psychological functioning. The highest need (the pointed tip on Maslow's triangle) is referred to as the need for self-actualisation.

Self-actualisation

Maslow has used a variety of different terms to refer to this level, such as *growth motivation*, *being needs*, *b-needs* and *self-actualisation*. During the self-actualisation level of need the individual will be able to function to their highest potential. Once engaged with the needs at this level, they continue to be felt. This is in stark contrast to the deficient needs level, whereby needs surface when they are not being met. The needs that are met during the self-actualisation level become stronger the more you feed them. Not surprisingly, only a small percentage of people operate at the self-actualisation level. In order for a patient to be able to achieve self-actualisation or be motivated to initiate change, their lower order needs to be fulfilled first.

Take Rejoice as an example. It would have been unrealistic for the community nurse to have put together a care plan requiring Rejoice to initiate change or just take her medication, seeing that there were many basic needs that needed to first be met.

It is important for a nurse to keep the self-actualisation needs level in mind. This will act as a constant reminder that many basic needs have to be met before a patient can become more in control of their own state of health. In the opening case study, many health professionals, such as the GP, attempted to help Rejoice, all of whom failed. It may have been the case that the actual basic needs of Rejoice were ignored in these attempts to help her. For example, the GP looked at the dignosis of depression and treated the biological origins of the illness rather than exploring possible psychosocial origins.

Maslow's hierarchy is also applicable to the nurse and their professional practice. In order for nurses to work effectively, they should also be aware of all

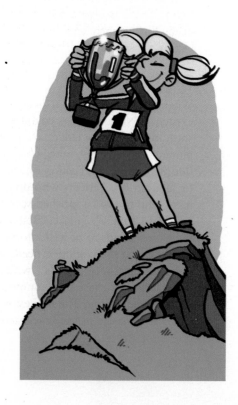

Think about this

The effectiveness and motivation of each individual is much like a chair. If there is one leg of the chair that is unstable or missing, then the chair will not be strong enough for someone to sit on it.

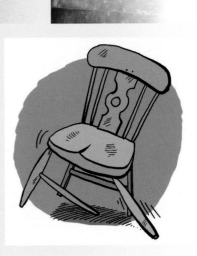

the basic needs, and ensure that they are being met. If they are not, then nurses should make them workable targets within their personal development.

This can be applied to patients, whereby if one level of need is missing, they can not be as effective as possible. For example, Rejoice felt insecure, lacked an identity because of having to give up work and did not have much contact with her friends or husband. This resulted in Rejoice not being as effective as she used to be, which led to a lack of motivation and enthusiasm on a daily basis in her role as a new mother.

Many health care professionals might feel frustrated when patients do not seem interested in changing their behaviour (Hunt, 1995). Other patients may not even attend appointments or follow the advice that the nurse has provided. Sometimes, simple information-giving is not enough. Instead, a different approach, such as addressing motivation, is needed to help patients achieve behaviour change (Hunt and Hillsdon, 1996; Miller and Rollinck, 1991; Prochaska *et al.*, 1994).

Many lifestyle behaviours are influenced by multiple internal and external factors, which are deeply ingrained. Stating that someone has to change will not motivate an individual (Hunt and Pearson, 2001). Instead, motivation itself may need to be addressed before initiating any proposed change that the patient will have to undertake.

Other models of motivation and change

When looking at patient motivation and initiating change, it is not only important to look at the present factors but preceding ones as well, before deciding on a course of action. Prochaska and DiClemente (1986) put forward the **stages of change model**, which indicates that change should be based on many factors. The stages of change model are depicted in Figure 3.2.

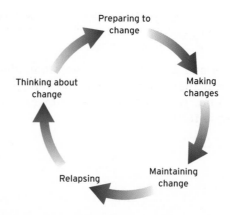

Figure 3.2 The stages of change model.
Source: Prochaska and DiClemente, 1986

In the case study below, the GP focuses on the symptoms presented during the consultation. According to Prochaska and DiClemente's (1986) stages of change model, any change that takes place should not be focused on the 'here and now'. Instead, many factors need to be taken into account. These can be seen in Table 3.2, which further elaborates on the stages of change model.

Case study

The GP has told Rwanda that she needs to stop smoking and lose weight immediately. The GP hands out a diet sheet and informs Rwanda to avoid the foods that are listed in the red column and instead eat more of the good foods that are listed in the green column. The GP ends the consultation by saying that the next time he meets Rwanda, he hopes she will have shed weight.

The stages of change model is a useful framework for a nurse when helping a patient initiate some kind of successful change. The model itself highlights the importance of many factors that contribute to the change process. Rwanda's GP did not take any of these factors into account. Nurses can use this model as guidance to assess the patient's current level of motivation and then select appropriate interventions that mirror the particular stage of change that they are in.

For example, has Rwanda attempted several times to maintain a healthy diet and give up smoking previously? As a result, it would be evident to a practitioner that the relapse and contemplation stage would have to be addressed. An appropriate intervention would look at the methods Rwanda used when attempting change and put more workable strategies in place. In addition to this, motivation may be another area that would need to be focused on, especially if Rwanda had just given up after several attempts. As a result she may have no confidence and very low self-esteem because of her lack of achievement at losing weight and giving up smoking. (See Chapter 6).

Stages of change	Rwanda in this stage
Pre-contemplation	Rwanda may not be willing to change for a number of reasons. These can range from her being unwilling to confront her eating and smoking behaviour, to not acknowledging that her present health behaviour is a problem that needs confronting.
Contemplation	The patient may be aware that her smoking and obese weight is a problem. However, Rwanda may have been reluctant to initiate any change because of fear of the sacrifices involved.
Preparation	During this stage, Rwanda may realise that changes need to take place. She will be preparing to make a change in the near future, but there is still anxiety attached to the proposed changes.
Action	Rwanda may be confident in beginning to make the change and this is reflected in her behaviour.
Maintenance	During this stage, Rwanda will make attempts to maintain the achievements and motivation level she had during the action stage. There will be a constant struggle with thoughts about relapsing. Lasts between six months to a lifetime.
Termination	This is the stage whereby Rwanda would have replaced her old habits with new ones. For example, meditating when stressed rather than smoking.
Relapse	This is not a stage of change but an outcome of action or maintenance stages. If Rwanda were unsuccessful in the action or maintenance change, then she would have to go back to the contemplation stage and seriously think about stopping smoking and losing weight again.

Table 3.2 Stages of change

Empowerment

The community nurse within the opening case study, attempted to *empower* Rejoice, so that she could regain control within her life. Rappaport (1984) defines empowerment as 'a means by which individuals gain some control or mastery over their lives'. The Royal College of Nursing has identified patient empowerment as a key aspect of nursing (RCN, 2007), which has been mirrored in the power shift from the practitioner to the patient (DoH, 2005a). (Refer to Chapter 16.)

A positive outcome of patient empowerment is the increased ability of the patient to become more active and independent within their management of illness and health (Hughes, 2004), rather than being dependent on carers.

Many initiatives have been set up to promote patient empowerment within the nurse–patient relationship. For example, the Department of Health (2001a), put together a document entitled *The Expert Patient: A New Approach to Chronic Disease Management for the 21st Century*. This document highlighted the need for the expert patient to be in more control of their self-care but at the same time recognised the importance of professional ongoing support surrounding the patient.

Promoting independence and control, especially for a patient who is managing a long-term illness, is important. This approach will reap many benefits such as increased patient control, the patient feeling that they are capable of participating in activities, not feeling that they are incapable, and distancing the patient from the learned helplessness and depression cycle. There are also benefits for the nurse who is supporting the patient, as the patient is less likely to become dependent for certain self-care activities that they are capable of doing for themselves.

Orem (1980) introduced the self-care model for nursing, which is a useful framework for a nurse to work within when attempting to empower their patients. The following self-care requisites form Orem's self-care nursing model:

- Maintenance of care associated with the elimination of air, water and food, e.g. supporting the patient when needing to go to the toilet, etc.
- Provision of care associated with the elimination of body waste, e.g. appropriate supporting facilities are in place to help the patient go to the toilet.
- Maintenance of a balance between activity and rest, i.e. the nurse ensuring that the patient has adequate rest as well as being active where possible.
- Maintenance of a balance between solitude and social interaction, i.e. a balance is provided by the nurse in the form of support and information as to how much to talk and when to rest.
- Prevention of hazards to human life, human functioning and human well-being, i.e. the nurse providing information on certain types of behaviour that could cause problems for the patient and their illness or act as a barrier when attempting to get better or managing their illness.
- Promotion of human functioning and development in social groups in accordance with human potential, i.e. nurse provides support for the patient to interact with individuals as well as providing information on social support networks that exist, such as the NHS Patient Advice and Liaison Service (PALS).

One criticism of this model is that it is largely needs based (Hughes, 2004).

An empowerment model that looks at the wider perspective of health promotion is provided by Labonte (1994), who identifies five empowerment strategies for health promotion which can be used at individual and community levels, as depicted in Figure 3.3 and Table 3.3.

One other model which relates to illnesses is the chronic disease self-management programme (CDSMP) (Cooper, 2001), which has now been incorporated in the NHS mainstream. This model was originally piloted and delivered to patients with conditions such as arthritis and depression. The model focused on drug and

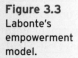

Figure 3.3
Labonte's empowerment model.

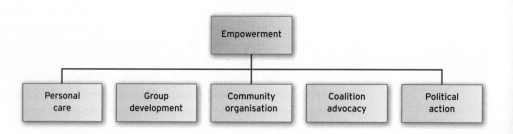

Table 3.3
Labonte's empowerment
model

Empowerment strategy	Example	Application to the case study of Rwanda
Personal care	Practice of activities that the individual personally initiates	Rwanda could be given appropriate literature that looks at weight loss and smoking which will begin to then enhance her control when losing weight and stopping smoking
Group development	Develop a sense of purpose with others	Make Rwanda aware that there are support networks, which will have members who also want to lose weight and give up smoking
Community organisation	Planned process that allows a community to use its own resources to accomplish goals	Rwanda with other service users may identify a gap where their needs are not met, such as a health weight forum, and work towards setting one up
Coalition advocacy	Organisations work together to achieve common goals	Rwanda could join a health loss group or smoking cessation group
Political action	Users of an organisation elect representatives to highlight the needs to others	Nurses could help Rwanda or her representative, if any need could be put into practice or examined in more detail

symptom management within these groups. Psychosocial consequences, lifestyle, social support, communication and other strategies were also addressed.

The outcome of this model was to develop five core self-management self-care skills for life:

- Problem-solving whereby patients are encouraged to think about current problems.
- Decision-making, which enables the patient to take ongoing action.
- Resource use, whereby patients are taught to collect appropriate and accurate material (especially with the wide use of the Internet), as well as informing patients about other networks of support that are available to them.
- Focusing on effective partnerships, where effective use and appropriate access of the health care service (DoH, 2001a) is looked at.
- Taking action, via coaching, promoting awareness and commitment to achieving goals, which can be done through reflection and teaching when looking at goal plans and revising them, so they are more realistic.

Think about this

By using the above empowerment and self-care models as guides, how did the community nurse attempt to empower Rejoice?

The research in focus box below highlights a study that looked at empowerment and how strategies are put into place for haematological cancer patients.

Research in focus

Bulsara, C., Ward, A. and Joske, D. (2004) Haematological cancer patients: achieving a sense of empowerment by use of strategies to control illness. *Journal of Advanced Nursing*, **13**, 251–258.

Background
The role empowerment plays through involving haematological cancer patients and their families in their treatment and care is undeniable. It encompasses the implementation of various strategies to achieve a sense of empowerment.

Aims and objectives
This study sought to identify core strategies used by cancer patients, regardless of their illness stage and prognosis, who exhibited a strong sense of empowerment in coping with their condition.

Design
A phenomenological approach, using an in-depth interviewing technique, was used to identify the common factors that patients and spouses believed could enable them to achieve a measure of control in managing their illness. These measures were referred to as coping strategies.

Methods
It was decided to conduct a purposive study and re-interview 7 of 12 patients who had previously participated in a pilot Haematology Shared Care project and who developed a high level of ability in coping with their illness. At the patient's discretion, spouses were invited to participate and to contribute to the interview. Three spouses participated in the interviewing process.

Results
Common strategies emerged regardless of the patient's stage of illness and prognosis. Informants identified the determination to remain in control of the illness and treatment side effects, having the support of family and significant others, illness acceptance and maintaining hope as crucial to their sense of empowerment.

Relevance to clinical practice
It is hoped that clinicians will gain a deeper understanding of the varied and numerous strategies used by cancer patients in coping with their illness. This understanding will ensure that by encouraging these strategies, patients and their families will be supported by health professionals to achieve a greater sense of empowerment. As this and other studies have shown, working alongside health professionals contributes to empowerment for both the cancer patient and significant others in their lives.

Patient advocacy

Part of empowering a patient is acting as an advocate for the patient. The importance of empowerment and advocacy within the nurse–patient relationship has been highlighted in a paper by the Royal College of Nursing, which states that 'a prime function of nursing is to empower clients to have more control over their lives' (RCN, 1995). This could be seen in the opening case study whereby the community nurse liaised with several support networks for new mothers on behalf of Rejoice.

Wheeler (2000) reviewed several studies and concluded there were three attributes of advocacy: **valuing, appraising** and **interceding**.

- *Valuing* is where the patient's advocate (the nurse), while providing expert care, maintains individualisation and humanity (Smith, 1979). Empathy, unconditional positive regard and congruency are all skills that will enable the nurse to respect the individuality of the patient.
- *Appraising*, a combination of informing, advising and educating (Wheeler, 2000). Kohnke (1982) highlighted the use of the nurse informing and supporting the patient, as the heart of patient advocacy. In the opening case study, the community nurse informed Rejoice about particular avenues that she could pursue. She also supported her in any new decisions she made when pursuing these avenues. Providing information, for example about implications of treatment, is an important aspect of appraising. This will hopefully result in the patient being in a position where they are equipped with the most appropriate information about their particular illness, treatment or surgical procedure.
- *Interceding*, which means that the advocate (the nurse) comes between parties and intervenes or mediates where necessary (Wheeler, 2000). Interceding may come into play when the patient is facing personal or health care service barriers. The nurse will act on behalf of the patient so that the barriers are overcome. This may be very much prominent with those patients who may have low self-esteem, are vulnerable (Copp, 1986) or do not want to challenge the health care provider. The community nurse in the opening case study could have interceded between Rejoice and her GP so that they could again pursue a healthy professional relationship as well as other social support networks, as Rejoice had very low self-esteem and could not find the energy within herself to talk to new groups of people.

Conclusion

The basic principles and concepts such as empathy, congruency and unconditional positive regard are key to the understanding of patient-centred care. By becoming familiar with these concepts and exploring them with further reading, a student nurse can become more confident when caring for a patient within a patient-centred environment.

Motivation is an area that resides within the humanistic psychology perspective and is important for a nurse to be aware of the basic models that exist when thinking about motivating the patient who may be finding it difficult to bring about change within their current behaviour patterns. Motivation models provided by Maslow, as well as other models that have been discussed in this chapter and the further reading, will be beneficial for a student nurse who may find it difficult to motivate their patient.

Related to the area of motivation are patient advocacy and empowerment which the nurse will encounter as part of their daily practice. Being aware of the literature that explores patient advocacy and empowerment will help the nurse to work confidently with the patient who may have low self-esteem.

Understanding the person as a whole before symptoms are treated forms the basic principle of humanistic psychology. In practice, the profession of nursing necessitates the care of the patient to be based upon patient-centred care and working within a therapeutic relationship, which are closely aligned.

Summary

- The humanistic psychology perspective is referred to as 'the third force' in psychology. The perspective strives to highlight a more holistic vision of both psychology and the understanding of the person from a holistic viewpoint.

- Carl Rogers (1902–1987) highlighted the importance of person-centred counselling, with empathy, unconditional positive regard and congruence being the three core components.

- Empathy is where the nurse will put aside her own way of experiencing and perceiving reality, preferring to sense and respond to the experiences and perceptions of her patient.

- Unconditional positive regard is whereby there are no conditions placed upon the nurse–patient relationship, which encourages warmth and acceptance of the patient.

- Congruence is where the nurse's or patient's inner feelings match their expression of verbal and non-verbal communication, which promotes genuineness.

- Abraham Maslow's (1943) five-stage hierarchy of needs model highlights that patient's basic deficit needs have to be met before a patient can think about growth needs, changing behaviour and eventual self-actualisation.

- Prochaska and DiClemente's (1986) stages of change model highlights the importance of the nurse not concentrating on the 'here and now' but acknowledging surrounding factors, when motivating or initiating behaviour change of a patient.

- A nurse will have a large part to play when empowering a patient so that they can gain more control over their lives. Performing the role of a patient advocate is one way a nurse can empower a patient.

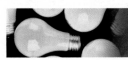 ## Check your understanding

1. How does empathy differ from sympathy? Which situation(s) between the nurse and the patient would require no empathy?

2. What are the three core conditions of the person-centred counselling approach? How can these be used when attempting to better understand the patient from a holistic perspective?

3. With the help of Prochaska and Diclemente's (1986) stage change model, put together an action plan for a patient who needs to lose weight. What stage is the patient at?

4. When initiating behaviour change or motivating a patient to help him or herself, what basic needs should be acknowledged to begin with?

5. What three attributes contribute to the nurse being an advocate and empowering the patient?

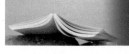

Further reading

Baldwin, M.A. (2003) Patient advocacy: a concept analysis. *Nursing Standard*, **17** (21), 33–39.

Hughes, S. (2003) Promoting independence: the nurse as a coach. *Nursing Standard*, **18** (10), 42–44.

Hughes, S.A. (2004) Promoting self-management and patient independence. *Nursing Standard*, **19** (10), 47–52.

Hunt, P. and Pearson, D. (2001) Motivating change. *Nursing Standard*, **16** (2), 45–52.

Morse, J.M., Bottorff, J., Anderson, G., O'Brien, B. and Solberg, S. (2006) Beyond empathy: expanding expressions of caring. *Journal of Advanced Nursing*, **53** (1), 75-90.

Murphy, B. and Manning, Y. (2003) An introduction to anorexia nervosa and bulimia nervosa. *Nursing Standard*, **18** (14-16), 45–52.

Newson, P. (2006) Loneliness and the value of empathetic listening. *Nursing and Residential Care*, **8**, 12.

Reynold, W.J. and Scott, B. (1999) Empathy: a crucial component of the helping relationship. *Journal of Psychiatric and Mental Health Nursing*, **6**, 363–370.

Watt-Watson, J., Garfinkel, P., Gallop, R., Stevens, B. and Streiner, D. (2000) The impact of nurses' empathetic responses on patients' pain management in acute care. *Nursing Research*, **49**, (4), 191–200.

Yegdich, T. (1999) On the phenomenology of empathy in nursing: empathy or sympathy. *Journal of Advanced Nursing*, **30** (1), 83–89.

Weblinks

Association for Humanistic Psychology	http://www.ahpweb.org/	Website that provides many links to other humanistic psychology websites. Also provides a historical overview of the perspective
John Rowan's Guide to Humanistic Psychology	http://www.johnrowan.org.uk/ background_humanistic.html	A website that provides in-depth theoretical content for humanistic psychology
Personality Test of Emotional Empathy	http://www.kaaj.com/psych/scales/emp.html	A look at articles written about emotional empathy, as well as measurements of emotional empathy

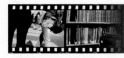

Media examples

Sister Act Whoopi Goldberg plays the part of a 'pretend' nun who empowers a group of children who had lost hope for their inspiring futures within academia and music.

Paul McKenna The last three years have seen a rise in the number of people attending the weight loss and confidence seminars that Paul McKenna hosts. His seminars, books, CDs, TV appearances (such as on GMTV), magazine features and DVDs are based on principles that enhance motivation and confidence for individuals who are struggling within particular aspects of their life. Have a look at his website http://www.paulmckenna.com/

Chapter 4

Anxiety and psychodynamic principles

Learning outcomes

When you have read through this chapter you should understand:

- How the principles within psychodynamic therapy can be applied to the patient and nurse relationship.
- Why defence mechanisms feature as part of the coping process of the patient.
- When patient anxiety occurs and how the nurse can communicate and care for the anxious patient accordingly.
- How communication with the patient is important in order to prevent the occurrence of defence mechanisms.
- When defence mechanisms benefit the patient and when they become a barrier to the patient's health and well-being.
- How recognition of defence mechanisms can make the nurse–patient relationship more effective.

Case study

Brian Grant is a 32-year-old man who has had treatment to eliminate gallstones, which have been causing him excessive pain. During his treatment Brian's health has deteriorated and he finds that most of his time is spent either managing his chronic pain or sleeping. Brian and his wife Emma are overjoyed to find that the treatment has been successful and that Brian will soon be discharged.

On the proposed day of discharge Emma begins to prepare for Brian's homecoming and phones the hospital to enquire about the time she should collect Brian. The staff nurse informs Emma that based on the arrival of a test result Brian cannot be discharged. The staff nurse insists that Emma should still come to the hospital though. While driving, Emma justifies Brian's further stay in hospital to herself. She reasons that he needs professional health staff to care for him until his physical health strengthens.

As soon as Emma arrives at the hospital, she is told that the consultant would like to discuss the test results with both Emma and Brian. The consultant informs them that the results have revealed that Brian has cancer of the kidney and that they will need to begin an aggressive course of chemotherapy immediately. Brain is distraught and begins to cry. The nurse touches Brian's hand and allows Brian to express his grief. Emma begins to ask many questions as to what treatment they can offer Brian. The nurse notices over the next few days that Brian rocks back and forth when comforting himself. Once the consultation has finished, Emma tells Brian that she needs to rush home, as she needs to make arrangements for his eventual discharge.

When Brian arrives home he is surprised to find how busy Emma is keeping herself. More concerning for Brian is that Emma has not embraced the subject of cancer, or even consoled him since his diagnosis. After several weeks of chemotherapy treatment Brian seems to be making good progress. The Macmillan nurse visits Brian and Emma to see how they are coping. The nurse is happy with Brian's progress and she can see a vast improvement in both his physical and mental well-being. Emma, on the other hand, appears exhausted and is constantly avoiding the subject of kidney cancer.

The Macmillan nurse visits Brian and Emma again, this time aiming to speak to Emma about her role as a carer. It becomes apparent to the nurse that Emma is very angry and short when kidney cancer is mentioned by the nurse. Emma also informs the nurse of how busy she is since Brian can no longer work. The Macmillan nurse can see that Emma does not want to talk about Brian's condition. The nurse's concern for Emma is further heightened by Brian's suggestion that there are enormous communication problems between them. The nurse hands over a leaflet, which explains the support that is available for carers.

Three months later and Emma has visited her GP with complaints of panic attacks and excessive palpitations of the heart. The GP is adamant that Emma is exhausted and highly anxious and suggests that Emma should take some time away from work. It is only when Emma is at home that she begins to face up to what has happened to Brian. Through this period she is highly emotional and for the first time since Brian's diagnosis, Emma begins to cry and talks to Brian about his kidney cancer.

Why is this relevant to nursing practice?

The opening case study exemplifies how people differ in the way they deal and cope with a new diagnosis. The psychodynamic approach provides an insight into how patients may deal with a situation of ill-health, which is a frequent occurrence within the field of nursing. In the case study above, Brian was a lot more accepting of the diagnosis of kidney cancer than Emma. The psychodynamic approach can be applied to help explain how individuals differ in their approach when accepting a loss or new or concurring illness, which can help a nurse tailor communication and care accordingly.

According to the psychodynamic approach, Emma dealt with the **anxiety** she had about Brian's illness by being in a complete state of denial over a long period of time. Denial is one of many different defence mechanisms that a patient may employ when dealing with anxiety. This chapter will look at the different types of defence mechanisms that patients could employ as part of their journey in accepting their loss or diagnosis.

It is important for a nurse to understand how and why such defence mechanisms are employed. In the case study above, Emma was in denial for a long period of time, which eventually resulted in her health becoming affected. This chapter will not only explore how defence mechanisms can become a barrier to an individual's well-being, but also how they can benefit the patient when coping with a new medical diagnosis. Differing illnesses create situations that determine if defence mechanisms will be beneficial or maladaptive for the patient's health and well-being. Accordingly, the nurse will need to adapt their communication with the patient. These issues will be explored in greater detail in this chapter.

The psychodynamic approach also highlights how individuals cope with anxiety. Anxiety and its possible impact on health is an important area to explore. This chapter will enable the nurse to consider what type of communication is warranted when dealing with anxiety. A consideration of this area is required for nurses who are at the forefront of helping patients within anxious situations, which are frequent occurrences within the nurse's working environment.

In the case study above Emma was in complete denial in relation to Brian's diagnosis of kidney cancer, even though she accepted that he was dependent on her because of ill-health. One avenue worth pursuing would be Emma's previous experiences with illness and how she dealt with those experiences. Many questions come to mind, such as has Emma had an experience of someone being diagnosed with cancer? Has a close family member or friend died as a result of cancer? Answers to such questions would clarify Emma's past experiences with cancer, which would affect how she deals with the present situation.

The psychodynamic approach highlights the importance of how we have dealt with past events, which influence our current behaviour. This chapter will help the nurse to explore a patient's previous experiences and their possible contribution to present anxiety states. This chapter will help the nurse acknowledge the impact that interpersonal communication can have not only on the alleviation but also the prevention of anxiety, an area in which the nurse will have a key role to play. The nurse will be better equipped to deal with anxious patients by being familiar with the psychodynamic approach, which explores anxiety and working with anxiety in a therapeutic relationship.

Communication skills themselves will not adequately equip the nurse to help the patient who may, like Emma, be in denial. Through acknowledging the psychodynamic approach in conjunction with counselling and communication skills (see Chapter 17), the nurse will become more confident and effective at targeting interpersonal communication at the appropriate level when helping an anxious patient.

The psychodynamic approach becomes even more relevant when looking at anxiety on a wider scale. Clearly the patient will be the obvious victim of anxiety. However, what tends to be ignored is the anxiety experienced by nurses, especially those who are new to the profession. By being self-aware of how anxiety and defence mechanisms can be used as a coping strategy, the nurse can become alert to how the care they provide can be affected when they become highly anxious or avoid certain areas within their practice by employing defence mechanisms (see also Chapter 3).

The psychodynamic approach

The **psychodynamic** approach explores how the mind (human psyche), especially the unconscious part of the human mind is responsible for everyday behaviour. This is reflected in Morris and Maisto's (2002, p. 445) definition of psychodynamic theory as:

> Seeing behaviour as the product of psychological forces that interact within the individual, often outside conscious awareness. The interplay of unconscious mental processes, determine human feelings, thoughts and behaviour.

Psychoanalysis, or *psychotherapy*, is the therapy that arises out of the psychodynamic approach which counsellors may use in practice. The aim of the therapy is to help the client gain a deeper insight into their behaviour. This is facilitated by recognising, exploring and understanding unconscious emotions and thoughts, which are believed to cause the surface problems. Nurses themselves cannot practise psychoanalysis or psychotherapy unless they are trained as a counsellor. However, the principles within this approach are useful for a nurse who may have to communicate with or confront a patient where the cause of the problem is not obvious, which will warrant some kind of exploration by the nurse.

In the case study above the nurse realised that Emma was in a state of denial about Brian's diagnosis of kidney cancer. This was a concern for the nurse as Emma had been in a state of denial over a long period of time. As a result of Emma being reluctant to talk, the nurse left leaflets that gave information about the counselling services available to Emma. The case study exemplifies how nurses are in a prime position not only to help patients who experience anxiety but also to refer patients to colleagues within counselling services. This case study also illustrates how a basic knowledge of defence mechanisms will enable the nurse to recognise when a patient may need help in alleviating their anxiety.

Sigmund Freud (1858–1939) was the pioneer of the psychodynamic approach. Freud practised as a medical doctor where he became fascinated by the possible influences that impacted on the working of the mind. In particular, Freud was interested in patients who presented physical or imagined symptoms for which there was no apparent physical cause. This is where Freud began to investigate the mind and how this could influence physical symptoms or imagined symptoms of the body. Freud began to use *hypnosis*, which could help patients reveal what was within their unconscious which, when explored, resulted in their physical symptoms.

Freud's initial work gave rise to the belief that all behaviour originates from previous experiences that reside within the unconscious mind. Freud referred to this as **psychic determinism**.

Sigmund Freud

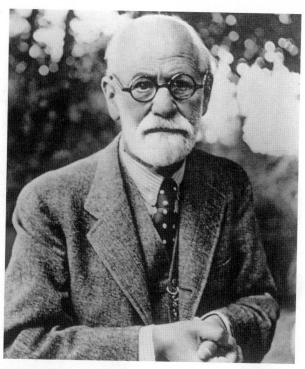

Mary Evans Picture Library/Alamy

Think about this

How would you explain the challenging behaviour of the patient? There are a number of explanations such as being distressed, anxiety about what is wrong with them, problems at home, not being attended to immediately. All of these answers result in a possible explanation of how previous experiences can influence current behaviour and thinking.

The explanation of the mind

Freud used the analogy of an iceberg to explain the different levels within the mind and how these can influence behaviour.

The **conscious** part of the mind is the first level at the tip of the iceberg, which deals with here and now experiences. Material that resides at this level does not cause any anxiety for the individual, as it is in conscious awareness and has no trauma attached to it. The **preconscious** part of the mind is the second level, which contains experiences, feelings and thoughts from the past that can readily be brought up into the conscious awareness without a problem: for example, a patient remembering the last time they visited the nurse for a routine check-up without any problems. The third and largest part of the mind is what Freud referred to as the **unconscious**, which contains thoughts, feelings, memories and emotions that the individual is not consciously aware of.

Previous experiences can result in anxiety. If such experiences have not been explored within the conscious awareness these episodes can be **repressed**

An iceberg, Freud's analogy for the human mind

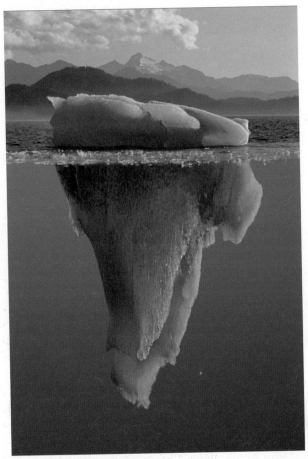

Alaska Stock LLC/Alamy

into the unconscious part of the mind. For example, if a patient had a previous hospital visit that was traumatic and the associated anxiety was not adequately dealt with by the patient themselves or by the health staff around them, this could result in the experience being repressed into the unconscious part of the mind. In the opening case study, Emma may have had many questions left unanswered, which would have contributed to her anxiety and the eventual repression of the diagnosis and her feelings about Brian's kidney cancer into her unconscious.

It is the unconscious part of the mind that motivates our day-to-day behaviour, feelings, thoughts and emotions. According to Freud, we can explore experiences that have been repressed into this level of the mind through hypnosis. By talking about them, experiences come into conscious awareness. This results in the alleviation of the symptoms initially being addressed. Freud referred to the exploration of the unconscious mind and bringing thoughts, feelings, memories and emotions into the conscious awareness as the **royal road into the unconscious.**

This forms the main premise of the therapy that arises from the psychodynamic approach. As stated above, nurses cannot incorporate psychotherapy into their practice when helping patients. However, there are many aspects of psychodynamic theory that the nurse can draw upon. First, anxiety can be prevented or minimised. Second, where anxiety or the mindset of the patient becomes a barrier to their present health and management of illness, the nurse should address these issues adequately by appropriate interpersonal communication. The section below explores anxiety in more depth and also explains why the consideration of anxiety is compulsory for effective nursing care.

Anxiety

Anxiety can be defined as 'a complex emotional state with apprehension and dread being the prominent features' (Kenworthy *et al.*, 1992) or simply as 'the experience of fear which has overtaken the sense' (Sanders and Wills, 2003, p. 1). Anxiety is explored within the psychodynamic approach as something that the mind deals with by repressing feelings and thoughts into the unconscious part of the mind.

The exploration of anxiety for a nurse is warranted, as admission to hospital can accentuate anxiety by disturbing the patient's normal life (Hughes, 2002). In addition to this, anxiety features as part of a normal coping process in response to a perceived threat (Sprah and Sostaric, 2004). Patients will tend to experience perceived threat during times of uncertainty, such as a diagnosis or medical intervention that they do not feel comfortable with. Hence, anxiety is a state that occurs frequently among patients. Familiarisation with this area and how to deal with and help an anxious patient is necessary for a nurse to take into consideration. Nursing policy documents from the United Kingdom Central Council for Nursing, Midwifery and Health Visiting (UKCC) (now known as the Nursing and Midwifery Council, NMC) have also emphasised the importance of interpersonal communication in determining outcome: 'communication is an essential part of good practice in nursing and is the basis for building a trusting relationship that will greatly improve care and help to reduce anxiety and stress for patients and clients, their families and their carer' (UKCC, 1996). Communication involves not only sharing information but also emotional support and care from the nurse (Dunne, 2005).

The consideration of anxiety by nurses is further necessitated by research that documents a link between anxiety and the patient's physical and mental health. Studies suggest that even though anxiety is a common and normal part of a coping response, it can have negative implications for the patient's health and well-being if it is prolonged. For example, Van Hout *et al.* (2004) carried out a study among older men in the Netherlands and concluded that those with depression and anxiety tended to have an increase likelihood of mortality. The negative impact of anxiety on health has been implicated in all age groups. For example, Weitoft and Rosen (2005) suggest that prolonged anxiety within any age group will be associated with general poorer health outcome.

The behavioural symptoms associated with anxiety include apprehension, uncontrollable worry, restlessness, panic attacks, avoidance of people and the constant reminder of illness (Sprah and Sostaric, 2004). Such behavioural symptoms can become problematic over a long period of time, as they will affect the quality of life of the patient.

Nurses are in a prime position when caring for patients to introduce strategies and tailor communications with patients that will prevent or minimise patient anxiety. Researchers such as Manthorpe and Iliffe (2006) see addressing anxiety as a key component of a nurse's role by stating that 'responding to anxiety symptoms is a part of the nursing role' (p. 29).

Anxiety and surgery

Patient anxiety is common when experiencing care within a hospital. Being aware of the contexts in which anxiety has the potential to occur can result in the nurse being better prepared to help the patient. One of the contexts in which patient anxiety is common is in patients who are waiting for surgery. Anxiety is common here for many reasons such as apprehension concerning anaesthesia, the operation itself, pain, discomfort and unconsciousness (Carr *et al.*, 2006). It has been found that the majority of patients who attend day surgery remain anxious when entering the hospital (Mitchell, 2005).

Mitchell (2000a, 2000b) provides the main themes which need to be addressed by the nurse when thinking about anxiety management with a patient undergoing surgery (see Table 4.1).

Table 4.1
Main themes of anxiety management

Intervention	Rationale
Differing levels of information provision	Too little information for the patient who desires a great deal can increase anxiety. Conversely, too much information for the patient who desires very little can also increase anxiety.
Promoting cognitive coping strategies	Constantly dwelling on the negative aspects of proposed surgical treatment can give a false impression of safety.
Therapeutic use of self	The close physical presence of the nurse is one of the most effective methods in anxiety management.
Providing a balance of control	Some patients desire more control over events than others. Therefore, in a health care system where the opportunity for such personal inclusion is often minimal, direct action is necessary.
Promoting positive self-efficacy	Some patients feel less able to cope with a surgical event than others. Encouragement in self-belief is therefore necessary, especially when recovery occurs at home.

(Mitchell, 2000a, 2000b).

Information provision

According to the Healthcare Commission (2005a) 42 per cent of day surgery patients in the United Kingdom are not offered a pre-assessment visit. This is in contradiction to studies that claim the majority of day surgery patients would like the information one to three weeks before surgery (Mitchell,

2000b). Within this study, no patient who was interviewed had a desire for information on the day of surgery.

The link between the provision of information and anxiety has been clearly documented (Mitchell, 2007). However, the amount of information that needs to be provided in order to ease anxiety differs according to each patient. The challenge for the nurse is to assess what level of information is appropriate for each individual patient (Stoddard *et al.*, 2005).

Think about this

How much information should be provided to the patient to ease their anxiety? Does this vary according to the patient's anxiety level? What other variables will contribute to the amount of information that needs to be provided in order for the patient's anxiety to be eased?

Castoro *et al.* (2006) demonstrated the differing requirements for information about surgery in their study which looked at 670 day surgery patients, 85 per cent of whom experienced some anxiety. Only 50 per cent required detailed information with further explanation on the day of surgery however.

Many of the differing information requirements and anxiety levels of patients can be explained to some degree by how the individual monitors their current state of health. According to Stoddard *et al.* (2005), patients classed as monitors are more likely to desire information than those with the coping style of a 'blunter' (do not monitor health closely). The key aspect of Stoddard's study demonstrates the importance of tailoring information to the coping style of each individual patient when aiming to reduce pre-surgery anxiety. This study implicates the importance when decreasing anxiety, of information-giving to patients according to their needs, in addition to the routine information that is provided.

Awareness should also be considered when determining how likely a patient is to absorb information. For example, when information in relation to a loss, future loss or new diagnosis is provided, patients will go through a grieving process (refer to Chapter 11). The initial stage of any grieving process will be one of **shock** and denial (the section below discusses denial in more detail). During these stages a nurse should be aware that information provided may not be fully attended to by the patient. Many interventions have been highlighted, such as audiotapes (e.g. Liddell *et al.*, 2004) and written material (refer to Chapter 5), which can ensure that the patient can utilise information after the consultation, so easing anxiety.

Discharge information provided by the nurse is also important when attempting to minimise patient anxiety. According to Henderson and Zernike (2001), discharge information should address information on pain management and practical issues surrounding recovery and wound management, as these areas that have been reported to correlate with high patient dissatisfaction if they are not addressed. Even post-surgery, patients may not be attentive to information that will be vital when at home. This is more so during day care surgery. For example, Dewar *et al.* (2003) found that day surgery patients felt unwell and were not able to absorb discharge instructions. Simplification of information should be sought at all times with such interactions (refer to Chapter 5).

Minimising anxiety is not the only positive outcome for the patient's health and well-being. In addition to this, information provision and how information is tailored to mirror the recipient's needs will also result in benefits such as a shorter stay in the hospital and a decrease in analgesia (Wicker, 1995).

Diagnosis and anxiety

Anxiety is something that is experienced at different levels which change according to the different phases of a terminal or chronic illness. Anxiety is likely to be highest when the patient is initially informed about their diagnosis or loss. Part of 'normal' coping features initial anxiety before this is replaced by defence mechanisms, such as denial. In contrast, if anxiety is experienced over a long period of time or is not dealt with appropriately, the transition to eventual defence mechanisms is more likely to be unhealthy. Individuals can vary as to the anxiety experienced.

Think about this

In the opening case study, Emma and Brian differed in their acceptance of the diagnosis of Brian's kidney cancer. This could have been the result of many contributing factors. It may be that Emma's initial anxiety was not dealt with appropriately, which may have resulted in an unhealthy transition to defence mechanisms, leading to Emma not talking about the diagnosis altogether. Is this a plausible explanation?

Straker (1998) suggests that these variations depend on whether patients have followed a healthy lifestyle or not. Those who have find it more difficult to come to terms with their diagnosis. Others may be highly anxious and fear death or dependency on others. Clearly, the anxiety state cannot last for long as defence mechanisms will be employed (discussed later in the chapter). A nurse can make a difference as to how questions and information are handled after the patient has spoken to the consultant.

The nurse should not assume that all the patient's questions have been answered by the consultant. For example, the patient may need the nurse to cover material again because they may not have been attentive during the consultation period. This is shown in research that suggests material may need to be repeated several times so that the patient will feel reassured (Latimer, 1998). This in turn will ensure that anxiety will not be exacerbated by too little information being provided or questions that have been unanswered.

Throughout the diagnosis of a terminal illness such as cancer, there will be many tests that will be carried out at the various stages of the illness. Anxiety will vary accordingly. Holistic care is important as sometimes the main focus can be on the medical intervention of tests and their outcomes alone. The nurse has a vital role in caring for and supporting the cancer patient emotionally and psychologically, and when supporting the patient's needs throughout this time (Walker, 2002).

According to Walker, it is important for nurses to understand what each test involves and what the patient is likely to experience. The nurse is then able to assist the patient in relation to informational, emotional and supportive needs, which will help minimise anxiety. According to Walker, the period before tests where an illness has yet to be diagnosed can be highly anxious and distressing for the patient, which can be helped by the nurse providing effective communication (see Chapter 17) and good information provision. Equally important is the family or key worker for the patient, who may also need their information requirements met so that their anxiety is not exacerbated. The opening case study demonstrates how a carer can be affected and how this concerned the Macmillan nurse.

In terms of informational and emotional support, the nurse should be aware of the social support networks that are available for the patient. A patient outside hospital often does not know whom to turn to, and can feel isolated in the experience of their diagnosis, which can lead to increased anxiety. The beneficial effect of social support on the anxiety levels of patients has been documented by studies. For example, Fridfinnsdottir (1997) found that among women with potential or actual breast cancer, those who had received effective emotional support reported less distress and made more adaptive coping responses.

Not only does the period during tests or medical interventions to establish a diagnosis result in a high state of anxiety, but the pre-admission period in general is also a highly anxious time for patients. Any situation embracing a highly sensitive and/or emotional topic will result in anxiety. For example, the pre-admission period for women undergoing gynaecological surgery can result in anxiety. As this area is laden with highly emotional and sensitive content, the nurse's role has expanded within gynaecological care to support the emotional needs of the patient. Nurses now play an important role in supporting and providing information for the patient (Walsgrave, 1999).

Sprah and Sostaric's (2004) literature review on the psychosocial coping strategies among cancer patients explains that the time when the patient is digesting information is when they may tend to overestimate the risks associated with the treatment and the likelihood of a poor outcome. Nurses will need to ensure that a balanced view and justification are provided by highlighting the positive outcomes of medical interventions and treatment. In the case study, the Macmillan nurse could have reiterated to Emma the purpose of the medical interventions and chemotherapy that would be taking place as well as the potential for a positive prognosis.

The enhancement of fear is common during an anxiety phase. For example, patients with head and neck cancers may worry about not being able to breathe (Sprah and Sostaric, 2004). Nurses can minimise fears by reassuring the patient, correcting information that may have been misinterpreted and suggesting relaxation techniques which could be included within a care plan (see Chapter 13). Emphasising relaxation will also have benefits for the patient on a long-term basis, as they will be less likely to associate fears with cancer and related interventions that take place in the hospital, e.g. vomiting or panic each time chemotherapy is administered (see Chapter 2).

The nurse's perception of death

Anxiety within a health context is not only prevalent among patients. Anxiety can also be experienced by nurses within the health environment, which can have implications on interpersonal communication and patient care.

There are many reasons as to why a nurse may become anxious. Studies by Farrell (1992) have found that many health care professionals tend to have high anxiety about the topic and experience of death, which can explain in part their unwillingness to talk to patients and families about death (refer to Chapter 11). If a nurse is aware of the possibility that this can occur, either by the use of self-awareness exercises (refer to Chapter 3) or by talking to a mentor about their feelings regarding death, communication will not be hindered by the nurse's unwillingness to discuss the topic openly with patients or their family and friends.

Wilkinson *et al.*'s (1998) study exemplifies how raising awareness of possible anxiety associated with death can improve how nurses communicate to patients about death. The researchers found that 90 per cent of nurses improved when comparing pre- and post-test scores on communication with patients about death. The other 10 per cent did not show any improvement or worsened as a result of training. When surveyed, nurses admitted that they did not want to get involved with the patients' concerns because it caused them too much stress. Researchers such as Dunne (2005) have suggested that health professionals need to develop communication and interpersonal skills so that they can help the patient disclose their feelings fully rather than use block and distance tactics, which hinder communication and most importantly increase anxiety both for the nurse and the patient.

If a patient is in the company of a nurse who avoids pertinent issues that should be discussed, then the patient may feel more anxious for a number of reasons:

- not having their questions answered;
- thinking that if the health professional does not talk about the issue then they should not;
- having informational and emotional support that is general as opposed to being individualised and patient-centred.

Anxiety and aggression

Any situation that results in the patient feeling that they have lost control or autonomy can result in anxiety, tension and aggression (McHale, 1999) (see Chapter 6). The hospital setting, in particular acute settings, can be stressful for patients, which can result in anxiety, loss of control, powerlessness and disorientation (Ferns, 2007). This can increase the probability of the patient becoming aggressive (Whittington *et al.*, 1996). By taking into account that a patient's aggressive behaviour could stem from feelings of anxiety, the nurse can help the patient appropriately.

Ferns (2007) distinguishes between experienced and inexperienced nurses when working with patients and aggression. According to Ferns, what distinguishes the two types of nurses is that experienced nurses are able to detect early patient deterioration. A less experienced nurse will tend to miss what an experienced nurse can see, which will result in the patient deteriorating and manifesting this deterioration as aggression.

Minimising anxiety is crucial when attempting to reduce patient aggression. Communication has been highlighted as one of the main contributors to anxiety and in turn aggression. Researchers have suggested that poor communication is a significant trigger to violent outbursts (Dolan and Holt, 2000). Patients, as well as family members, need to be kept in continual dialogue especially with interventions that will result in any kind of delay, may have side effects or cause any confusion. Any of these examples can result in increasing anxiety.

At the same time, relatives may become frustrated if they have to wait a long time to see medical staff, for tests to be carried out and results obtained or wait for a bed to become available for the patient (Lyneham, 2000). Continual contact and communication with the family and the patient can result in questions being answered and confusion decreasing. This will result in a decrease in anxiety, which will, in turn, result in a decreased probability of frustration and aggression.

Think about this

In the opening case study Emma appeared to be very angry when she replied to the Macmillan nurse. What could have arisen during previous communications between Emma, the nurses and consultant which could have resulted in Emma becoming angry over the following months?

Personality structure: the id, ego and superego and the employment of ego defence mechanisms

Personality structure

According to Freud, there are three components of personality, referred to as the **id**, **ego** and **superego**. The id is the primitive part of the personality which is in existence as soon as a child is born. This is based on the **pleasure**

The id, ego and superego

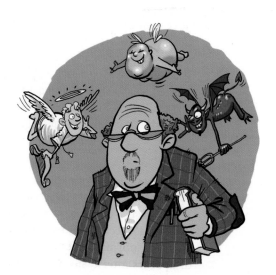

principle, which drives the thirst for satisfying needs immediately. For example, a child during their earlier years will cry when hungry, irrespective of the time or how busy the parent could be. The id becomes moulded as the child matures but still exists as a less dominant force.

The second component of personality is referred to as the superego, which contains morals and rules within society. The superego emerges as soon as the parents and other surrounding figures begin to teach the child what is right and wrong. Freud suggested that the superego comes into existence between 3 and 5 years of age and develops through maturation. The prime role of the superego is to prevent the gratification of the id's immediate needs by observing the circumstances and the rules that operate.

The third component of personality is referred to as the ego, which is based on the reality principle. The ego mediates between the id's demands and the superego's wishes which clash and can have the potential to cause tension and anxiety. As a result of the tension and anxiety that are produced by the clash between the id and the superego, the ego will judge if the need can be met. If this is not the case, then the ego will repress the needs and their associated feelings, thoughts, desires and wishes into the unconscious part of the mind with the use of **ego defence mechanisms**.

Ego defence mechanisms are employed by the ego when there is conflict between the id and superego, which gives rise to anxiety and tension. The ego employs the defence mechanisms in order to reduce tension and anxiety by repressing feelings, thoughts and emotions into the unconscious part of the mind. Hough (2002) states that 'ego defence mechanisms protect the individual against painful anxiety and ensure that the ego is not overwhelmed'. It was Sigmund Freud's daughter, Anna Freud, who explored defence mechanisms and the different types of defence mechanisms that can be employed by an individual when reducing anxiety.

Ego defence mechanisms and catharsis

There are many defence mechanisms which can be employed by the ego when reducing anxiety. A nurse who is familiar with the different types of defence mechanisms can help a patient within the context of interpersonal communication to move forward psychologically. A patient who employs a defence mechanism will signal to the nurse that the patient is enduring anxiety that is masked by a defence mechanism. Nurses who are aware of defence mechanisms can then tailor communication so that patients feel comfortable to talk about their feelings. This is referred to as **catharsis** (refer to Chapter 17) where an individual is able to discharge their emotions, feelings and thoughts. Below is an exploration of the types of defence mechanisms that can be held by an individual.

Denial

Denial is one type of defence mechanism that can be defined as 'the refusal to acknowledge the existence of a real situation or the feelings associated with it' (Freud 1961). More specifically aligned to health practice, denial manifests itself as a 'mechanism of denying the presence of illness and medical diagnosis. It is normally activated after the first stages of shock, and usually disappears after a short time' (Kreitler, 1999). As reflected in the definition, denial is part of a normal coping process and is featured within many of the grief framework models that are available (see Chapter 11).

Employing denial

Denial itself can be healthy to a certain extent within the short-term. For example, patients who have been diagnosed with a terminal illness or patients and family that have been given shocking or bad news may employ denial as a coping response during the short-term period, which will be beneficial for the individual. Davidhizar and Newman Giger (1998) cite an example of terminal illness, where denial can be advantageous in providing hope by alleviating the painful external reality of sickness and allow courage to assist the endurance of unreasonable suffering.

Within grief work models, denial is cited as the most common reaction or response during the earlier stages of grief work. Kubler-Ross (1969), who explored patients and their families' experience of loss, found that denial provided a way of coping in the short term while allowing the patient to organise more effective defence strategies and providing some time before the patient or family members have to begin to adjust to the loss. In the main the advantage of patients employing denial over a short-term period is that it will reduce anxiety (Sprah and Sostartic, 2004). This will help the patient become more comfortable when adjusting to their present state of ill-health or loss rather than enduring long-term anxiety which has negative implications for their health.

Davidhizar and Newman Giger (1998) suggests that nurses must recognise that denial may be the only way of coping with the unimaginable. Common verbal reactions of a patient in denial can be: 'no it can't be me', 'you must have the results mixed up', 'I'll be fine' and 'my partner is just unwell, he does not have kidney cancer'. Open communication and being attentive when listening to a patient talk about their feelings and emotions are highly beneficial during this stage. During active listening the nurse should not interrupt, share personal stories, change the subject or offer platitudes (Clearly and Gifford, 1990) (see Chapter 17 for further elaboration on attentive listening).

A patient in denial will tend to withhold information that they are not comfortable talking about. Nurses will be able to recognise this by noting disparities between the verbal and non-verbal behaviour of the patient. For example, in the opening case study Emma stated that she was fine but the nurse could see that this was not the case because as soon as the nurse asked her how she was coping, she began moving frantically around the room and keeping busy, rather than being relaxed and mirroring 'I'm fine' through her non-verbal communication. This contradiction is known as **incongruence,** which can indicate the defence mechanism of denial or other defence mechanisms being employed by the patient (refer to Chapter 3 for further elaboration on congruence and incongruent behaviour).

Denial as a problem

Clearly there are many advantages for the patient who may employ denial during the early stages of their coping process. However, denial can be maladaptive rather than adaptive for the patient's health and well-being in different contexts. A patient with a diagnosis of a chronic illness who is given medication and discharged immediately is one example when being in denial can be problematic for the patient. Being in denial can have implications for compliance to medication and interfere with ongoing treatment (Sprah and Sostaric, 2004), such as missing appointments. A nurse can play a vital role in ensuring that this particular patient is facilitated and invited by the nurse to explore their anxieties in relation to the newly diagnosed illness. At the same time, family members of the patient will also need to be attended to, especially if they will be the main carer or social support for the patient when at home.

Think about this

In the case study is it evident that Emma has difficulty coming to terms with Brian's diagnosis of kidney cancer? What could the discharge nurse have covered with Emma so that she could have coped better and in turn prevented Emma from being in a state of denial over a long period of time?

Employing denial during the early stages of an acute illness such as myocardial infarction, can also be detrimental for the patient. Mumford *et al.* (1999) have suggested that delays in seeking medical assistance after the onset of severe chest pain can contribute to delays in the patient's hospital admission and thrombolysis, which results in the increased likelihood of longer-lasting effects of myocardial infarction on the body. More worryingly, the study found that those patients with prior ischaemic heart disease (74 per cent of patients) presented longer delays than those who did not have any history of heart disease.

Researchers have suggested that denial impacts on the individual delaying seeking help, as the recognition of symptoms may be ignored or explained with non-cardiac rationalisations. Mumford *et al.* saw this as the defence mechanism of **displacement** (refer to section below for detailed account of displacement) taking the place of denial. Studies like Mumford *et al.* and earlier studies such as Simon *et al.* (1972) have found that patients who employ denial when enduring chest pains that are related to potential heart disease will tend to engage in non-therapeutic activity such as arranging clothes for the overnight stay or contacting friends, before calling the ambulance service.

Nurses can make a difference by informing angina patients about the possible implications of denial during the early stages of an ischaemic heart attack. In addition to this, nurses should stress the importance of seeking help in relation to any symptoms that are experienced, rather than finding other explanations or engaging in activity that distracts the individual from seeking help. The nurse also needs to further stress to patients who have already experienced an angina attack that symptoms should not be underestimated after a first heart attack.

Factors that enhance denial, which impact on the delay of accessing health services among patients, can result from the following: past experiences with health services, expectations, and social and cultural influences (Tod *et al.*, 2001). Tod's study identifies social influences that encourage denial as largely stemming from cultural sources such as having a fierce outlook on independence rather than dependence, which increases the likelihood of brushing pains away. Nurses need to reinforce the importance of symptoms and address issues that relate to the patient's perception of dependence, which can especially be prevalent among men.

Denial can also become a problem for the patient who employs this defence mechanism over an extended period of time. Denial then becomes a barrier to the patient being able to accept their current state of health, loss or diagnosis. Literature supports the notion that nurses can prevent this from occurring by working through grieving stages with a patient. For example, Field and Payne (2003) reiterate the importance of working through grieving stages where patients are encouraged to disengage from their relationship to the dead person. This in turn prevents the patient from employing denial over a long period of time.

Nurses should also encourage and facilitate the patient to talk, especially about their feelings, anxieties and perception of their loss, illness or matter at hand. Not doing so will further encourage the patient into denial which will have long-term implications for the patient's physical and mental well-being. Communication (see Chapter 17) is therefore important within the nurse–patient relationship in the prevention of prolonged denial. Booth *et al.* (1996) illustrated how the nurse's communication can have an impact on whether the patient talks about their feelings. Booth concluded from a study of hospice nurses ($n = 41$) that blocking behaviour was evident in nurse–patient interactions when patients disclosed their feelings. Nurses need to avoid blocking behaviour when patients are disclosing their feelings and thoughts, since disclosing feelings is necessary for the patient to move out of denial.

Think about this

Both Brian and Emma have experienced denial in relation to Brian's kidney cancer but for differing lengths of time. Emma had an unhealthy coping process (with prolonged denial) compared with Brian. Can you think how communication with patients in the hospital can influence the coping processes of individuals such as Brian and Emma? What could have been carried out differently so that Emma could have found it easier to cope with Brian's illness?

Nurses need to work with, rather than override, any denial defence mechanism. The first step for a nurse will be to establish the extent of denial in the patient. According to Baile *et al.* (2000), open-ended questions such as 'what is your understanding of the reasons we did the scan?', will allow the nurse to assess the extent of denial. The nurse can then determine what the patient needs to know as well as clarifying any misunderstanding. Dunne (2005) advocates communication skills such as empathy and open-ended questioning as being core components of the facilitative relationship between the nurse and the patient in denial. Literature suggests that nurses should work with, rather than confront, patient denial. Houldin (2000), for example, states that instead of confronting denial it is better to support the patient and discuss issues of concern to them, which they will then be able to think about at their own pace. Houldin further maintains that direct confrontation of patient denial will only result in the increased use of this defence mechanism. One way that a nurse can work with denial is to highlight positive aspects of the patient's current coping mechanism and build on them, which will result in the patient moving forward.

When working with a patient, a useful question for the nurse to ask is 'is the defence mechanism helping the patient to cope at the moment?' If denial is not affecting current medication-taking behaviour because they are in hospital or are in long-term stay within the hospital, then the nurse may need to step back and provide the patient with some space, but at the same time be attentive to the patient when they do begin to discuss their feelings. However, when denial is affecting compliance with necessary appointments or medication, then denial needs to be confronted (Straker, 1998). In the case study above, while Brian was in hospital the nurses allowed him some space to be in denial for the first couple of days. At the same time they also began exploring his feelings. They began to tackle these after a couple of days in preparation for his being discharged from hospital.

Denial does not necessarily manifest itself in patients who are in hospital or who need to contact the NHS because of ill health. The defence mechanism of denial can also become apparent in individuals who may not have ill-health but have a differing state of health, such as pregnancy. Below is a research in focus box which explores denial in relation to the acceptance of pregnancy among young women.

Research in focus

Wessel, J. and Buscher, U. (2002) Denial of pregnancy: population based study. *British Medical Journal*, **324**, 458.

Introduction
The prevalence of denial of pregnancy, a woman's lack of awareness of being pregnant, is not reliably known. Few studies describe large numbers of cases, but descriptions of 27 and 28 patients at a single obstetric hospital led to estimates of one denied pregnancy per 300-600 pregnancies. However, these numbers were determined within a more or less random observation period and are lacking an epidemiological relevance.

Methods and results
Between 1 July 1995 and 30 June 1996 we asked all 19 obstetric hospitals and five obstetrics and midwives' practices in the Berlin metropolitan area to report cases of women who were not aware of being pregnant and did not have a doctor's diagnosis of pregnancy during the first 20 weeks, or more, of gestation.

Altogether 62 women did not realise they were pregnant until after 20 weeks' gestation. On the basis of 29 462 deliveries during the study period, we determined that 1 in 475 (95 per cent confidence interval 370 to 625) pregnancies were denied by the woman.

In 37 women pregnancy was diagnosed before the birth; in the remainder, the diagnosis was made during labour. In 12 deliveries (1 in 2455 (1429 to 5000) births) a viable foetus was born without the woman having realised that she was pregnant until she went into labour.

Conclusion

The common view that denied pregnancies are exotic and rare events is not valid. Denial of pregnancy may put both mother and foetus at risk.

The ratio of one denied pregnancy in 475 births is based on complete reporting within a large region (all births in Berlin metropolitan area during one year) and is representative for the total population of a German federal state. In all of Germany in 1995 and 1996 there were about 770 000 deliveries per year; on this basis we calculate that in about 1600 births the mother would not have been aware of her pregnancy at 20 weeks' gestation, or later, and each year 300 women would not have realised they were pregnant until going into labour.

As the completeness of recruited cases could not be determined, the true rate may be higher. Also, though cases were determined prospectively, the period of 'non-awareness' was determined from information supplied by the woman after she became aware of her pregnancy.

It cannot be stated whether the results are generally applicable outside Berlin. However, ratios determined earlier for a small German city of Celle (1:357) and for Berlin (1:275–586) compare to those in this study. Furthermore, a ratio of 1:400 in the large Austrian city of Innsbruck indicates a comparable frequency of denial of pregnancy across different sociodemographic regions.

Other defence mechanisms

Denial is one of the most commonly employed defence mechanisms. There are other types of defence mechanism that nurses need to be aware of so that they can recognise and tailor information accordingly, in order to provide the best care possible.

Repression is a defence mechanism where 'unacceptable feelings, thoughts and emotions are pushed into the unconscious' (Hough, 2002). According to Freud, any traumatic incidents encountered are usually repressed into the unconscious and can then manifest themselves in enormous anxiety or, as Lyonfields (1993) suggested, constant worrying. For example, a patient displaying high levels of anxiety when seeing a needle would be explained from the psychodynamic perspective as stemming from earlier negative experiences with injections which were repressed rather than explored.

Extreme reactions as well as high anxiety displayed by a patient can be indicative of repressed thoughts and feelings which are closely aligned to the present context. Nurses should invite the patient to talk about their current anxiety and further facilitate disclosure of information which explores the anxiety.

Repression is a defence mechanism that is often cited by those who work with victims of child sexual abuse where victims of abuse cannot remember large parts of the ordeal several years later. Andrews *et al.* (2000) carried out a systematic survey of British psychologists describing their experiences of recovered memories among clients. They revealed that reported forgetting for a variety of sexual and non-sexual traumas occurred in 40 per cent of incidents. Research suggests that focusing on ways of thinking such as hopelessness, worthlessness and, in turn, enhancing personal meaning are preferable to changing the way a person is currently thinking within the therapeutic setting (Power and Brewin, 1997). Irrespective of the type of defence mechanism being used, nurses who are finding it difficult to move the patient forward from their current way of coping through such defence mechanisms may find it more achievable to focus on current thinking patterns and assign personal meaning to what is occurring.

Think about this

Taking the example of Emma in the opening case study, the nurse could have facilitated Emma into thinking about how her current actions affected her on a day-to-day basis. In addition to this, the importance of the carer and how they can be affected could also have been explored. Taking time out for herself would have been another avenue that could have been pursued, which could possibly have influenced Emma's feelings of worthlessness and lack of control over Brian's illness.

Regression is another type of defence mechanism. During times of stress and anxiety the individual will regress to an earlier childhood state which is comforting. In the case study above, Brian displayed regression during the initial stages of his diagnosis of kidney cancer. Regression enabled Brian to retreat to a childhood state by rocking backwards and forwards, which provided a comforting feeling. Nurses should be aware that regression extends not only to adults but to children as well. For example, older children may suck their thumb.

Displaying regression should be indicative to the nurse that the patient is experiencing anxiety and is coping by comforting themselves. This may help the patient initially, especially when adjusting to a new diagnosis of a differing state of ill-health. At the same time, when patients display behaviours indicative of regression, nurses should again aim to reduce patient anxiety by offering appropriate information, asking the patient what they currently understand and in turn correcting misunderstandings. This provides an invitation for the patient to disclose how they currently feel and why. Gaining such disclosure can be helped with communication and counselling skills as well as the humanistic principles. Finally, the patient should be provided with information and coping strategies which encourage relaxation. In the above case study the nurse caring for Brian observed that the patient was coping by regressing and in turn tailored her support and information accordingly. A nurse who is not aware of regression could result in the patient's anxiety not being explored, which will further heighten anxiety. This could have further negative implications for the patient's mental and physical well-being.

Projection is another type of defence mechanism where the individual attributes their own unacceptable thoughts, feelings and impulses on to another person. For example, a patient who may dislike a nurse, but cannot deal with the feelings of dislike, could project by openly accusing the nurse of disliking the patient. Nurses need to be aware of projection and, as in the example cited, not to take the feelings of a patient personally. Projection could even be extended to not liking the present state of ill-health, but these feelings could be projected on to health care staff.

Reaction formation is a defence mechanism where the individual may conceal his or her true feelings by behaving in the opposite way. The defence mechanism of reaction formation can be employed within many contexts. For example, it is not uncommon for a patient to have a loss of control when staying in hospital or when being given a diagnosis. Loss of control as well as accompanying feelings, such as loss of esteem, worth and security, can result in the patient concealing these feelings by either portraying to the nurse that they are fine or possibly by portraying aggression. Research supports that such factors that could lead to an outburst of aggression. For example, Ferns (2007) highlighted factors such as fear, pain and anxiety as variables that tend to be closely linked to aggression.

As well as calming the patient down, communication with the patient is important so that aggression is not further aggravated and the contributing factors can be explored. This has been supported by Hines (2000) who found that poor communication undermines patient confidence and leads to confusion, which in turn can result in aggression. When communicating with a patient and attempting to explore why they had an aggressive outburst, communication, according to Potter and Perry (2006), should have four main aims: to establish positive relationships, to give factual information, to determine needs and to optimise the use of resources.

Think about this

Emma greeted the nurse in an angry manner and proceeded to be very short with her. If the nurse was to apply reaction formation as an explanation to Emma's behaviour, what were the feelings that Emma concealed in relation to Brian and his diagnosis of cancer?

Displacement is also referred to as 'kick the cat syndrome'. This is where energy such as anger, frustration or hostility is displaced on to a non-threatening object or person. There has been much literature and highly publicised cases of carers and the unacceptable care or abuse towards elderly patients (refer to Chapter 10). Although there are many factors that contribute to such unacceptable behaviour, one plausible explanation can be the employment of displacement. Research has highlighted that the stress of caring is often identified as a trigger for elder abuse (Wieland, 2000). However, more recent research has suggested that there is no link between the stress of caring and abuse (Action on Elder Abuse, 2004).

Nurses need to be aware of displacement and how carers can displace their anger or frustration on to others. Nurses need to equip themselves with information regarding appropriate support mechanisms and who to contact when dealing with stressful situations. These can be used by the nurse themselves and as informational support when liaising with other health workers and carers at large. At times, awareness can give rise to the individual acknowledging displacement, which results in positive steps being taken to deal with the precipitating factors that are producing feelings such as anger, frustration, etc. According to McGarry and Simpson (2007), nurses have a central role to play when recognising and preventing abuse through a multi-agency approach.

Rationalisation is where an individual justifies their own behaviour or provides excuses for their own shortcomings, which serve to avoid criticism, condemnation or disappointment by others. In the above case study, Emma is the main carer as well as provider within the home since Brian's commencement of treatment for kidney cancer. Emma has been avoiding conversations that involve anything in relation to the kidney cancer diagnosis or how Emma may be feeling about Brian. Emma may use rationalisation; excusing her avoidance of emotional subjects as a result of being too busy, just like other carers who must also be very busy.

Human beings will employ such defence mechanisms in order to alleviate anxiety. This means that it is not only patients who employ defence mechanisms, but nurses can also employ such tactics during times of stress. Barre and Evans (2002) are among many researchers who have outlined how the defence mechanism of rationalisation can be employed by nurses who are working with suicidal or self-harming patients. According to Long and Reid's (1996) study, nurses tended to use rationalisation as a form of protection against anxiety they themselves experienced. The researchers proposed that nurses need to be able to question their own beliefs about suicide, death and other life issues in order to practise nursing in a less defended way (refer to Chapter 3 on self-awareness).

Think about this

How would a nurse help Emma, who may have employed rationalisation, so that conversations in relation to Brian's kidney cancer and how Emma feels could be explored? Would this help Emma to disclose, and come to terms with, Brian's diagnosis of kidney cancer earlier?

Conclusion

The psychodynamic approach brings forth several areas that are valuable for nurses to consider. The main areas such as anxiety and defence mechanisms feature day to day as part of a coping process of patients who attempt to deal with being in an environment that brings stress and anxiety uncertainty regarding the future or even temporary loss of control within their life. Nurses need to be familiar with such areas so that appropriate communication and care can be offered. Tailoring communication and care accordingly, being able to recognise the diverse components that contribute to the patient's coping process and if it is helpful or not to the patient's well-being, will enable the nurse to offer care that is not-only patient centred, but also moves the patient forward both mentally and physically from their present mindset.

At the same time the psychodynamic approach highlights how nurses can employ defence mechanisms and react in certain ways within an anxious situation, which can influence the care they provide. Poor quality care, low patient-centredness and patients' concerns not being adequately addressed may result from the nurse employing defence mechanisms.

Summary

- Sigmund Freud (1858–1939) pioneered the psychodynamic approach which explores how the mind (human psyche) is responsible for everyday behaviour. Psychotherapy or psychoanalysis is the therapy that stems from this approach.

- According to the psychodynamic approach, all behaviour originates from previous experiences which reside within the unconscious mind. Freud referred to this as psychic determinism.

- The three levels of the mind are referred to as the conscious, preconscious and unconscious. The third level forms the largest part of the mind and contains repressed feelings and thoughts that influence day-to-day behaviour, which the individual is not consciously aware of.

- Personality consists of the id, ego and superego. These are in constant conflict, which results in tension and anxiety. As a result the ego employs defence mechanisms so that thoughts are pushed into the unconscious, which then provides conscious relief for the individual.

- Anxiety is a complex emotional state with both apprehension and dread being common features. Anxiety is common within the health setting and can be seen readily in contexts where individuals are faced with death, a new diagnosis, waiting to be given a confirmed diagnosis, surgery and the hospital itself.

- Effective interpersonal communication that meets the patient's needs and recognition of patient anxiety and how to help the patient decrease anxiety are vital components when caring for patients.

- Defence mechanisms should be worked with rather than overridden by a nurse. The beneficial effects of defence mechanisms change depending on several variables, which differ among patients.

- Denial, repression, regression, projection, reaction formation, displacement and rationalisation are all types of defence mechanisms that a patient could employ when experiencing anxiety.

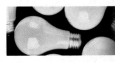

Check your understanding

1. Exploring factors that are contributing to anxiety, as well as disclosure, is helpful in ensuring that feelings and thoughts are not repressed into the unconscious part of the mind. The communication that occurs when the individual is facilitated to disclose their thoughts and feelings is referred to as what?

2. Name three types of defence mechanism, and give examples of how a patient could employ these when experiencing anxiety.

3. Name the three levels of the mind and describe what is contained within them.

4. What part of the personality employs defence mechanism and what are the advantages and disadvantages of patients employing defence mechanisms?

5. List four things that a nurse should address when caring for a patient who is experiencing high anxiety.

6. What variables contribute to defence mechanisms becoming maladaptive for the patient?

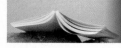

Further reading

Bond, M. and Perry, J.C. (2004) Long-term changes in defence styles with psychodynamic psychotherapy for depressive, anxiety and personality disorders. *American Journal of Psychiatry*, **161**, 1665–1671.

Ortega, A.N. and Alegria, M. (2006) Denial and its association with mental health use. *The Journal of Behavioural Health Services and Research*, **32** (3), 320–331.

Russell, G.C. (1993) The role of denial in clinical practice. *Journal of Advanced Nursing*, **18** (6), 938–940.

Telford, K., Kralik, D. and Koch, T. (2006) Acceptance and denial: implications for people adapting to chronic illness: literature review. *Journal of Advanced Nursing*, **55** (4), 457–464.

Weblinks

Simply Psychology	http://www.simplypsychology.pwp.blueyonder.co.uk/psychodynamic.html	Saul McLeod's A level psychology website. This website has one section which gives an in-depth account of the psychodynamic approach and defence mechanisms written for newcomers to the psychodynamic approach.
Freud's Museum Website	http://www.freud.org.uk/	An in-depth account of Freud, his work around psychoanalysis and his research as well as a look around his house and his life. There is a substantial amount of information within the education section which looks at dream interpretation.
Gerard Keegan and his Psychology Site	http://www.gerardkeegan.co.uk/resource/funteaching.htm	A look at the psychodynamic perspective with extensive multiple choice questions. Also complemented by other perspectives within psychology.
Patient Plus	http://www.patient.co.uk/showdoc/40002439/	A look at anxiety, anxiety care and measurements of anxiety within the context of the health environment and illnesses.

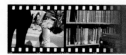

Media example

Ally McBeal A humorous look at the conflict and tension experienced between the id and the superego and how this impacts on day-to-day behaviour.

Chapter 5

Cognitive psychology

Learning outcomes

When you have read through this chapter you should understand:

- How an understanding of memory can help the nurse increase the probability of patients remembering health instructions.

- How nurses can effectively give information to patients.

- How to work with dementia patients effectively.

- What cognitive behavioural therapy is and how nurses can apply cognitive behavioural strategies when helping patients.

- The differing problem-solving strategies that exist for both patients and nurses.

- How to communicate with patients who have a sensory deprivation.

- How individuals reason and think.

- How perception theory promotes holistic care.

Case study

Stewart Horne is a 48-year-old man who has a history of mild depression. Within the past year, Stewart has found it difficult to manage his depression. This has been coupled with panic attacks and a dramatic decrease in weight. After much persuasion from his wife, he has decided to attend an appointment with his GP. After two appointments, the GP concludes that irrespective of the medication that is being prescribed to Stewart, his physical and mental health is still deteriorating. Stewart's GP refers his patient to the community mental health nurse.

After two meetings between the community mental health nurse and Stewart, it is also apparent to the nurse that Stewart's depression is becoming worse. After a discussion with Stewart the nurse realises that the patient has had many different types of medication prescribed to him over the years, which has caused him confusion. After asking Stewart about his daily drug routine, the nurse discovers that he has become confused with his medication instructions. The nurse addresses Stewart's confusion over his medication by collecting all his current medications and telling him which medications he should not take, as well as when to take the correct medication. The nurse tailored the new drug regimen to Stewart's daily lifestyle. The nurse also provides cues for the patient so that he does not forget to take his medication.

The nurse begins to address Stewart's panic attacks by identifying triggering factors. Over the next couple of sessions, Stewart and the nurse identify triggering factors and manage to eliminate or control the factors. As a result, Stewart has now begun to have fewer panic attacks.

The community mental health nurse informs the GP in a letter that the patient has dramatically improved in both his mental and physical health. The nurse indicates that Stewart's mental and physical deterioration was a result of confusion over his medication, being in a mindset of continual negative thinking and helplessness, feeling confused and distressed in many situations, and a visual impairment, of which Stewart was not aware. The nurse also described the interventions and referrals that were used when helping Stewart. These included a revision of his medication, cognitive behavioural therapy and strategies for adjustment to his sensory impairment. The letter finally concludes that Stewart does not need to see the community mental health nurse any more, as his panic attacks and depression have dramatically decreased. Stuart has regained full control of his life. He has begun to manage his depression, panic attacks and sensory impairment with success.

Why is this relevant to nursing practice?

There are many strands within cognitive psychology that are relevant to the practice of nursing, some of which have been exemplified in the opening case study. The first area that has been highlighted is the patient's medication-taking behaviour; Stewart was not adhering to his medication routine (see Chapter 16). There are many questions that arise in relation to Stewart's lack of adherence to his medication. Was Stewart confused with his previous medication-taking instructions? Was the information delivered in a way that ensured Stewart understood? Did Stewart attend to the information when it was being provided? Or simply, had Stewart over time forgotten or become confused by the instructions that were initially provided?

The nurse also used cues and tailored Stewart's medical regimen to his lifestyle. Cognitive psychology explores on the area of **memory** and how to avoid forgetting information, which will be looked at within this chapter.

The case study shows how Stewart lost an enormous amount of vision as well as having an increase in depression. Both visual reduction and depression can bring about sensory impairment or cognitive reduction, which can influence the patient's day-to-day behaviour. With the use of cognitive psychology, an exploration of what needs arise as a result of one or more sensory impairments will be undertaken.

The area of **perception** and its importance when providing holistic care to the patient will be looked at. The community mental health nurse ensured that she took as much information as possible about Stewart, rather than just looking at his presented symptoms, when putting together the care plan. Familiarity with the area of perception will raise the nurse's awareness of how important holistic care is in practice, as at times what is presented and perceived during the initial interaction is not sufficient information.

The community mental health nurse was faced with Stewart's symptoms of severe depression. In order to help him, the nurse had to problem-solve, to the end goal of helping Stewart get better. Problem-solving, as well as thinking and reasoning, will be considered within this chapter, as this is something that nurses will participate in on a daily basis. Familiarity with possible problem-solving strategies will enable the nurse to effectively solve problems at a much quicker pace and more confidently.

The community mental health nurse worked within a framework that stemmed from cognitive behavioural therapy when identifying triggering factors that resulted in distress. Frameworks and principles from cognitive behavioural therapy are useful for nurses when attempting to find explanations or identify triggering factors to challenging behaviour or, as in Stewart's case, distress. Such frameworks help to identify factors and guide how to better manage or even avoid such factors for the patient's health and well-being.

Cognitive psychology

Ulric Neisser (1967) entitled his book and at the same time coined the term **cognitive psychology**. He defined it as the study of how people learn, structure, store and use knowledge.

Cognitive psychology is the branch of psychology that is concerned with the study of mental states and processes such as problem-solving, memory and language. The cognitive psychology perspective is different from previous approaches on two fronts. Firstly, this perspective suggests that data that is **introspective** (an individual's recalled information) is not scientific, i.e. cannot be tested or measured. This is what the psychodynamic perspective is largely based on (see Chapter 4). Secondly, cognitive psychologists focus on mental states as being important in determining and predicting behaviour, which behavioural psychologists do not consider. Instead, behaviourists propose that only behaviour that is observable can be studied. Cognitive psychologists in contrast, suggest that a large part of behaviour that is not observable, e.g. memory, is equally important.

Cognitive psychology explores the area of memory and attention. Knowledge of these areas will enable the nurse to ensure that information is provided in a way that will decrease the probability of the patient forgetting or becoming confused, once the initial health instructions have been provided.

Memory

How successful the patient is in managing or recovering from an illness or state of ill health will be determined to some degree by how the patient retains information within their memory. How the nurse communicates health information is key to this. Research suggests that good communication is the cornerstone of health education and giving information effectively (Partridge and Hill, 2000). Why patients such as Stewart forget initial instructions that have been provided can partly be explained by ineffective information-giving exchanges. An effective information-giving session with a patient will involve the nurse being familiar with how memory works and how to prevent the patient forgetting information.

Memory is the process of encoding, storing and retrieving information. **Encoding** refers to the active process of inputting stimulus information into a form that can be used by memory stores. **Storage** refers to the process of maintaining information in memory. **Retrieval** involves the active process of locating and recalling information, which is held within the memory store. During any of these stages information being processed can be distorted or forgotten. The following section explores how a nurse can ensure that the patient processes information effectively, so that forgetting or confusion is less likely to occur.

Models of memory

Atkinson and Shiffrin (1968) put forward one of the first memory models within cognitive psychology known as the **three-stage memory store model**, or *multi-store memory model* (see Figure 5.1). The model proposes that there are three distinct stores within memory, beginning with the initial stage of when information is received to the processing and retention of information.

The **sensory memory store** is the first store within the memory model which receives information from different **sensory registers**. Auditory and visual sensory channels are the commonly used ones. The sensory memory store continually receives information from the senses (Cowan, 1988); however, only a small amount of this is actually processed. Unless material is given attention or revisited, the material will fade rapidly i.e. be forgotten. Cowan (1988) referred to this as **masking**, where new information replaces old information immediately.

Sensory memory and attention

As information that is received within sensory memory can be lost immediately, the nurse has to ensure that the patient is attending to the health information that is being provided. Broadbent (1958) refers to the process of attention as a **filtering process**. Stimuli that meet certain requirements are more likely be attended to, and last longer, within our sensory memory than stimuli that do not meet such requirements. Information that is familiar and understandable to the patient is less likely to be filtered out.

Recognition and understanding of information that is being provided to the patient can be a problem when the information is complex or new.

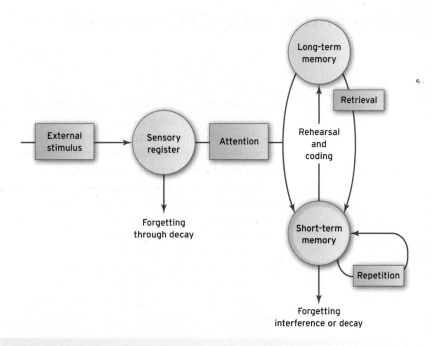

Figure 5.1 A diagram of the multi-store memory model

Source: Morris, Charles G.; Maisto, Albert A., *Understanding Psychology*, 6th Edition, © 2003, Pg. 203. Reprinted by permission of Pearson Education, Inc., Upper Saddle River, NJ

Information can be made familiar and understandable to the patient with the use of everyday examples, as well as making the medical information simpler. In the opening case study, the community mental health nurse simplified the patient's drug regimen by collecting all his medication and then providing instructions in relation to his daily routine.

The number of distractions that the individual faces can also explain attention and how much information is received. Cherry (1966) explained this in his **cocktail-party phenomenon.** The theory explores how a person can attend to a single talker among a background of noise and other conversations (Arons, 2005). Cherry found that the talker's pitching their tone of voice slightly higher, as well as expressing interest when talking, would ensure that the person would listen to this particular conversation rather than others around them.

Within the hospital setting there are many environmental distractions. Busy wards, high levels of background noise and a lack of privacy can impair learning (Caress, 2003). These distractions are difficult for the health professional to eliminate (Janseen *et al.*, 2000). The patient's attention can also be impaired by internal distractions such as pain, fear or anxiety. Referring to the patient by name throughout the conversation as well as acknowledging any internal distractions will encourage the patient to pay as much attention as possible to the nurse.

Effective written and verbal information

Information-giving that is delivered in as many formats as possible will be more likely to be attended to and registered within the sensory memory channels. For example, research has shown that most patients do not read a leaflet from start to finish, as leaflets do not vary in how information is portrayed (Kools, 2006). A simple way of delivering information in different formats is to use written material to complement verbal information. This will not only simplify verbal health information but also make information easier to understand and further engage the patient.

Research has supported the benefits of using pictures in addition to written and verbal information to increase the chances of getting the patient's attention, engaging with the patient, enhancing patient comprehension, increasing patient recall of information and making the patient more likely to adhere to health instructions (Houts *et al.*, 2005). This method does not necessarily require the use of extra funding or resources.

Leaflets in waiting rooms can be used in an interactive way. For example, highlighting a page or paragraph or sticking a Post-it™ note to the most relevant sections within the leaflet will increase the likelihood of the patient engaging with material or can act as a reminder when outside the hospital. This was seen in the opening case study, where the nurse collected all the medications that Stewart was taking and then had a information-giving session to revisit his medical regimen. Since Stewart was confused about his medications, the nurse could have used a variety of written information, such as leaflets or charts, to complement verbal information.

Research highlights the link between delivering information in differing formats and positive patient satisfaction outcomes. Spinks (2003) found that patients who were waiting for colonoscopy procedures and had received both verbal and written information on the procedure had a better understanding of the procedures than those who had just been given written information. These patients were also more confident in making a decision about the procedure than those with just written information. This is supported by Nickiln (2002), who stated that the role of a nurse must incorporate the provision of written material that reinforces the spoken word and compensates for the information that is forgotten at a verbal consultation.

Researchers have also highlighted the importance of using other aids to complement verbal information giving between the nurse and patient, which can enhance the amount of information the patient retains. For example, Scott *et al.* (2006) recommended aids such as written material, videotapes and audiotapes of the consultation, which enhance retention of material.

The use of pictures in addition to verbal or written material has also been shown to be advantageous when recalling information, especially for those who have **low literacy skills.** According to the United Nations Development Program (UN, 1999), the United Kingdom has the highest percentage of low literacy skills – estimated at 21.8 per cent – in comparison with other industrialised countries. The use of pictures within material would benefit the high percentage of low literacy patients.

Delp and Jones (1996) exemplified the beneficial effects of pictures on the patient's comprehension, recall and adherence to health instructions. 234 patients who came into the emergency room with lacerations were included in the study. After recovering from treatment, but prior to discharge, patients were given printed instructions for caring for their wounds at home. Half were randomly given just text. The other half received the same text plus pictures that illustrated the information in the text.

Subjects were phoned and interviewed three days later. They were asked if they had read the instructions (attention). If they had, they were asked a series of questions about information in the handout (recall) and also what they had done to care for their wounds (adherence). The researchers found those who received the handouts with pictures more likely to read the written material. They were also more likely to remember what they read and follow the instructions than those who had read the text alone. Most importantly, the study found that those with low literacy especially benefited from the addition of pictures to text. See Table 5.1.

A literature review carried out by Levine (1987) showed that children can benefit from additional aids such as pictures, as they tend to prefer stories with pictures. Also, audiovisual presentations are rated as more enjoyable and interesting if accompanied by pictures when providing health information to children.

Pictures are not a necessity in order for information to be effective. Written information complementing verbal health information can also result in enormous benefits. This was exemplified by McDonald *et al.* (2004) who found that patients who were attending surgery for hip and knee replacement surgery were less anxious if they received written information in addition to verbal health information than patients who had verbal information alone. The findings have been further supported by studies that have shown written information decreases anxiety among advanced cancer patients (Gaston and Mitchell, 2005).

Written information is not beneficial for all patients, however, for example, patients who have an intellectual disability. Strydom and Hall (2001) tested a specially designed information leaflet intended to improve the knowledge of psychotropic medication in patients with intellectual disability. Fifty-four patients were recruited and received either verbal medication information from a nurse or psychiatrist, or verbal information plus an information leaflet. It was found that medication knowledge and understanding in patients was significantly lower in the intervention group (the group that received both verbal and written information). The researchers noted that leaflets could confuse patients who have a cognitive disability.

	Text plus cartoons (%)	Text alone (%)
Table 5.1 Effects of text alone versus text plus cartoons on patient attention, recall and adherence		
Read instructions (attention)	98	79
Answered all four wound care instructions correctly (recall)[a]	46	6
Adherence to wound care instructions[a]	77	54
Less than high school education: adherence to wound care instructions[a]	82	45

N = 234.

[a] analysis only included patients who read instructions.

Source: adapted from Delp and Jones (1996).

Short-term memory

Short-term memory is the second store within Atkinson and Shiffrin's (1968) three-stage memory store model. It is also referred to as **primary memory** (Waugh and Norman, 1960). The short-term memory store consists of information that we have received from the sensory registers. This store has two primary tasks: to store new information briefly and to work on that information. An analogy of short-term memory is of a working desk where information is either discarded (decay), stored or worked on (where material is attended to and revisited frequently). Hence, short-term memory is also referred to as the **working memory** (Baddley and Hitch, 1974).

Capacity of short-term memory

How long material lasts in short-term memory is dependent on what you do with the information. Working on information within this store increases the likelihood of it being retained. The capacity of the short-term memory is limited to a range of between five and nine pieces of information or material that have been attended to (e.g. listened to or read) at any one time. This can be vastly increased with a technique referred to as **chunking** (Miller, 1956).

Miller explained the technique of chunking with the phrase 'the **magical number seven plus or minus two**'. The technique of chunking enables more information to be taken into the short-term memory store and increases the likelihood of information being remembered. If a person was asked to have a look at the numbers below for a couple of minutes and then recall them, an average recall would be five to nine digits.

4	5	6	6
6	9	1	1
1	0	1	0
1	1	9	9
3	2	9	0
1	1	9	4

However, if the digits were grouped together into 'chunks' and have meaning attributed to them, recall would be better.

1914   WW1
1903   First flight by the Wright brothers
1066   Battle of Hastings
1969   Neil Armstrong is first man on the moon
1945   Beginning of the NHS

Chunking numbers into something that is meaningful means that more information is remembered, despite still working within the capacity of short-term memory.

Applying chunking

By using the principle of chunking, patients' recall of health information and instructions can be far superior to that of patients not using chunking. When chunking information it is important to take into consideration that patients are more likely to remember the first thing that has been stated, which is referred to as the **primacy effect**, and the last thing that has been said, the **recency effect**. Nurses should therefore attempt to provide the most important information chunk at the beginning and end of information-giving sessions.

A nurse can chunk a verbal consultation by breaking up information with open questions (see Chapter 17). This will also ensure that the patient understands the previous chunk of information. Another advantage is that breaking information into chunks with questioning will enable the nurse to clarify information that the patient may not have understood. In addition, this further supports the patient-centred model and encourages patient empowerment (see Chapter 3).

Think about this

Health promotion leaflets are an example of chunking that is used within written material. The paragraphs and subheadings break the text into chunks of information.

Rehearsal of information

Information lasts only up to a few seconds within the short-term memory store, unless it is worked on. Information can be held for a longer period of time using the method of **rote rehearsal** (also called maintenance rehearsal) (Greene, 1987). This technique simply involves repeating information over and over again out loud. This technique is very useful where the information is complex or new to a patient. One way of applying this technique is to ask the patient to repeat what has been said as well as referring back to the important information throughout the verbal exchange.

Audiotaping a consultation is one way to increase the likelihood that a patient will rehearse information and in turn recall health advice and instructions, especially within an emotional context. The benefit of taping a consultation is two-fold: the audiotape can be played back when the patient is more accepting of their diagnosis and it also acts as a method of information rehearsal .

On average 80 per cent of patients who listened to an audiotape of their medical consultation rated it as useful or very useful (Thomas *et al.*, 2000). There are many other benefits of audiotaping a consultation. These include increasing patient satisfaction with treatment (Bruera *et al.*, 1999), reducing anxiety and depression (Thomas *et al.*, 2000), increasing patient–practitioner partnership (Schapira *et al.*, 1997), increased patient recall (Scott *et al.*, 2006) and helping patients share information about their medical condition with people in their support network (Ong *et al.*, 2000). It has also been found by numerous studies that any misunderstandings or distractions, such as anxiety, which detract from the recall of information, can be reduced with audiotapes of the consultation that can be taken home and can be heard again (see Research in focus box below for the advantages and disadvantages of audio-taping consultations). The community mental health nurse could have taped the cognitive behavioural framework session, which would have helped Stewart when working within this framework later on by himself.

Research in focus

Liddell, C., Rae, G., Brown, T.R.M., Johnston, D., Coates, V. and Mallett, J. (2004) Giving patients an audiotape of their GP consultation: a randomised controlled trial. *British Journal of General Practice*, **54**, 667–672.

Background
Providing patients with an audiotape of their medical consultation has been a relatively common practice in oncology clinics for some years. However, broader generalisability of the technique has yet to be examined.

Aims
To investigate the efficacy of providing patients with an audiotape of their consultation in a general practice setting.

Design of study
Randomised controlled trial: 95 experimental participants, 85 controls.

Setting
Routine surgeries run by two general practitioners (GPs) in two different health centres.

Method
All participants attending GP appointments were eligible for inclusion. Patients were followed up by telephone 7–10 days later.

Results
More than half (61 per cent) of the patients who received a tape listened to it. Among listeners, 64 per cent rated the tape useful or very useful. Twenty-four per cent noticed information not heard in the consultation. Half of the listeners (46 per cent) said that their understanding of the consultation improved after listening to the tape. Half of the listeners (48 per cent) shared the tape with others, of whom 71 per cent found sharing helpful or very helpful. However, 21 per cent of those who shared the information with others found this unhelpful or very unhelpful, suggesting that patients may need to be briefed on the potential risks of sharing. At follow-up a week later, it emerged that being given a tape had no effect on adherence with GP's advice, nor on anxiety about conditions.

Conclusion
Providing patients with an audiotape of their GP consultation was positively rated by many patients. Although there were no detectable clinical effects at follow-up, the technique merits further evaluation in general practice.

Encoding and interference

Verbal information is encoded phonologically (by sounds) for storage within the short-term memory store (Baddeley, 1986). Similar-sounding information can result in confusion when recalling (Sperling, 1960). Recommendations for the gold standard of how health information shoud be given states that information should be 'brief, simple education, linked to patients' goals' (BTS and SIGN, 2003).

Researchers have suggested that information needs to be conveyed in a clear way and that complex medical jargon should be avoided (Carthey, 2006) to prevent patient confusion. According to Gibson *et al.* (2002), patients tend not to understand information because either it is too complex or they cannot read it. Gibson also highlighted another reason why patients may not be able to recall information and, in turn, change their health outcomes; patients may not appreciate the relevance of information to their situation or not realise the link between two pieces of information, e.g. smoking and high blood pressure.

Simplification of information also includes clarification of preliminary points such as an appreciation of bodily functions in relation to the illness rather than just the illness alone (Caress, 2003). Hence, attributing meaning to information is highly beneficial to the patient when understanding information. In the case study above, the community mental health nurse had a revised information-giving session with Stewart where his medication was discussed in a simple format and made relevant to his lifestyle.

The **levels of processing** model postulated by Craik and Lockhart (1972) further highlights the relationship between attributing meaning to information and the enhancement of recall of information. According to this model, the more elaboration that is sought for information, the deeper the understanding and increased recall. This is based on the **elaborative rehearsal** technique, whereby there is active processing of items within the short-term memory store in order to code information for the long-term memory store. Material may be processed in various ways, ranging from an emphasis on sensory characteristics (visual appearance, sound) to a focus on the **semantic** content (meaning of information).

Linking information back to a person can be one way of enhancing meaning, for example, by linking prescribed medication or proposed behaviour change to the person's everyday life. In addition to this, patients need to be given the opportunity to discuss their expectations and have questions answered. Kerrell (2001) recommended that parents of autistic children have ongoing support by referral to other appropriate bodies, as well as having expectations and questions dealt with by the nurse. This would result in more meaning being ascribed to the information provided rather than receiving information in isolation. In the case study above Stewart was clearly confused with his medication-taking, which may have been as a result of medications that were prescribed in isolation to one another.

Long-term memory

Long-term memory is the component of memory that retains information over relatively long periods of time (hours, days, weeks or longer). Information is transferred into long-term memory via methods such as rehearsal, attracting meaning and creation of links to information already held within long-term memory. During this process it possible for forgetting or confusion to occur, as previous information that the patient holds can interfere with the new information. Knowledge of interference is useful so that a nurse can ensure it does not occur.

There are two kinds of interference: **retroactive interference** and **proactive interference**. Retroactive interference happens when new material interferes with information already in long-term memory. This can occur on a day-to-day basis, e.g. remembering a new telephone number, only to find an old one cannot be recalled. Proactive interference occurs when information already in memory interferes with new information. In practice when providing new information, a concerted effort needs to be made with patients to establish their knowledge base and what they already know through the aid of questions. In the likelihood that information could be influenced by interference, acknowledgement of previous information and providing new information in light of this would be appropriate. This is what the community mental health nurse did with Stewart. She could see that his lack of adherence to medication was a result of medical instructions provided interfering with one another, which resulted in Stewart's being confused.

Glintborg *et al.* (2007) encourage health practitioners to discuss the use of prescription medication within the background of previous medication as well as the patient's interpretation of previous instructions. The nurse may only have the information that the patient provides about their previous or current medication. If this is the case and the nurse is unsure about the administration or medications that the patient should be taking in relation to 'other' illnesses, information should be sought from district nurses, general practitioners or pharmacist (Foss *et al.* 2004). This will ensure that present prescribing of medication advice is carried out in light of what the patient already has to reduce confusion.

Alteration of information over time is known as **displacement.** If it has been a while since the patient has taken medication, the nurse should ask the patient what they know from previous experience, and then relate new information to the existing information that the patient has.

Something that practitioners do not have control over is forgetting that is dependent on situational factors. Environmental cues can often act as an aid to remembering. This is known as **context-dependent learning.** For example, in a health-care setting, remembering would be related to hospital smells and setting. Nurse prescribers can aid the patient by attempting to link information to the home environment where they will be taking their medication. In addition to this, **state-dependent learning** is guided by internal cues. Remembering is enhanced by being in the same emotional state that occurred during learning. For most patients this would be heightened anxiety. This would work for patients who need to take medication before a certain anxiety episode. In comparison, for those patients whose state of ill health has to be managed over a long period of time, calming a patient and easing their anxiety before providing instructions is good practice.

Think about this

Health information may have been provided to Stewart previously when he was highly anxious or very unwell, which may have resulted in confusion when he had to recall the instructions. The community mental health nurse decided to revisit Stewart's medication instructions but not at the initial meeting, where anxiety could have been high. In wards where this is not possible, taking a few minutes to calm a patient before providing instructions will be highly beneficial to the adherence behaviour of the patient.

Schemata and faulty thinking

A **schema** is a mental script, which guides individuals and influences how they perceive and interpret events around them based on previous experiences. When we receive information, we locate it within a schema (Launder *et al.*, 2005). This saves time and energy through use of an already established knowledge base. However, information may not be correct or may be limited, which can result in **stereotyping** and faulty thinking (see Chapter 6 for social bias and stereotyping). Stereotyping is a cognitive framework whereby characteristics are attributed to an entire group of people (Cunningham, 1999).

Some nursing stereotypes from the media or previous experience with other health professionals could influence the way the patient interacts with the nurse. These stereotypes tend to be perpetuated by inferences made from nursing uniform (Alford *et al.*, 1995) (also see Chapter 6). According to Launder *et al.* (2005), this can cause problems when patients have pre-existing ideas about their medication and illness and are given new information. Moreover, information can be distorted to fit the present schema. The nurse should ensure that preconceived ideas and beliefs are explored fully with the patient before new information is provided, which also enhances patient-centred care. Price (2006) states that being patient-centred and sensitive is based on a rich understanding of the patient (see Chapter 3).

Techniques for improving the retention and recall of information

Mnemonic devices are a way of providing artificial links and meaning to meaningless information when learning or listening to new information. The more links made, the higher the probability that these will remain within the long-term memory store. See Table 5.2 and Figure 5.2 for examples.

Table 5.2
Mnemonic devices

Mnemonic principle	Definition	Example in practice
Elaboration and the keyword mnemonic	Converting names of drugs into meaningful words that sound similar or even making the words active	The more meaning that is attributed the more likely that this would be recalled
Association	Giving meaning to a word or name which then must be attached to something	Selecting a context with commonalities where possible: e.g. sleeping tablets placed by the bed, using visualisation, which reinforces the commonality with interaction
Link system	Associating things remembered with each other	Good to use with patients who have been diagnosed with a chronic illness and have to change their lifestyle. Link behaviour to everyday lifestyle (as shown in the case study above)
Story system	Advantage over the link system is that the flow of the story will allow the remainder of the list to be retrieved, whereas the link system will lose all the information if one link has been lost	A useful strategy to give to patients so that they can take it away with them
Loci system	Derived from a system within Ancient Greece, it is based on the principle of mentally positioning things to remember in a well-known room, e.g. making a speech looking at certain points in a room	Particular parts of the patient's house could be associated with medication-taking
Rhyming peg words	Rhyming meaningless words or numbers (see Figure 5.2) with established words	One is bun Two is shoe...

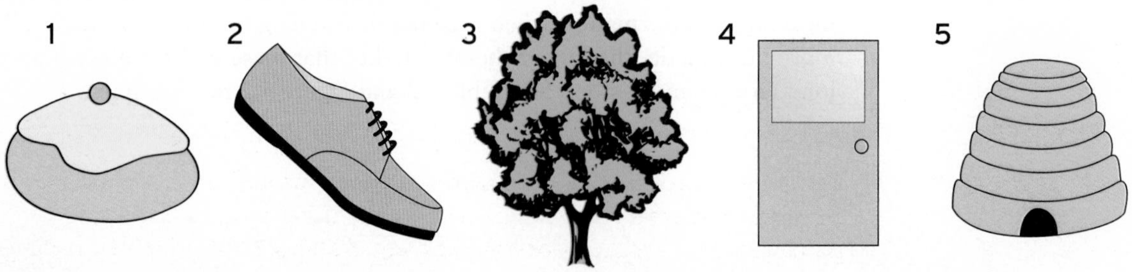

Figure 5.2 A child's chart of rhyming peg words, showing numbers up to five with names associated with them

Dementia

According to the 2001 census, there are 775 200 people who live with dementia in the Unied Kingdom, with a predicted increase to 870 000 by 2010 (Alzheimer's Society, 2004). Dementia tends to affect the elderly, with about 1 in 20 over 65 years of age having dementia. This increases to 1 in 3 over the age of 90 (Gow and Gilhooly, 2003). However, dementia also affects those who are not elderly; 18 000 people with dementia are under the age of 65 (Alzheimer's Society, 2004). As older people are primary users of health care (Victor *et al.*, 2000), and dementia can be as a result of particular illnesses such as Down's syndrome (Kerr, 1997), it is likely that all branches of nurses will at some time come in contact with patients who have dementia. Archibald (2003) suggests that nurses within acute care will have a number of patients with dementia to care for (see also Chapter 6).

Symptoms of dementia include the loss of recent memory (Cunningham, 2006) as well as other reduced cognitive abilities (Lowery *et al.*, 2000), which can result in the hospital experience being stressful and frightening for the patient. Nurses should be aware of the area of dementia and the psychosocial aspects of the condition, so that nursing care is sensitive to the needs of the patient (Cunningham and Archibald, 2006).

Patients with dementia tend to have a decreased ability to filter unwanted noise, which may lead to confusion (Harrington, 1998). A calm environment around the patient is recommended (Kerr, 1997). In a hospital environment within particular wards or at certain times a calm environment may not be possible. If this is the case, the nurse should make a concerted effort to keep the patient engaged. This can be facilitated by maintaining eye contact, referring to the patient's name throughout the interaction and keeping information simple and jargon-free. Consideration should also be taken of the environmental surroundings, as certain environmental factors, as well as the environment being unfamiliar to the patient, could result in the patient becoming confused, frightened or aggressive (Cunningham, 2006).

Nurses are limited as to the extent they can control the environment around the dementia patient. There are a number of steps a nurse can take however, such as keeping the routine and staff team around the patient much the same. If there is a new staff member, they need to be introduced to the patient. Constant reminders will also act as cues for dementia patients. For example, even though meals may have arrived, the patient will have to be told that it is time to eat, if they have not touched their food.

The Royal College of Psychiatry states that the following points can help reduce patient confusion (Timms, 2001):

- external aids;
- imagination;
- organisation;
- exercise the brain (dependent on the patient).

The consideration of environmental factors, which can contribute to the dementia patient's confusion, is even more important with the elderly and patients who have a **sensory impairment**. Pollock (2003) highlights simple things such as modern toilet signs (see picture) coupled with poor lighting that result in confusion and challenging behaviour.

Easy to get confused?

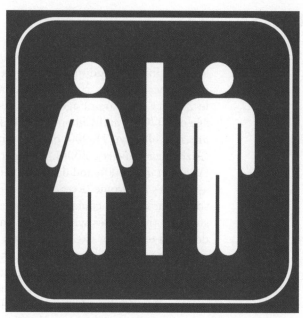

Watergate Creative/Alamy

Marshall (2005) suggests that personal belongings of the patient placed around the hospital bed can help prevent disorientation. Patients can be further helped by the compilation of a patient profile, which enlists what the patient is familiar with (Archibald, 2003). This will help nurses who may not know the dementia patient, as well as being helpful when talking to the patient about past experiences, which dementia patients do not have difficulty with.

Cunningham (2006) recommends that in order for nurses to successfully manage challenging behaviour, the nurse should be able to identify triggering factors to the behaviour, which can then be prevented from occurring in the future. The **ABC model** can be used as a tool to identify factors and prevent challenging behaviour occurring in the future (see section on cognitive behavioural therapy below). Stokes (2000) refers to a simple chart (see below) that should be filled in each time behaviour occurs that is challenging or causing distress. The chart will enable the nurse not only to identify triggering factors, but also to see possible patterns that may be emerging over time.

Dates	Antecedent	Behaviour	Consequence

Source: Stokes (2000)

Sensory impairment

Sensory impairment refers to the reduction or loss of one or more senses of a human being. Having a sensory impairment can be as a result of being born with an impairment. For the large majority of people however, sensory impairment stems from an illness that tends to be associated with increasing age (Kane, 1999). It has been estimated that within the United Kingdom there are 20 million registered blind or partially blind people, 90 per cent of which are 60 years of age or over (RNIB, 2002). This demonstrates the increasing probability of sensory impairment with advancing age. States of ill-health, such as suffering from a stroke or congestive heart failure are two examples that can result in sensory impairment.

Patients with sensory impairment may seek help for a range of health needs and states of ill health, which will result in care being sought from every branch of nursing. This is a topic with which every nurse needs to be familiar. Many surveys have been carried out exploring the communication between sensory impaired patients and nurses, with findings that do not make comfortable reading. For example, a national survey carried out by Hines (2000) found that the inability of hospital staff to communicate effectively with hearing impaired patients was a national problem.

Miller (2002) suggests that in order for nurses to communicate effectively with patients who have a sensory impairment they need to understand sensory loss. Chives (2003) found a difference between nurses who attended visual awareness programmes compared with those who did not, with the attendees having more positive interactions with and more effective clinical care of visually impaired patients.

If a patient has a sensory loss it does not necessarily mean that they have complete loss of that particular sense. For example, of those who are registered blind, very few will have total loss of vision. A large majority may retain some sort of visual function or reduced vision, although everyday life may still be difficult (Chives, 2003), especially since those who have recently had a sensory impairment will have large adjustments to make.

There can be a tendency for health professionals as well as carers to discourage independent functions that the sensory impaired patient can still perform. One researcher maintains from her own personal experience after having had a hearing (sensory) impairment that there were many changes in the way nurses (her colleagues) responded. She noted that, compared with the time when she did not have her hearing impairment, colleagues and people in general tended to talk to her in a patronising way, and individuals were more likely to talk at her as well as shout.

Fitzgerald and Parkes (1998) explain such a response as resulting from a sympathetic response. Reasons for a sympathetic response can stem from the nurse not knowing much about the sensory impairment. Fitzgerald and Parkes maintain that a nurse who takes time with the patient will tend to overcome this kind of response.

Taking time with a patient who has a sensory impairment will enable the nurse to encourage the strengths of the patient and work on weaknesses. For example, congestive heart patients who have undergone surgery and stroke treatment will tend to have reduced cognitive abilities compared with how they were before the state of ill health. Recognising this will firstly change the nurse's interaction with the patient and, secondly, means the patient can begin to work on these abilities so that they begin to feel in control rather than helpless.

Knox (1998) states that rehabilitation goals for sensory impaired patients are to motivate patients (refer to Chapter 3) and recognise their strengths and limitations so as to encourage the patient to regain control. In the opening case study the nurse took into account that as a result of severe depression, Stewart may need longer to process information that was provided.

Those patients who have recently had a sensory impairment will be experiencing loss and will, to some extent, be grieving about their loss. This resembles the reaction and grieving process that individuals have as a result of bereavement (refer to Chapter 11). Fitzgerald and Parkes (1998) exemplified this with their findings from a survey carried out with patients who were visually impaired. Fitzgerald found that patients tended to experience the following:

- all patients experienced shock and disbelief with common statements including 'this cannot be permanent';
- weeping was also common with all patients that were interviewed;
- 83 per cent of patients had a preoccupation with their visual past;
- 97 per cent of patients longed to see things that they previously could see;
- 70 per cent of the patient sample experienced high anxiety coupled with tearfulness frequently;
- all patients experienced anger at some point;
- 85 per cent of patients experienced depressive episodes after tearfulness;
- those experiencing depression reached the final stage of acceptance and resolution. These patients had high self-esteem and also self-sufficient behaviours in place.

Acknowledging that a patient with a recent sensory impairment may be experiencing any of the above will help the nurse to engage with the patient appropriately.

Cognitive behavioural therapy

Cognitive behavioural therapy (CBT) comprises both cognitive and behavioural principles. It was pioneered by Beck (1976) and Ellis (1994), who are both renowned figures within counselling and psychotherapy. The cognitive aspect concentrates on our thoughts, assumptions and beliefs, which the therapy challenges when they become maladaptive to the patient's well-being. The behavioural aspect concentrates on the change of behaviour.

Clinical psychologists, as well as other cognitive behavioural experts, tend to advocate cognitive behavioural therapy being used only by nurses who have undergone an accredited diploma in cognitive behavioural therapy (Oldham, 2007). However, nurses will often find they need to identify causative factors for particular behaviours and, here, frameworks within cognitive behavioural therapy are helpful for effective identification of such factors. Other proponents suggest that when a nurse works within a collaborative therapeutic relationship with the patient, this warrants the use of CBT skills (O'Brein, 2001).

Any situation or context where the patient has negative thoughts, hold beliefs or schemata that are irrational and maladaptive to their health and well-being requires the nurse to challenge such beliefs. CBT principles are recommended routinely with disorders and illnesses that encompass anxiety and depression (Curran *et al.*, 2006). CBT has been shown to be effective within mental health nursing with patients who have mild to moderate depression (NICE, 2004). More general examples of the application of CBT include patients experiencing post-traumatic stress, trauma or general distress (Child-Clarke, 2003). This exemplifies how CBT can be applied to many settings within which the nurse has an important role to play.

ABC model

The ABC model (Ellis, 1977) is a framework that nurses can work within when challenging a patient's beliefs, thought patterns, assumptions and inferences about themselves or events around them, which may impact negatively on their well-being. This model is from the **rational emotive** therapy strand of cognitive behavioural therapy. The model links to cognitive psychology as negative *schemata* of the patient are challenged. Schemata are the mental structures used to organise knowledge within long-term memory, which influences a person's intepretation of information and subsequent behaviour. Within the framework, the nurse will attempt to change the mental script of the patient so that new ways of thinking will result in a change in behaviour. The ABC model will allow the patient to explore the causative factors of their current thinking and think about the implications of their behaviour. As a result, alternative viewpoints that do not result in negative consequences the patient's health and well-being will be sought. The model works in the following way, where each letter represents a stage within the model.

- *A: Activating event or experience*: The patient, with the help of the nurse, could explore triggering factors in this initial stage, which impact upon the current behaviour. For example, Stewart may have held the belief that he was never going to get better. The nurse could explore where this belief stemmed from, e.g. past experience with depression or other illnesses, other people, situations that Stewart has been in, loss of control and low self-esteem.
- *B: Beliefs about the event*: Exploration of both irrational and possible rational beliefs. For example, the nurse helping Stewart could have explored statements such as: 'I could end up not getting better' (not a good belief), 'I need to get better so that I can feel better' (good belief).
- *C: Consequence:* Exploring the consequences of unhealthy negative emotions. For example, if Stewart continues to believe that he will not get better he will lead a lifestyle that will result in further deterioration of his mental and physical health.
- *D: Disputing:* Disputing, questioning or challenging irrational beliefs. The nurse will dispute the cognitive, emotional and behavioural aspects of the patient's current thinking. In Stewart's case the nurse could state to the patient that he could actual make steps in getting better.
- *E: new Effect:* Exploring the alternate rational belief and the implications on feelings (healthy) and behaviour (self-helping actions).
- *F: Further action:* acting against the irrational belief. For example, Stewart's becoming more active and adhering to medication resulted in his realising that it is not that hard and he can have control over his health.

This model does not necessarily have to be applied just within a mental health setting. Patients who have the following cognitive thought patterns will benefit from this framework:

- irrational thoughts and 'distortions of reality';
- black-and-white or all-or-nothing thinking;
- filtering;
- over-generalisation;
- emotional reasoning;
- faulty cognition;
- learned helplessness;
- hopelessness;
- no control.

Froggatt (2001) outlines the many benefits the patient can receive when the ABC model is used. Firstly, a patient will have their self-awareness raised regarding the link between their emotions and behaviour and their cognitions, such as beliefs and thinking, which they aim to be in control of. Secondly, the nurse can also demonstrate to the patient how beliefs can be uncovered, which will be beneficial for patients who may not see the link between their current irrational thought patterns and behaviour. Thirdly, the nurse can use this model to teach the patient how to challenge their irrational beliefs when they are not within professional health care, which acts as a vital coping strategy for patients. For example, the next time Stewart begins to feel low, he may be able to identify triggering factors and avoid them. Finally, getting a patient to act against their beliefs will result in their actually feeling the benefit and realising the impact their cognition or thinking patterns have on their behaviour.

Think about this

There are many diets on the market that people buy when they want or have been told to lose weight. The most successful diet programmes tend to be those that have cognitive behavioural therapy as part of the programme. Dieters will then have cognitive and behavioural strategies at their disposal when there is a likelihood of relapsing. The therapy also helps dieters who have an all-or-nothing mentality where the therapy helps the individual to realise that a relapse does not mean another failed diet attempt.

Perception and holistic care

Human beings use perception to make sense of what they see around them. The area of perception is useful for a nurse. There are basic principles within this area that can help nurses understand how interactions can be influenced by how individuals are perceived. The area also has theoretical underpinnings which can help the nurse to explore holistic care. Take a look at Figure 5.3. What can you see?

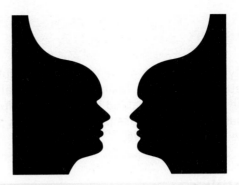

Figure 5.3 Perceptual illusion.

Making sense of what we see

The visual process that has taken place when you look at Figure 5.3 is referred to as the **top-down process**. According to **Gestalt psychologists**, the top-down approach is how perception works overall in that we strive to see things as a whole so that they are meaningful. The reverse to this is known as the **bottom-up process**, which is used in the visual process whereby receptors in the retina recognise shape and colour alone. When a visual stimulus has no meaning, we tend to make sense of the object by seeing the picture as a whole, with the help of previous learning and experiences. In the words of the Gestalt psychologist Max Wertheimer (1880–1943), the whole is greater than the sum of its parts.

The process by which we structure the input from sensory receptors is based on an overarching principle of **perceptual organisation** (Baron, 2001). Perceptual organisation allows us to perceive shapes and forms from incomplete and fragmented stimuli. As human beings we strive to have consistency, by filling in gaps. Table 5.3 gives examples of laws that exist within perceptual organisation and how they relate to holistic care.

Table 5.3
Laws of perceptual grouping

Laws of similarity	Tendency to perceive similar items as a group	The community mental health nurse could have put together an ineffective care plan had she based it on the diagnostic label of depression alone. This can lead to stereotyping with no room for individuality of the patient.
Laws of closure	Tendency to perceive objects as whole entities despite the fact that some parts may be missing or obstructed from view	Assessing Stewart on the basis of what he presented to the community mental health nurse alone rather than probing the patient further.
Laws of figure and ground	Tendency to look at the obvious figure	A patient with challenging behaviour may be labelled as disruptive. However, when the triggering factor has been identified, the patient may be distressed rather than disruptive.
Laws of simplicity	Tendency to perceive complete pattern in terms of simpler shapes	Providing health information in a simplistic format.

Think about this

The community mental health nurse used the principle of figure and ground when putting the care plan together for Stewart. Taking into consideration Stewart's current lifestyle, history of medication and perspective enabled the nurse to help Stewart in the most effective way possible. Had the nurse based the care plan on Stewart's presented symptoms alone the care plan would not have been as effective.

Problem-solving

Problem-solving is relevant to the day-to-day practice of the nurse who will encounter many problem situations and will have to attempt to find solutions. Researchers have stressed the importance of problem solving in caring for patients (Price, 2003). An example of problem-solving as part of the caring relationship can be seen in the opening case study where the community mental health nurse had to reach an end goal of reducing the severity of Stewart's symptoms of depression.

Problems can be solved either from an **algorithm** problem-solving approach or a **heuristic** approach. Algorithms tend to be used when there is an obvious end goal and where the same rule can be applied. For example, multiplication of numbers has the same rules that do not change. The problem is that in many situations, the nurse is confronted with problems that tend not to have straightforward solutions, which warrants the use of heuristic problem-solving strategies. Schmieding (1999) suggests that a problem that at first may seem to have an obvious solution tends to require complicated thought processes. For example, in the case study above, the treatment of Stewart's depression were not as simple as treating his symptoms with medication. Stewart was clearly confused about his medication instructions as well as his negative state of mind. Table 5.4 gives examples of heuristic strategies that can be used by nurses when helping patients as well as by the student nurse when attempting to understand a problematic scenario.

According to Taylor (1997) understanding problems can be aided by group discussion. Price (2003) further supports this by recommending that understanding a problem is enabled when a number of different practitioners combine their styles (see Chapter 4 for multi-disciplinary team work). This flexible approach is also important when using the strategies above, as one approach should not be used as a rule of thumb for every scenario. These strategies are effective when used in a flexible and creative manner that meets the unique needs of each problem.

Conclusion

Effective patient-led management of illness, following health instructions/advice or the patient attempting to enhance their health and well-being are all, to an extent, dependent on how well the patient can recall information. Cognitive psychology unravels the variables that influence retention and recall of information, as well as how the nurse can provide effective

Table 5.4
Heuristic strategies

Heuristic problem-solving strategy	Application in practice
Trial and error: systematically eliminate possible solutions until the correct or workable one is found. Is the least effective and most time consuming.	Can be effective for patients who are not anxious and have resources available to them, e.g. the patient's having control over the elimination of particular foods when attempting to identify trigger factors for their migraine.
Hill climbing: a directed approach where you begin at the bottom of the hill and steadily work towards the solution while re-evaluating each step. Only workable when the nurse attends to the patient on a regular basis.	The community mental health nurse in the opening case study would have set strategies for Stewart to try as part of the ABC model. The patient would then feed back to the nurse about how he felt and whether it was achievable.
Sub goals: breaking a problem into smaller more manageable pieces.	The community mental health nurse took the approach of tackling each problem individually rather than tackling everything together.
Working backwards: work backwards from the problem. Can be a good starting point and has the advantage of not straying away from the problem and the end goal itself.	The community mental health nurse could have used this strategy to begin with when putting together the care plan for Stewart. This would have guided the nurse by working backwards from the presented symptoms.

information-giving. By taking such variables into account, the nurse is not only able to enhance the probability of patient wellness or effective illness management, but also to become more dynamic and effective in their information-giving.

Communication in the hospital as seen in this and other chapters is problematic within the surroundings of the health care environment combined with the heightened anxiety of the patient. Coupled with this, nurses may have to communicate and care for patients with a sensory deprivation that they may have had prior to the current treatment or that has stemmed from their current state of health or medical intervention. Being aware of what can confuse a patient with a sensory deprivation will ensure that the nurse is being active in making information as simple as possible and decreasing the anxiety of the patient.

Problem-solving is something that both patient and nurse will engage in on a day-to-day basis. Being aware of possible problem-solving strategies will help both the nurse and the patient to make plans that are more effective in reaching end goals.

Summary

- Atkinson and Shiffrin (1968) put forward the three-stage multi-store memory model to explain how memory works, which consists of sensory memory, short-term memory and long-term memory.

- According to Broadbent (1958), stimuli that meet certain requirements during the sensory memory stage are more likely to be processed within memory while other material is filtered out.

- Miller (1956) described the principle of chunking, which refers to the process of converting meaningless information into meaningful units, which increases the capacity of short-term memory.

- Rehearsal, mnemonic techniques and elaboration enhance memory.

- Retroactive and proactive interference can cause confusion to the patient when new information contradicts existing beliefs and experiences. Cognitive schemata, which are referred to as mental scripts, can also act as barriers to new health information.

- The law of perceptual organisation results in individuals making sense of what they can perceive with the help of their existing knowledge and experience which can overlook the details of new material.

- Caring for sensory impaired patients gives rise to a number of considerations, these being the dependency versus independence argument as well as the grieving process that the patient has to go through when accepting the loss or reduction of the functionality of one or more senses.

- Dementia patients will have their day-to-day memory affected. Tailoring communication and addressing needs accordingly is a necessity, which will ease the confusion and anxiety of the patient.

- The ABC model (Antecedents, Behaviour, Consequence) originates from the perspective of cognitive behavioural therapy/rational emotive therapy, which is the framework to help identify trigger factors to present behaviour.

- Heuristics are strategies within problem-solving used to solve problems that do not have an obvious answer. Strategies include: trial and error, hill climbing, means-end analysis and working backwards.

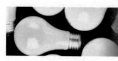

Check your understanding

1. Atkinson and Shiffrin (1968) put forward the three stage-memory model. Describe the three memory stores and how forgetting can occur at each stage.

2. Describe the two types of interference and explain three strategies a nurse can implement to prevent patients becoming confused or forgetting information.

3. Name three patient variables that need to be taken into consideration when providing written material.

4. List four types of problem-solving strategy that fall under the term heuristics.

5. Describe the ABC model and how this can be used in practice.

6. List five factors that a nurse needs to take into consideration when caring for a patient who has a sensory impairment.

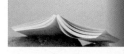

Further reading

Caress, A.L. (2003) Giving information to patients. *Nursing Standard*, **17** (43), 47–54.

Curran, J., Machin, C. and Gournay, K. (2006) Cognitive behaviour therapy for patients with anxiety and depression. *Nursing Standard*, **21** (7), 44–52.

Houts, P.S., Doak, C.C., Doak, L.G. and Loscaizo, M.J. (2005) The role of pictures in improving health communication: a review of research on attention, comprehension, recall and adherence. *Patient Education and Counselling*, **61** (2), 173–190.

Kools, M. (2006) A focus on the usability of health education material. *Patient Education and Counselling*, **65** (3), 275–276.

Nickiln, J. (2002) Improving the quality of written information for patients. *Nursing Standard*, **16** (4), 39–44.

Weblinks

Encyclopedia of Psychology	http://www.psychology.org/links/ Environment_Behavior_Relationships/Memory/	An array of weblinks to cognitive psychology and specifically to memory literature
The Magical Number Seven, Plus or Minus Two: Some Limits on Our Capacity for Processing Information by George A. Miller	http://www.well.com/user/smalin/miller.html	This site is dedicated to the work of George Miller's work on chunking. His original article can be found here
NeuroMod. Online Memory Improvement Course	http://memory.uva.nl/memimprovement/eng/	Online memory improvement course which has an in-depth look at mnemonic techniques
Wadsworth. Cognitive Laboratory 2.0	http://coglab.wadsworth.com/	Various experiments and demonstrations. You need to register before viewing the material
Illusions Gallery, University of Massachusetts Lowell. David T. Landrigan	http://dragon.uml.edu/psych/illusion.html	Examples of perceptual organisation illustrated by many examples of illusions
AAFP: Family Practice Management	http://www.aafp.org/fpm	Looking at effective health practitioner and patient communication

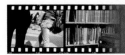

Media examples

Hear No Evil See No Evil A film that takes a humorous look at how people have to function in extreme cases with a sensory deprivation.

Finding Nemo A cartoon portrayal of a fish that has a three-second memory span.

Chapter 6

Social psychology

Learning outcomes

When you have read through this chapter you should understand:

- The processes that are involved in inter-group behaviour when working as part of an inter-disciplinary team.
- What makes the nurse an effective team member.
- How the perception of nurses' and patients' self has an impact on behavioural and health outcomes.
- How assertiveness can be used within a professional relationship.
- The importance of self-awareness and reflection for improving nursing practice.
- How nurses can avoid stereotyping and labelling patients.
- How a nurse can initiate attitude change and use persuasion within a professional relationship.
- How to help a patient who may appear aggressive.

Case study

Ava Richards is a 32-year-old patient who has been admitted to hospital after collapsing. The health care team have carried out routine blood tests and found that Ava is pregnant. She has also been found to be severely anaemic and suffering from exhaustion. While taking Ava's medical history, it was revealed that she was diagnosed with the HIV virus four years ago. The consultant has decided that Ava will need to stay in hospital until her immune system strengthens. She becomes frustrated and angry.

Nigel Tackett is a nurse on the ward who has been in frequent contact with Ava. This is Nigel's first post since qualifying as a registered nurse. He has been working for two weeks.

Two weeks later and the multi-disciplinary team have arranged a meeting to discuss whether Ava is ready to be discharged. The multi-disciplinary team consists of Nigel, Nigel's mentor, who is the senior staff nurse on the ward, the consultant, a social worker and community nurse. The consultant informs the team that he is happy to discharge the patient. He asks the rest of the team if there are any concerns; there is a general consensus that Ava can be discharged.

Nigel feels that a couple of points still need to be addressed before Ava can be discharged. The patient is adamant that she does not want her partner to know about her HIV status, which Nigel thinks could cause problems. Nigel is also concerned about Ava's pregnancy, as her partner is overjoyed but Ava wants to terminate the pregnancy. As a result, Nigel is concerned about Ava's future state of health, as there are particular issues that still need to be addressed by a counsellor or other support groups. Despite the concerns Nigel has, he does not voice them during the meeting. Reflecting on the meeting, Nigel wishes he had commented on the issues he felt needed addressing. Over the next couple of weeks, Nigel's guilt about not expressing his concerns increases. Nigel has begun to be preoccupied by the same thought patterns on a daily basis. This has resulted in his beginning to lose confidence when communicating with patients and other members of the ward team.

Nigel's mentor has noticed the difference in Nigel's behaviour. She has noted many absences in team meetings and she decides to talk to Nigel. It is apparent from the interaction with Nigel that he has lost enormous amounts of confidence and will just agree with the senior staff nurse's comments. With persuasion, Nigel confides in his mentor and explains the situation surrounding Ava and how he wished he had expressed his concerns during the team meeting. The nurse reassures Nigel that it is not uncommon for newly qualified staff to feel uneasy when expressing their concerns within a team setting. However, the nurse wishes that Nigel had spoken to her much sooner so that he was not preoccupied with negative thoughts that affected his work and personal life. The nurse encourages Nigel to attend future team meetings and assures him that his contribution will be valued. In addition to this, the nurse reassures Nigel that she will contact Ava's GP and discuss the possibility of arrangements being made for a community nurse who specialises in HIV/AIDS care to visit Ava.

The nurse ends the meeting by suggesting to Nigel that he takes ten minutes away from the ward to reflect on this particular incident and how he dealt with it. The nurse insists that Nigel should speak to her tomorrow with any thoughts so that they can move forward and begin to restore Nigel's confidence as a nurse.

The following day both Nigel and the senior staff nurse conclude that Nigel has to work on his assertiveness skills. The senior staff nurse decides to send Nigel to a two-hour assertiveness skills workshop. In addition to this, the senior staff nurse reassures Nigel that Ava's GP has arranged an appointment with Ava so that they can monitor her current state of health and how she is coping with her situation. The senior staff nurse is also impressed with the reflective cycle tool that Nigel has used when looking back at the situation. Nigel comes to the realisation that, irrespective of not having much experience, his contribution is seen as valuable, which has now enhanced his confidence.

Why is this relevant to nursing practice?

This case study highlights the possible dynamics that can occur when a nurse holding a new post begins to work in practice within multi-disciplinary teams. A nurse beginning a new post or placement may meet many obstacles. The first obstacle that was apparent in the case study above was Nigel's lack of contribution to the multi-disciplinary team meeting. Working as part of a multi-disciplinary team involves many group dynamics; differing perspectives as well as communication skills need to be taken into account. Group dynamics and teamwork constitute an area that social psychologists explore and that will be considered within this chapter.

Another theme that is documented within the case study is assertiveness. Nurse Nigel was not assertive within the team meeting. A nurse needs to know how to assert themselves so that they can communicate information to colleagues as well as patients.

It was apparent from this case study that Nigel began to feel guilty and wished he had approached the incident in a different way. Not expressing his views during the team meeting resulted in his losing confidence, which began to affect his day-to-day behaviour at work. The area of self-perception, social perception and self-esteem will be explored, since confidence is required not only in meetings but also when carrying out day-to-day duties with patients.

The senior staff nurse encouraged Nigel to reflect on the incident and see what he could learn from the experience. Reflection is important when a nurse is developing within their profession, but just asking a nurse to reflect will not ensure a good reflection process. This chapter will consider some useful reflection tools, as well as self-awareness, that are important when being objective about your own experience and useful for nurse portfolios.

Dealing with patients who may have particular states of ill-health can result in different attitudes that can be held by family members and the health care team. In the above case study, it was clear that Ava was afraid of informing her partner about her current HIV status because of the stigma attached to HIV and AIDS, especially regarding expectant mothers. The area of stigma and, in particular, attitudes and stereotyping, will be looked at in this chapter. Nigel himself did not have a problem or hold any judgements about Ava. However, a nurse in a similar situation may have questions that they may ask themselves which could influence the care that they provide. For example, is Ava selfish for not telling her partner? Is she an awful person? Such questions can easily result in bias within the care that is provided and the label can become permanent with many members of the team, which clearly did not occur in the case study above. Work regarding the '**unpopular patient**' explores attributions or explanations that health care staff make about patients based on behaviour observed in the hospital, labels given and their implications. All of this will be explored in this chapter.

Social psychology

Social psychology has been defined as 'the scientific investigation of how the thoughts, feelings and behaviour are influenced by the actual, imagined or implied presence of others' (Allport, 1935). Research within this area is based on behaviours that are observable. When exploring behaviour that is not directly observable (such as attitudes), social psychologists believe that some can be inferred through observable behaviour.

What makes social psychology *social* is that it deals with how people are affected by others who are physically present or who are imagined to be present. In the case study above, Nigel's behaviour (lack of expression) and conformity to the general consensus that the patient should be discharged was influenced by the presence of the multi-disciplinary team. Topics within social psychology, such as group dynamics, the influence of groups on individual behaviour and conformity within groups, will be considered.

Think about this

Would Nigel have expressed himself differently had there been only himself and the senior staff nurse within the meeting? Would this have differed had the meeting consisted of the same individuals but Nigel had worked there for several years? The actual or implied presence of others has the potential to strongly influence our behaviour. How true is this?

In the case study above, nurse Nigel began to lack confidence (or **self-esteem**) as a result of his experience during the team meeting. The theme of self-esteem links with several other areas, such as perception of the **self** and **social perception** (how you think others perceive you). This area is important for student nurses to take into consideration as being placed within a new area can bring many uncertainties in relation to how competent the individual is, which can affect the self-esteem of a training nurse. At the same time, patients with a particular diagnosis or undergoing treatment will also experience uncertainty, which will affect their self-esteem. Being familiar with strategies that have been used to enhance self-esteem will be highly beneficial for nurses.

Linked to self-esteem is the area of **self-awareness** and **reflection**. Nigel reflected on his experience with the use of a reflective tool. This involves assessing oneself objectively and learning from previous incidents so that future practice can be improved. It is vital that nurses learn from both previous negative and positive incidents and learn from such experiences. This chapter will highlight the reflective frameworks and self-awareness tools that are available.

Another area within social psychology is **attribution theory**. It is part of human nature to attribute an explanation for the behaviour of an individual. This can have negative implications when an explanation for a patient's behaviour is incorrect. The implications that stem from attributions are **stereotyping** and **labelling**, which a nurse should be familiar with so that they are not distracted from the individualised care that they strive to provide.

Nigel thought that his lack of expression within the team meeting was noted by the team, which gave rise to his questioning his competency as a nurse. Those who are new to the profession of nursing may not know how to assert themselves without offending colleagues. The area of professional **assertiveness** will be explored, which will enable the training nurse to assert themselves correctly and confidently within their work.

Groups

A group can be defined as:

> two or more individuals in face-to-face interaction, each aware of his or her membership in the group, each aware of the others who belong to the group, and each aware of their positive interdependence as they strive to achieve mutual goals (Johnson and Johnson, 1987, p. 8).

In the case study above, Nigel did not contribute to the multi-disciplinary team meeting. Effective teamwork is important to ensure that the patient is given the most appropriate care and treatment that is available. As a result of Nigel's silence, certain areas in Ava's case went untreated.

The benefits of effective teamwork are sizeable. Effective teamwork can contribute to:

> reduced hospitalisation time and cost, increased patient safety, improved patient health and innovations in patient care as well as enhanced staff motivation and wellbeing (Borrill and West, 2002, cited in RCN, 2006).

By becoming familiar with how an individual is influenced by groups as well as principles that are recommended to enhance group work, a nurse can begin to become aware of their conduct within a group environment and will be able to follow the steps to becoming an effective team member.

Presence of others: does it improve or impair behaviour?

The effect of others on behaviour was the subject of the first study carried out in social psychology by Norman Triplett in 1898. Triplett observed people cycling and found that people cycled faster when surrounded by other cyclists than when cycling alone. This was later referred to by Allport (1920) as **social facilitation**, which refers to an improvement in performance resulting from the mere presence of individuals or a passive audience. On the other hand, just as behaviour can be improved by the presence of others, behaviour can also deteriorate, which is referred to as **social inhibition**.

According to Zajonc (1965), social facilitation (better performance) is more likely to occur when a task is easy or has been rehearsed many times. In contrast to this, social inhibition is more likely to occur when a task is not easy or well learned. During the latter, impaired performance occurs, as you are more likely to think about making a mistake. In the case study above Nigel was in a new team and it was the first time he had participated in a multi-disciplinary group, which resulted in his behaviour (expressing himself) being impaired. The presence of other, more established members of the groups resulted in social inhibition of Nigel's behaviour, which affected his confidence to speak within the meeting (refer to self-esteem section later in this chapter).

Think about this

If Nigel was involved in a similar multi-disciplinary group meeting but had been working within his post for three years, would the outcome have differed? What would be more apparent – social inhibition or social facilitation as a result of other members of the group being present on Nigel voicing his concerns?

Group socialisation

Any effective working group will go through a developmental sequence, which Tuckman (1965) described in his five-stage developmental sequence (Table 6.1). According to Major (2002), the most obvious flaw that

Table 6.1
Tuckman's five-stage developmental sequence

Developmental stage?	Aim of stage	What happens during this stage
Forming	To negotiate a shared framework of expectations and objectives. Referred to as the familiarisation stage.	Debate and identify common goals. Discuss ground rules and shared expectations. Address whether external challenges are being met. New members are integrated and team dynamics negotiated if necessary.
Storming	To identify discrepancies and understand 'self' (can be thought about individually, then brought to the team). Members know each other well enough to start working out disagreements and discrepancies.	Discuss how different professional disciplines will be acknowledged. Explore expectations of self and that of the team. Will expectations hinder or further progress the team's objectives? Work through disagreements about goals and practices.
Norming	To develop affiliation and openness. Having worked through the disagreements, cohesion, consensus and a common sense of identity and purpose emerge.	Cohesion, common identity and purpose emerge. Team accepts each member's role. Team prepared to take responsibility.
Performing	To fully function. Group works smoothly as a unit with shared norms and goals and good morale and atmosphere.	Group works as a unit sharing the same norms and goals. Energy directed towards problem-solving tasks. Monitor and evaluate ongoing work.
Adjourning	The group dissolves because it has accomplished its goals, or because members lose interest and motivation and move on.	Once goals have been met the group can disperse.

Source: Tuckman (1965)

contributes to ineffective teamwork within health care is when the forming stage of Tuckman's (1965) developmental model has not occurred. This was evident in the case study as Nigel was not present during the initial team meetings. Nigel's possible contribution to the team was further hampered, as the senior staff nurse did not brief Nigel. Major also suggests that communication barriers, such as withholding information, can result in a 'them and us' scenario. This was evident in the case study above, where Nigel felt that he could not openly discuss his concerns with a team who were already established in terms of their agenda for Ava.

Working in a multi-disciplinary team

Multi-disciplinary teamwork is essential to successful care and the answer to workforce pressures (Naish, 2004). According to the Royal College of Nursing, effective teamwork is essential to delivering patient-centred care, which forms one of the five visions of the future nurse (Naish, 2004). Multi-disciplinary teamwork has also been implicated as being crucial to patient care and outcomes (Smith, 1998, p. 115).

There are different types of multi-disciplinary teams. To begin with there are integrated nursing teams, which have been defined as:

> a team of community based nurses from different disciplines, working together within a primary care setting, pooling their skills, knowledge and abilities to provide the most effective patient care within a practice and the community it covers. (HVA, 1996)

Integrated nursing teams include nurses working within adult, child, mental health, learning disability, public health and specialising within specific areas. In addition to this, an integrated nursing team could also include health care assistants and auxiliary nurses as well as health visitors, school nurses, family

A multi-disciplinary hospital team.

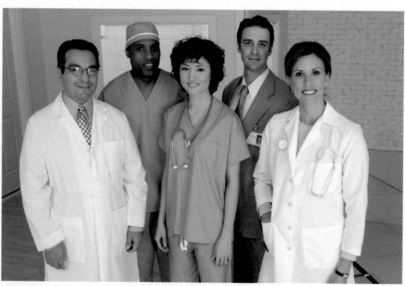

© Comstock/Corbis

health nurses and those for whom public health activities constitute a major part of their role (Flying Start, NHS, 2007).

Other allied health professionals that a nurse could work with on a multi-disciplinary team come from disciplines such as occupational therapy, speech and language therapy, physiotherapy, podiatry, art therapy, dietetics, orthotics, orthoptics and diagnostic and therapeutic radiography. Other team members could include doctors, support staff, administrators, managers, social workers, voluntary agencies, pharmacists and student nurses. It is important for a newly qualified nurse to be familiar with the other disciplines. For example, Nigel could research the other team members' roles.

Communication among differing team members is paramount and the key to effective teamwork (Webster, 2002). In expanding organisations where technology is growing in importance, and departments are merging into larger sections, it is important for a nurse to be aware of and monitor their communication with others.

Media reports have clearly highlighted what can go wrong when communication within multi-disciplinary working relationships is not effective or closely monitored. This was seen in the media coverage of the Bristol Royal Infirmary Inquiry (2001), where there was an investigation of the high mortality rates in a paediatric surgical unit. The inquiry was set up in 1998 investigating the period between 1984 and 1995. It was identified that communication was strained among differing health disciplines. The report encouraged more open communication between health professionals, NHS management, patients and the public.

Research carried out with nurses working as part of a multi-disciplinary team has found effective communication to be key to effective teamwork and decreasing the probability of mistakes being made. For example, Nestel and Kidd (2006) explored nurses' perceptions and experiences of communication in the operating theatre. They found that nurses felt a lot of frustration with the inadequate communication that took place between the surgeon and the nurse. The study concluded that documentation as well as active listening was essential to effective teamwork, which was largely absent.

In the case study above, written information was largely absent, which resulted in confusion as to what the team had discussed previously. In addition to this, Nigel was asked if he had any concerns but there was no elaboration or invitation for comments to be made, which is important if **two-way communication** is to occur (see Chapter 17). Even though Nigel had much to say about Ava as a result of his frequent contact with the patient, he was unable to express this because of the situation he was in. Nurses play a vital role in the continuity of patient care, are more emotionally involved and more in touch with the day-to-day needs of the patient. However, they may not voice this when in meetings (Coombs and Ersser, 2004). The researchers suggest that nurses need to voice their concerns through being honest and open within meetings.

By acknowledging barriers that can exist when working as part of a multi-disciplinary team, the manager of the team, as well as team members such as nurses, can prevent them from occurring. Webster (2002) highlights the following factors that can act as barriers to multi-professional working:

● Dominance by any one profession can be seen as producing a professional hierarchy, which is counter-productive to teamwork.

- 'Tribalism' refers to individual practitioners who are over-protective of their roles and responsibilities for service provision.
- 'Playing the game', whereby the nurse or other professions will put across their perspective in such a way that a doctor can dress it up as their own.
- Difficult to work with conflict situations, e.g. enforced hierarchies or role dominance.

Think about this

Which figure was completely dominant during the meeting in the opening case study? Did this result in lack of open discussion about Ava? Did tribalism exist among the team when discussing Ava during the discharge meeting?

Role clarity is another ingredient for effective teamwork, especially when teams comprise members from several differing health disciplines. According to Whyte (2007) confusion of roles can result in individual members questioning how they fit in, which can result in the individual team member being undervalued. Secondly, resentfulness can set in when there is a dominance of one profession over others. Health care practice is now moving away from traditional professional hierarchies to a model where nurses work 'together' rather than alongside one another to achieve effective multi-disciplinary teamwork (Lewis and Allen, 2003).

In the case study above, Nigel was confused by what each member of the team contributed to the discussion, as he was not briefed in advance. As a result of not knowing what perspective each team member represented, Nigel may have undervalued his own possible contribution as a new member of the team. In addition to this, there was a lack of discussion with the end decision regarding Ava. According to Foden and Preston (2001), working collaboratively as a team is largely dependent on working closely together, to establish and agree explicit common aims, acknowledge the complementary nature of expertise, communicate successfully, negotiate all decisions and actions, act honestly and be flexible.

It was clear that the end decision was not reached with negotiation and any such negotiation that may have occurred previously was not acknowledged within the meeting. In turn, this impacted on Nigel who did not 'act honestly' and express what he needed to. The end result was that Nigel lost his confidence and that Ava may have been discharged too early or without the support she needed.

Conforming in groups

In the opening case study, members of the team all agreed with the end decision, which was reached without any discussion. Nigel also agreed with the rest of the team, even though he had concerns regarding the patient being discharged without appropriate support. In essence, Nigel conformed to the rest of the group. **Conformity** can be defined as 'a deep-seated private and enduring change in behaviour and attitudes due to group pressure' (Hogg and Vaughan, 2002, p. 246) (see Chapter 16 for further explanation).

Asch (1952) in his classic study of conformity set out to explore how people use other people's behaviour to determine a correct or appropriate response. Asch (1951, 1952, 1956) invited male participants to take part in a study that they thought was about visual discrimination. Five to nine participants were seated around a table and were asked individually which of a set of comparison lines matched the standard line (see Figure 6.1). There were 18 trials. Individuals called out their answers publicly and randomly. In reality there was only one participant, the rest were confederates who were told to give the obvious wrong answer. The naïve participant was always second to last to answer. Asch found that 25 per cent of participants remained independent and provided the correct answer irrespective of the obvious wrong answer given by the majority of the group. However, 50 per cent of participants tended to conform to the majority mistaken answer.

When Asch further probed participants as to why they gave an answer publicly that they knew was wrong, the explanations were even more intriguing. They all felt some confusion and self-doubt about their answer in comparison to the rest of the groups', which soon evolved into fear of disapproval, feelings of anxiety and even loneliness. Different reasons were given for yielding to the group, which ranged from thinking that perception may have been inaccurate, to not wanting to 'stand out' from the crowd. A small minority even reported that they saw the line the same way as the group did and believed that this was the correct answer.

In the above case study Nigel conformed to the rest of the group who all agreed with the decision. The pressure to conform was heightened as Nigel was not an established member of the team and wanted to be accepted by his new colleagues. This is common for many student nurses out on their first placement who want to fit in with the established teams. However, a nurse needs to understand that when there is a concern for the patient that needs to be addressed immediately, this needs to take priority, which may at times break the conforming vision of the group.

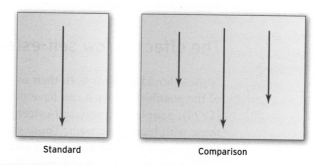

Standard   Comparison

Figure 6.1 Asch's study of conformity.

Perception of self and self-esteem, and inter-group behaviour

Self-esteem influences how a nurse will conduct themself within their practice, as well as influencing how a patient will manage or recover from their present health experience. Self-esteem has been defined as 'the individual's perception of themselves' (Randle, 2003, p. 396), and **professional self-esteem** as 'the self-evaluative beliefs that nurses hold about themselves' (Randle, 2003 p. 396). It is important for nurses to be aware of the area of self-esteem and the potential impact it can have on their day-to-day behaviour, motivation and perception of events around them.

It is apparent throughout the case study that Nigel began to lose confidence when contributing to team meetings. This eventually spread into other areas of his personal and working life. By the end of the case study, he felt that his contribution at any level was not valuable. Nurses who begin a new placement or, as in Nigel's case, a first-time position as a registered nurse will find that they will strive to identify with the group that they are working with. This has been referred to as **social identity**. There are several consequences of nurses identifying with a group and attempting to establish themselves as a member of the group. The major outcome is the effect on the defining level of self-esteem.

Self-esteem is affected when identifying with an established group because of a process that takes place that is referred to as **social comparison**. Social comparison is the 'process of comparing one's behaviour and opinions with those of others in order to establish the correct or socially approved way of thinking of being' (Hogg and Vaughan, 2002, p. 133).

Part of the identification process will involve the student nurse comparing their competencies and knowledge to those of other nurses. This could result in the dampening down of confidence and self-esteem, since comparison with experienced nurses will result in the acknowledgement of what student nurses cannot currently do. This has been demonstrated in a study carried out by Begley and White (2003) who interviewed Irish nursing students about their experiences during placement. It was found that self-esteem tended to be low for student nurses, especially when negative feedback was given on placement. However, the study also found that nurses' self-esteem tended to increase as their course progressed and when they were near to the completion of their registration.

The effect of low self-esteem

Nurses should monitor both their own and their patients' self-esteem because of the possible impact it can have on the individuals. According to Campbell (1990), people with low self-esteem tend not to be as highly motivated as those with high self-esteem. Those with high self-esteem tend to capitalise on their positive features and pursue success, whereas those with low self-esteem try to remedy their shortcomings. For a student nurse and a patient, motivation is important. In the case study above, Nigel's enthusiasm and motivation for his day-to-day job began to be affected by his low self-esteem.

Other effects of low self-esteem, outlined by Britt *et al.* (1997) include performing less well, a decline in productivity, less assertiveness, lower

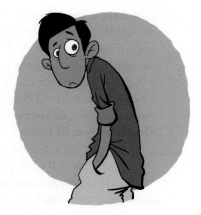

self-expectation, increased susceptibility to stress, lower job satisfaction, less commitment and lower levels of enthusiasm. In the case study above, Nigel began to show signs of low self-esteem by undervaluing himself. This feeling would have the potential to ultimately affect patient care and the patients' well-being.

Patients and low self-esteem

Patients who are facing a new situation or health dilemma may be uncertain, which can hamper self-esteem. It is vital that a nurse is aware of the patient's current state of confidence so that self-esteem can be addressed as part of a care plan. This in turn will ensure that the patient's motivation is at an appropriate level when managing their current state of health. Below are a few examples of differing health issues where self-esteem needs to be addressed.

Incontinence can result in a reduced sense of well-being (Braslis *et al.*, 1994). Immediate post-operative functioning also appears to result in a decline in self-esteem (Fan, 2002). For example, Moore and Estey (1999) found that coping with surgery was extremely stressful and affected the quality of life of prostate cancer patients and their spouses. This in turn affected their confidence and self-esteem. Self-esteem can also be affected when conditions of the skin are visible to others around the individual. According to Peters (1999a), people with low initial self-esteem tend to lose further confidence, the ability to use coping mechanisms and, in turn, motivation to care for their skin. This results in the skin condition dominating the patient's life.

States of mental ill-health, such as depression, tend to include low self-esteem as part of the onset of the illness. How self-esteem is addressed during treatment can make a major difference to how severe a depressive episode will be or how likely the individual will be to cope with the depressive episode. According to Kelly *et al.* (2007) depressed individuals with a high baseline level of self-esteem were more likely to gain positive aspects from a depressive episode and recover quicker when self-esteem was addressed as part of their recovery, compared to those with a lower level of self-esteem.

Eating disorders such as anorexia nervosa have causative factors, the main one being low self-esteem. Low self-esteem has a central part to play in the onset of such an eating disorder. According to Strober (2000) an eating disorder such as anorexia nervosa or bulimia nervosa is usually masking deep problems with self-esteem, and reaching the 'ideal' body shape as shown in the media means severe weight loss. The sufferer sees this as a success in improving self-esteem and gaining control over their environment but it has the opposite effect, as the ideal body shape set by the sufferer is not realistic.

Lower self-esteem can also be seen when a person is labelled as having a learning disability. Thomson and McKenzie (2005) interviewed 40 adults with a learning disability and 40 without and found that when a learning disability individual compared their skills and abilities with other individuals who did not have a learning disability, self-esteem was likely to be low. On the whole it was found that those with a learning disability tended to have lower self-esteem than those who did not have a learning disability. This was a sample that did not include those individuals who were enduring depression or experiencing a mental illness, as rates of low self-esteem are likely to be high in this group (Cooper and Bailey, 2001).

The importance of addressing self-esteem is also evident in areas where health promotion has to be addressed, especially within the area of sexual health. Evans (2004) highlights the holistic perspective nurses should embrace when promoting safer sexual practices within a young patient population. One of the core areas that Evans highlights within this holistic approach is the area of self-esteem and, in particular, low self-esteem. This needs to be addressed because of the potential link between high self-esteem and practising safe sex. Evans suggests that individuals with low self-esteem tend to generally disregard themselves, which will result in a lack of confidence when initiating the use of condoms within a relationship.

It is apparent from the above section that self-esteem is something that needs to be addressed when putting together a care plan for patients. In the case study above, Ava could not disclose her HIV status to her partner, which is clearly an ethical matter. The issues of low self-esteem, fear of rejection and being confident enough within her relationship to disclose such information are clearly points that should have been addressed before her discharge.

Think about this

How can the low self-esteem of a patient be enhanced? What are the possible avenues that can be taken to enhance self-esteem for a newly qualified/student nurse?

Enhancing self-esteem

According to Higgins's (1987) **self-discrepancy theory**, we have three types of self-schema: actual self (how we currently are), ideal self (how we would like to be) and ought self (how we think we should be). Any large discrepancies when comparing the actual self with the ideal, or ought, self will result in low self-esteem. It is important to address discrepancies and work on being more realistic. For example, a patient who may be classed as 'obese' and has been instructed to lose weight will be successful only if their ideal or ought self is realistic. This can be the same for newly qualified nurses (such as Nigel) or student nurses out on placement. Being realistic as to what is expected from yourself as a newly qualified nurse or a student nurse will result in a healthy self-esteem level. Setting goals that are unrealistic will negatively affect self-esteem. The unrealistic ought, or ideal, self can be seen in patients who have been diagnosed with anorexia nervosa. These patients tend to set high standards (weight ideal) for themselves, which result in continual self-criticism when they are not achieved (Blatt, 2004). Addressing such high expectations and making them more realistic is an important area to address when caring for such a patient.

Empowerment (refer to Chapter 3 for an in-depth exploration) is another area that a nurse can focus on when attempting to enhance the self-esteem of a patient. For example, Evans (2004) highlighted the need for nurses to address empowerment when educating young individuals on safer sex practices within relationships. Negotiation and communication were highlighted as being key to facilitating empowerment and, in turn, the self-esteem of the individual. In the case study above, after the meeting the senior staff nurse and Nigel highlighted assertiveness (see below for a section on assertiveness) and public speaking as two of the key areas that Nigel should be working on.

Spending time with a patient addressing confidence and providing reassurance is a way of enhancing self-esteem. Peters (1999b) found that the amount of time that the nurse spent with a patient addressing psychosocial issues surrounding dermatological (skin) conditions was important for the enhancement of their self-esteem. In the case study it was apparent that, apart from Nigel, other members of the team had not spent any extensive period of time with Ava. Had other members of the team spent time with the patient, they would have soon come to the realisation that other issues, such as Ava not wanting to disclose vital information to her partner, were areas where she needed reassurance. Comfort and encouragement by the nurse have been seen to be just as important as communication priorities when attempting to enhance self-esteem in cancer patients (Jakobsson *et al.*, 1997). Referring a patient to other support groups or further specialised help is also important and can help the individual's self-esteem (Buchanan, 2001).

Positive feedback should also be taken into consideration when working with a patient who has low self-esteem. Positive reinforcement and rewards such as praise have been linked to improving self-esteem (Logan, 1985). Building on a small attainable goal and praising the patient can result in enhanced self-esteem and confidence to tackle other goals. Positive feedback and praise are also important for nursing students and newly qualified nurses. This two-way beneficial effect was shown by Huberman and O'Brien (1999) who found that positive reinforcement was one of the factors that resulted in improvements in the work of therapists and in the progress of patients in mental health. The senior staff nurse, during her meeting with Nigel, praised him on his process of self-evaluation and the concern he had for Ava, which would have begun the process of enhancing his confidence levels as a nurse (also refer to Chapter 2).

Addressing possible comparisons an individual makes is also important when attempting to enhance self-esteem. Thomson and McKenzie (2005) highlight the importance of tackling issues such as attitudes, labelling and comparison of skills among learning disabled patients when attempting to enhance self-esteem in these particular individuals (see sections later in the chapter for attitudes and labelling).

Behavioural and cognitive coping strategies have also been seen as helpful for patients attempting to gain control, especially after surgery. For example, Fan (2002) found that for cancer patients especially after surgery, using behavioural and cognitive coping strategies resulted in an improvement in emotion, quality of life and self-esteem (see Chapter 13 for coping and Chapter 5 for cognitive behavioural therapy).

Self-awareness

Self-awareness is important for nurses to master since it allows them to develop, reflect and learn from experiences, as well as to be able to identify obstacles that could hinder the care that they provide for patients. Marks (1997) suggested that clinical staff are reluctant to deal with emotional states such as anxiety and depression because they feel they lack the necessary understanding and skills to deal with them competently. Moreover, nurses may avoid situations that mirror experiences within their own personal lives, which could result in avoidance behaviour that they may not be aware of. For example, a nurse who has experienced a recent family death could experience enormous anxiety when caring for dying patients, which could in turn result in the nurse not being able to provide care for the dying patient effectively (see Chapter 11). By being self-aware a nurse can work on limiting behaviours.

Much of the research that centred around the importance of self-awareness within nursing was carried out during the 1990s. There was a consensus of results; to care for a patient effectively, a nurse firstly needs to understand their 'self' and become self-aware (e.g. Burnard and Morrison, 1998). Later research that has looked at the relationship between self-awareness and different aspects of nursing care supports such research. For example, Burnard (2002) found a positive correlation between the nurse's level of self-understanding and their openness and honesty in interactions with others. Further beneficial outcomes of practising self-awareness among nurses have been identified by researchers who have suggested that the more self-reflective the nurse, the more likely it is they will be able to appreciate the emotional connection with patients. More recently, self-awareness has also been documented as being important when the nurse attempts to keep a professional distance within the nurse–patient therapeutic relationship (e.g. Dowling, 2006) (refer to Chapter 3 on empathy).

Self-awareness can be defined as 'a state in which one is aware of oneself as an object, much as one might be aware of a tree or another person' (Duval and Wicklund, 1972). Much of self-awareness is about finding out about one's self. This includes how we conduct ourselves and the impact of our behaviour on others. According to Cook (1999, p. 1293), self-awareness also involves becoming aware of one's personal characteristics such as values, attitudes, prejudices, beliefs, assumptions, feelings, personal motives, competencies, skills and limitations.

We are unlikely to be self-aware at all times. However, certain situations will result in self-awareness. A student nurse who is aware that their mentor is observing them will be self-aware. Nigel was self-aware within the team meeting as a result of concerns about how other members of the team perceived him and responded to him. The examples above demonstrate **objective self-awareness**, which tends to occur in situations where we are aware that 'others' are observing us or assessing our skills.

Think about this

Think back to a time you were being observed, for example in a play, production, driving test, presentation, exam or on placement. How did you feel?

Common feelings individuals have when objectively self-aware include sweaty palms, heart palpitations, hearing one's voice shake, etc. Self-awareness, or having someone observe you performing a new skill or competency, can result in behaviour being impaired because energy is invested in focusing on being observed, rather than the task at hand. This effect diminishes however. After having been observed on several placements, the nurse will be familiar with being observed in their day-to-day tasks and impairment of performance is less likely to occur.

Individual self-awareness can also bring about feelings of uneasiness when assessing or reflecting on one's own behaviour. However the individual will continually employ self-awareness, so being self-aware will become less daunting over time. In the case study above, Nigel was asked to reflect on the incident, which he did by using a self-awareness tool. This enabled him to reflect appropriately as well as assess his own behaviour and impact on the situation in the best manner possible.

The **Johari window** (Luft, 1969) is an example of a self-awareness tool. According to Luft, there are certain parts of our personality that are open to all, others that are open just to us and others that are not even open to the ourselves. The Johari window attempts to raise awareness of these aspects (see Figure 6.2).

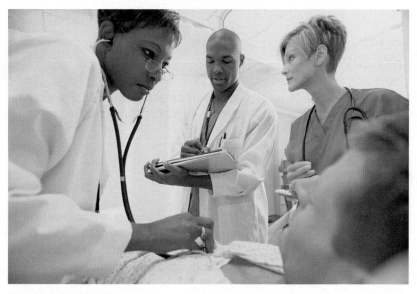

© Comstock Select/Corbis

1. The *public area*: This is the self that is known both by the individual and others. For example, Nigel and those within the team meeting knew that Nigel was a newly qualified nurse.
2. The *hidden area*: This area contains characteristics or aspects of ourselves that individuals around us are aware of but we are not fully aware of ourselves. For example, the senior nurse revealed to Nigel that he seemed unhappy at work. As far as Nigel was concerned he was conducting himself as normal.
3. The *unknown area*: This includes things about the self which neither others around us or we ourselves are not aware of. Raising awareness of this area can be complex, as this is the hidden part of ourselves which usually manifests itself within the unconscious and subconscious part of our personalities (refer to Chapter 4). Being aware that symptoms (e.g. continual headache, panic attacks) are usually triggered by other factors enables you to become aware of, and work on, such factors.
4. The *private area*: This contains aspects of ourselves that we are aware of but keep hidden from others, e.g. hidden away from professional practice. This is acceptable unless the nurse begins to find it hard to work, or if patient care becomes compromised. For example, another nurse may have avoided Ava because of her HIV status, which was something that a family member died of. If the nurse did not inform anyone, they would have worked under enormous emotional stress, which would not have been the case if the nurse had informed a colleague.

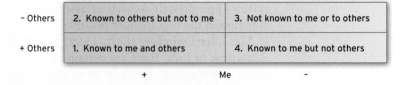

- Others	2. Known to others but not to me	3. Not known to me or to others
+ Others	1. Known to me and others	4. Known to me but not others
	+ Me -	

Figure 6.2 Johari window.

Source: Joseph Luft, *Of Human Interaction* (1969), Mayfield Publishing Company, reproduced with permission of The McGraw-Hill Companies

Think about this

Do you think this is an effective tool when attempting to aid a student nurse raise awareness of himself or herself as a professional nurse? Is this a useful tool to use with patients?

Reflection

Reflection and self-awareness are interlinked. In the above case study, Nigel used a **reflective framework model,** which enabled him to reflect more effectively. Without knowledge of reflective framework models a nurse may not be able to get the best outcome from their reflective experience.

Reflection is key within nursing as 'qualified nurses should be competent reflective practitioners' (An Bord Altranais, 2000). Reflection enables the individual to go beyond merely describing incidents within practice and instead learn from the incidents and experiences that they have been involved in or have observed. The nursing portfolio is a prime example of reflection; incidents are filed in a manner that requires the student nurse to reflect and learn from their experiences (Joyce, 2005).

The act of reflection has several benefits for a new student nurse. Firstly, reflection allows you to critically analyse practice to uncover underlying influences, motivations and knowledge (Taylor, 2000). Secondly, the reflective process allows the student nurse to apply theoretical constructs to practice, which enables them to bridge the gap between theory and practice (Bulman and Schutz, 2004). Thirdly, the enhancement of knowledge, skills and learning within nursing practice is dependent on the reflective skills of the nurse (McMullan *et al.*, 2003).

Reflective framework models enable the process of reflection to be carried out in an effective manner, as they direct the individual to ask appropriate questions. Such models are especially useful for novice reflectors, as they encourage deeper levels of reflection and learning within their practice (Hilliard, 2006). Gibbs's (1988) reflective cycle is one of the basic reflective framework models that are introduced to student nurses (see Figure 6.3).

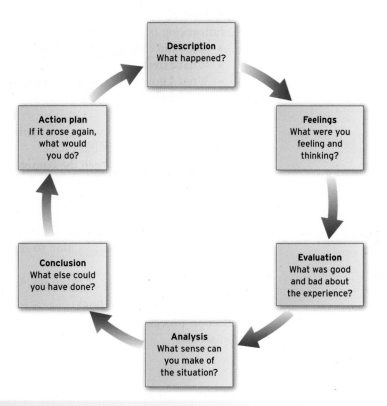

Figure 6.3 The Gibbs reflective cycle.

This resource was produced using material developed by the Learning and Skills Development Agency

Think about this

How would nurse Nigel apply Gibbs's (1988) reflective model when looking back at the incident concerning the team meeting and his contribution? Remember the cycle should enable Nigel to see what he has learned from the incident and how he would change his behaviour within a similar situation.

Gibbs's reflective cycle is circular and never-ending, which should enable the nurse to see that, for any incident, there is always room for improvement. For nurses who prefer a model that poses actual questions when reflecting, they can use Johns's (1995) model of structured reflection:

1. Incident (description)
2. Key issues
3. Reflection
   - What was I trying to achieve?
   - Why did I intervene as I did?
   - What were the consequences of my actions for the patient, myself and the people I work with?
   - How did I feel about this experience when it was happening?
   - How did the patient feel about it?
   - How did I know how the patient felt about it?
4. Influencing factors
   - What internal factors influenced my decision-making and actions?
   - What external factors influenced my decision-making and actions?
   - What knowledge did, or should have, influenced my decision-making and actions?
5. Alternative strategies
   - Could I have dealt with the situation better?
   - What other choices did I have?
   - What would have been the consequences of these other choices?
6. Learning
   - How can I now make sense of this experience in light of past experience and future practice?
   - How do I now feel about this experience?
   - Have I taken effective action to support others and myself as a result of this experience?
   - Has this experience changed my ways of knowing in practice?

According to Hilliard (2006), once a nurse becomes more confident in their reflection process they can then find innovative ways to fit their own reflection process.

Assertiveness

The opening case study demonstrates factors that cause a lack of assertiveness, as well as consequential factors that can result from a lack of *assertiveness*. Studies suggest that on the whole, nurses tend to be non-assertive (e.g. Martin

Who is assertive and who is passive?

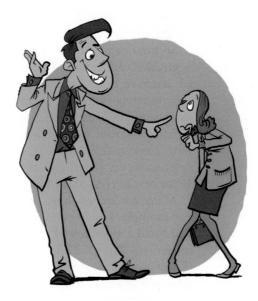

et al., 2000). Many plausible explanations have been offered for why there is a lack of assertion among nurses who work collaboratively with other health practitioners. The most frequently cited explanations include that nurses just want to get on with their jobs, traditional hierarchical power structures in health care settings, i.e. the doctor and nurse working relationship, deter the nurse from being assertive (Benton, 1999) and the nurse's working environment, which can encourage or discourage assertiveness (e.g. Timmins and McCabe, 2005). Not being able to identify the appropriate level of assertiveness and distinguish this behaviour from aggression (e.g. Rakos, 1997) is another common explanation for the lack of assertiveness among newly qualified and student nurses.

Assertiveness enables you to express yourself with confidence, without the inappropriate use of aggressive, passive or manipulative behaviours (Bishop, 2000). When being assertive it is important for the individual to see themselves as being of worth, while at the same time valuing others equally (Bupa, 2004). Assertiveness can often be confused with aggression. This can happen when the individual is passionate about something or needs particular issues addressed immediately. The hurried or passionate viewpoint of the individual may come across as being aggressive. On the other hand, like nurse Nigel, an individual can be perceived as being passive. There are many reasons for this, e.g. low self-esteem, being a new member of the team or not being briefed appropriately. Another reason that is widely documented is that practitioners such as nurses may not be equipped with the assertiveness skills they need within professional practice. Nurses need to be assertive when acting in the patient's best interest (Morris, 2004).

When someone is aggressive, they tend to ignore the rights of the other person. This distinguishes aggression from assertion. According to Paterson (2000), aggression is a short-lived strategy. Aggression will result in others not listening to the individual, as well as loss of respect. On the other hand, **passiveness** is when an individual ignores his or her own rights (Lawton and Stewart, 2007). For example, an individual may find it hard to say 'no' or, like nurse Nigel, be unable to express themselves fully, which will result in a loss of confidence. Being passive tends to be associated with stress, an over-burden of work and loss of respect.

So how can a nurse be assertive without being perceived as passive or aggressive? According to Underman Boggs (2003) there are four components of assertive behaviour: being able to say no, asking for what you want, appropriately expressing thoughts and feelings and being able to initiate, continue and terminate interaction. More specifically, Chenevert (1996) refers to a list of assertive rights. These include the right to: be treated with respect, have a reasonable workload, have an equitable wage, make mistakes and be responsible for them, give and receive information as a professional and act in the best interest of the patient.

Many researchers have reviewed assertiveness skills that can help nurses. For example, Lawton and Stewart (2007) reviewed the work of Smith (1975) and listed a summary of techniques that can enhance assertiveness in district nurses (see Table 6.2). In addition to these techniques, it is important to use 'I' statements, as opposed to 'you' or 'them' statements, which can be misinterpreted as attributing blame or being aggressive. The 'I' statement will also ensure that the individual is not being passive but instead is being honest and is taking responsibility for their actions. Preparation is also key to being assertive within team meetings (Lawton and Stewart, 2007). For example, had Nigel asked to have been briefed with minutes of earlier meetings, he would have been more fully prepared and been more assertive with his views and concerns regarding Ava. He would also have been familiar with the proposed agenda of the team.

Attitudes and persuasive communication

Attitudes are important for patients and nurses. Patient attitudes affect their understanding and following health advice. Attitudes are crucial for nurses when providing care that is unconditional and non-judgemental (refer to Chapter 3). Attitudes are learned predispositions to respond in a consistently favourable or unfavourable way towards a given object, person or event (Fishbein and Ajzen, 1975). More recent definitions have highlighted attitudes as comprising 'cognitive, affective and behavioural components, which are all basic to human experience' (Hogg and Vaughan, 2002). Acknowledging and

Table 6.2 Assertiveness techniques	Technique	Description
	Saying 'no'	Broken record technique. Repeat 'no' back to the person. With each repetition the goal is to stay calm, keep the same tone of voice and avoid giving in to pressure.
	Fogging	Coping with criticism from colleagues. Listen closely to what the person is saying and acknowledge that there may be some truth in it.
	Negative assertion	Accept that you have made a mistake and agree with the criticism.
	Negative inquiry	Follow up the perceived criticism with a specific prompt to find out about the criticism.

raising awareness of how attitudes are formed, influenced and changed can enable the nurse to communicate and care for a patient in a way that is non-judgemental, as well as being able to change the attitudes and, in turn, behaviour of the patient.

According to Festinger's (1957) **cognitive dissonance theory**, when an individual takes in two bits of information that are contradictory the individual experiences *cognitive dissonance*. Human beings strive towards consistency at all times, so the state of cognitive dissonance creates tension in the individual. As a result, they will strive to reduce tension by aiming to make bits of information consistent. This can be done by ignoring new information, which can cause problems when the new information is important. For example, a nurse may ignore a test result that does not fit with a patient's current diagnosis. Another way of making information consistent is to change a behaviour, so that behaviour and information become consistent. In the opening case study Ava smokes and has been advised by nurse Nigel to give this up because of her pregnancy. Ava may minimise the discomfort of smoking and being pregnant by giving up smoking. Alternatively, she could have disregarded the health advice and literature that Nigel provided.

The area of attitude change concentrates on the source of information, the actual message and how it is communicated which influence whether a patient is more likely to change their attitude and in turn their behaviour. Hovland *et al.* (1953) pioneered this work and believed that at the heart of attitude change is **persuasive communication**. Persuasive communication is determined by certain factors associated with the source of communication (nurses perceived expertise and trustworthiness), the message itself (message appeal to logic or emotion, complexity of the message) the recipient of the communication (who is more easily persuaded and who is not) and the channel of communication.

In light of Hovland's model of persuasive communication, Clark (1999) suggests the following points are important for nurses to take into account when using persuasive communication to change patient attitudes:

- When the sender is perceived as being credible, experienced and trustworthy the message is likely to be more persuasive.
- A message is more effective when seen as relevant to the audience and is vivid and personal.
- Health information, particularly that which induces fear, should be accompanied by practical advice about what to do.
- Patient participation in a health promotion strategy will significantly enhance retention of the message.
- Media campaigns act as a trigger to action, which are more effective when supported by interpersonal pressure.
- Most persuasive forms of communication take place when there is personal interaction between communicator and recipient.

Message framing

How a health message is explained will determine how likely it is that a change of attitude will take place. Health messages can be framed in terms of the benefits of engaging in the health behaviour (gain frame) or in terms of the costs of failing to engage in the behaviour (loss frame) (Mann *et al.*, 2007). The type of frame (loss or gain) that is chosen when communicating a health message will influence how likely the patient is to adhere to the nurse's advice and, in turn, be persuaded to change their attitude.

Think about this

Will a high or low fear message be effective when communicating with a patient about their unhealthy lifestyle?

The type of framing that will be most effective will depend on the health behaviour that is being addressed. Detweiler *et al.* (2007) set out to explore how best to motivate an individual to use sunscreen. In the study, beach-goers were either given a leaflet that emphasised the good things that would happen (gain frame) if sunscreen were used or one that emphasised the bad things that could happen (loss frame) if sunscreen was not used. Within the leaflets were coupons that could be redeemed on sunblock products. It was found that 71 per cent of those that received the gain message redeemed their coupons, in comparison with only 53 per cent of those who received the loss message. Detweiler concluded that, in this instance, gain framing worked best for sunscreen use and preventative health behaviours in general. Loss frames worked best for detection behaviours such as screening. This can be seen in the study carried out by Meyerowitz and Chaiken (1987), who looked at the detection behaviour of breast self-examination (BSE). Four conditions were used in the study. Subjects were given a pamphlet which contained either a loss frame (decrease in survival being emphasised), gain frame (increase in survival emphasised), neutral frame or no pamphlet. It was found that those subjects that received the loss pamphlet, reported in engaging in BSE significantly more than subjects in the other three conditions. Also, those who received the loss pamphlet were more likely to see themselves carrying out BSE in the future.

Other research has highlighted the framing of messages in accordance to the motivation level of individuals. This was explored by Sherman *et al.* (2006) who randomly allocated 74 undergraduate psychology students to either a gain-framed or a loss-framed flossing pamphlet. It was found that those with an approach orientation (more likely to engage in instructed health behaviour) flossed more after reading the gain-framed article. Participants who had an avoidance orientation (less likely to engage in instructed health behaviour) flossed more after reading a loss-framed message. Tailoring messages according to the individual's psychological characteristics has been proven to be more effective than presenting framed messages according to the type of health behaviour, i.e. prevention or detection. Health messages that are tailored to an individual's coping style have also been found to be far more successful in the increasing health behaviours than when messages are not matched with coping styles. For example, Piehota *et al.* (2005) explored coping styles and framing messages among women. They found that when mammography messages matched to whether the patient had a monitor (women who are constant monitors of their own health) or blunter (those who ignore health information and signs of changing health) coping style, attendance of mammography was encouraged more effectively than if the message was mismatched.

Nurses' attitudes

The attitude a nurse holds towards a patient and their state of ill-health will determine the type of emotional, physical, informational and psychological help the patient will receive from the nurse. A positive, as opposed to a negative or neutral attitude, will result in the patient having all their needs met. In the case study above nurse Nigel spent an enormous amount of time with Ava. As a result, there were many things that Ava disclosed to Nigel of which the team were unaware. This is a clear example of a nurse who holds a positive attitude towards the HIV and AIDS virus and will provide the care and appropriate support that is required without judgement.

There will be instances where negative attitudes may be held, which stem from personal experience. The replacing of negative attitudes with positive ones is essential for nurse professionals. Research studies that enhance knowledge are effective in changing negative or neutral attitudes to positive ones. For example, Sidley and Renton (1996) conducted a study that looked at accident and emergency nurses and their attitudes towards patients who attempted to commit suicide. It was found that those with a sound knowledge base about this client group and a greater familiarity of risk assessment procedures were more likely to have positive attitudes. In turn, these nurses were more likely to provide the necessary support for these patients and were able to liaise with appropriate teams more effectively. May (2001) suggested experienced staff with positive attitudes should act as role models for newly qualified staff to enhance positive attitudes.

Many studies have examined the types of attitude that are held by nurses towards particular illness, as well as explanations as to why such attitudes are held. Diverse explanations have been found. For example, Cole and Abel (2000) examined nurse attitudes towards AIDS within an emergency department. They found that the emergency nurses in the study held the most positive attitudes towards working with patients who had acquired the HIV/AIDS virus through a blood transfusion and the least positive attitude towards someone who acquired AIDS through intravenous drug use. Nurses themselves may not be aware of the attitudes they hold towards particular states of ill-health until they reflect on the care that they have provided for the patient (see sections above on reflection and self-awareness and Chapter 3 on conditional positive regard).

The research in focus box later in the chapter highlights a study where the importance of experience, information and education when promoting positive attitudes is revealed.

Stereotyping

The concept of stereotyping originated from the work of Lippman (1922). Schneider (2004) defines stereotyping as: 'qualities perceived to be associated with particular groups or categories of people' (p. 24). There has been a tendency to suggest that stereotyping is negative because of the conclusions that are made about individuals from simplified information, which does not allow room for diversity and individuality. Sterotyping is not necessarily negative, however. Individuals stereotype when they have to make sense of the world around them with the limited information that they have. They provide a useful shortcut to classify people and events into pre-existing **mental schema** (Byrne and Byrne, 1992) drawn from personal experiences. In a health setting, these may be past experiences with consultants and nurses, as well as other sources of information, e.g. media portrayal of health professionals.

The problem with using a limited amount of information is that there is an enormous amount of generalisation. All members of the group being represented, e.g. nurses, are assumed to share similar characteristics. Think about the diversity there is among nursing students and how many factors, such as gender, age, socio-economic status, education, experience and regional upbringing, vary within this category. Generalisations are problematic when they are applied to every person within a particular group (Schermerhorn *et al.*, 2004) and do not allow for diversity. For example, nursing is perceived traditionally as a female occupation even though there are many male nurses.

Stereotyping and labelling

Labelling a patient according to their illness or disability can result in the patient being perceived, treated and expected to behave in a certain way. This can have a negative impact on the care that is provided for the patient. For example, the strengths of a person are likely to be clouded by their diagnosis and labels (Finlay, 2005) as well as their individuality not being recognised. Thomson and McKenzie (2005) drew attention to the implications of labelling an individual who has a learning disability. They found that treating a patient according to the label of 'learning disability' resulted in the patient being viewed, treated and supported differently. Nurses should counteract this by not caring for the patient according to their diagnosis alone but by paying attention to the individual qualities of the patient and treating them accordingly.

The 'good' and the' bad' patient

Labels that concentrate on a diagnosis differ from the labels that are used by nurses to make social judgements about patients. A vast amount of literature over the past 40 years has highlighted how health professionals tend to categorise patients by applying a range of labels and evaluations beyond the diagnostic label (Kelly and May, 1982). Again this undermines the uniqueness of the individual patient and contradicts the ethos of patient-centred care (see Chapter 3).

Stockwell (1972) carried out a study exploring the use of labels that are used with patients when making social judgements and found that nurses tended to care for 'popular patients' more frequently than 'unpopular patients'. Stockwell's work had a large impact on raising awareness within nursing after the publication of her book, *The Unpopular Patient*, which has been widely cited. According to Stockwell's work, patients with characteristics such as being demanding and not following what the nurse had to say were perceived as unpopular and were less likely to have the attention that they needed. Patients who were polite, followed what the nurse said and were clean were viewed as popular and were more likely to receive attention and care from nurses.

More recent research has supported the work of Stockwell. For example, Finlay (2005) carried out a literature review which explored the labels of the 'good' and the 'bad' patients, and summarised the commonly cited characteristics which categorised patients in these groups (listed in Table 6.3). Such categories can have negative implications for patient care as patients soon become stigmatised and start responding accordingly, and as a result their problems are aggravated (Goffman, 1963). Within psychology this is referred to as the **self-fulfilling prophecy**, where individuals behave as they are treated or expected to behave.

There are times where phrases are used loosely when talking about a patient. For example, 'she's demanding', 'watch him, he challenges everything' or 'he is a right one'. Such phrases can result in other colleagues providing care that is based on preconceived ideas. Such labels are not condoned in good nursing practice. Nurses need to be aware of how such terms can easily be applied and their negative implications for patient care. Assigning the label 'bad' or 'difficult' may be as a result of the need to distance oneself emotionally from the patient in order to cope with workload (Smith, 1992). Labelling a demanding patient as 'bad' may help the nurse to justify reducing the attention they give them.

Holyoake (1999) carried out a survey questioning nurses about favouritism with patients. Holyoake illustrates prime examples of patients who are favoured and those who are not. For example one nurse in the study stated that, 'I always leave the aggressive patients to Angela because she's good with them'. Other examples have been cited where nurses are not aware that they favour patients. For example, one nurse stated that, 'I like working with depressed patients because I think that I have the right attitudes' but later said 'I would never have a favourite patient because it is totally unethical'. This study clearly exemplifies how easy it is to label and categorise patients without actually realising it is happening.

Table 6.3

Characteristics of 'good' and 'bad' patients

Good patient	Bad patient
Cooperative	Demanding
Appreciative of their treatment	Uncooperative
Cheerful	Ungrateful
Uncomplaining	Make staff feel ineffective
Allow staff to practise their skills/or specialities and they usually improve	Patients with the potential for poisoning
	Anxious patients
Patients with health-seeking behaviour	Violent patients

Source: partly adapted from Finlay (2005)

Finlay (2005) draws attention to the importance of reflecting on one's own conduct when caring for patients (see reflection section) with the aid of the following questions:

- Would we mind the patient knowing that we perceive them as difficult? If we do mind, what does this indicate?
- What intentions lie behind evaluating someone as difficult? Are we trying to express our own uncertainty or are we alerting others to the complexities of the problems involved? Are we being derogatory?
- What is implied by the label 'difficult'? That is, are we representing the person as being uncooperative, as having many problems, as being an interesting and challenging case or as taking more time than we can commit to?
- Does representing someone as 'difficult' have any damaging consequences? For instance, are they likely to be discharged or denied treatment? Might they behave in a more difficult way in response to such evaluations? Or might this offer an opportunity to help them because they become more aware of their behaviour and ultimately become more reasonable?
- Can anything be learned from becoming aware that we are representing someone as difficult? What does it tell us about ourselves and our relationship with the difficult person?

Research in focus

Rondahl, G., Innala, S. and Carlsson, M. (2004) Nurses' attitudes towards lesbians and gay men. *Journal of Advanced Nursing*, **47** (4), 386-392.

Background
During the past decade, official policy and Swedish legislation have strengthened the legal rights of homosexuals and demanded tolerance for this group. There is evidence in the literature that homosexual patients have experienced negative attitudes and poor-quality care from nurses and may be unwilling to disclose their sexuality because of fears of discriminatory treatment.

Aims
The aim of this paper is to report a study that investigated the attitudes of nurses towards lesbians and gay men and nurses' beliefs about the causes of sexuality.

Method
The study had a descriptive, comparative design. The Attitudes Toward Homosexuality Scale was used, along with Causes of Homosexuality Questionnaire. The participants were registered nurses and assistant nurses from one infectious disease clinic in central Sweden (response rate 67%, n = 57), and students enrolled in a university nursing programme and in upper secondary assistant nurses' training (response rate 62%, n = 165).

Results
In general, participants expressed positive attitudes (62%). Nurses expressed the most positive attitudes, whereas the assistant nursing students expressed the least positive attitudes. A minority of the sample (30%) expressed neither positive nor negative attitudes. The most common belief about the cause of homosexuality was that it was congenital. Those who held this belief

expressed more positive attitudes towards homosexuality than those who believed that homosexuality was acquired. Limitations of the study were that the sample was relatively small and not randomly selected.

Conclusion

This study demonstrated that attitudes have improved towards homosexuals compared with earlier international studies, although more needs to be done to increase the positive attitudes among the staff and students with neutral attitudes (neither positive nor negative attitudes) to enhance the well-being of homosexual persons. General education about homosexuality is a necessary beginning to make homosexual patients visible, which is an important aspect of practical nursing ethics.

Aggression

In the opening case study, the senior nurse informed Nigel about the aggression Ava displayed when she administered medication to her. Aggression can be defined as 'the intentional infliction of some form of harm on others' (Baron and Byrne, 2000). Violence or physical assault is defined by the Department of Health as 'The intentional application of force to the person of another without lawful justification, resulting in physical injury or personal discomfort' (Counter Fraud and Security Management Service Division, 2003). The definitions that exist for aggression seem to imply some form of intent. This may be the case for many aggressive acts; however, when looking at aggression within the health care environment, 'intent' cannot be applied in such a liberal manner to the majority of the aggressive acts performed by the patients.

Think about this

Think about Ava, as well as patients within your branch of nursing. What precipitating factors could result in the patient becoming aggressive? The following should be given consideration:

- Hospital environment
- Illness
- Side effects of medication
- Events that have occurred prior to seeing the nurse

There are many precipitating factors that can result in a patient being aggressive. A nurse should be aware of these factors, as well as being familiar with the origins of aggression so that the challenging behaviour can be dealt with in the most effective manner.

How common is aggression?

The Health and Safety Executive (2007) indicate that health care workers are up to four times more likely to experience work-related violence and aggression than other workers. Nurses are three times more vulnerable to violence and aggression than other health care personnel (Kingma, 2001). Within nursing itself, accident and emergency and mental health areas have the highest rates of violence and aggression (Nolan *et al.*, 2001; Wells and Bowers, 2002). Nursing staff are more likely to experience aggression from patients with whom they have direct contact (Hesketh *et al.*, 2003).

Theories of aggression

The **Frustration–aggression hypothesis** (Dollard *et al.* 1939) explores how aggression is caused. It postulates that aggression has origins in some frustrating event or situation. A patient who is unwell or is in hospital may experience many factors that could result in frustration, which could lead to aggression.

Think about this

What factors could have resulted in Ava becoming frustrated? Can frustration result in aggression? What factors do you think result in patients becoming frustrated?

Proponents of the social learning theory have suggested that aggression is dependent upon the learning process (Miles and Carey, 1997). Bandura (1977) was the most famous supporter of this view and highlighted the importance of observational learning or modelling. Observing an aggressive role model can result in aggression (see Chapter 2). The idea of learning by direct experience was based on Skinner's concept of operant conditioning, where behaviour can be maintained by rewards or punishment. In vicarious learning, a behaviour can be promoted or inhibited through the observation of another individual receiving a reward or punishment for performing the behaviour.

Think about this

What role can the media have in enhancing or minimising aggressive tendencies? Can television programmes such as *Casualty*, which at times portrays aggressive incidents, influence patients? Does aggression result from how individuals have been rewarded and punished as children? What about patients who have predominantly been in prison settings and have continually observed others around them being aggressive? Are they more likely to interact in an aggressive manner when in a difficult situation with a nurse?

Illness and aggression

In the case study, Ava pushed the senior staff nurse because of the excessive pain and discomfort that she was enduring. It has been widely acknowledged that aggression can be a result of physical pain, distress or mental health problems (Budd, 1999). Ferns (2006) suggest that violence and aggressive acts that are carried out maliciously against nursing staff should be differentiated with unintentional, disorientated acts which can result in physical injury.

The following list highlights factors that may predispose patients to becoming violent (from Drury, 1997; Keely, 2002; Saines, 1999; Whykes, 1994; Wing *et al.*, 1998; adapted from Ferns, 2006).

- Head injuries, cerebrovascular accidents, cerebral pathology, organic brain dysfunction or clinical brain injury.
- Hypoxia.
- Seizures, frontal, temporal or limbic epilepsy.
- Psychiatric disorders, hallucinations, depression, anxiety, stress reactions or personality disorders.
- Side effects of prescribed medication.
- Intoxication.
- Drug overdose.
- Drug or alcohol withdrawal.
- Age considerations, e.g. senility, dementia, adolescence, childhood disorders, conduct disorders, hyperkinetic disorders, autism or learning disability.

Particular ward settings and patient diagnoses can increase the likelihood of aggression. For example, nurses working within intensive care units are more likely to experience unintentional aggression from confused, hypoxic or delirious patients (Whittington *et al.*, 1996). Dyer (1995) compared the lived experiences of intensive care patients with Amnesty International's (1973) *Report on Torture*. The study demonstrated how a patient's experiences within the intensive care unit could include dehumanisation, lack of personal control, sensory overload from equipment alarms and bright artificial lights, lack of sleep, experiences of painful procedures, chemical or physical constraint and a loss of dignity, all of which were linked to frustration and a possible aggressive outcome.

Even though the likelihood of aggression is high within such an environment, a nurse can manage aggression through his or her communication with the patient, by accommodating the triggering factors of frustration for the patient. Dyer (1995) listed the following factors as lessening the negative effects of acute care and, in turn, decreasing the probability of an aggressive episode:

- Orientate the patient to the environment and the time.
- Make the environment comfortable, for example, patient position, lighting and heating.
- Talk to patients and give more than minimal instructions. Encourage two-way communication.
- Good communication skills, for example, active listening, eye contact, appropriate use of closed and open questions, calm, confident and relaxed voice and giving information and appropriate encouragement.
- Avoid depersonalising the patient.
- Ensure effective assessment and management of pain and sleep.
- Use a humanistic personal approach (see Chapter 3).

Further studies have demonstrated that communication is key to the management of aggression. Webb and Hope (1995) draw attention to patients prefer the fact that nurses who are friendly, warm and sympathetic take time to care, listen to worries, teach about their conditions and relieve pain. This is the approach nurses need to take when minimising assault (Ferns, 2007).

Mental health and aggression

The incidence of aggression and violence in acute mental health settings is on a par with that in accident and emergency units (National Audit Office, 2003).

Lowe (2000) has reviewed research concerning aggression and violence within psychiatric intensive care units, and has found that a small number of patients are involved in a high percentage of the violent incidents. This is something that needs to be taken seriously due to the frequent occurrence of aggressive events of which nursing staff are often the victims (James *et al.*, 1990). Lowe (2000) listed aggressive incidents by diagnosis (see Table 6.4). The prevention and prediction of violent incidents are vital to take into consideration when being prepared for a possible occurrence of aggression. The patient's illness and state of health, as well as the environment that the patient is in, should be taken into account when assessing and predicting the likelihood of aggression. A multi-factorial approach has been recommended when approaching aggressive situations (e.g. Beech and Bowyer, 2004; UKCC, 2002). The multi-factorial approach takes into account several levels, such as the staff team, staff attitudes, the environment and organisation, which all have to be integrated when understanding the aggressive patient (see section above on attitudes).

A government-supported campaign of Zero Level Tolerance (Department of Health, 1999) has been embraced by 96 per cent of primary care trusts within the United Kingdom. The emphasis is on health care staff working in safe environments, as well as documenting aggressive incidents. In conjunction with the multi-factorial approach, patient aggression can be managed without the patient's care being compromised. (Refer to Chapter 4 for a section on anxiety and aggression.)

Attribution

The opening case study centred on a multi-disciplinary team meeting regarding the discharge of patient Ava. During the meeting the members of the team may have attempted to explain Nigel's lack of contribution. The explanations could have ranged from Nigel being a new member of the team, to not being confident, to not wanting to contribute to the team. The process of assigning a cause to one's own or others' behaviour is referred to as **attribution**.

Table 6.4
Distribution of aggressive incidents by diagnosis

Diagnosis	Patients involved	Patients not involved	Total
Schizophrenia	17	56	73
Personality disorder	9	9	18
Bipolar affective disorder	14	20	34
Drug-induced psychosis	8	12	20
Schizo-affective disorder	6	8	14
Other	3	8	11
Total	57	113	170

Source: adapted from Lowe (2000).

Theories of attribution

There are a number of theories that explore attribution. Heider's theory of naive psychology (1958) is based on three main principles:

1. Our own behaviour is influenced by motivation, e.g. I am feeling good so will begin my exercise regimen today; as a result we tend to look for causes and reasons for others' behaviour in order to discover their motives.
2. We try to discover stable personality traits and enduring qualities within people or situations that cause behaviour so that we can predict behaviour.
3. Explanations for behaviour tend to fall in one of two categories. The first is **internal (dispositional) attributions** where behaviour is attributed to internal factors. For example, the senior staff nurse may have attributed Nigel's lack of contribution at the team meeting to his being introverted and generally not confident as an individual. The second is **external (situational) attribution** where behaviour is attributed to external or environmental factors. The senior staff nurse reasoned that Nigel did not express his views within the team meeting because of his position as a new member within an already established team where other team members were more assertive.

Another theoretical model that explains attributions is derived from the work of Kelley (1967, 1973). It is referred to as the **covariation model**. According to Kelley, people behave like scientists as they attempt to identify factors that co-vary with the behaviour and then assign that factor a causal role. This decision is based on three classes of information:

1. Consistency information (whether Nigel conducts himself in this manner at every meeting or only sometimes).
2. Distinctiveness information (whether Nigel does not contribute to every team meeting or only this one).
3. Consensus information (no members contribute or only Nigel).

Table 6.5 demonstrates what types of attribution are made as a result of considering the consistency, distinctiveness and consensus of a person's behaviour.

Biases in attribution

Social psychologists have found that individuals tend to attribute behaviour to internal rather than external causes, even when external causes are apparent. This has been referred to as the **fundamental attribution error** (Ross,

Table 6.5
Types of attribution

Consistency	Distinctiveness	Consensus	Attribution
Low			Discounting (search for a different cause)
High	+high	+high	External (attribution to the stimulus)
High	+low	+low	Internal (attribution to the person)

Source: adapted from Hogg and Vaughan (2002)

1977) or **correspondence bias** (Gilbert and Malone, 1995). In the case study, the senior staff nurse as well as the other members of the team could have made a fundamental attribution error if they attributed Nigel's lack of communication within the team meeting solely to Nigel's personality.

Many studies have found the fundamental attribution error can easily occur within health care practice. Bromley and Emerson's (1995) study is one example. Fundamental attribution error was looked at in relation to patients who are perceived by nurses to have challenging behaviour. The researchers found that nurses tended to attribute challenging behaviour to factors such as the patient's internal mood. As a result, the help provided will not address environmental causative factors, such as lack of satisfaction with medication, staff or the ward itself, which could cause frustration within the patient. Other studies have documented that as a consequence of the fundamental attribution error, inappropriate responses are given to patients (Carr and Kurtz 1991), which result in the patient receiving care that does not meet all their needs.

Raising nurses' awareness of the possible consequences of the fundamental attribution error for patient care has been shown to decrease the use of the error when explaining the behaviour of patients. Studies have found that training and education have a big part to play in reducing fundamental attribution error within practice. This was documented by McKenzie *et al.* (2004), who found that learning disability nursing *students* were more likely to attribute challenging behaviour to internal psychological state or mood than nurses who explored the fundamental attribution error through progressive training; these nurses were more likely to have a balanced view where they took into account both internal and external explanations of the patient's behaviour.

Think about this

How can the fundamental attribution error apply to patients who will not justify their unhealthy behaviour, e.g. smoking, drinking heavily, which they have been advised by the nurse to stop?

Conclusion

Social psychology highlights and enables the nurse practitioner to explore many aspects of nursing practice. This perspective can help the student nurse to be aware of their own professional practice and how they can develop from their experiences with the help of self-awareness tools. In addition to this, the student nurse can explore interactions that occur among nurses and other multi-disciplinary team members, which enable the nurse to present themselves and learn from their interactions in the best way possible. This will improve not only their competencies as a nurse but also their nursing portfolio in general.

Theories and models within social psychology also enable the nurse to explore how readily patients can be labelled, grouped and stereotyped and how nurses can have preconceived ideas, which are not condoned within the practice of nursing. Raising awareness of this will enable the nurse to ensure that it does not occur in practice.

Helping a patient who may appear or actually be aggressive is something with which every nurse will have to become familiar. The social psychology approach enables the nurse to understand the factors that can result in aggression. By being familiar with factors that are linked to aggression, the nurse can form strategies to minimise or prevent aggressive outbursts from occurring.

Overall, the social psychology perspective postulates theories as well as strategies that help a nurse develop within their practice, excel in teamwork and, most importantly, provide care to the patient with an understanding that is not judgemental in any way.

Summary

- Social facilitation leads to an improvement in performance as a result of others being present. By contrast social inhibition results in a deterioration in performance.

- An effective group will go through a developmental sequence, described by Tuckman (1965) as forming, storming, norming, performing and adjourning.

- Multi-disciplinary teamwork is essential to successful care. Such teams include integrated nursing teams and teams working with different health professionals. The Bristol Royal Infirmary Inquiry (2001) highlighted what can go wrong when working within and across multi-disciplinary teams.

- Self-esteem and professional self-esteem are the evaluative beliefs that nurses hold about themselves, which influence behaviour, motivation and care that is provided. Social identity and social comparison have the potential to affect the level of self-esteem.

- Low self-esteem is common among patients undergoing surgery, being given a new diagnosis or having medical interventions and tests carried out to confirm or establish a diagnosis. It is also common in patients who experience depression or loss of control within their life. Higgins suggests that low self-esteem is a result of a discrepancy between the actual and ideal or ought self.

- Self-awareness is important for nurses to master as it allows the nurse to develop and reflective effectively and be able to predict potential problems before they occur. The Johari window (Luft, 1969) is a self-awareness tool that can be used in practice. Objective self-awareness can be experienced when the individual is aware that they are being observed.

- Reflection is a key skill, as nurses should be competent reflective practitioners. The process enables the nurse to go beyond just describing events. Reflective framework models such as Gibbs (1988) enable the reflection process to be carried out effectively.

- Assertiveness enables an individual to express themselves with confidence and without the inappropriate use of aggressive, passive or manipulative behaviours. Assertiveness is encouraged within nursing. This is in stark contrast to passiveness, where an individual ignores his or her own rights.

- Cognitive dissonance is an unpleasant state where two pieces of information are inconsistent. As a result individuals strive to make information consistent by ignoring some information or carrying out behaviour that is contradictory to the health advice that has been given. Cognitive dissonance plays a central part in attitudes and persuasive communication. The way a message is framed, e.g. emphasising loss or gain impacts on patient health behaviour.

- Stereotyping has been defined by Schneider (2004) as 'qualities perceived to be associated with particular groups or categories of people'. Labelling is where individuals are treated according to a label, e.g. a diagnosis, and can also result in assumptions being made about the individual's feelings, thought and behaviour which originate from the label. These have negative consequences within nursing practice as Stockwell (1972) showed in her 'unpopular patient' research. One of these consequences is the self-fulfilling prophecy where individuals begin to behave according to the way they are expected to behave.

▶

● Aggression can be defined as the intentional infliction of some form of harm on others (Baron and Byrne, 2000). The frustration-aggression hypothesis (Dollard *et al.*, 1939) explores how frustration can result in aggression. There are many factors within the hospital setting and the care of the patient that can result in frustration and eventual outburst of aggression if not addressed.

● Attribution occurs when causes or explanations are provided to explain behaviour. Internal attributions occur when causes stem from the individual themselves whereas external attributions occur when causes are assigned to the environment. The fundamental attribution error (Ross, 1977) occurs when causes are attributed to internal factors alone and obvious external factors are ignored.

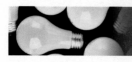

Check your understanding

1. Define attributions and explain how the nurse can make an error when attributing a cause to a patient's behaviour.

2. List four things that a nurse can do in practice when working in team to prevent the unpopular patient labelling occurring.

3. Explain how patient aggression can occur.

4. Describe different types of message framing and explain how they are important within persuasive communication.

5. Name and describe the stages outlined by Tuckman (1965) that a group will go through.

6. Give three patient scenarios where self-esteem can be low. What can a nurse do to enhance the self-esteem of the patient or ensure that the effects of low self-esteem are kept to a minimum?

7. Describe each of the stages that feature within Gibbs's reflective framework model and apply to a chosen incident in practice.

8. Which inquiry highlighted what can go wrong within and across inter- and multi-disciplinary teamwork? List three things that result in good teamwork.

9. Define and distinguish between assertiveness and passiveness within nursing practice. Which of the two is beneficial for the development of the nurse and why?

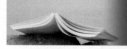

Further reading

Ferns, T. (2007) Factors that influence aggressive behaviour in acute settings. *Nursing Standard*, **21** (33), 41–45.

Foden, P. and Preston, E. (2001) Teamwork: it's the way forward. *Nursing Times*, **96** (44), 39.

Hilliard, C. (2006) Using structured reflection on a critical incident to develop a professional portfolio. *Nursing Standard*, **21** (2), 35–40.

Lawton, S. and Stewart, F. (2007) Assertiveness: making yourself heard in district nursing. *British Journal of Community Nursing*, **10** (6), 281–283.

Sherman, D.K., Mann, T. and Updegraff, S. (2006) Approach/avoidance motivation, message framing, and health behaviour: understanding the congruency effect. *Motivation and Emotion*, **30**, 165–169.

Timmins, F. and McCabe, C. (2005) How assertive are nurses in the workplace? A preliminary pilot study. *Journal of Nursing Management*, **13** (1), 61–67.

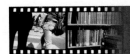

Weblinks

The Bristol Royal Infirmary Inquiry	http://www.bristol-inquiry.org.uk/	A look at the inquiry as well as recommendations.
Mountain State Centres for Independent Living	http://www.mtstcil.org/skills/assert-intro.html	The website provides an extensive coverage of assertiveness exercises and tips on assertiveness.
Rose NHS	http://www.rose.nhs.uk/Working_in_the_NHS/ Working_as_a_health_professional_in_the_NHS/ Team_work_in_the_NHS/index.html	A website dedicated to teamwork within the NHS. This site provides information on policy and resources that are related to working within a diverse range of health teams.
The University of Texas Counselling and Mental Health Centre	http://www.utexas.edu/student/cmhc/booklets/ selfesteem/selfest.html	Large amount of information on self-esteem as well as a look at enhancing self-esteem.
Gerard M. Blair: Groups	http://www.see.ed.ac.uk/~gerard/Management/ art0.html?http://oldeee.see.ed.ac.uk/~gerard/ Management/art0.html	A look at groups, group work and team dynamics.
Support 4 Learning	http://www.support4learning.org.uk/sites/ support4learning/education/learning_styles.cfm	A look at learning styles and models.

Media example

It's a Boy Girl Thing (2007) A film looking at the stereotypical gender roles that people are expected to conform to daily.

Part 2
Psychology across the lifespan and cultures

Chapter 7

Child development and health care

Learning outcomes

When you have read through this chapter you should understand:

- How children's cognitive development has been characterised by both Piaget and Vygotsky.

- Erikson's staged personality development and its application to chronic illness in adolescence and young adulthood.

- How children define and perceive health and illness and how this can be related to the stages of cognitive development.

- How an understanding of child development can be applied to a child's health and illness.

- How children react to medical and surgical procedures and how this changes across the lifespan.

- How psychological interventions can be used by the nurse with children to reduce the anxiety and stress associated with various medical procedures.

- How a knowledge of developmental processes can enhance the development of programmes designed to improve health behaviours in children.

Case study

Mrs Dahlia Patel had to rush to hospital with her middle child – Roshi – who is 5 years of age. Roshi had fallen over and cut her head open on the concrete during a playground incident at her primary school. Mrs Patel has three children in total, with a daughter of 14 being the eldest (Soha) and the youngest being an 11-month-old son, Gabe.

After falling while playing, Roshi was whisked to hospital by her mum with a deep cut to her forehead. Owing to the position of the wound it was decided that it needed to be stitched in order to close it successfully. Both Roshi and Mrs Patel were extremely and visibly anxious and Mr Patel was rushing to the hospital from his work to support them both. However, when Mrs Patel realised that she would have to decide whether her daughter would have either a local or general anaesthetic (because of the high levels of distress and anxiety) before the stitches then she became more anxious and insisted that the nurse wait until her husband arrived. When Mr Patel did arrive he cuddled Roshi and held her hand while she had three stitches inserted in her forehead under local anaesthetic. However, Roshi was distraught and cried throughout the whole procedure despite the health care staff considering it a relatively minor procedure.

The Patel family are close knit. Mr Patel works as a dentist in a local practice and his wife stays at home to care for Gabe and the other two children. Soha has been doing well at school – she would like to move into a business career when she finishes her education. Mr and Mrs Patel are, however, becoming worried about Soha's health. She has started going out with friends at the weekend and Mr Patel is sure that he can smell cigarettes and alcohol on her breath. Furthermore, her diet appears to have deteriorated so that she prefers to eat chips and burgers and is only having small portions of fruit and vegetables (certainly not achieving her five portions a day). Her parents are worried about her because it appears that she is developing a range of poor health habits. They are also worried since Soha experiences epileptic seizures and has done so since the age of 11. Her **complex partial seizures** are occurring on a weekly basis and occasionally (perhaps every 6–8 weeks) she has a secondary generalised **tonic-clonic seizure**. Not surprisingly, her parents are worried about her health behaviours and the consequence it has on both her epilepsy and her long-term health.

Soha does not see what all the fuss is about and wants to be left alone as she says it 'is her life anyway' and feels that her behaviour is perfectly adequate and like the rest of her friends. There is certainly more family strife at the moment – in previous years the family got on extremely well and the Patels were a model of family life.

Why is this relevant to nursing practice?

This case study has relevance to nursing practice on a number of different levels. The nursing of children offers a unique challenge – it cannot simply be seen as dealing with small adults. Furthermore, the stage of development of the child influences the nature of the issues that may arise, the presentation of the form of problem, and the nursing intervention and psychological care that will have to be implemented. The case study highlights such issues: Gabe is 11 months old and is at one stage of development. Roshi, the middle child, is 5 years old and can be viewed as in another stage of development. Finally, Soha is in her teens and in the middle of adolescence. According to some psychological theories, each of the Patel children is in a different stage of social, **cognitive** and individual development. Although the specific description of the nature of this development may differ among theories it is apparent that children's understanding of health changes over time and that the age of the child impacts on the approach that the nurse should take.

Think about this

Consider the three ages of the Patel children: what sorts of health behaviour and understanding of health and illness would you expect from them?

Child cognitive development

Children are not merely small versions of adults. Although this statement looks rather simplistic and obvious, it was not until the 1930s that the view of the child as a miniature adult began to be challenged. Prior to this period it was assumed that children thought in the same way as adults, but had less knowledge simply because they had less experience. Jean Piaget (1896–1980), a Swiss psychologist, was instrumental in changing this perspective. He argued that children did not simply learn through a behavioural process of punishment and reward (see Chapter 2) but that children's minds developed over time – not smoothly but in qualitatively different stages. At certain points children's thinking 'takes off' and moves into completely new areas and capabilities. These transitional stages take place at about 18 months, 7 years and 11–12 years. Each of these corresponds to certain stages of child development. Before these ages, children are incapable – irrespective of how intelligent they are – of understanding things in certain ways.

Hence, the suggestion is that an important role of development is children's increasing capacity to understand their world. Furthermore, they cannot undertake certain tasks until they are cognitively mature enough to do so. There are several theorists who propose that this development occurs in stages, and the nature of these has an impact on health care. During this chapter, these theories will be presented and how the child's stage of **maturation** influences their health, illness, behaviour and the care they should receive from health care professionals will be discussed.

Piaget's stages of cognitive development

Piaget suggested that there were four stages of **cognitive development** and that movement through the stages is **invariant**.

The sensorimotor phase

The first of Piaget's stages is the **sensorimotor** period which lasts for the first two years of an infant's life. During this time, the child is exploring and discovering the relationship between their own body and the outside environment. The infant relies on seeing, touching, sucking and feeling – using their physical sensory abilities to explore the environment and in this way learn things about themselves and the environment. Hence the term used by Piaget to describe this stage – sensorimotor – because intelligence is manifested by sensory **perceptions** and motor activities. Through a series of interactions with the environment the child explores and experiments and comes to discover that the external world is separate and distinct and not merely an extension of themselves.

Infants, at this stage, develop important understandings. Firstly, they appreciate that an object can be moved by a hand (concept of causality) and develop the notions of displacement and events. Furthermore, an important discovery by the child during the latter period of the sensorimotor stage is the concept of '**object permanence**'. This is the awareness that an object continues to exist even when it is not in view. For example, infants will lose interest in a toy when it has been covered by a cloth or hidden by a piece of paper (see picture). The child has not yet mastered the concept of object permanence – they do not appreciate that the toy still exists when it has been covered. After a child has developed object permanence (by about 8 months of age), when a toy is covered the child will actively search for the object, since they appreciate that the object continues to exist.

Object permanence is distinct from memory – babies can usually recognise and respond to their mother by the third day of life. However, they will not cry when left by their mother at this age – the mother is 'out of sight and out of mind'. When object permanence has been developed, if the mother leaves the child then they will show signs of distress – **separation anxiety**. This is because the child now appreciates what he has lost – his mother! However, there is some more recent evidence to suggest that object permanence occurs earlier than Piaget suggested and that this may be more closely related to separation (see subsequent discussion on Bowlby).

Another indication that object permanence has been achieved is the baby's enjoyment of games such as 'peek-a-boo', which demonstrates that just because the parent/guardian is out of sight she is still there and can be recalled by moving the hands or sheet out of the way.

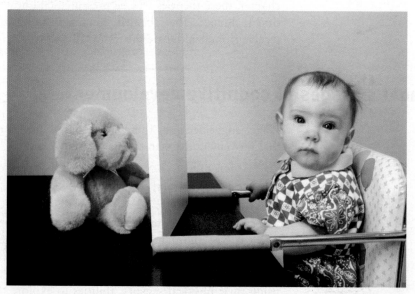

Doug Goodman/Science Photo Library

The pre-operational stage

The **pre-operational stage** occurs from 2 to 6 years of age, and is the second stage in Piaget's stages of cognitive development. During this stage the child learns to use symbols such as language. Children do not yet understand concrete logic, but are adept at using concrete symbolism (are able to use an object to represent something, for example a stick as a gun) and are still **ego-centric** – they are unable to take the point of view of others.

One of the techniques used by Piaget to confirm his theory was the three mountains task. Children are shown a scene (three mountains) and then asked to recognise a picture of the scene from where they are sitting – they can correctly do this. When children are then asked to select a picture that shows what someone else would have observed when looking at the scene from a different viewpoint they cannot do so – invariably children select a scene showing their own view. They cannot do this, according to Piaget, because they are egocentric. However, subsequent research has indicated that if the child is allowed to walk around a three-dimensional model they find the task easier. As we will see later, this highlights the need of the nurse to use concrete rather than abstract language in order to explain any procedures.

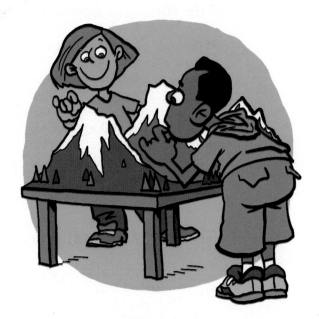

Another well-known group of experiments to demonstrate cognitive development in children devised by Piaget were the so-called **tests of conservation**. For example, in one experiment children are shown equal amounts of liquid poured into two identical containers which is then transferred into a different-shaped cup – for example a tall thin cup or a short wide cup. Children are then asked which cup holds the most liquid: they invariably select the cup that appears the fuller despite the fact that they have seen the same amount of liquid poured into the different shaped cups. Piaget conducted a number of similar experiments on conservation of number, length, mass, weight, volume and quantity. Piaget found that few children showed any understanding of conservation prior to the age of 5.

An example of one of
Piaget's tests of
conservation

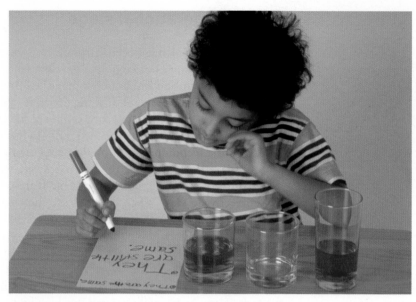

© Laura Dwight/CORBIS

The concrete operational stage

Piaget suggested that between the ages of 7 and 12 the **concrete operational stage** is reached. During this stage, the child begins to think logically and organise thoughts more coherently. However, they can only think concretely – i.e. about actual physical objects – rather than handle *abstract* reasoning. This stage is characterised by the loss of egocentric thinking and they begin to think of others and appreciate that their actions have an impact on both themselves and others.

At this stage the child has the ability to master most conversation experiments, and begins to understand reversibility (i.e. the ability to see physical transformations and then imagine reversing them so that the change is cancelled out).

The formal operational stage

The fourth and final stage is the formal operational stage which begins at approximately 11–12 years of age and continues into adulthood (however, Piaget does suggest that some people may never reach this stage of cognitive development). The formal operational stage is characterised by more abstract thinking – the ability to formulate hypotheses and systematically test them out in order to address clear problems. For example, children can answer abstract problems about 'What would happen if …' or understand the finer meanings of death and dying (see later in this chapter).

Movement through the stages

Piaget suggests that there are five interrelated factors that allow movement through the stages:

● *Maturation*: Physical (and especially neurological) growth and change.

- *Physical experience*: interaction with objects in the environment.
- *Logico-mathematical experience*: creating relationships between objects, experiences and ideas.
- *Social transmission*: the communication of information about concepts – particularly from other children.
- *Equilibrium*: This last factor occurs when maturation, experience and social transmission come together in order to build **mental schema** (i.e. mental representations of concepts, ideas, etc).

Relatively recently there has been criticism of Piagetian research which suggests that this theory underestimates children's reasoning abilities, partly because of the limited consideration that it gives to the social context of children's understanding and behaviour (Carey, 1985). That is, it neglects the wider world and how children learn from others and their environment.

Think about this

How can knowledge of Piaget's developmental stages be used when dealing with a child in a health care context?

Vygotsky's social development theory of learning

Another theory of child cognitive development is that of Lev Vygotsky (1896–1934) who proposed the social constructivist theory of learning, suggesting that social interaction influences cognitive development. Vygotsky suggested that development is a continual, life-long process, rather than a set of stages with a predefined end point which is reached in early adolescence. According to Vygotsky, this process starts at birth and continues until death and cannot be defined by stages owing to the complexity of development.

Vygotsky suggested that social interaction and social learning leads to cognitive development. He deemed this the **zone of proximal development** which he defined as 'the distance between the actual development level as determined by independent problem solving and the level of potential development as determined through problem solving under adult guidance or in collaboration with more capable peers' (Vygotsky, 1978). In other words, a task under adult guidance or with peer collaboration can be better achieved than those attempted alone.

The concept of the 'zone of proximal development' has been extremely influential in education – from primary school through to higher education. For example, it has been used to encourage group peer tutoring, where those with better skills help those with weaker skills. Bruner (1983) has used the term '**scaffolding**' to highlight how the more knowledgeable 'teacher' modifies the amount of help required by the child on the basis of the child's response so that the child develops and learns more.

Applying this to health, illness and health care suggests that some children may have a better understanding in some areas because of opportunities to engage socially with others and receive guidance. This may be why children with chronic illnesses may be more advanced developmentally in their knowledge about the illnesses and associated procedures (e.g. drugs, treatments and consequences). For example, a child with a chronic illness may appear 'wise beyond their years' because of the eloquence and knowledge with which they speak about their condition and its treatment – a result of the interaction with others concerned with the condition.

Think about this

How would a self-group for children help with their understanding of their conditions? How can this be related to Vygotsky's theory of development?

Overall, therefore, various theories of cognitive development would suggest that, not surprisingly, the child's knowledge and understanding have to be taken into account when preparing them for health-related interventions – whether these be surgical, medical, behavioural or gaining consent for treatment. On the basis of Piaget's conceptualisation then it could be predicted that children's understanding relates to their cognitive developmental stage (roughly equivalent to their age). Vygotsky, in contrast, would suggest that understanding will differ according to social experience and opportunities to interact with others. The key thing, Vygotsky proposes, is to find out what the child understands already and to build on that.

Erikson's theory of personality development

Another theory we should briefly consider is that of Erik Erikson (1902–1994) who explored **personality** development (rather than cognitive, or thinking, development). He suggested that there are eight unique stages in human personality development, beginning at birth and extending to late adulthood. At each stage different psychological (or social-emotional) crises occur. In order for a successful adult personality to emerge, the individual must resolve each of these conflicts. The success or otherwise of these resolutions depends on the emotional quality of the individual's social environments.

In brief the eight stages (and crises) are as follows:

- *Stage 1*: Trust versus mistrust (infancy). Responsive and sensitive parenting is required in the first year of life otherwise a mistrustful and sceptical teenager will result who, as a consequence, may reject the suggestions of perceived authority figures such as nurses.
- *Stage 2*: Autonomy versus shame and doubt (toddlerhood). A toddler's independence needs to be supported or they could grow into a teenager without a basic sense of responsibility. Hence, dealing with a chronic illness may then become problematic because of a lack of the control necessary to provide good self-care.
- *Stage 3*: Initiative versus guilt (preschool years). The world needs to be full of rich experiences and positive guidance during the preschool years in order to acquire a sense of curiosity, ambition and empathy.

- *Stage 4*: Industry versus inferiority (school-age years). If the child experiences limited success at school then they can develop into somebody who feels incompetent and inferior and their options may be limited.
- *Stage 5*: Identity versus role confusion (adolescence). During this stage, the teenager should demonstrate a range of behaviours in order to develop positive development as a competent adult.
- *Stage 6*: Intimacy versus isolation (early adulthood). People should develop close relationships and those who are successful will develop good relationships in the future. If not then they are likely to develop emotional isolation and depression.
- *Stage 7*: Generativity versus stagnation (adulthood). During this stage we focus on our career and family. Those that fail during this stage will feel unproductive and uninvolved in the world.
- *Stage 8*: Integrity versus despair (old age). This stage involves a reflection on past life. Those feeling unsuccessful will feel their life has been wasted and will experience regrets and despair.

Erikson argued that successful adaptation is a consequence of successful accomplishment of the eight stage tasks. For example, in the first year of life the baby needs to develop a trusting relationship with another person, usually the mother; if a relationship is established, that is considered to be a successful outcome.

Think about this

How could Erikson's theory be applied to the adaptation of Soha to her illness? How could it be applied to others with a chronic illness (e.g. epilepsy) developing at different ages?

Attachment

Close relationships with the mother (or other primary caregiver) of the child are essential for successful development (and indeed survival in humans) and consequently studies of **attachment** (and separation) have taken a number of forms in psychology. The early behavioural approach to the study of attachment was to take an **operant conditioning** perspective (see Chapter 2) and viewed the attachment process occurring because the mother provided essential reinforcement for the child in terms of food and comfort. However, a classic animal experiment by Harlow (1959) suggested that this was not an adequate explanation. During this experiment rhesus monkeys showed a preference for soft physical contact with an inanimate object even if it did not deliver milk. Furthermore, these experiments demonstrated that female monkeys that had no previous experience of receiving mothering made poor mothers subsequently. These studies demonstrated that attachment is an important prerequisite for normal social development, although more recent work suggests that this attachment does not have to be to the mother; it is the sensitivity and responsiveness of the relationship that matters most for development.

Harlow's research: an infant rhesus monkey cuddles an artificial mother

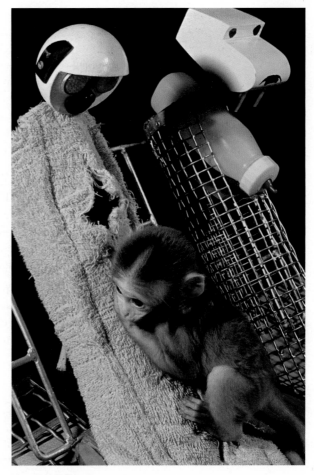

Time & Life Pictures/Getty Images

The name most associated with studies of attachment is that of John Bowlby (1969) who noted that babies exhibit a number of behaviours that have a survival value, since the behaviours ensure that the parents (or caregivers) support their basic needs. For example, crying, babbling and smiling reinforce the parents' behaviours and clinging, and suckling (whether gaining milk or not) encourage the mother to protect the child. Bowlby's theory is based on an interactional model which, as the name suggests, proposes that attachment is dependent on the interaction between the mother and the child rather than being simply dependent on either the infant's or the mother's behaviour. For example, a depressed mother may not respond appropriately to a child's behaviour. Similarly, a premature child may not produce appropriate responses that will elicit an adult attachment response.

By the age of 7–12 months, Bowlby noted 'separation anxiety' in babies in as much that they become distressed in the absence of their mother. Before the 1960s mothers were asked to leave their children in hospital and stay away. This was because children became distressed every time their mother was asked to leave – so the logic was get them to leave just once! As a result of various studies (notably the seminal studies of the Robinsons during the 1950s) from the 1960s onwards, studies suggested that children's units reverse their policies, and now mother's are encouraged to stay (if possible) during the duration of the child's admission.

Think about this

What do Bowlby's studies suggest for the care of children with a chronic illness, particularly those who require considerable time in hospital? How does this alter with the age of the child?

Cognitive development and an understanding of illness

How does an understanding of the developmental stages proposed by Piaget relate to child's concepts of health and illness? Previous research has linked Piaget's stages of cognitive development to children's beliefs about illness (Bibace and Walsh, 1980). From a nursing and health care perspective, research on children's understanding of illness can help generate age-appropriate explanations of illness by children. This is especially pertinent in nursing settings as children may display unnecessary fear, guilt and anxiety before receiving treatment for illness (Myant and Williams, 2005). The reasons for this should become clear if we consider the early stages suggested by Piaget and how these to relate to a child's understanding of illness.

- *Pre-operational stage (2–6 years)*: At this stage children are seen as having limited logic and are highly egocentric. Consequently, children's beliefs about illness are vague with fear and often superstitious. They cannot grasp the finality of death, for example. Myant and Williams (2005) reported that those children in the pre-operational age answered 'don't know' about the understanding of illness or linking it to some behavioural factors.
- *Concrete operational stage (7–12 years)*: At this stage logical reasoning ability develops and children begin to understand that ill-health and death have biological causes. They appreciate the links between thinking and ill-health and the link between the biological causes and the symptoms. Myant and Williams (2005) found that those children between the ages of 9 and 10 gave definitions of health related to absence of illness, whereas those 11–12-year-olds moved away from illness-related definitions based on health related behaviours (an interesting link with definitions of health covered in Chapter 1 can be made). They also begin to recognise the risks (in the short term) of their own behaviour and the impact that this may have on their illness/health. In contrast, the long-term outcomes of their behaviour are understood less (Eiser, 1997). However, by the end of this stage children begin to understand that death is final and they begin to understand their own mortality.

Mental illness and child development

Understanding the distinction between mental and physical illness appears to develop progressively (Buchanan-Barrow *et al.*, 2005). However, Buchanan-Barrow *et al.* (2005) suggest that understanding the causes and consequences of mental and physical illness does not progress developmentally and that the 'representation of physical illnesses are established in early childhood' but not for mental illness. For example, all children from the age of 5 described the cause of a cold as being caught and needing to see the doctor or rest as a consequence. In contrast, the understanding of mental illness was developmentally different. Younger children considered mental illness to be 'caught', while, for example, older children considered dementia to be 'something wrong with her brain'. Similarly, with anorexia, the older group were more likely than the young or the middle groups to respond that 'it's to do with how she thinks and feels' (young = 43 per cent; middle = 43 per cent, old = 76 per cent; Buchanan-Barrow *et al.*, 2005, p. 18). There was a similar pattern of development of the understanding of the different consequences of mental and physical illness. Overall this suggests that children develop an understanding of health and illness (particularly mental illness) as their own experience grows (Buchanan-Barrow *et al.*, 2005).

Admission to hospital

When a child enters hospital they are removed from their safe home environment to an environment that is both unusual and frightening (see Chapter 18 for further details of the stresses and strains of entering hospital). Furthermore the child may not be able to associate the illness with the hospital and the need and expectation of getting better. This lack of understanding and inability to communicate much may result in the child believing that entering hospital is a punishment, which leads to psychological distress and disturbance. Roshi, for example, was rushed to hospital because of her fall and consequent injury. Many children that come to the A&E department, like Roshi, require a brief but painful procedure. This pain, coupled with the stress and anxiety associated with entering the hospital, can make the whole experience considerably more unpleasant for the child. This may, of course, impact on the child's behaviour so they become stressed and uncooperative. Therefore, the nurse has an important role to play in reducing the negative consequences of hospital emergency admission.

Think about this

What sort of behaviours do you think Roshi would present when she enters hospital, and how should the nurse deal with these?

As we have noted, the child entering hospital through the A&E department can be stressed, anxious and upset and the nurse has an important role to play in reducing the negative consequences of the emergency admissions, which may also have long-term psychological consequences (Williams, 1995). When we look at the individual child we need to consider the child's stage of development as suggested by Piaget. For example, Roshi is 5 years of age and therefore in the pre-operational phase. As we have seen, during this phase, children have difficulty in distinguishing real from unreal and events are often seen as magical and surreal. Children of this age are more likely to be concerned with surface features of illness or injury – an explanation of why children (Roshi included) often insist on plasters or bandages even though these may not be required.

If we apply Piaget's theoretical framework in preparing Roshi for the suturing it is essential that the nurse both chooses and uses appropriate words and phrases in order to improve understanding: for example, using short sentences and simple explanations, and describing the injury/treatment in terms of how it would affect the child herself. The nurse should also closely observe the child to review the non-verbal messages that they may be expressing. Furthermore, the nurse should encourage the child to express their own feelings about the planned care and the injury itself.

If we apply Vygotsky's approach we would predict that the child's understanding will be based on the nature and extent of their previous experiences. Hence, it is not simply a consequence of the age of the child. In this case Roshi had not been to hospital before but her dad is a dentist and hence she was used to seeing masks and gowns. Furthermore, the theory suggests that the nurse should 'scaffold' information – build on the current information, knowledge and understanding of the child.

The role of the family

Obviously Mr and Mrs Patel have a role to play with their daughter during her time in the A&E department. Reviews of the literature have, not surprisingly, revealed that the parents of children entering hospital experience intense stress and feelings of helplessness when their children undergo minor (as the nursing and medical staff may see it) procedures (e.g. Brennan, 1994). Lack of understanding about the upcoming procedures, uncertainty with the environment and uncertainty over the injury/illness and its treatment are some of the major factors contributing to parental stress. The Patels were encouraged to remain with Roshi throughout her stay in the department for a number of reasons. At the most basic, parents can provide the necessary information required by the nursing and medical staff in order to help the child with the injury or condition. They can also provide nurses with an insight into the child's individual needs, fears and coping behaviours and help to identify ways in which they can help their child. However, there may also be some negative consequences of the parents remaining. Young children are often perceptive of their parents' behaviour and feelings, so they could pick up on either anxiety and fear, or the complete opposite. Hence, the nurse should spend some time with the parents reassuring them and ensuring they fully understand the situation in order to reduce their anxiety and fears – especially as these could be transmitted to the child. Furthermore, the nurse should be aware of the important role that parents play in management of a child's illness – it has been shown that it is the parents' perception of their child's health and well-being that has the greatest influence on the utilisation of health care services (Varni *et al.*, 2001)

Obviously the role of the parent in caring for their child when admitted to hospital is important but should be fully negotiated – parents have to be involved but have to agree to be involved. Some parents may not be able to help and then feel guilty and helpless if the nurse (or some other health care professional) presses them to become involved.

Think about this

What role do Roshi's parents have in increasing or decreasing her anxiety? What role has Mrs Patel played in increasing the anxiety? How could the nurse help Mrs Patel, and consequently her daughter?

Admission to hospital

When entering a hospital, therefore, it is essential to provide information for both the child and the parents in order to reduce the anxiety associated with the admission. Programmes for preparing parents and children for admission should include (Siegel and Conte, 2001):

- information provision;
- encouragement of emotional expression;
- establishment of a positive relationship between child and staff;
- providing the parents with information; and
- encouraging the development of **coping strategies**.

It is important to include the parents when devising the type of information presented since reducing anxiety in the parent can result in better coping for the child, and consequent quicker recovery and better outcomes. Chambers *et al.* (2002) report that those children whose mothers had been better prepared cried less and recovered more quickly following minor surgery. Furthermore, the relationship between the child and the parent has been implicated in the child's experience of hospitalisation (Carson *et al.*, 1991), being related to three factors: separation (or not) from the parent, the quality of the parent–child relationship and the behaviour of the parent in the situation. If a parent stays with the child, there is a strong relationship between the child and parent, and the parent is supportive and non-anxious, then the child responds better to the hospitalisation (Siegel and Conte, 2001). The link between such behaviours and those observed by Bowlby (as described above) is evident.

Think about this

How can the work of Bowlby be applied to the separation anxiety expressed by mothers/ children during hospitalisation? What relevance has this for nursing?

The experience of pain

As we have noted in Chapter 14, the experience of pain is complex and associated with psychological, social and biological factors. The experience, understanding and interventions aimed at reducing pain are similarly complex. How these differ between adults and children is important and has been the focus of many studies. Gafney and Dunne (1986) suggest that children's understanding of pain develops over time in accord with the cognitive development stages of Piaget. They found three categories of response which matched the pre-operational, concrete and formal operational stages. Subsequent research by Harbeck and Peterson (1992) supported this contention that there was a developmental continuum of defining (and reporting) pain.

There is evidence to suggest that children are less likely than adults to receive adequate analgesia in some hospital interventions because of the adult's conceptions of pain and their understanding of the children's pain. For example, Sahinler (2002) notes that there is a series of myths associated with childhood pain including:

- children do not feel pain;
- children do not remember pain;
- **analgesics** can do more harm than good;
- addressing and treating pain takes too much time;
- pain builds character;
- children are at increased risk for addiction to **narcotics**.

In terms of fear of pain, Albano *et al.* (2001) suggest that fear of death, serious illness and pain emerges only in later life (13–18 years) but that this is different for those children that have experienced pain, surgery or some form of health problem in early childhood.

The experience of pain can be influenced by many different factors (see Chapter 14) but is strongly influenced by understanding and communication including the non-verbal cues provided by significant others (Cohen, 2002). Chambers *et al.* (2002) highlighted that a child's experience of pain and fear may reflect the anxiety and fear in the mother, and consequently can impact upon the recovery from surgery.

McCarthy and Kleiber (2006) developed a model of **psychosocial** factors associated with pain, and how parents can influence these factors, for either better or worse (see Figure 7.1). For example, looking at the social factors highlighted in the model, there is extensive evidence that toddlers and pre-school-aged children (particularly under 8 years of age) demonstrate the most behavioural distress and pain during medical procedures. Similarly, evidence suggests that girls display more expressive responses such as crying and clinging and may report more pain, whereas boys use different forms of behaviour and report less pain (McCarthy and Kleiber, 2006; Rudolph *et al.*, 1995).

Other variables indicated in the model include procedural variables such as the difficulty of the procedure – for example, the more attempts at stitching or inserting a cannula, the greater the distress in the child and increase in anxiety. Obviously the ability of the nurse (or other health care professional) with these procedures is also considerably important and a lack of experience and skill can increase anxiety and, consequently, pain.

The family and, in particular, the parents can play an important role in their child's experience of pain (Chambers *et al.*, 2003). Parental variables that can affect a child's response include their ethnicity, their child's sex (parents are more likely to use distracting activities with girls), previous experience and belief that the intervention will be helpful, parenting style and parental anxiety.

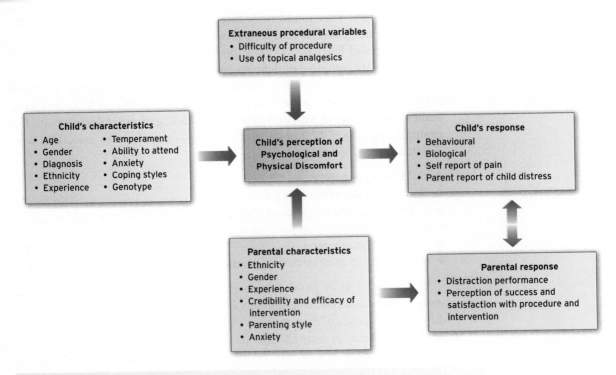

Figure 7.1 Model of factors influencing children's responses to painful procedure.

Source: McCarthy and Kleiber (2006)

Think about this

Explore the case study – what factors could influence Roshi's experience of pain? What methods could be used to reduce anxiety and pain in Roshi?

Reducing pain in children

Since the mid-1980s, health care professionals have begun to recognise the importance of reducing pain and emotional distress during medical and surgical procedures in children through non-pharmacological methods. Such interventions include those procedures used before (e.g. providing education), during (e.g. **distraction**) and following the procedure (e.g. positive reinforcement). Although preparation can decrease anxiety associated with the unknown and unexpected, it does not teach the child coping strategies to use during the stressful procedure (Jay, 1988).

There are a number of ways of using non-pharmacological methods to improve pain management in the child including: explanation of the procedure using age-appropriate pictures, diagrams and language; touring the facilities if the procedure is planned; watching a DVD of the procedure (in adolescents), and playing through a procedure with dolls or a demonstration on a doll for younger children. A number of interventions have been found helpful for children during painful procedures including distraction (Sander Wint *et al.*, 2002), **controlled breathing** (Lal *et al.*, 2001) and **imagery** (Pederson, 1995). Each of these interventions involves helping the child focus attention on something other than the painful procedure and can, therefore, be more simply described as a distraction technique.

Distraction

Distraction is a form of psychological intervention that takes attention from an unpleasant stimulus by redirecting the subject's attention or by actively involving the subject in the performance of a diversion task (Fernandez, 1986). Distraction involves capturing the child's attention and focusing it away from the stressful situation and towards something more pleasant. There are a number of advantages to using distraction: it requires little training, is easy to apply, requires little specialist equipment, and is familiar to most. Furthermore, distraction may be particularly appealing to parents because it requires little practice and can be incorporated into play. However, it should be noted that the most effective distraction technique is interactive, varied and engages the child's motor responses (Dahlquist *et al.*, 2002). Examples of distracters used with children are picture books, talking, music, party blowers, kaleidoscopes, pop-up books, blowing bubbles, looking for hidden objects in the room, counting out loud, handheld computer games, imagining fun and exciting things, or quiet and relaxing scenes. There is now considerable research that supports the contention that distraction can reduce pain and distress (e.g. Manimala *et al.*, 2000).

Parents as coaches

Getting parents to act as 'distraction facilitators' or 'distraction coaches' is an appealing development – it takes the pressure off the nurse and other health care staff, and it allows for the parent and family to be actively involved with their child and their treatment. Parents sometimes report feeling like 'spare parts' since they want to remain with their children but do not what to do (e.g. Simons *et al.*, 2001). When involving parents it is important for the nurse or the health care professional to provide some guidance to the parent. The parent may provide reassurance and guidance to the child rather than distraction (Cohen *et al.*, 2002). However, parents can learn how to distract their children cheaply and quickly and they can start to use it almost immediately and in a variety of situations. Thus, distraction is a versatile, inexpensive intervention that parents can use to help their children during stressful events and it benefits both the child and the parent.

Kleiber *et al.* (2001) reported that parents were able to learn distraction techniques and to perform such techniques with their children quickly and easily during intravenous line insertion. Other studies have reported on the use of parent distraction on child distress and pain during child immunisation. Results have indicated that child distress scores were significantly better for treatment groups (e.g. Blount *et al.*, 1992), verbalised pain was decreased (Manimala *et al.*, 2000) and self-reported pain was lower (Cohen *et al.*, 1997).

Think about this

What techniques could the nurse, or the parents use with Roshi in order to reduce her anxiety and pain while she has her stitches inserted?

Children's response to illness

Eiser (1990) identified three major factors in children's response to illness. The first factor is related to the degree to which the illness is life-threatening and disruptive to daily routine. The second factor is related to understanding the cause of the illness, with better understanding leading, not surprisingly, to better adjustment and coping. The third and final factor is the support received from the family in terms of both open communication and expressiveness.

When providing information about the illness and the treatment, there are several factors that have to be considered by the nurse. Firstly, children differ in the amount of information they want and this may vary according to the type of medical procedure and how long the child has experienced the illness. For example, those children that have had an illness for some time may prefer more information about the interventions and consequences of the illness and the treatment (Siegel and Conte, 2001). Furthermore, the amount and type of information provided by the nurse will vary according to the age of the child and the stage of development they are at. The medium through which the information is presented will also differ. Finally, the information should match the preferred coping style of the child.

A number of surveys have indicated that there may be psychosocial adjustment problems in children with chronic medical conditions (e.g. Gortmaker *et al.*, 1990). There may be a number of contributing factors to this increased risk – the severity of the condition, duration of the condition, the social physical and emotional impairment, the perceived stress and the negative life events (Immelt, 2006). However, psychosocial factors can influence the impact of the chronic illness-coping strategies, **social support** and perceptions and **illness behaviours** (Butz, 1995).

Think about this

How would you suggest Soha be helped to cope with her illness?

Improving adjustment to childhood chronic illness

Studies have indicated (Immelt, 2006) that a key method for improving children's adjustment may be the perception of both the parent and the child of the illness. Maternal worry and maternal perception of the impact of the disease on her family have been shown to be the strongest predictors of maternal reported psychological adjustment. However, others involved with the child, whether these be health care staff or extended family, can also have a significant impact on the child's adjustment to their illness.

Nurses are increasingly regarded as among the most important care providers for children with chronic conditions and their families (Balling and McCubbin, 2001). As such, they are in a position to teach, guide and promote the empowerment of these children. They can deal with the routine care associated with the chronic condition – routine monitoring, medication administration and so on – and are also available to provide guidance to both the child and the parent to help them adjust to the chronic illness.

Immelt (2006) suggested that the nurse's role (along with other health care professionals) should emphasise positive characteristics of both the condition and the individual child. For example, to try to promote positive self-perceptions in important domains for school-aged children, asking about favourite activities, favourite subjects, best friends, games, holidays, pets and so on may be just as valuable to the child's long-term adjustment as asking the child about their condition, their treatment and medication regimes. Obviously if the nurse listens to the parents then useful information can be gleaned about the condition and how it impacts on the individual and the family. Similarly, those families that are not functioning can be identified and helped. Nurses can develop and encourage access to psychologically based interventions and these can promote adjustment to the long-term condition (e.g. Chernoff *et al.*, 2002; Drotar, 1997; Ireys *et al.*, 2001). More importantly, useful information on managing the disease and how family adjustment can be promoted can also be provided.

Children's adherence to treatment

Chapter 16 highlights the poor levels of concordance with treatment (the terminology associated with **concordance**, **adherence** or **compliance** is outlined and discussed in Chapter 16) and this can range across both conditions and forms of treatment. The level of non-adherence has been estimated to lie between 25 and 50 per cent (approximately 60 per cent over-using and 10 per cent under-using) depending on the type of population studied and the method used for study (Riekert and Drotar, 2000). A significant proportion of patients do not follow medical advice and this may be related to the lack of understanding/recollection of the medical consultation. Influential factors include presenting information that is too detailed or in a manner that is too technical for either the parent or the child to understand and digest. This may be further confused by the health care professional if they do not check the understanding of the child or the parent. Obviously there are other variables that influence the recall of medical information and the willingness or ability to act upon the medical advice – for example the nature of the interaction, the trust of the child/parent holds in the health care practitioner, the patient's/parent's beliefs about the illness, the treatment involved and how it was explained and so on (see Chapters 1 and 16).

For children with a chronic illness, adherence to a medical regiment is of key importance and it is essential that the value of the treatment is stressed to the child, but without increasing anxiety and worry. In terms of improving adherence in children DiMatteo (2000) made a number of recommendations:

- The nurse should ensure that the child and parent fully understand what they are being asked to do: better knowledge and understanding equate to better adherence.
- If the parent or child lacks knowledge about the treatment then adherence is likely to be poor.
- The health professional needs to understand the commitment of both the child and the parent to the treatment.

There is a need to reduce the barriers to adherence. This may involve practical help in developing a routine, or in developing coping resources. This may necessitate the development of links between family, school and the health care settings (Rand, 2002). Obviously, the younger the child, the greater the need for developmentally appropriate parent–child partnerships (e.g. in terms of who should be responsible for and administer the medication) and the nurse should be aware of this.

Think about this

How can Soha's adherence to treatment be improved? How would the approach you use with Soha differ if she were younger?

Biopsychosocial model of adolescent development

Adolescence is a transitional developmental period between childhood and adulthood. This stage in development can have considerable biological, psychological and social role changes and probably more of such changes than any other stage of life except infancy (Lerner *et al.*, 1999). Given the magnitude of such changes, it is not surprising that there are also significant differences in the types and frequency of health problems during adolescence compared to childhood (Rutter, 1980a). An organising framework for understanding adolescent adaptation and adjustment is shown in Figure 7.2.

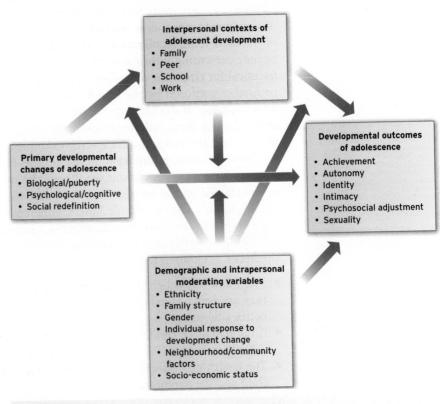

Figure 7.2 Framework for understanding adolescent development and adjustment

Source: Holmbeck and Shapera (1999)

Health during adolescence

Adolescence is a key time for the development of positive health behaviours (e.g. diet and exercise), along with the emergence of health risk behaviours (e.g. smoking, unsafe sex practices and drug use). Thus, the period of adolescence is a good time for primary prevention.

Furthermore, the major causes of ill-health during adolescence are different from those in adulthood so it is important to develop specific targets and intervention practices in order to improve mortality and morbidity. Finally, in an adolescent with a chronic illness the transition from childhood to young adulthood is of key importance for disease implications in later life.

Primary prevention in adolescence

During adolescence the goal of primary prevention is to intervene to alter health risk behaviours *before* they have begun. Given the difficulty in changing engrained negative health behaviours it is better to prevent the risk behaviours from developing in the first place. The major causes of adult mortality (e.g. cancer, heart disease and stroke) have many risk factors associated with behaviours, for example smoking, alcohol use, exercise and dietary habits (see Chapter 12). Such behaviours usually begin and are established during adolescence (Chassin *et al.*, 1996).

From Figure 7.2 we can note that the important others involved with the adolescent include the family, peers, school and work environments – all of which offer the opportunity for preventative interventions. However, some of those listed may be more amenable to interventions than others. For example, peer relationships within the school environment may be one particular focus. A number of exemplary school-based prevention programmes exist that have targeted a variety of adolescent health behaviours, including the prevention of smoking, alcohol use, drug use and early sexual behaviour, and health problems due to poor diet and exercise habits, sexual behaviour, HIV risk reduction, pregnancy, cigarette and marijuana use, alcohol use, exercise promotion and cardiovascular health. Hence, some studies have suggested that improving peer relationships may prove beneficial in improving health behaviours and, for example, recruiting non-smoking adolescents to act as health educators/promoters among their smoking peers (Garrison *et al.*, 2003).

Developmental considerations when considering interventions

When attempting to define target interventions it is important to select appropriate age ranges because of the developmental changes that occur throughout childhood. For example, it could be argued that smoking/obesity, etc. prevention should be directed towards 11- and 12-year-old children and their families for several reasons. First, the body image of children of this age is more malleable as are attitudes towards eating and illness. Hence, although adolescents may struggle with a negative body image and unhealthy eating patterns, the body image of younger children may be more flexible and prevention more likely to succeed (Kater *et al.*, 2002). Secondly, from the age of 11 or 12, children become more autonomous in their health-related self-management behaviours (Pradel *et al.*, 2001). There is also some indication that children's health **locus of control** (see Chapter 1) is at its maximum during the transition into adolescence (Cohen *et al.*, 1990). This is, of course, in line with Piagetian cognitive developmental theory. At the stage of 11 or 12, children are entering the 'formal operational' stage (Piaget, 1972) and are developing the skill of abstract thought. Consequently, children at this cognitive stage can begin to imagine the potential consequences (both positive and negative) to a specific health behaviour, which as a result allows them to assume a more internal locus of control.

What should be remembered about Piaget's cognitive stages is that although most children reach each of the stages by the specific ages suggested, not all do. Hence, although most children reach the formal operations stage by the age of 11 or 12, not all children will automatically move to this stage as they biologically mature. However, in constrast, some estimates suggest that only about a third of children enter this stage by the age of 12 years (Kuhn *et al.*, 1977). Consequently, it could be argued that the developments of theory-based interventions (e.g. using the **transtheoretical model** – see Chapter 15) aimed at preventing health-damaging behaviours (e.g. poor diet, smoking, alcohol) may be problematic for many 11- and 12-year-olds since they are unable to think abstractly about 'change' and to consider the possible outcomes of the situation. This being said, however, these issues can be addressed by ensuring age-appropriate language in any intervention obtaining examples from children on how they would change their behaviour.

A final concern is that the negative consequences of poor health behaviour may be too far in the future for a pre-formal operational child to imagine (e.g. imagining long-term lung cancer or heart disease as a consequence of smoking). Children may therefore need some definite and immediate examples for them to consider before they will make their change in behaviour. To deal with this the nurse could ask the child to provide personally relevant examples to ensure they understand the concepts being introduced. It is also important to focus on issues that are most important to children at this age such as body image (e.g. smoking gives you bad skin and makes you smell when kissing).

Think about this

What sort of language and methods would you use to try and promote healthy behaviours in children such as Soha and Roshi?

Involving the family

Parental involvement in any child health programme is essential (Trost *et al.*, 2003). One reason for this is that poor health behaviour tends to 'run in families' – children who smoke are more likely to have parents who smoke, or obese parents tend to have obese children, for example. It would be counterproductive to try to implement intervention programmes for children if the parents are modelling or supporting unhealthy lifestyle behaviours such as overeating, smoking or not exercising. Parents also play an important role in accessing such positive health behaviours, for example removing poor food

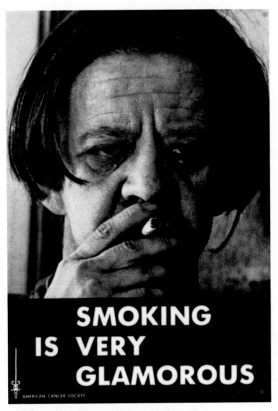

Image courtesy of The Advertising Archives

choices from the home, increasing the child's access to physical activities, or engaging in family leisure-time physical activities. Parents can also be involved in **behavioural methods** to reward their child's efforts at building healthy behaviours by reinforcing healthy choices – fitness regimes, or healthy eating for example (Faith *et al.*, 2001).

Overall, the research literature has suggested that outcomes for any health-based intervention are considerably better when both parents and children are targeted and reinforced, compared with when the child is targeted alone, particularly when obesity prevention programmes are considered (e.g. Faith *et al.*, 2001). Such programmes will involve a range of activities including:

- getting started: goal setting, self-efficacy;
- changing health behaviours;
- charting and monitoring goals;
- having fun working towards health goals;
- health basics (e.g. information on consequences of poor diet, five-a-day fruit and vegetable consumption, or smoking/alcohol abuse consequences);
- self-monitoring of progress;
- maintaining improvement.

Think about this

How could your knowledge of child development be used to devise a programme to improve health behaviours of all the Patel children? Ensure that you involve both Mr and Mrs Patel.

In conclusion, therefore, the development of changing health behaviour intervention packages must be guided by the cognitive development stage of the child, and an understanding of Piaget and other child development theorists is both essential. Furthermore, the involvement of the child's wider social environment particularly the family is important and essential for the success of any intervention.

Death and dying and the child

Irrespective of age, every child will have a perspective on death gathered from a range of experiences whether from real-life experiences or as depicted in the media (e.g. cartoons, films and books). The family's perception of death and dying and their associated fears and anxieties are also important for defining the culture for the child, along with possibly transferring some misconceptions and fears about death and dying. Hence, as has been emphasised throughout the chapter, the family must be worked with by all health care professionals involved in the care of the child. Furthermore, when dealing with a terminally ill child, the individualisation of care is of key importance (probably more so than in any other area of nursing). However, the developmental age of the child is important for their thinking and processing of information about death and dying. For example, we can apply Piaget's stages to a child's concept of death and dying:

- *Sensorimotor stage (0–2 years)*: An infant will have no real concept of death. However, they will react to separation from parents, painful procedures and alterations in care routines. Therefore, a dying child will require consistent physical and emotional care and the maintenance of an established routine (which can also be important for parents).
- *Pre-operational (2–6 years)*: Again, death has little meaning for the toddler although they pick up anxiety from the emotional responses of those around them and become sad, depressed or fearful. The terms 'death' or 'forever' have no real meaning and death is not seen as a permanent condition. Concrete language has to be used and the terms 'sleep' and 'passed away' should not be used as they can be misconstrued. Towards the end of this stage, death begins to be seen as something to be feared (a view picked up from their parents). However, death is still not seen as permanent but is viewed as reversible (as in cartoons).
- *Concrete operational (7–12 years)*: During this stage, children begin to understand the concept of death more clearly – that it may be permanent, irreversible, universal and inevitable. Fear of the unknown, loss of control and separation from family and friends can be the school-aged child's main sources of anxiety and fear. It is important to be honest and open with the child in order to provide consistent and accurate information.
- *Formal operation/adolescence (12+ years)*: Adolescence is a time of identity, independence and relationship establishment. During this period an adolescent may begin to feel immortal or exempt from death and hence, with the realisation of their forthcoming death a terminal adolescent may no longer belong or fit with their peers or communicate effectively with those closest around them (i.e. their family). Consequently, they may want to discuss death with a friend or someone other than a parent or member of their family. The nurse needs to encourage communication in any manner.

Research in focus

Brewer, S., Gleditsch, S.L., Syblik, D., Tietjens, M.E. and Vacik, H.W. (2006) Paediatric anxiety: child life intervention in day surgery. *Journal of Pediatric Nursing*, **21** (1), 13-22.

Background

Considerable research over the past 60 years has indicated that young children undergoing anaesthesia and surgery have reported having significant emotional reactions following their surgical experience. The aim of this study was to use children's drawing as a self-report measure of anxiety before and after an intervention programme aimed at preparing children for elective surgery.

Method

Participants: The intervention group consisted of 80 children who received a formal pre-operative preparation process. The non-intervention group consisted of 62 children was escorted into the waiting room where there were simple diversionary materials such as films and books. All children and parents received standard pre-operative information by the nursing and support staff during the admission process and were provided with developmentally appropriate reassurance about the surgery and the recovery process.

Procedure: Permission to participate was obtained from parents. Children and families were then taken to a private room and each child was administered the CD:H instrument (Clatworthy *et al.*, 1999) which was designed to assess hospitalised children's anxiety. A child is asked to draw a picture of a person in the hospital upon admission and post-operatively. The drawing is assessed on a number of levels (e.g. position of the person, length of person, facial expression, and number of colours used) with different levels of anxiety being apparent dependent on the features of the drawing.

The intervention consisted of children and their families taking a 20-minute tour of all the relevant areas of day surgery as well as providing developmentally appropriate explanation of the surgery process for the children. The nurse explained the purpose of the holding area, the location of the surgery room, and where and when the separation from the parents will take place. A room equipped with actual medical equipment was then used to prepare each child and his or her family for the surgery process. Children were given opportunities to explore and rehearse with the relevant equipment and questions were answered and misconceptions addressed.

Results

The study showed that children receiving the intervention had less anxiety following surgery than those who did not receive the intervention. This supports previous research that psychosocial preparation for elective surgery reduces anxiety. Interestingly, the authors reported that children between 8 and 11 years had greater anxiety without preparation due to their greater ability to process cognitive information. This age group relates to Piaget's concrete operational period in which children are less egocentric, more logical and have the ability to project others' experiences on to themselves. They understand and are impacted by what they have observed in their environment. Thus, medical situations witnessed within the family or on television increase their anxiety levels. Children aged between 5 and 7 years are intuitive thinkers who focus more on personal perceptions rather than objective principles.

Implication

The findings of this study imply that children benefit post-operatively from pre-operative preparation prior to surgery inasmuch as when children are prepared for surgery, their coping ability increases and anxiety reduces. Nurses can therefore reduce a child's anxiety level, which may improve both the child's and parental anxiety. Preparing families for the surgical experience not only reassures parents but also provides them with the knowledge to support their child through the surgical process. A collaborative approach between nursing and the family should improve overall patient outcomes. All these variables support that children in different cognitive stages need to be prepared based on their developmental level.

Conclusion

This chapter has demonstrated that children cannot be viewed simply as 'small adults'. The way that children develop psychologically can have an impact on the way the individual child views their illness and their health, both immediately and in the long term. Nurses can use this knowledge to improve the care they provide to children both in an acute setting with childhood illness, and in a public health setting to maintain positive health behaviours and hence prevent illness. Furthermore, the role and value of the parents and wider family have been outlined and nurses can use this valuable resource to improve the care provided to children.

Summary

- There are a number of age-related changes in children's understanding of health, illness and pain.

- Children's experience of treatment, nursing and hospitalisation can be positively influenced by the supply of appropriate information and by considering parental interactions.

- The family and social context can impact on children's perception of pain and their quality of life.

- There are a number of non-pharmacological techniques that can be used by nurses in order to reduce pain and distress in the child undergoing treatment.

- Addressing unhealthy lifestyle health behaviours during childhood has many positive benefits and during particular childhood stages interventions may have better chances of success.

- Changing health behaviour during childhood requires a different set of skills than changing adult health behaviours.

- Health behaviour change interventions should use age-appropriate language and techniques.

- The involvement of the child's parent and wider family is important in any programme aimed at improving the child's health behaviour.

- Adherence to treatment is a major issue for children's health services.

- Attempts to understand and improve adherence have used different psychological models of behaviour.

- Methods that help children and their families to understand health-related information improve subsequent adherence.

- Children have a differing perspective on death, depending on their stage of development.

- It is important to individualise care and communication when dealing with a terminally ill child

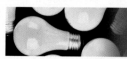

Check your understanding

1. How can Piaget's stage theory help with nursing children aged from 2 to 12 years?

2. How can Erikson's theory be applied to an adolescent coping with a chronic illness?

3. Discuss the importance of cognitive maturation during childhood.

4. Discuss the application of nursing care to the several stages of emotional and psychosocial development according to Erikson.

5. What developmental considerations have to be taken into account when attempting to change children's health behaviour?

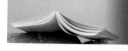

Further reading

Beale, E.A, Baile, W.F. and Aaron, J. (2005) Silence is not golden: Communicating with children dying from cancer. *Journal of Clinical Oncology*, **15**, 3269-3631.

Christ, G.H. and Christ, A. (2006) Current approaches to helping children cope with a parent's death. *CA: A Cancer Journal for Clinicians*, **56**, 197-212.

Immelt, S. (2006) Psychological adjustment in young children with chronic medical conditions. *Journal of Pediatric Nursing*, **21** (5), 362-377.

Trost, S.G., Sallis J.F., Pate, R.R., Freedson, P.S., Taylor, W.C. and Dowda, M. (2003) Evaluating a model of parental influence on youth physical activity. *American Journal of Preventative Medicine*, **25**, 277-282.

Williams, P.G., Hombeck, G.N. and Greenley, R.N. (2002) Adolescent health psychology. *Journal of Consulting and Clinical Psychology*, **70** (3), 828-842.

Weblinks

The Jean Piaget Society	http://www.piaget.org/	The Jean Piaget Society is an international, inter-disciplinary society with a membership of scholars, teachers and researchers interested in exploring the nature of the developmental construction of human knowledge. A rather dry website that presents information on the Society and some background on Jean Piaget.
Learning and Teaching site	http://www.learningandteaching.info/learning/piaget.htm	The Learning site provides a brief overview of part of the field. This link takes you to a brief overview of Piaget and his work. A useful site, however, for the range of information it contains not just on Piaget but also on such topics as behaviourism, humanism and other topics covered in this text. Primarily for teachers, a useful background set of information.
Dreams come true	http://www.dctc.org.uk/	A charity whose aim is to fulfil the dreams of terminally ill children.

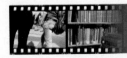 **Media examples**

Mask (1985) Peter Bogdanovich's engrossing film is based on the life of Rocky Dennis who suffered from a chronic facial deformity. The film depicts his relationship and the tumultuous but always loving relationship he shared with his mother. The movie succeeds in proving the importance of maintaining a positive attitude despite life's adversities.

Reflections on Childhood Cancer: A Book of Poems Access at: http://www.ukccsg.org/poems/reflections.pdf. An anthology of poems described as 'moving, inspiring, touching, sad and often humorous - in short the emotions expressed are common to the path that patients and families take on the cancer journey'. Although specifically about cancer, the range of emotions expressed are fully and frankly described and offer a window on the views of children, parents and their carers on chronic illness in childhood.

Chapter 8

The impact of social group on health

Learning outcomes

When you have read through this chapter you should understand.

- How society can be stratified.
- The evidence linking social class and health.
- The explanations for the link between social class and health.
- The biological and social differences between the sexes.
- The link between gender and health.
- The relationship between ethnicity and health status.
- Psychosocial factors involved in inequalities in health.
- How nurses have to alter their practice to take into account the influence of these social factors on health.

Case study

Stan is a 63-year-old school caretaker who is widowed and lives alone in a council flat. He has three grown-up children but they all live away from home. He rarely sees his children and grandchildren (he has seven) any more, other than at Christmas. They live many miles away in a different part of the country – not one of his relatives lives locally. His mother and father died from heart attacks many years ago and Stan has often considered returning to his native Jamaica where his brother and sister still live.

Stan works on a part-time basis at the local school where he has been employed for 15 years. He likes his job, although is finding it somewhat stressful at the moment due to a new headteacher who has insti-gated a number of changes to his routine. He is finding it tiring dealing with the continuous problems at the school and the increasing number of children being rude to him. He is also finding that his home life is stressful – the flat is damp and the neighbourhood is becoming more unpleasant.

Stan is an affable person and likes to socialise with his friends in the local pub. He is partial to 'a pint or two', especially on darts nights. Stan is a smoker who would not consider trying to give up because he believes that 'we all have to die from something' and he finds that it helps him to cope with the stresses of his work and his home life. His diet is poor, consisting of a breakfast 'fry-up' at the local café before he starts work, a sandwich at lunchtime and an evening meal either from the local take-away or a ready meal from his local convenience store.

Stan started to suffer chest pains recently and went to see his GP since he was worried about having a heart attack (not only did his parents die from a heart attack but his wife also died from one three years ago). He was admitted to hospital and is referred to you for advice. Medical assessment has revealed that Stan is having angina attacks and these may be the precursor of a serious heart attack. Indeed the consultant physician noted that 'it is not a matter of if but when he has a serious heart attack'. Obviously his health is being adversely affected by his health behaviours – his smoking, lack of exercise, alcohol consumption and diet is not ideal by any stretch of the imagination! Also Stan has some stresses in his life – his work and housing and the fact that he has limited contact with his family. However, he does appear to have some good friends, although this is often associated with his drinking and smoking.

When you meet with Stan it is evident that he will find it difficult to change his behaviours and there appears to be a communication gap between you. He does not seem to appreciate the seriousness of the situation and has difficulty in understanding the medical terms the doctor used when describing his condition. You press on and let Stan know, in no uncertain terms, that he has to change his behaviour, or else he will die. Stan finally appreciates this but you are unsure whether he will actually change any of his behaviours.

Why is this relevant to nursing practice?

You will notice that Stan has become ill and possible causative factors are his health behaviours: his smoking, his diet, his alcohol consumption and his lack of exercise. How can these be explained: why does Stan act in such a way? Furthermore, Stan was having difficulty in communicating with the nurse and doctor (or perhaps, more properly, the nurse and doctor were having difficulty communicating with Stan). What factors can contribute to these poor health behaviours? What may underlie the communication diffi-culties? What can be done to overcome some of these?

One of the factors that may underlie these issues are the basic characteris-tics of Stan: he is a man (rather than a woman!), he could be described as working class (rather than middle or upper class) and he is from the Afro-Caribbean (rather than from any other) ethnic group. All of these social factors may impact upon health and communicating with the health care professional. This chapter will explore these social factors and examine how they can be measured, how they can contribute towards illness and poor communication and what the nurse can do to improve the health of individual clients and patients within these groups.

Introduction

There are many different groups in society and our health will be influenced by the group we are in. For example, there are a range of groups to which Stan can be classified: social class, sex/gender and ethnicity. Some people have claimed that these social variables are, in fact, the key factors in whether we live or die and that medical variables pale into insignificance when compared with these. This chapter will explore the validity of this claim and explore its relevance for nursing. Furthermore something can be done to improve the health of those in different groups and the nurse and health care professional will play a key part in these improvements. It is essential, therefore, that in this chapter we explore some of these social differences and the focus will be on three areas of **social stratification** – social class, sex/gender and ethnicity. How does health differ among the social classes? How can these differences be explained? What relevance is this for the nurse and health care professional? What about sex: who is the healthiest, men or women? How can the health differences between men and women be explained? What about ethnic groups? How does health differ among these groups? How can we help to improve the health of all these social groups?

Stratification of society

Research into society seldom considers it as a whole and more usually considers the position of a group (or groups of people) within society. In this way individual members of society can be categorised into different groups. For example, you can classify people according to their:

- sex;
- level of education;
- social class;
- left- or right-handers;
- age group;
- ethnic group.

Categorising people can involve simple **nominal** groups such as right-handed or left-handed or you can stratify **society** into groups with a clear order, such as small, medium or large. There are a number of simple ways of stratifying society. Some types of stratification are easy to apply (e.g. age bands) whereas others are more difficult and contentious (e.g. social class). There is another difference between these forms of stratification. In the case of sex, ethnic group or left/right-handers there is no order: you cannot sensibly argue that one is 'better' or 'higher' in the classification system than the other. This is an example of horizontal stratification. In the other cases, social class or education for example, you can rank the groups in order: for example, in terms of number or level of qualifications, or income or some ephemeral quality of social class – this is a system of vertical stratification.

Although there are a number of ways in which society can be stratified in this chapter we will explore just three areas that clearly affect Stan: social class, sex/gender and ethnicity.

Think about this

How do you think these variables can impact on health? How does being a man impact on Stan's health? Does it matter that Stan is in the lower social class for his health? If so, how? What about ethnicity – how does this influence health?

Defining and measuring social class

The definition of social class has been provided by the seminal Black Report (Townsend and Davidson, 1982) which first clearly stated the link between health and social class in modern society. This definition is the one used whenever social class is referred to in this chapter:

> Segments of the population sharing broadly similar types and levels of resources, with broadly similar styles of living and (for some sociologists), some shared perception of their collective condition.

In essence, different classes have differential power to access material resources: homes, cars, white goods, electronic goods and so on. Although this is a solid definition it does not really take us any further forward when discussing what social class is and how best to measure it. In light of this, we have to explore how social class can and has been measured. It will not be a surprise that there are a number of different methods for measuring social class. These methods can be broadly broken down into either subjective or objective methods and either can be used, depending on the situation or the research being carried out. However, it is not surprising that all methods have both positives and negatives associated with them but it is worth exploring these in more detail.

Firstly, in the subjective method, you simply ask what social class people think they are in. Although this has been used in the past, there are a number of problems with this approach since it lies too much on self-perception rather than any objective measure of social class. Previously in the 1950s, for example, many people would simply state they were in the 'middle class' since there was an aspiration to such. In contrast, these days many people have a form of reverse snobbery and describe themselves as 'working class'. Very few people in either era describe themselves as 'upper class'. This raises a separate issue – that of terminology. If we ask people 'Do you think you are working class?', then many may agree. However, if we ask 'Do you think you are lower class?', then relatively few may agree, despite both being similar in the stratification.

The objective method, in contrast, uses a range of measures such as occupation, car ownership, unemployment, income, postcode, education and so on. These are all indicators that can be objectively measured. It is these measures that have been the ones most frequently used in the research.

The two most widely used measures are both based on occupation: the Registrar General's Standard Occupation Classification and the Socio-Economic Groups (SEG). Although both of these methods have been supplanted by another method (which will be discussed later), it is worth outlining these older methods in the first instance since much of the previous research has relied on these methods (in particular the Registrar General Classification system) and many health care workers still use it as a shorthand for classifying people.

The Registrar General's Standard Occupation Classification measurement was employed in the census from 1901 until relatively recently. It is based on the occupation of the individual head of the household (usually defined as the man – it was defined in less enlightened times!) who is classified into one of six groups, given in Table 8.1.

Table 8.1
Registrar General's Standard Occupation Classification

Class	Title	Examples
I	Professional	Lawyer, doctor, university professor
II	Intermediate	Farmer, nurse, office manager, health care professionals
III(NM)	Skilled non-manual	Cashier, secretary
III M	Skilled manual	Machine fitter, miner, bus driver
IV	Partly skilled	Postman (sic), traffic warden
V	Unskilled	Labourer, messenger, window cleaner

There are a number of problems with the Registrar General's system. Firstly, as has been hinted at, the role of women is minimised and the relevance of women as 'breadwinners' or the value of dual-income families is underplayed. Secondly, some of the classes are not internally homogeneous – a top flight corporate lawyer will earn considerably more than a university lecturer, for example. Furthermore, some of the jobs themselves may not be homogeneous – a farmer could relate to both a small farm-holder and a large industrial farmer. The occupations were thus classified according to status of the profession rather than the income. Finally, it does not deal with housewives/husbands, students or the unemployed very well.

In order to overcome some of these difficulties, the socio-economic groups listed below were developed by attempting to increase the number of categories into which individuals could be assigned. It was not based on status, rather it was based upon similar occupations:

1. Employers and managers in central and local government, industry, commerce – large establishments.
2. Employers and managers in central and local government, industry, commerce – small establishments.
3. Professional workers – self-employed.

4. Professional workers – employees.
5. Intermediate non-manual workers.
6. Junior non-manual workers.
7. Personal service workers.
8. Foreman and supervisors – non-manual.
9. Skilled manual workers.
10. Semi-skilled manual workers.
11. Unskilled manual workers.
12. Own account workers (other than professional workers).
13. Farmers – employers and managers
14. Farmers – own account.
15. Agricultural workers.
16. Members of the armed forces.
17. Occupation inadequately described.

However, again it was rather subjective and offered little more than an extension of the RG's system. In order to overcome these difficulties a new government social classification system was developed: the National Statistics Socio-Economic Classification (NS-SEC). This new method of classification was used in the 2001 census. The NS-SEC is an occupationally based classification but has rules to provide coverage of the whole adult population (see Table 8.2).

Table 8.2
The National Statistics Socio-Economic Classification Analytic Classes

1	Higher managerial and professional occupations
1.1	Large employers and higher managerial occupations
1.2	Higher professional occupations
2	Lower managerial and professional occupations
3	Intermediate occupations
4	Small employers and own account workers
5	Lower supervisory and technical occupations
6	Semi-routine occupations
7	Routine occupations
8	Never worked and long-term unemployed

Think about this

In what situation(s) would finding out about somebody's social class be useful? You want to find out what social class Stan is in. How would you go about this? What sort of questions would you ask, and what considerations would you take into account when gathering the information?

The link between social class and health

It has long been recognised that social class does impact on health and illness. For example in Bethnal Green (an area in the East end of London) in 1839 the average age of death was as follows (cited in Davey-Smith *et al.*, 1992): 'Gentlemen and persons engaged in professions, and their families 45 years; tradesmen and their families 26 years; Mechanics, servants and labourers, and their families 16 years.' This suggests that there was a relationship between the level of profession and mortality – the higher up the social scale, the longer the life expectancy. More recent evidence has also suggested that there is a relationship between social class and health. Indeed, the evidence presented has indicated that there is a social gradient in health and death in all societies (Marks, 2005; Schnittker, 2004) such that those in the lower social classes have a poorer health status than those in the higher social classes (van Rossum *et al.*, 2000).

Just as there are a number of ways of measuring social class, however, there are a number of ways of measuring health (see Chapter 1) and it is important to explore each of these definitions in turn and how they relate to the social class–health gradient. If we look at **morbidity** in the first instance we find that there is a direct relationship between social class and ill-health. For example, Blaxter (1976) concluded that: 'Even if examination is confined to the more stringent and objective condition of handicapping chronic illness, prevalence rates in Social Class V ... are well over twice the rate ... reported in Class I.'

Recent evidence has also supported this claim. For example, the Welsh Health Survey (National Assembly for Wales, 2001) found that manual groups had two to three times the rate of non-manual groups for symptoms of angina, breathlessness, persistent cough and phlegm. Similarly, the adult dental health survey of 1988 found that the proportion of people from class I was with no natural teeth was much lower than in the other classes, although classes IV and V had shown improvements in recent years. Indeed, whichever survey is examined a similar picture emerges: the lower the social class, the higher the rate of morbidity. As Benzeval *et al.* (1995) concludes: 'People who live in disadvantaged circumstances have more illnesses, greater distress, more disability and shorter lives that those who are more affluent'.

As indicated from the Benzeval *et al.* (1995) quote, mortality also reveals some disparities between the classes. The way of examining mortality is to calculate the standard mortality ratio (SMR). If the figure is above 100, then the death rate is higher than average, if it is lower than 100 then the death rate is lower than average (see Chapter 1). Alternatively, we can explore the life expectancy. Here, we find a significant difference between the social classes. Recent census data (ONS, 2001a) have suggested that, overall, there is a 7.4 year gap for men between professional and unskilled groups, and 5.7 years for women (see Figure 8.1). That means that those in the unskilled group are dying over 7 years earlier than their counterparts in the professional groups. If we examine the causes of death by different illnesses, we get a similar picture – with those in social class V (e.g. labourer) having a higher SMR than those in social class I (e.g. lawyer) – see Table 8.3.

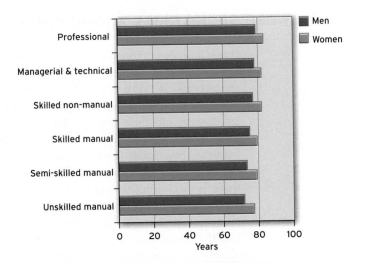

Figure 8.1 Life-expectancy according to different groups.

Source: ONS (2001b)

Table 8.3
SMR according to cause of death by social class

Cause of death	| SMR					
	I	II	III (non-manual)	III (manual)	IV	V
Males						
Ischaemic heart disease	69	81	102	106	110	137
Lung cancer	42	62	78	117	125	175
Cardio-vascular accident	61	70	88	105	114	171
Bronchitis	34	49	84	109	134	208
Car accidents	64	75	79	101	114	175
Pneumonia	34	49	80	89	121	211
Suicide	86	78	94	84	110	190
Females						
Ischaemic heart disease	41	55	69	106	119	152
Breast cancer	107	103	105	100	99	94
Cardio-vascular accident	61	70	88	105	114	171
Bronchitis	33	54	71	100	119	165
Car accidents	76	89	102	63	94	114
Pneumonia	37	51	67	86	110	140
Suicide	77	81	79	55	176	184

Think about this

Examine Table 8.3. What does it say about the relationship between social class and health? Why is there an inverse (i.e. opposite relationship) for breast cancer? Another example (not in Table 8.3) is skin cancer, which is reported more in social class I/II rather than IV/V. Why would this be?

The proportion of stillbirths and deaths of children under one year of age per 1000 live births also reflects a relationship between social class and health (Table 8.4). For example, there are twice as many stillbirths in social class V than in social class I (the most recent statistics can be found at www.statistics.gov.uk).

Table 8.4
Stillbirths/deaths and social class

	Stillbirths	Infant deaths
I	3	6
II	3	5
III (NM)	4	6
III (M)	4	6
IV	6	8
V	6	11

Think about this

Consider the last time you were in a clinic. Did you notice any differences in the types of patient that you saw? Did you think they were from a certain social group – did men outnumber women? Did those in the lower social classes outnumber those in the upper social classes? Were any particular ethnic groups particularly over represented?

Mental health and social class

The evidence thus far presented suggests a strong link between social class and physical health (e.g. Banks *et al.*, 2006; Marks, 2005). Numerous studies have reported such a relationship and these have been found year on year. However, what about the evidence linking mental health and social class position? How strong is the evidence for such a relationship?

There is a strong relationship between psychotic disorders and socio-economic position: people in the lower social class have higher rates than those in the upper social classes (Fryers *et al.*, 2005). Furthermore there is also indication that there is a link between lower class and common mental health disorders (e.g. anxiety and depression; Fryers *et al.*, 2003). This relationship can be accounted for by social drift: as the disorder takes hold, the person is unable to hold on to their job and subsequently moves down the social position. However, this cannot be the complete picture, especially with the more common disorders where people may be more capable of holding down permanent positions.

The evidence linking social class position and neurotic disorders has been mixed. Dohrenwend (1990) in a review of the international literature reported an inconsistent picture. Similar, unclear findings have been reported by Meltzer *et al.* (1995) and Erens and Primatesta (1999) in the United Kingdom. Both were large-scale government-funded studies, yet one (Meltzer *et al.*) found occupational social class to be a strong predictor while the other (Erens and Primatesta) did not. However, these studies used occupational status as a measure of social class. When other studies were explored that have used more complete measures of socio-economic status a clear relationship exists (Fryers *et al.*, 2003, p. 229): 'Common mental disorders are significantly more frequent in socially disadvantaged populations' and these disadvantages 'produce a significant amount of suffering and dysfunction in working aged adults' (Fryers *et al.*, 2003, p. 236).

Similarly, there is considerable evidence linking unemployment and suicide behaviour (Preti, 2003). Indeed, there appears to be a strong association between unemployment levels and the extent of suicide in the population (Blakely *et al.*, 2003). Although there is some indication that this may be related to socio-economic status, it is probably more than this. For example, unemployment can impact on the social interaction individuals have with others at both the community and individual levels. Whitely *et al.* (1999) and Preti (2003) suggest that measures of social fragmentation can predict the risk of death by suicide and alcohol-related diseases.

Therefore, whatever form of evidence is explored the picture is the same: those in social class IV/V (the lower working class) have more illness – both physical and mental – and die younger from a range of illnesses than their compatriots in social class I/II. What can explain this difference in health status? This will be discussed in the next section.

Explaining the social class health differences

The Department of Health's Research Working Group on Inequalities in Health (DHSS, 1980) – which has become known as the Black Report – suggested four types of explanation for the social class differences in health.

The *artefact explanation* suggests that observed social class differences in mortality may be an error in the process by which they are measured (i.e. an 'artefact' of the measurement procedure). In short, this explanation suggests that since it is difficult to measure both social class and health, how can we demonstrate any link between the two? Although this explanation has some immediate appeal there are some arguments against this being the sole explanation, the strongest being simply the weight of the evidence from a number of sources suggesting a link between social class (however measured) and health (however measured).

Another suggestion is the *social/natural selection explanation* which suggests that the healthy are more likely to move up the social classes and the unhealthy move down. There is some good evidence for this, and it does appear to make sense. For example, an individual who is chronically sick or disabled may move down the social scale since they are unable either to find employment or are under-employed (i.e. they are more qualified than their current employment would suggest). However, some studies have found that health inequalities exist in people who have not moved social class, for example in the retired. These two explanations were dismissed relatively easily and cannot be the whole story behind the health inequalities. There were two major explanations, however, that have merit and are considered the leading contenders.

Behavioural/cultural explanations suggest that social class differences in health are a consequence of the behaviours that people *choose* to engage in. Thus health differences emerge because the lower social groups have adopted more dangerous and health-damaging behaviour than the other social groups. Thus those in the lower class *choose* not to eat well, *choose* to smoke more cigarettes, *choose* to drink more and *choose* not to exercise. Everyone would probably agree that these are behaviours that may damage a person's health but how does this explanation stack up? Are those in the working classes more likely to engage in damaging health behaviours? For example, Stan does not exercise (other than darts), he smokes, drinks and eats the 'wrong' food. With *smoking* data suggest that there is a class difference in smoking, with a greater proportion of those in the lower social classes smoking and this can be seen over a number of years (percentage smoking); see Table 8.5.

The relationship between social class and coronary heart disease (CHD)/lung cancer can be explained, in part, by these differences in smoking habits and so it does seem to provide evidence that there is a more prevalent behaviour that can lead to morbidity and death in the lower social classes (see Figure 8.2). However, just because there is a social class gradient in smoking does not indicate that this is the only explanation. Davey-Smith *et al.* (1994) found a social class gradient in health in those who had never smoked. The other question that has to be posed is, why do people smoke? Why is the smoking behaviour greater in the lower social classes? We will return to these questions later in this chapter (and related issues are explored in Chapter 12).

The other information that can be drawn from Figure 8.2 is that those in the lower social classes have not taken up the no-smoking message as frequently as those in the upper social classes. Studies have shown that smoking

Table 8.5
Smoking and socio-economic group

Socio-economic group	Men	Women	Average
Professional	20	18	19
Intermediate	27	25	26
Manual	32	31	32

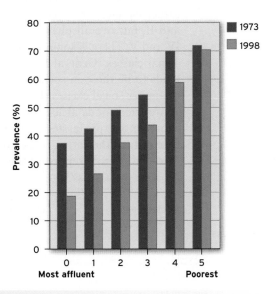

Figure 8.2 Cigarette smoking by deprivation in Great Britain (1973) and (1998).
Source: ONS (1973, 1998)

levels have remained virtually unchanged among those in the poorest groups (Dorsett and Marsh, 1998; Jarvis, 1998; Marsh and McKay, 1994). Obviously there are different possible explanations as to why this might be:

- The middle/upper classes have been targeted by health promotion campaigns. The lower/working classes have not.
- The middle/upper classes are better able to act on the advice given in health promotion campaigns.
- The middle/upper classes have a more extensive choice of how to behave.

Whatever the explanation, however, it is apparent that there is still some work to be undertaken in order to reduce the level of smoking in the working classes (de Meyrick and Yusuf, 2006).

Think about this

How would you encourage people to stop smoking? How would your advice differ between clients in the working and middle classes?

Another behaviour that may differ according to social class and which could impact on health status is physical exercise. In terms of *exercise*, the most popular leisure time activities – walking and swimming – have been examined in the General Household Survey (2001). This survey suggests that the professional groups have the highest participation rates in both walking and swimming as leisure activities (Table 8.6).

It must be noted that this is leisure time activity rather than amount of physical activity. Obviously those in the working classes tend to have more physically demanding jobs and hence they do more activity than their professional counterparts. Hence, in terms of health behaviours the evidence is rather inconclusive – leisure time activity is greater in those in social classes I and II, but overall physical activity may be greater in those in social classes IV and V. There is some evidence that there is a difference in *diet* between the social classes (General Household Survey, 2002). Table 8.7 indicates that it tends to be those in social classes IV/V who have a poorer diet than those in the upper social classes (I/II). For example, 60 per cent of those in social class V ate fried foods at least twice a week compared with only 34 per cent of those in the professional group. These proportions were almost exactly reversed for the eating fresh fruit at least once a day – with only 35 per cent of social class V reporting this on a daily basis compared to 60 per cent of those in social class I.

Table 8.6
Exercise and social class

Social class	Walking (2 miles+)	Indoor swimming
I	30	16
II	23	11
III NM	22	12
III M	17	7
IV	15	7
V	12	3

Table 8.7
Food consumption and
social class

Food type and frequency of consumption	I (%)	II (%)	IIINM (%) (non-manual)	IIIM (%) (manual)	IV (%)	V (%)
			Social class			
Drinks soft drinks once a day or more	24	31	38	37	40	39
Eats fried food two or more times/week	34	43	43	49	60	57
Uses skimmed or semi-skimmed milk	73	69	68	60	52	52
Eats oil-rich fish less than once a month	17	26	36	36	42	45
Eats wholemeal bread	22	14	10	8	6	6
Eats fresh fruit once a day or more	60	54	45	44	34	35
Eats cooked green vegetables five or more times a week	52	45	37	36	30	32
Eats raw vegetables or salad two or more times a week	59	55	43	39	32	41

Alcohol consumption differs among the classes, although the relationship is a little complex. When the data are examined, it appears as if the proportion of heavy drinkers is greater among non-manual than manual groups. That is, the lower social classes are drinking less than their higher social class counterparts. However, this is probably because the higher social classes were drinking a couple of glasses of red wine with their meals throughout the week rather than binge drinking at the weekends. When the dangerous form of drinking – binge drinking – is examined, the difference is the other way around: the manual and unskilled workers have a higher rate (see Haustein, 2006, for a review).

The behavioural explanation: is there a *choice*?

As we have seen, there is a difference in the health status between those in the different classes and this maps to a certain extent to their health behaviours. So is it just the 'wilful ignorance of the working classes' that leads to their ill-health; that is, they chose to smoke, drink and so on, so they have to suffer the consequences? In contrast, some argue that the decision is not simply about the choices that people make, it is about the fact that there is no choice for those in the lower/working classes. In order to deal with stresses of their lives (which are more impoverished and therefore more stressful than their middle/upper class counterparts) individuals have to use methods that are known to them, that work for them and that are available to them.

Hence, it is argued that people smoke, drink and eat poorly because it is easy and relatively cheap. (Although people may disagree with this given the price of cigarettes. It must be remembered, however, that smoking is relatively cheap, is easy, is easily transportable and is regarded as the 'norm' in certain sections of society.) Furthermore, Siahpush and Carlin (2006) report that financial stresses increase smoking behaviours and result in greater relapse after stopping smoking. People are not *choosing* to indulge in these behaviours, but are *forced* into them because of where they live and the circumstances that they have to deal with. In short, the middle/upper classes have the luxury of a choice: the working classes do not (as exemplified in the case study).

Case study

Jane is a teacher and has just returned from a day's work teaching in a special needs school. She has had a stressful day at school and decides that she will have some time to herself before collecting her own children. She decides that she needs to go to the gym and get rid of her stress. She pops off to the local gym, where she is a member, and attacks the step machine with vigour. She then has a dip in the jacuzzi for ten minutes before she is ready to collect her children. This has taken her an extra hour and a half but she can afford the extra costs of the childminder.

Now consider a similar scenario. Jackie returns home after a stressful day working in the local shop where some local teenagers have been giving her a hard time and constantly harassing her. The owner of the shop has only just returned from the cash and carry and asks Jackie if she can work later. Unfortunately she has to say no as her children are being looked after by a neighbour and who is only willing to look after them for half an hour each day. When she collects her children they add to her stress and she sends them upstairs with a packet of sweets to play in their rooms. For the first time all day Jackie has some time to herself and decides to relax. She sits down with a cup of tea, a TV soap opera and a cigarette.

Think about this

Make a list of those activities that the middle class mum could do (e.g. go for a swim) and those that the working class mum could do (e.g. smoke). Who has the greater 'choice'? Is it a choice for the working class woman to smoke? Or is it her only choice?

The final explanation offered by the Black report was the *materialist explanation* which concentrates upon hazards inherent in society and to which some people have *no choice* but to be exposed. Thus those with a lower socio-econimic status (SES) are exposed to more unhealthy environments. For example, they do more dangerous work, have poorer housing, have fewer resources available to secure the necessities for health and are unable to use the health services. Hence, the whole structure of society is involved. For example:

- Income is a central factor: if and when money is short the essentials will be covered first (e.g. rent and rates) whereas the basis necessities for health (e.g. heating and balanced nutrition) may be the first to go.
- Housing has been implicated in the health of the poorer classes. Numerous factors come into play; the stress of living in poor conditions, the dampness, the pollution experienced, heating (or rather lack of it) may all have an impact on health.

● Several studies have indicated the way in which lower-income families attempt to reduce the stresses of living on low wages: sweets are used to comfort the child since they are quick and easy; breast feeding may be abandoned earlier to give more time to other family members (e.g. Dubois and Girad, 2006; Kelly and Watt *et al.*, 2006); smoking can ease tension and be used as a coping mechanism (e.g. Prus, 2007). All these go against the advice provided by health professionals.

It was the materialist approach that the Black Report adopted and suggested needed be addressed by the Government. However, more than 30 years after the publication of the documentation very little has been achieved with regard to improving the material conditions of those in the lower social classes. Indeed, there was some evidence that, for a number of years, the health inequality gap has continued to increase (Shaw *et al.*, 2005).

It can be argued that there is limited impact that nurses and other health care professionals can have on materialist underpinnings of health inequalities. However, some other relevant factors may contribute to the social class divide and need to be considered in day-to-day practice. Some of these factors can have a direct impact on the health, and the treatment that some individuals will receive. Addressing these factors may help improve inequalities in health. The first of these that needs to be considered is the so-called 'inverse care law'.

The 'inverse care law' was a concept first noted by Tudor-Hart in the 1970s: 'The availability of good medical care tends to vary inversely with the need for the population served' (Tudor-Hart, 1971). Tudor-Hart was a GP based in the South Wales valleys and reported that those most in need of health care received it the least. Hence, those in the lower social classes with the poorer health had less access to health care than those in the middle–upper classes. It could be argued that the middle classes living in a leafy suburb do not need as many health care facilities as those living in a large, urban run-down environment, yet it is suggested that they actually enjoy more and better services. This is not simply a historical issue – a similar pattern of need and provision has been found by Shaw and Dorling (2004). They reported that an inverse care law relationship existed between the need for care and availability of medical practitioners, dentists and other health professionals. They also suggested that it is just not a matter of *quantity* of services, but also of *quality*. That is, those in the middle class areas receive not only more but better services than those in the working class areas.

Furthermore, different groups tend to define health and illness differently. The upper and middle classes are more likely to place a medical explanation on their ill-health rather than another form of explanation (see Chapter 1). Hence, they are more likely to go to their GP with an illness, and seek out effective medical interventions. In contrast, those in the working classes are more likely to respond to more local '**folk definitions**' of health and illness. In response to these forms of definition, advice will be taken from a friend or member of the family rather than medical treatment, which means that it may be less likely to be successful. If a person defines health as 'getting through the day' as it is suggested that the working class does, then they are less likely to request an appointment than those who define it more symptomatically.

The inequalities do not end there: studies have found that the average consultation time for class I is 6.1 minutes compared with 4.7 minutes for class V. Similarly, the material presented in the consultation can differ. Those in

Think about this

Think about how you interacted when you were speaking to individuals from the working, middle and upper classes. How did your behaviour and language change? If it did not change, should it? If it did change, should it?

social classes I and II get more (and therefore better?) information than those in social classes IV and V: 'Patients visiting GPs in disadvantaged areas may not be receiving the same high quality of care as patients in more advantaged locations' (Furler *et al.*, 2002). Finally, it has also been suggested that higher social classes are more likely to be referred to specialists for more intensive and specialised treatment.

Think about this

Consider all the material presented above about the relationship between social class and health. What could you, as a health care professional, do to try to reduce the health care inequalities? How would your interactions differ according to the social class of the individual patient/client?

Psychosocial factors underpinning the social class–health relationship

Other than the lifestyle factors already discussed, there are potential psychological factors that can underpin the social class–health relationship (see Adler and Snibbe, 2003). Extensive data suggest an important role of personal control and mastery in the social class–health gradient. Lower social class brings fewer opportunities for control and hence those individuals in lower social class levels report less mastery and control than their higher class counterparts. Perceived control is also related to health outcomes, and may influence health (e.g. Lachman and Weaver, 1998), and control in the work environment appears to be particularly important. Control may be missing in the lower class occupations.

Lower SES (lower social class) environments may also diminish optimism and foster hopelessness and hostility. Furthermore, negative cognitions and affective states increase as SES decreases (e.g. Gallo and Matthews, 2003) and therefore may be important in heart attacks and cardiac deaths (Fiscella and Franks, 1997). Hostility and anger are likewise potent predictors of mortality and morbidity (see Chapter 13), and among some groups they mediate the relationship between SES and cardiovascular functioning (Gump *et al.*, 1999). Finally, optimism–pessimism predicts such health outcomes as recovery from coronary bypass surgery and onset of AIDS in HIV-positive men (Adler and Snibbe, 2003).

Gender and health

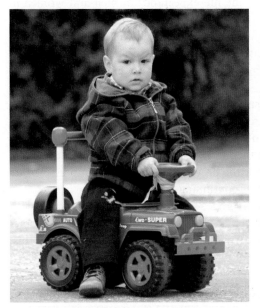

Profimedia International s.r.o/Alamy

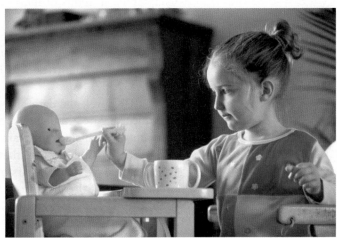

Picture Partners/Alamy

Look at the pictures above and write down a series of words that describe the boy and then a series of words that describe the girl.

Consider how parents and adults in general change their behaviour on the basis of their child's sex. How does this influence the way children develop and, how is an individual's gender developed? Consider how parents change their reactions in line with the sex of their child; what about health care professionals? Do they alter their behaviour in light of the sex of the child? How can this influence the treatment and care that they provide? These questions will be explored in this section of the chapter.

It is worth, at the outset, highlighting the difference between 'sex' and 'gender'. Sex is the biological underpinning – our genetic make-up. Gender, on the other hand, is more socially constructed – it is more concerned with how we think and behave (WHO, 2006). Hence when talking about sex we will talk about males and females or man and woman. Alternatively, when we talk about gender we talk about masculine and feminine. Thus, it is possible to be a 'masculine' female (i.e. a woman who acts in a 'typically' masculine manner) and similarly it would be possible to be a 'feminine' male (i.e. a man who acts in a 'typically' feminine manner).

Think about this

What does masculine mean? How does a 'typical' man act? What about feminine? How does a 'typical' woman act? How does this relate to health care? Is it possible to describe how a 'typical' male or female acts? Or is this stereotypical? Can you recall a 'typical' masculine and feminine patient – how do you think they behaved? How do you think this affected their health?

The relationship between sex and health has been explored in a number of different ways depending on how health is defined and measured (see Chapter 1). In terms of mortality, the life expectancy of men and women in various countries is presented in Table 8.8. There is a consistent difference between men and women, with women consistently living longer than men. This is true from the poorer countries with low life expectancies (e.g. Nigeria) to those richer countries (e.g. France) with higher life expectancies (WHO statistics, 2007).

At a UK level, the data also support this view, with women living longer than men. Figure 8.3 demonstrates the differences in life expectancy between men and women since the start of the century (Office for National Statistics, 2004). It is possible to note that the life expectancy of both men and women has increased by some 3 years over the previous 20 years – an impressive rate of improvement that looks as if it is continuing.

In 2001 a baby girl could, on average, live to 80.4 years compared with 75.7 years for a baby boy. However, as we have seen, simply because somebody is alive does not mean that they are healthy! It is much more than this, so we have to explore the illnesses of men and women – their morbidity.

Table 8.8

Life expectancies in different countries

Country	Male life expectancy	Female life expectancy
France	75.9	83.5
Albania	67.3	74.1
Denmark	74.8	79.5
USA	74.6	79.8
Canada	77.2	82.3
Nigeria	48.0	49.6
China	69.6	72.7

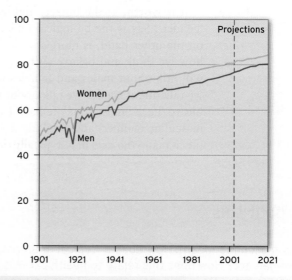

Figure 8.3 Life expectancies for men and women.

Source: www.statistics.gov.uk

The General Household Survey (2002) suggests that a greater proportion of women (35 per cent) have a long-standing illness than men (34 per cent), although the difference is relatively minor. This is a common pattern – 22 per cent of women report a limited long-standing illness compared with 20 per cent of men. Looking at acute illnesses, 16 per cent of women report an acute illness compared with 14 per cent of men. These figures impact on the number of restricted activity days in the previous year, with men experiencing 31 such days compared with 34 for women. These data suggest that women have a higher rate of morbidity than men. So, at this stage there is a paradox – men die younger but women have more illness.

There are a number of explanations proposed explaining the link between sex and health. In essence, these can be broken down into two different categories (biological versus social) and each of these has implications for the health care professional (Mackenbach, 2005). At the most basic, some have suggested that the difference in health status between men and women is related to genetic difference. Although at first glance this would appear to be a sensible explanation, there are some arguments against it. The strongest argument against its simply being a genetic link is the fact that there are countries where there is a different pattern: men live longer than women, and women get ill less frequently than men. So it cannot be simply a genetic explanation and there must be some other factors involved.

Another explanation is that the major reason for the difference in health status between the sexes is due to variation in the way children are socialised (i.e. brought up to be a man or a woman). For example, friends at school and at home influence the way that children develop: boys may be more likely to act tough and play with guns and action men. In contrast, girls may be more likely to play 'house' or with dolls. This stereotypical development can lead to the development of mainly 'masculine' boys and 'feminine' girls (Courtenay, 2000a). This may be reinforced by the media. For example consider the poster of the Tarzan film on the next page. How are Tarzan (the male) and Jane (the female) represented in the poster? This reinforces the way in which women are seen and are expected to behave in society. All of this suggests that girls may be brought up to be submissive and dependent and boys to be tough and macho.

Think about this

Consider the ways in which boys and girls are socialised. How do you think that these can impact on health? Is there anything about men having to act 'tough' that will impact on their health? Can you think of a person whose health you think has been damaged because of the way they act – in either a 'masculine' or 'feminine' manner? What about Stan? How has being a man influenced his health? How can the way you treat a child in clinic influence the way they perceive themselves and their gender?

The way that children are brought up can impact on the way they behave and this is one of the major reasons proposed for the difference in increased mortality in men. In a large, although now somewhat dated, review, Waldron and Johnston (1976) suggests that over three-quarters of the difference can

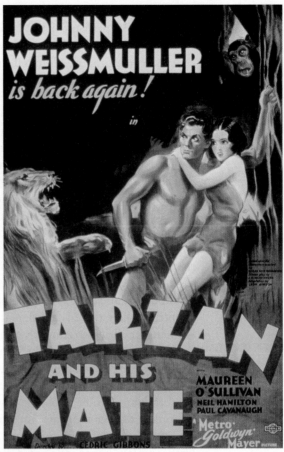

The Picture Desk

be accounted for by these behaviours and Courtenay (2003) suggests that health behaviours are the major determinant of excess mortality. What types of behaviours maintain or impair health? Obviously a simple list can be drawn up of those unhealthy behaviours: smoking, drinking alcohol and the protective health behaviours such as exercise and a good diet. It is suggested that males indulge in health-impairing behaviour (more than 30 different forms of health-damaging behaviours) more frequently than women, that women take more care of their health and that this is all due to socialisation (Courtenay, 2000b, 2003).

Smoking has been considered a predominantly male activity for a number of years and the data seem to confirm this (see Figure 8.4). However, the graph indicates a couple of key facts. Firstly, the proportion of men that smoke is higher than women and this has been the case for a number of decades. However, the rate is coming closer together, that is the proportion of women smoking is decreasing at a slower rate than men. If we also look at the rate of smoking according to different age bands then we find that at the younger age bands more girls than boys are smoking. This means that in years to come the rate of smoking for men and women will be equivalent which could ultimately have a negative impact on women's life expectancy (Emslie *et al.*, 2002; ONS, 2001a).

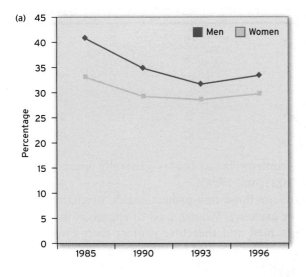

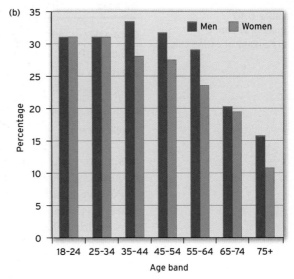

Figure 8.4 Percentage of men and women smoking.

Think about this

Why do men and women smoke? Is it that men try to look 'macho' whereas women try to look 'cool and sophisticated'? How would this information impact on the way you try and prevent children from smoking? Or encourage adults to give up?

There is a similar difference in eating and drinking habits between the sexes. For example, let us take two simple examples (drawn from the General Health Survey, 2002) to demonstrate this difference. Table 8.9 shows a healthy behaviour (the frequency of eating fresh fruit and vegetables) and indicates that women eat healthy foods more frequently than men (Courtenay, 2000b, 2003). If we look at the converse – the frequency of eating chips – then it can be noted that men eat more unhealthily than women (Table 8.10). Hence it would appear as if men are not following the 'healthy eating' guidelines to the same extent as women are. This is a very simplistic overview but it indicates that there are differences in eating behaviours between the sexes. Again, it indicates (as does smoking and alcohol use) that men's behaviour is

Table 8.9 Healthy eating (fruit and vegetables)	All ages	Men	Women
	More than once a day	14	22
	Once a day	25	30
	5-6 days a week	5	5
	2-4 days a week	23	22
	Once a week	13	9
	1-3 times a month	10	6
	Rarely or never	11	7

Table 8.10
Unhealthy eating
(frequency of eating chips)

All ages	Men	Women
Once a day or more	5	2
5-6 days a week	5	3
2-4 days a week	41	29
Once a week	24	26
1-3 times a month	15	21
Rarely or never	10	18

less than ideal and that women's behaviour is generally more positive (Courtenay, 2000a, 2000c, 2003; Shi, 1998).

Positive health behaviours are those that protect health, or guard against illness (e.g. healthy eating or exercise). Women tend to engage in more positive health behaviours than men and therefore protect their own health (Courtenay, 2003). Data from the General Health Survey (2002) tends to support this. For example, Table 8.11 presents information on taking vitamins and other supplements according to sex.

Table 8.11
Vitamin and supplement
consumption

All ages	Men	Women
Do not take supplements	85	74
Vitamins	8	15
Fish oils	7	9
Iron supplements	1	3
Calcium	0	2
Other minerals	1	3
Other supplements	3	7

All of these differences tend to indicate that men do not look after their health as well as women do. Indeed, Courtenay (2000a, p. 1386) explains that the data indicate:

> the prevalence of risk behaviours among adults is more common among men than women for all but three of fourteen (non sex-specific) behaviours, including smoking, drinking and driving, using safety belts, getting health screenings and awareness of medical conditions.

This suggestion, that there is a greater tendency for men to engage in behaviour that puts their health at risk, can be traced back to the socialisation of the child.

Another major difference that may be related back to such socialisation patterns is the proportion of suicides, with men having a much higher rate than women. The Department of Health website (www.dh.gov.uk) suggests the following (rates per 100 000 population) in terms of deaths from suicide:

	1993	1994	1995	1996	1997	1998
Men	15.0	14.7	14.9	14.2	13.8	15.5
Women	5.2	4.9	4.9	4.8	4.7	4.8

There are many reasons why men commit suicide more frequently than women and some of these can be related to socialisation. Firstly, boys are socialised to take on the protector and breadwinner role. When they cannot achieve this role as men then depression and other mental health problems may result. This may lead to severe and chronic depression and, ultimately, suicide. Furthermore, Farrell (1994) suggests that the traditional role of men as supporters and protectors mitigates against their seeking help for their problems and suggests that 'suicide is the only symptom without chance of solution' (p. 123).

Additionally, boys are socialised to be more aggressive. Hence when they come to attempt suicide they use more 'forceful' and 'aggressive' methods (for example, gunshots, drowning or hanging) whereas women use less aggressive methods (for example, overdoses) where the chances of recovery are much higher. Pritchard (1995) points out that men are more likely to use car exhaust or hanging while women are more likely to use self-poisoning. Hence, more women may attempt suicide than men (i.e. have higher rates of para-suicide), but men are more 'successful' than women.

The roots of these behaviours are in the socialisation of the child and can be seen quite clearly. However, there are other health behaviours that can also be related back to the socialisation process: for example, when people become aware of their symptoms, how they acknowledge these and how on the basis of this they seek out assistance from health care professionals.

Women are more likely to acknowledge their symptoms than men. They will seek help when they get a symptom whereas men are more likely to ignore the symptoms and carry on as usual. This may relate to socialisation as young children – boys are brought up to be tough and macho so when they fall over they are told to get on with it, whereas girls may be given a cuddle and more affection when injured and so they are not afraid to express their feelings and their symptoms.

Seeking medical help

Women tend to go to the doctors more frequently than men and this is backed up by recorded statistics (Galdas *et al.*, 2005). Although this can be explained, to a certain extent, by the additional visits as a result of pregnancy and gynaecological problems, this is not the whole answer and there are some other considerations. Some of them have been discussed – the stoicisms of the men, for example (Courtenay, 2000c, 2001). But more importantly, there are considerations that are relevant to the nurse practitioner (Seymour-Smith *et al.*, 2002). Strong (1979), for example, explored the medical practitioner (paediatrician) consultation with a visiting parent:

Doctor: Now this is the new patient.

Nurse: It's the father who's come up with him today.

Doctor: Uh-huh. I wonder why it is always the father?

Later ...

Doctor: What was the weight at birth?

Father: Seven and a half pounds.

Doctor: Gosh, you've got a good memory! I expect mothers but not fathers to remember. Seven and a half pounds you think.

When women go to visit the doctor or deal with a health care practitioner it is more likely that they will be:

- medicated more;
- have procedures performed on them more;
- get further consultations more;
- be labelled as 'sick' more.

Thus women are medicated more often than men, have procedures performed on them more often than men, end up in doctors' offices and hospitals more than men, and eventually come to believe that the symptoms they are experiencing are actually indicative of illness or disease. For example, Verbrugge (1980) reported that urinary, eye or ear problems in women were more likely to be reported as 'sickness' and receive treatment than exactly the same conditions in men. Hence, health care practitioners tend to be influenced by the sex of the patient. The argument is that health practitioners differentially interpret, diagnose and treat identical symptoms in males and females.

Think about this

Remember the last consultation you had with a patient: do you think it would have been different if the person you were seeing was a different sex?

Ethnicity and health

Stan is from Afro-Caribbean origin: how does this impact upon his health? As with the other social variables we have explored, there is evidence to suggest that the different ethnic groups have different health status. The first important point is that it is impossible to say 'ethnic minorities have poorer health' since the term ethnic group covers a multitude of individuals and a range of different ethnic groups (Rassool, 2006). It is likely that some of those groups, will have better health status than the indigenous population, some will have the same and some will have worse. We can break it down by different ethnic groups, as shown in Figure 8.5. Pakistani and Bangladeshi men and women in England and Wales reported the highest rates of 'not good' health in 2001 (ONS, 2001a).

So why should this be? One reason may the health behaviours of the different groups and, in particular, smoking and drinking patterns. When these are explored, data reveal that Bangladeshi men are the most likely group in England to smoke cigarettes (44 per cent), followed by White Irish (39 per cent) and Black Caribbean men (35 per cent) and this compared to 27 per cent of the general population.

Although very few Bangladeshi women smoked cigarettes, a relatively large proportion (26 per cent) chewed tobacco. This method of using tobacco was also popular among Bangladeshi men (19 per cent), but they tended to use it in conjunction with cigarettes. This example highlights a discreet behaviour that can lead to health problems. Chewing tobacco may lead to specific forms of cancer, which may be found only in the Bangladeshi population.

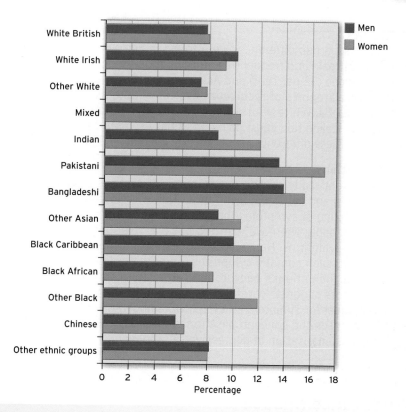

Figure 8.5 Ratings of health according to ethnic background, April 2001, England and Wales.

Source: ONS (2001b)

Research in focus

Rhee, H. (2005) Racial/ethnic differences in adolescents' physical symptoms. *Journal of Pediatric Nursing,* **20** (3), 153–162

Background

In order to provide appropriate care it is important that patient-centred care is developed and implemented. Obviously, this may be based on **race** or **ethnicity** and it is important to review the ethnic group health concerns of interest. This study sought to explore the prevalence of certain physical symptoms in different ethnic groups and to examine the extent to which SES and psychological problems explain the differences in reporting physical symptoms in children and adolescents.

Method

Participants: This was a longitudinal study that explored the data from a nationally representative sample of some 200 000 adolescents drawn from 132 schools. The age ranged from 11 to 21, with the mean being 16 years of age, with an approximately 50:50 split of males and females.

Measures: The study focused on 10 physical symptoms: headache, stomach ache, musculoskeletal pain, fatigue, feeling hot, cold sweat, sore throat, urinary problems, dizziness and chest pain. Depressive symptoms were assessed using a 20 item questionnaire (the CES-D: Aseltine *et al.*, 1994). Demographic information on income and ethnicity were also recorded.

▶

Results

Significant group differences were found in five symptoms: headache, musculoskeletal pain, feeling hot, chest pain and frequent/painful urination. Hence, white participants had the highest prevalence of headache (32 per cent) and Asian groups the lowest (16 per cent). The results demonstrated that the overall reports of recurrent physical symptoms in adolescents differed by their racial/ethnic backgrounds. White youths showed a higher tendency to headaches and musculoskeletal pain whereas feeling hot, chest pain and urinary symptoms were more frequent among minority groups. Some of these differences could be explained by SES differences between the groups.

Implications

The present study contributes to nursing practices by highlighting the differences in ethnicity in describing and reporting symptoms. This is important for a number of reasons. Firstly, it may be the reporting of symptoms that is most important rather than the actual experience of the symptoms. Secondly, there were strong positive relationships between depressive symptoms and all 10 physical symptoms. Hence, it is suggested that there is a need for a depression screening when reviewing such somatic symptoms. Thirdly, the findings suggest that nurses have to take cognisance of the patient's background rather than simply focusing in on the physical symptoms. As the authors suggest: 'careful consideration of the race/ethnicity ... can be an important first step in the quest for symptom relief' (p. 161). Importantly, this study suggests that there are significant differences in the conceptualisation of health between different ethnic groups (see Chapter 1) and that the somatisation of depressive symptoms may similarly differ between ethnic groups.

Substance misuse

White Irish men (58 per cent) and women (37 per cent) were more likely than any other ethnic group to drink in excess of government recommended guidelines (i.e. no more than three to four units per day for men and two to three units per day for women). After the White Irish, Black Caribbean (27 per cent of men and 17 per cent of women) were most likely to drink above the guidelines. Less than 10 per cent of men and women from the Pakistani, Bangladeshi and Chinese groups drank more than these recommended amounts on their heaviest drinking day. Very few Indian women exceeded the guidelines (5 per cent) but 22 per cent of Indian men drank above this level (Figure 8.6).

Evidence from a number of studies has indicated that drug abuse within black and minority groups, particularly among South Asians is lower than the white population (Ramsey *et al.*, 2001). However, there are indications that drug abuse is greater among young black and ethnic minority women (NTA, 2003). Although the substances misused were similar between different ethnic groups there were indications that there were differences between classes of substances and mode of consumption by different ethnic groups (Sangster *et al.*, 2001) which may be related to cultural characteristics of the ethnic groups.

Think about this

Consider Stan again: how can his health be influenced by his ethnic status? Why do you think there are differences between those in different ethnic groups?

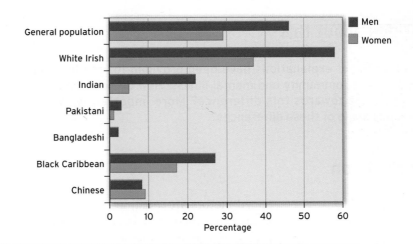

Figure 8.6 Adults drinking above recommended daily alcohol guidelines: by ethnic group and sex, 1999, England.

There may be more to the differences in health status, however, than just health behaviours and there are specific issues facing those from the ethnic group, for example cultural differences, health care practitioner interactions and the experience of racism in the health service. Both of these major issues will be explored more fully in Chapter 9.

Ethnicity and mental health: a case for treatment?

Psychotic disorders, which include schizophrenia and other delusional disorders, are relatively infrequent, with research suggesting that about 1 in 200 (0.5 per cent) people in the United Kingdom being affected (Nazroo and King, 2002). Similar research has highlighted that Black Caribbean people are three to five times more likely than White people to be admitted to hospital with a first diagnosis of schizophrenia. However, it is important to note that there are differences within each community, with individual differences outweighing group differences in extent and importance (Fernando, 2002). The picture is also mixed for other ethnic groups with, for example, Indian and Pakistani people having higher rates of psychotic symptoms but, in contrast, people from Bangladesh had a lower rate of symptoms than their White counterparts.

In contrast to this work in the United Kingdom, epidemiological work in the Caribbean does not suggest an increased risk of psychosis in the indigenous Caribbean population. Consequently, it is likely that Black Caribbean people are treated differently in the United Kingdom. Furthermore, many black people fear mental health services because they associate them with other more obviously coercive agencies such as the criminal justice system (Sivanandan, 1991), and African Caribbean men may be ten times more likely to be sectioned than their white counterparts (Mind, 2002; Reid-Galloway, 1998).

Think about this

A number of explanations have been provided for the link between those from the African-Caribbean community and mental illness. How do you think the health and social services can contribute towards this difference? More importantly, what do you think you could do to reduce some of these differences?

Conclusion

Social factors are a major factor impacting on our health and some have argued that these may be more important that individual psychological or biological variables. The social position of an individual, the sex of the individual and their ethnic status all impact on health – whether this be physical or mental. The nurse and health care professionals in general have to appreciate the social context of the individual and the impact that this can have on their health status.

Summary

- Social class can impact upon our health significantly.

- Social class is underpinned by a series of behaviours and expectations that can hinder health.

- There is a difference in the life expectancy between men and women.

- Men acknowledge their symptoms less than women.

- There may be a bias in health care practitioners with them treating women as 'sick' and 'ill' rather than men.

- Boys are socialised to be 'masculine' and this has consequences for their health.

- There is a difference in health status among ethnic groups. This can be explained, in part, by the health behaviours of the different groups.

- There are specific issues facing members of the ethnic minorities – racism and cultural awareness issues in the NHS.

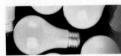

Check your understanding

1. What is the main influence on gender development?

2. How does socialisation influence health status of both men and women?

3. How can social class can impact on health?

4. How can the nurse influence health care that is dependent on social class, gender and ethnicity?

5. How can and should the nurse alter their behaviour in light of social class, gender and ethnicity of the individual patient?

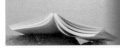

Further reading

Courtney, W.H. (2000) Construction of masculinity and their influence on men's wellbeing: a theory of gender and health. *Social Science and Medicine*, **50**, 1385–1401.

Hayes, B.C. and Prior, P.M. (2003) *Gender and Health Care in the UK. Exploring the Stereotypes.* London: Palgrave.

The Health of Minority Ethnic Groups (2001) *Health Survey for England 1999.* London: TSO.

Weblinks

Gender and health group at Liverpool University
http://www.liv.ac.uk/lstm/research/gender_health.htm

Department of Health Inequalities
http://www.dh.gov.uk/PolicyAndGuidance/HealthAndSocialCareTopics/HealthInequalities/fs/en

World Health Organization Gender and Health
http://www.who.int/gender/en/

Ethnicity and Health website from the University of Wolverhampton
http://www.be-me.org

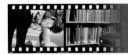

Media examples

Fight Club (1999) Note the concept of masculinity that runs throughout this testosterone-filled film – no wonder men die younger!

Vera Drake (2004) What this movie shows is not only the average life of a 'lower class' family but the options forced on them that were different from those in the higher brackets of society.

The Royle Family (TV sitcom) An exaggerated view of stereotypical lower class behaviour.

Chapter 9

Cultural awareness and transcultural issues

Learning outcomes

When you have read through this chapter you should understand:

- How the nurse, patient and health organisation culture can impact on patient experience and outcome.

- How different health beliefs can influence a patient's health behaviour and understanding of their own health state.

- How different religions and faiths impact on how the patient expects to be treated within the health care context.

- How to communicate appropriately with patients who may hold health beliefs that differ from the biomedical approach.

- How a nurse can enhance and practise cultural awareness and culturally competency appropriately.

- How transcultural-nursing framework models such as the ACCESS model can be used.

- How to work with both personal and professional translators effectively and without the patient feeling uncomfortable.

- How non-verbal communication can vary across cultural groups and how these can impact on the care and communication the patient receives.

Case study

Mr Rafiq Saddiqui Mohammed is a 68 year old Bengali Muslim. He has just had an angina attack as a result of hypercholesterolaemia; a high content of low-density lipoprotein (LDL). His two daughters Zara and Ashifa accompany him to hospital. The consultant has asked the nurse to advise Mr Mohammed on changes he will need to make to minimise his chances of another attack. The nurse has booked a translator for the consultation as Mr Mohammed does not speak fluent English.

The nurse asks the translator to inform the patient that if he is to prevent another angina attack as a result of hypercholesterolaemia, his smoking and dietary behaviours have to change. The translator relays the information to the patient only to find that Mr Mohammed cannot understand what she is saying. The translator concludes that Mr Mohammed can only understand and speak Sylheti. This is not a language the translator is trained in. The nurse is dismayed as she mistakenly believed that there were many commonalities among the Indian subcontinent languages. The nurse is then left with no option but to ask Mr Mohammed's daughters to translate the information to him.

However, neither of the daughters is fluent in Sylheti and they both have difficulties when translating and explaining medical terms. The difficulty for the daughters increases when they are asked to translate information and health advice that challenges their father's current lifestyle. The daughters become apprehensive and, although they relay the information, they do not state the importance of it. Throughout the consultation the nurse informs the daughters of what to tell Mr Mohammed by talking directly to them.

Mr Mohammed gets angry and tells his daughters that he has had enough in the hospital. As far as he is concerned the hospital cannot identify the cause of his illness. Mr Mohammed believes that only a spiritual healer can help him. In addition, it is also a Friday. Friday is prayer day for Muslims and Mr Mohammed is not aware of any prayer rooms or washing facilities. As a result he urges his daughters to get him out of the hospital. At the same time Mr Mohammed nods to the nurse signalling to her that he understands the health advice he has been given. The nurse gives one of the daughters a follow-up appointment so that they can monitor his progress over the coming weeks. The nurse also gives them a leaflet written in Sylheti so that Mr Mohammed can read more about the link between behaviour and angina attacks. With that, the family leave and make arrangements to see a spiritual healer. Over the next few weeks their father does not amend his health behaviours and his condition worsens. As a result the daughters feel enormous guilt about not emphasising the importance of the nurse's advice during their translation.

Why is this relevant to nursing practice?

There are many issues that stem from this case study, which are central to the area of culture and communication. The overarching theme of culture within nursing practice is mirrored within the *Nursing and Midwifery Council code of professional conduct: standards for conduct, performance and ethics*, which states that:

> You are personally accountable for ensuring you promote and protect the interests and dignity of patients and clients, irrespective of gender, age, race, sexuality, economic status, lifestyle, culture and religious and political beliefs. (Nursing and Midwifery Council, 2004, p. 4, para. 2.2)

Within practice there will be a diverse range of patients with various levels of understanding of the English language. Patients may come from many different religious backgrounds, and may have health beliefs that diverge from the **biomedical** viewpoint. Mr Mohammed could not speak fluent English and therefore a translator was booked for his appointment. Unfortunately though, the nurse had mistakenly assumed that the translator could speak all the Indian subcontinent languages. However, there is enormous dialectal **diversity** across and within ethnic cultural groups. In this case the translator could not speak the dialect of Sylheti and the nurse asked the daughters to conduct the translation. Although the daughters spoke some Sylheti, they were not fluent. The nurse's mistaken assumption that all family members were fluent in the language hindered communication. These issues of diversity and the impact of **stereotyping** will be examined within this chapter.

The roles of **translators** are paramount within the NHS, especially within Primary Care Trusts (PCTs) that have an ethnically diverse patient population. There are many rules surrounding the use of translators, which student nurses will not be aware of when they first begin their training. In the opening case study, the nurse maintained eye contact with and spoke to both of the daughters, rather than maintaining eye contact with Mr Mohammed. This is a common mistake made by nurses who do not know how to work with a translator in the most effective way. For example, eye contact should have been maintained with Mr Mohammed. This chapter will look further at the role of the translator and how the nurse can make the best use of their services so that the best patient outcome is achieved without any problems, miscommunication or misunderstanding.

The case study exemplifies the role of differing health beliefs within the health care context and the potential problems that can arise if a nurse does not take these into account. In this particular instance, Mr Mohammed did not see any worth in the biomedical standpoint, but instead preferred to see a spiritual healer. Patients, irrespective of their religious and ethnic cultural backgrounds, may not necessarily hold the same health beliefs as the one that they are receiving care within. Within this case study, the nurse did not pursue the possible exploration of a differing health belief. The nurse used the family members to translate, which further inhibited any insight to the patient's differing health belief as information was not being fully disclosed. Different kinds of **health beliefs**, and how to explore and work with a patient who may be holding them, will be explored within this chapter. Health beliefs consist of many variables, one being cultural, which influences health behaviour. The case study illustrates what can happen when a differing health belief is not addressed within a care plan. This chapter will outline questions that a nurse can use when addressing differing health beliefs (see Chapter 15 for an in-depth look at how they work).

Another assumption made by the nurse was that if Mr Mohammed could speak and understand Sylheti fluently, he could obviously read it. However, many first-generation immigrants from developing countries (those individuals who migrated to the United Kingdom), may not be literate within their own mother tongue, even though they may be able to speak their language fluently. Even though leaflets are translated into several languages, patients may not be able to read them. This is another area that will be pursued and the exploration of how the nurse can overcome such obstacles will be looked at.

The case study is an example of the type of patient you may care for in practice; someone from an ethnic minority, has a health belief different from the biomedical viewpoint and lives his day-to-day life according to the principles of his faith. Mr Mohammed is a Sylheti-speaking Muslim. For Muslims who follow the Islamic faith, Friday is the most important day of the week, as it is prayer day. The nurse in the opening case study did not ask Mr Mohammed about prayer day. In return Mr Mohammed did not mention anything to the nurse. As a result, the patient assumed that there were no facilities for prayer in the building. Religious beliefs will be explored in this chapter, as it is important to have a basic understanding of the many religions that exist.

The need for the nurse to be aware of a patient's religious, cultural and health beliefs, and the way to explore and work with these beliefs when caring for a patient, is the main focus of **transcultural nursing.** Transcultural nursing can be defined as:

> A formal area of study and practice focused on comparative holistic culture care, health, and illness patterns of people with respect to differences and similarities in their cultural values, beliefs, and lifeways with the goal to provide culturally congruent, competent and compassionate care.
> (Leininger, 1997)

The UK has a diverse and dynamic population, so awareness of transcultural nursing issues are vital for practice. According to Gerrish *et al.* (1996), Le Var (1998) and Peberdy (1997), Britain is regarded as one of the most ethnically diverse countries in Europe. According to the last census in 2001, the size of the minority ethnic population in England and Wales was 7.9 per cent (4.6 million); see Table 9.1 for a breakdown (Office for National Statistics, 2001).

Table 9.1
Population size 2001
England and Wales:
ethnicity

	Population count	%	Minority ethnic population (%)
White	54 153 898	92.1	N/a
Mixed	677 117	1.2	14.6
Asian or Asian British			
Indian	1 053 411	1.8	22.7
Pakistani	747 285	1.3	16.1
Bangladeshi	283 063	0.5	6.1
Other Asian	247 664	0.4	5.3
Black or Black British			
Black Caribbean	565 876	1.0	12.2
Black African	485 277	0.8	10.5
Black Other	97 585	0.2	2.1
Chinese	247 403	0.4	5.3
Other	230 615	0.4	5.0
All minority ethnic population	4 635 296	7.9	100
All population	58 789 194	100	N/a

Source: adapted from ONS (2001a)

Since the UK 1991 census there has been an increase in people from ethnic minorities living in the UK. The amount has risen from circa six per cent (3 million) to nine per cent in 2001 (ONS, 1991; ONS, 2001). These growth figures may not seem particularly large. However, they can be misleading, as ethnic minority groups tend to reside within 'close-knit' communities. In certain parts of England minority groups are now becoming ethnic majorities. Even if a nurse is not working with a diverse ethnic or religious population, an awareness of transcultural nursing is still essential because of the differing health beliefs individuals may hold.

Because of the complex nature of diversity, it is a key issue within the exploration of transcultural nursing. Diversity is a result of a number of factors, including religion, culture and geography. These variables result in subtle differences within ethnic and religious minority, and majority, groups. The role of diversity within ethnic and religious minority and majority groups will be explored in depth in this chapter. Take, for example, Mr Mohammed and the translator. The nurse made an assumption that the translator, who was Indian, could speak the same language as Mr Mohammed. However, this was not so. The case study further exemplified diversity as neither of Mr Mohammed's daughters could speak her father's language fluently. Hence, 'Diversity across and within ethnic groups has resulted in the need for health care workers such as nurses to deliver culturally sensitive and culturally appropriate care' (Narayanasamy, 2003, p.185).

The requirement for nurses to study culture and transcultural nursing during pre-registration courses has been highlighted in various studies. These studies have found that the health needs of ethnic minorities are not always being adequately met (Chevannes, 1997; Fletcher, 1997; Gerrish, et al, 1996; Gerrish and Papadopoulos, 1999; Le Var, 1998; Narayanasamy, 2003; 2003; Papadopoulos et al, 1998 and Serrant Green, 2001).

To date, pre-registration nursing courses have made encouraging steps in highlighting transcultural nursing. However, there is still a need for further improvement. For example, Narayanasamy (2003) conducted a survey of 126 post-registration nurses and found that, despite having completed a pre-registration programme, these nurses still expressed a need for further education in order to meet the cultural needs of their patients.

This chapter will provide nurses with the first basic stepping stones into the area of transcultural nursing.

Culture

Defining culture

Anthropologists have provided numerous definitions of **culture**. Among these, the most famous and most often cited definition is Tylor's definition in 1871: 'That complex whole which includes knowledge, belief, art, morals law, custom and any other capabilities and habits acquired by man as a member of society' (Tylor, 1920, cited in Leach, 1982, pp. 38–39).

Andrew and Boyle (1995, p. 10) view culture as consisting of four overarching characteristics:

1. Culture is learned from birth through the process of language acquisition and socialisation. From society's viewpoint, socialisation is the way culture is transmitted and the individual is fitted into the group's organised way of life.
2. Culture is shared by all members of the same cultural group: in fact, it is the sharing of cultural beliefs and patterns that bonds people together under one identity as a group (even though it is not always a conscious process).
3. Culture is an adaptation to specific activities related to environmental and technical factors and to the availability of natural resources.
4. Culture is a dynamic, ever-changing process.

Diversity and culture

Andrews and Boyle's (1995) last characteristic of culture being 'dynamic and forever changing' has been echoed by other studies. Henley and Schott (1999, p.3) state that culture is not genetically inherited, nor is it fixed or static but in fact changes in response to new situations and pressures. This can pose a problem for nurses who read resources to gain insight into other cultures and religions. As a result of the dynamic nature of culture, and the huge diversity between cultural and religious groups, what has been read may be outdated. Furthermore it may encourage stereotypical views of everyone within a particular cultural group as having the same health beliefs. For example, even though Mr Mohammed and his two daughters all followed Islam there were clear generational differences in their fluency of Sylheti.

Culture has an important influence on many aspects of people's lives, including rituals, language and health beliefs. The case study demonstrated how culture influenced the health beliefs of Mr Mohammed: he interpreted the cause of his angina attack as something that only a spiritual healer could cure. This led to Mr Mohammed ignoring the fact that smoking played a role in his angina attack. More importantly it resulted in him ignoring the fact that smoking could contribute to a recurrence. However, his two daughters knew that the smoking behaviour was a contributing factor but also agreed to take him to a spiritual healer. This is an example of a number of contributing factors that can influence health-related beliefs and behaviours.

Helman (2001, p. 3) lists these 'other' influences as:

- individual factors (such as age, gender, size, appearance, personality, intelligence, experience, physical and emotional state);
- educational factors (both formal and informal and including education into a religious, ethnic or professional sub-culture);
- socio-economic factors (such as social class, economic status, occupation or unemployment, and the networks of social support from other people);
- environmental factors (such as the weather, population density or pollution of the habitat, but also including the types of infrastructure available, such as health facilities).

Culture needs to be seen within the current context. For example, Mr Mohammed who is a first-generation Muslim, clearly has health beliefs that differ from those of his daughters. They are second-generation Muslims who were more inviting of the biomedical approach. However, this case study does not necessarily mean that every first-generation ethnic minority will support an opposing health belief model compared with their younger counterparts.

Think about this

Think about how many influences you have that make up the health beliefs you hold today. Are these different from when you left school? Your reflection process could involve different educational influences, friends, family, 'sayings', e.g. 'an apple a day keeps the doctor away' and resources, e.g. the Internet, books, journals and the media.

The different cultures that operate when you care for a patient

Think about this

Before reading the following section, think about Mr Mohammed and the consultation with the nurse. How many cultures were operating here?

De Santis (1994) identified three possible cultures that are dominant when caring for the patient: **organisational culture,** which you are working within; **patient culture,** that you will be interacting with and **nursing culture.**

Nursing culture can have an impact on the outcome of the nurse–patient relationship. In the case study above, the nurse mentioned the 'smoking cessation officer'. However, the nurse failed to elaborate on the role of the smoking cessation officer and how they can actually facilitate a person to give up smoking. In addition, the nurse consultation was not patient-centred. The nurse should have attempted to assess what Mr Mohammed understood by the terms 'angina' and 'hypercholesterolaemia' by using open-ended questions (refer to Chapter 17).

There will be medical terms and words, sometimes abbreviated, that will be understood by nurses, but alien to those who have not had any medical training. This can cause problems when the patient is attempting to understand their current health state. The use of such terms within the nurse–patient relationship is referred to as **medical jargon.** Simplification of information and awareness that there will be terms that will be unfamiliar to the patient is a good starting point within transcultural nursing. The negative effect of the use of medical jargon is increased if the patient cannot speak fluent English.

The following terms and acronyms are used by nurses on a daily basis:

- handover
- last offices
- ECT
- crashed
- not pu'd
- catheter
- the rounds
- ADHA

According to Castledine (1998), jargonistic language is inappropriate to use with the patient, as it may be misunderstood as using professional language. It is important to use language that is fully understood by the patient. This will ensure that the patient feels understood. The nurse should attempt to make the patient feel comfortable enough to explore any complex information, in order to ease concerns and anxiety. This is even more important when talking and caring for patients who do not speak fluent English.

Think about this

To further raise awareness of how easy it is to use nursing jargon, think about either yourself on first placement, or your previous medical encounters as a patient. How many examples of situations can you cite where you have heard terms used by trained nurses and consultants that were unfamiliar to you? This will raise your awareness as to the diversity within nursing culture.

Organisational culture

As shown in the case study above, although the nurse booked a professional translator, the translator was inappropriate for the needs of her patient. Every hospital will have resources such as professional translators (see working with a translator section for more detail). In addition to this, there are many rules that operate within the organisation that the nurse has to work within. For example, a patient coming into the hospital can become easily confused within an environment that is unfamiliar to them. This confusion can stem from signs in the hospital (see picture) to certain names that are attributed to wards. Further confusion can stem from the protocol that the nurse has to follow.

Signs in hospital: how confusing are these?

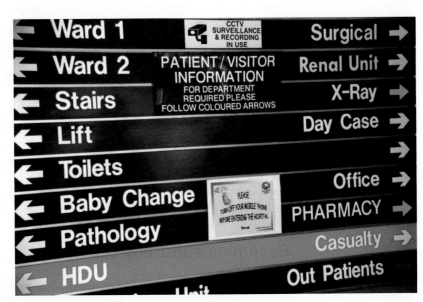

Shout Pictures

Think about this

What aspects of the hospital environment would seem unfamiliar to a patient who does not visit the hospital regularly?

Signs intended to help direct patients around the hospital can often seem alien. On your first placement, you may feel, or have felt, disoriented at the unfamiliar environment around you.

Patient culture

The patient who comes into the hospital brings with them their own culture, which influences how they perceive their current symptoms. This could conflict with the treatment that they are receiving, which is based on the biomedical approach. In the case of Mr Mohammed, the patient interpreted his heart attack symptoms differently to the nurse. This was seen when he did not value the opinion that smoking contributed to, or could possibly contribute to, another heart attack. Instead, the prevailing health belief for Mr Mohammed stemmed from the **supernatural health belief model**, from which he believed that he had been cursed and that only a spiritual healer could cure him.

Think about this

What can a nurse do in order to be able to fully explore the health beliefs of their patient in the most effective way?

In the opening case study, it was clear that the nurse made no attempt to explore the religious or cultural beliefs of Mr Mohammed and his family. In order to begin the process of becoming **culturally competent**, and in turn provide the best possible care for the patient, it is important to recognise that the patient brings religious and cultural beliefs. These values could influence their health beliefs and how they interpret their health state. Nurses need to develop knowledge and competence in order to be effective in meeting needs related to cultural beliefs and practices (Ayer, 1997; Gerrish and Papadopoulos, 1999; Le Var, 1998; Narayanaxamy, 2002; Papadopoulos and Lees, 2002). The section below highlights the process that is required when developing the knowledge and competence required from nurses working with diverse patient groups.

Becoming culturally competent

In order for a nurse to become culturally competent and explore the patient's health, cultural and religious beliefs with confidence, the following information can help. However, this is only a starting point in the process of becoming culturally competent as a nurse. A nurse who says they have learned everything about the diverse patient population they work with is a nurse who has stopped becoming culturally competent, because they have stopped learning about their continually changing patient groups.

Religious beliefs

Having knowledge about prevailing religions and faiths is a good starting point. However, it is important to remember that there is enormous diversity within religious groups. Stereotyping and generalisation of the patient can result when the individual is assumed to think about health in a particular way based on the religion they represent. This has been illustrated by Hong and Kale (2003) who state that when attempting to understand different beliefs and lifestyles, a risk of over-simplification and stereotyping can result.

Take for example the definition of culture above, which encompasses enormous diversity. For example, age, education and generation all result in variety in the way individuals live. In the case study above, Mr Mohammed and his two daughters are all Muslims. Friday is prayer day for Muslims and Mr Mohammed required adequate washing facilities and a place to pray. However, his two daughters do not pray on a Friday as they usually have other priorities and as such did not require washing facilities. There is a generational difference between Mr Mohammed and his two daughters in their practice of the Islamic faith.

Below are introductions to the differing religious and faith beliefs that you may encounter in practice. When reading these, you need to take into consideration that there is enormous diversity within the religious and faith groups. At the same time, nurses who work with patients who come from various religious backgrounds need to make themselves familiar with the basic beliefs of the religion concerned, in order to care for a patient and recognise their possible spiritual and cultural needs (Neuberger, 1994a).

Jehovah's Witnesses

Case study

Nathan, a 43-year-old man, has been admitted to hospital with a dangerously low blood count. He has been accompanied by two of his friends from the Jehovah's Witness Church, who refer to one another as 'brother'. The nurse informs Nathan that he has to have a blood transfusion immediately, or else he could be faced with the possibility of severe weakness to his body. The nurse also informs Nathan of alternative blood products but states that they will not be effective as the original proposed blood transfusion. Nathan and his two brothers refuse all of these. The nurse documents on paper that blood transfusion has been refused.

Think about this

Has the nurse followed the correct procedure when working with a patient who has refused a blood transfusion? Is there anything that the nurse could have done better?

American Charles Taze Russell founded the Jehovah's Witness religion in the 1870s and there are about 125 000 Jehovah's Witnesses in the United Kingdom (Simpson, 2002). The most important implication for a nurse when dealing with a patient who is a Jehovah's Witness is their refusal of a blood transfusion, as documented in the above case study. However, the Jehovah's Witness religion has enormous diversity within it. For example, there are patients like Nathan who refuse red blood cells, but others who will accept blood proteins such as Factor VIII. Pregnant women who are rhesus-negative may not accept immunoglobulins (Simpson, 2002).

Many Jehovah's Witnesses will accept such procedures as intra-operative blood salvage and post-operative blood salvage from drains (cell saver), as well as haemodilution techniques. To make such procedures acceptable, tubing should be visible to show the diverted blood is still in contact with the patient, as tubing is seen as an extension of the circulatory system (Simpson, 2002). However, some Jehovah's Witnesses may refuse all blood transfusions, including stored autologous blood. They also refuse red cells, white cells, plasma and platelets. They may elect to receive fractions of these components, such as albumin, clotting factors, immunoglobins, interferon and haemoglobin-based oxygen carriers (Simpson, 2002). A group of Jehovah's Witnesses, known as the Associated Jehovah's Witnesses for Reform on Blood (AJWRB), is currently seeking to reform the organisation's position on blood products.

The nurse in the above case study suggested to Nathan that there were alternative blood products. However she failed to inform him what these were. The nurse also failed to document in full that the patient was given the option of the blood transfusion, as well as other blood products, all of which were refused. This fully completed document should have also been signed by the patient. In a scenario such as this, informing the patient in as much detail as possible and documenting the discussion is vitally important. If the patient's health further deteriorates, or the patient become unconscious, there is then written documentation of the patient's consent. This can then be shown to family members or external parties if required.

Baptised Jehovah's Witnesses often carry an advanced medical directive/release document, instructing health care professionals not to give blood transfusion under any circumstances and releasing hospitals of the responsibility for damage caused by the refusal of blood. Problems could arise if this is a verbal instruction, without any written documentation (Simpson, 2002).

The nurse in the case study should have put a wristband on the patient to alert other staff that the patient is a Jehovah's Witness. Patient confidentially is important within such a scenario. The fact that the information given to the patient and his refusal of a blood transfusion took place in front of two friends, who were also Jehovah's Witnesses, did not ensure possible full disclosure of what the patient really wanted. It is important to carry out such a consultation in private as well as keeping information as confidential as possible.

Rastafarianism

Case study

Nurse Richard has been taking care of patient Jim, who has been in hospital for three days. Jim is Rastafarian. He decided several weeks ago to heal his bleeding ulcers naturally. However, because of his refusal of a blood transfusion, the body has become very weak. As a result, Jim was admitted to hospital. Jim is adamant that he still does not want a blood transfusion. Nurse Richard holds the patient in high regard, as he is very pleasant and well mannered. The patient refers to nurse Richard as 'brethren', which Richard thought was an offensive term, until he asked the patient, who clarified the term as meaning 'brother'. Jim has weakened over the past six days and on the seventh day in hospital has become unconscious. Nurse Richard is frustrated at the constant refusal of blood transfusion, which has weakened the patient's body, all of which was documented and signed by the patient when conscious. Nurse Richard holds Jim's hand and thinks about how frustrating it was not to give him a blood transfusion so that he could get better. At the same time, he admires his continual belief in natural healing.

Rastafarians evolved with the teachings of Marcus Garvey (1887–1940), who worked to promote the interests of people of African decent and grew in strength as an alternative to the western colonial influence. This was displayed with the 'Back to Africa' campaign, the roots of which lie in Ethiopia and Jamaica. There are 1 000 000 followers worldwide, with rapid growth occurring from 1975 to the present (Mack, 1999). No exact numbers have been published for the number of Rastafarians living within the United Kingdom; however it has been suggested that sizeable communities reside within London, Leeds, Manchester, Birmingham, Liverpool, Bristol and Nottingham, with estimates that six out of every ten Jamaicans follow the Rastafarian way of life (Baxter, 2002).

Rastafarians believe in the natural healing process. Patient Jim was clearly adamant that he did not want a blood transfusion, so much so that even when he became very weak, he put his belief down in writing, irrespective of the prospect of his health becoming worse. Rastafarians regard the body as the temple of God, which should be protected from contamination (Baxter, 2002). This can range from eating only the most natural food that is fresh and pure, referred to as *Ital,* to the prohibition of pork, alcohol and predatory fish. In relation to medication, herbal remedies are opted for, along with the belief that the body can heal itself. Medical procedures and treatments are viewed as invasive because of the interference with God's plans (Baxter, 2002). Such beliefs differ among Rastafarians. As a result the nurse should individualise care and communicate as much as possible with the patient to assess what their particular beliefs are in regards to medical intervention as well as dietary requirements. In the case study it was clear that Jim lived his day-to-day life with the principles of Rastafarianism; this may not be the case for other Rastafarians.

A distinguishing feature of Rastafarians is the dress code, which is characterised by uncut hair that is grown into dreadlocks and beards for men. However, the nurse should be aware that patients might choose to have dreadlocks as a fashion choice, rather than being a Rastafarian follower.

As shown in the case study, nurse Richard was at first confused as to why the patient referred to him as 'brethren'. Fellow members are referred to as brethren (men) and sistern (women). It is clear that the patient also held nurse Richard in high stead, hence referring to him as brethren. Nurse Richard also kept communication very open, by asking the patient what 'brethren' meant. When working with a patient who uses terms or acronyms that are not familiar with the nurse, it is usually to ask the patient, good practice which will clarify any misunderstanding that could occur.

Christianity

Case study

Anna is with her son in hospital, who has been ill with leukaemia for two years. He is now falling in and out of consciousness. The consultant has informed Anna that they will not resuscitate her son, but will let him die peacefully. Anna has decided to inform the minister of the church to come in to baptise her son. She has also attached a religious picture to her son's bedclothes and has put rosary beads by the side of her son. Anna is praying constantly. The priest performs the Holy Communion. A couple of hours later, Anna's son is dead.

Think about this

Is it typical for a Christian parent to baptise their child when facing death, or are there many variations as to what Christian parents would do?

It is estimated that there are seven million practising Christians in the United Kingdom and many more who would describe themselves as Christian (Henley and Schott, 1999). The case study above shows a mother who follows the Roman Catholic strand of Christianity, as exemplified by the religious picture pinned to the bed and the rosary beads. Within Christianity, the core belief system and the reading of the Bible are the same, but they are modified and interpreted differently, depending on the branch of Christianity. There are many different branches, including the Church of England, Catholicism, Orthodox Christian, Presbyterianism, Methodism, Pentecostalism, Seventh Day Adventism and many others (Christmas, 2002). Hence, there is enormous diversity within the Christian faith, depending on the branch of Christianity that is practised.

Christians behave differently at times of stress and death, depending on what branch of Christianity they reside within (Neuberger, 1994a). In this particular case study, Anna wanted her son to be baptised by the local priest, so that he could be admitted into the Christian community before his death. However, baptism varies depending on each person and family. In addition, the rosary beads and the picture pinned to Anna's son's bedclothes, are evidence of Roman Catholicism. The type of symbolic religious jewellery and pictures brought in for the sick patient depend again on the particular branch of Christianity the individual/family believe in. According to Neuberger (1994a), sensitivity and care is needed at all times, as sometimes individual items are brought in that are of monetary value but may not be safe within the hospital environment.

Holy Communion, also referred to as 'the sacrament of the sick', is significant for those who are Christian Roman Catholics. The Holy Communion tends to be carried out by the priest for those patients who are dying. The sacrament of a piece of bread and wine is given to represent the body and blood of the Lord Jesus, which signifies remission of sins. It is important for a nurse to keep all channels of communication open, as well as informing the family that they are free to invite a local priest, if they are not happy with the chaplain service within the hospital.

There is also enormous diversity with regards to family planning. The Roman Catholic Church forbids artificial contraception, sterilisation and termination of pregnancy on the grounds that it interferes with God's natural law (Schott and Henley, 1996). Generational differences result in a mixed view on contraception and abortion and older practising Christians are more likely to object. However, this is changing as a result of greater freedom and choice of the individual (Christmas, 2002). Nurses must be aware of these differences and accept that the younger Christian cohort will still have individuals who oppose abortion and contraception. However, other factors may take precedence as to the eventual decision that is taken. For example, many Catholic women will agree to a termination if the baby has a congenital abnormality or if they have been subjected to rape (Holland & Hogg, 2001; p.52).

Buddhism

Case study

Joe is a follower of Buddhism. He has been admitted into the mental health ward with severe anxiety and depression. The nurses are alarmed to find that Joe is still refusing to take medication. However, despite his severe depression, Joe is managing to wake up during the early hours of the morning to meditate and carry out deep breathing exercises. His state has improved slightly but the consultant and nurses are still going to inform the family that he needs medication.

Think about this

How can the nurses break down the communication barrier, so that they can work more effectively with Joe?

There are about 500 000 Buddhists living in the United Kingdom, with many groups and sects (Northcott, 2002). The followers of Buddha should be thought of as 'individuals', as the religion has no single creed, authority or scared book, but are united in their recognition of Siddhartha Gautama, an Indian Prince who became the Buddha, or enlightened one (Northcott, 2002). Buddhism is a way of life. The cornerstone of Buddhist living is meditation. As shown in the above case study, Joe meditated, as he believed that by meditating, he could find peace and hopefully eradicate his symptoms. Research presented to the 2001 annual conference of the Royal College of Psychiatrists found that using **Vipassana** (Buddhist meditation) as a therapy, did benefit prisoners and people who had mental health problems (Northcott, 2002).

In this case study, the mental health nurse is frustrated with Joe because he is not willing to take medication. However, at the same time the nurse does acknowledge that Joe wakes up early in the morning and is active with his daily meditation routine. A problem highlighted in this case study is the refusal to take medication, which the nurse justifies as a Buddhist belief. This is a stereotype popularly held with respect to the Buddhist way of life. Buddhist thinking recognises mental health problems as arising from a hectic life and imbalanced diet. As a result Buddhists see meditation as a way to inner calm. However, they are also willing to accept medical treatments that are advocated.

In this scenario the nurse should have communicated with Joe about the importance of medication in managing depression. It was clear to the nurse that medication had been refused over a long period of time. A possible solution could have been to invite the Buddhist chaplain, lay advisor or elder of the Buddhist community to be present when addressing the issue of medication and Buddhist beliefs with Joe (Northcott, 2002).

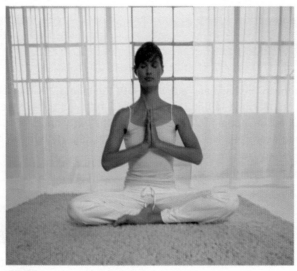

© Adrianna Williams/zefa/Corbis

Judaism

Case study

Penuel Katz was born a week ago but has been kept in hospital due to respiratory problems. He has shown improvements within the last day and his mother has been informed by the nurse that they hope to discharge her son in the morning. Devorah is relieved that she is returning home as she has not eaten properly during her stay in hospital. She had explained to the nurses that she is an Orthodox Jew who can only eat kosher meat. Much to her amazement the staff ordered her vegetarian meals cooked in the hospital. Also, the nurses did not understand why Devorah informed them a 'Mohel' would be coming into the hospital to perform circumcision. The nurses did not appreciate why this needed to be done so soon, particularly as baby Penuel was just beginning to grow stronger.

It is estimated that 300 000 Jews live in the United Kingdom, the majority (200 000) in London (Collins, 2002). There is enormous diversity within the Judaism religious group, which can be observed firstly with the overarching divisions within the religion. Orthodox Jews comprise modern orthodox Jews who have integrated into society while still observing Jewish law. In comparison, ultra-orthodox Jews live separately and dress in a traditional fashion.

Devorah, the mother of the child in the above case study, is a modern orthodox Jew, who lives her daily life according to Jewish principles. For example, Devorah will eat only kosher meat, which is characterised by the way it is slaughtered. Offering an alternative such as a vegetarian meal, or a meal cooked in the hospital, which has been prepared with hospital cutlery, is not appropriate for Devorah. However, there are many diverse laws that relate to kosher food, so it is advisable to ask patients about their particular customs (Collins, 2002).

It is customary within the religion of Judaism to carry out circumcision on baby boys, usually when they are 8 days old (Collins, 2002). In this particular case study, Penuel could not be circumcised immediately because of his respiratory problems. However, the Mohel (who is an expert in carrying out circumcision) was aware of this and had continual contact with Devorah; they both decided that before Penuel went home he should be circumcised. The nurses should have communicated openly with Devorah as to circumcision practice, so that no misunderstanding and negative connotations to the practice could occur. The Mohel would also have been happy to speak to the nurses.

Hinduism

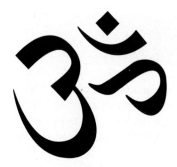

Case study

Akshay Kumaria is a 36-year-old man who has been in a severe car accident and as a result has had both of his legs amputated. The consultant has advised the immediate and extended family that, despite the operation, Akshay's internal organs have become severely infected and are slowly beginning to fail. He only has a matter of a couple of hours. Soon after he dies, the nurse finds it strange that the family take Akshay's hand, so that he touches several coins. In addition, there is a *diva* (lamp which is ignited by ghee and lit), by the side of Akshay. There is also the constant smell of incense. Akshay's wife has informed the nurses that she does not believe in any of these rituals, but it is the wish of the elders to carry out these practices before death, or when the individual has just died.

Hindus first came to the UK in the 1920s (Deaken, 1970). The UK witnessed a further influx of Hindus at the end of the Second World War as a result of a labour shortage. Hindus make up a large proportion of the Indian ethnic minority (ONS, 2001). There is enormous diversity within the Hindu religious group arising from different countries of origin, castes and generations. For example, in the case study above Mrs Kumaria did not really believe in the rituals being conducted by the elders in the family.

The touching of coins is symbolic of the dying person's generosity as the coins are then distributed to the poor. Not being able to carry out such a ritual can cause enormous distress. The lighting of the *diva* and incense sticks is indicative of the family and priest praying within a religious environment. The praying by the priest is important for the dying, or the recently deceased, as this ensures the soul is helped smoothly to transmigrate into another body (Jootun, 2002). Belief in karma, the soul and rebirth are core to any Hindu. Rebirth of the soul is believed to be necessary until it is completely purified and can join the cosmic consciousness (Radhakrishnan, 1968).

In terms of dietary requirements, there is again enormous diversity. Hindus who practise their religion daily will not touch any meat products, as vegetarianism is regarded as an indication of spirituality (Jootun, 2002). This varies according to how the Hindu's daily life is influenced by their religion. It is important for a nurse to ask each individual patient. An overall prevailing belief system is that of food being classified as hot or cold in terms of their effect on the body and emotions (Henley, 1983). An imbalance of hot or cold foods can disturb the body's energy equilibrium and lead to ill-health (Jootun, 2002). This has implications to what the patient can eat depending on their state of health.

Sikhism

Case study

Rajvinder Kaur is an 18-year-old female patient who has been admitted to hospital with severe bipolar depression. There has been enormous anger in the family who were distraught to find that Rajvinder's *kirpan* (a small sword worn on the body) has been removed from the patient and not given back. In addition, the patient's religious book (*Nit Nam*) was moved several times by the nurses, without washing their hands.

Along with Hinduism, Sikhism is another religion that completes the 'Indian' ethnic minority group. There are about 300 000 Sikhs living in Britain, many of whom settled here in the 1950s and 1960s (Kur Gill, 2002). Again within this religion, there is enormous diversity in how people live according to the Sikh religion. In the case study above, Rajvinder is a baptised Sikh, as she wore a *kirpan* (sword). A baptised Sikh will always wear the fiveKs, which are never to be removed: *kara* (steel bangle), *Kesh* (uncut, unshaven hair), *kangha* (small wooden comb), *kirpan* (small sword wrapped in a cotton garment which is worn under clothing) and *kaccha* (unisex undershorts). In the above case study, the sword was removed, which is forbidden for baptised Sikhs. If the nursing team thought that Rajvinder was in danger of her own life, then this should have been discussed immediately before the removal, so that no problems would have occurred. A symbolic picture of a sword that could have been worn as a necklace would have been suitable as a replacement.

The religious book, *Guru Granth Sahib*, or readings from the *Guru Granth Sahib (Nit Nam)*, are to be kept by the side of a person who is unwell. It is compulsory for it to be by the side of a baptised Sikh. It is also compulsory to wash hands before touching the religious book. A baptised Sikh will not consume food that has meat or eggs in it and beef is forbidden for both Sikhs and Hindus. However, this again varies for non-baptised Sikhs, where eggs and meat (apart from beef) may still be consumed.

Islam

The opening case study showed Mr Mohammed, a Muslim, in hospital. Many Muslims follow the religion and live their lives according to the teaching of Islam (Henley, 1983). According to the 2001 Census 1.8 per cent of the UK population were Asian Muslims (ONS, 2001). There were 1.6 million Asian Muslims in the UK in 1991 and the population is predicted to increase to 2 million by 2010 (Akhtar, 2002). There are two main branches within the Muslim group: Sunni Muslims and Shia Muslims.

Muslims do not have a universal language as their mother tongue depends on their country of origin. In the case study above, Mr Mohammed spoke Sylheti. This dialect is characteristic for some Bangladeshi Muslims. However, other Bangladeshi Muslims speak Bengali. Muslims whose origins are in Punjab (Mirpur District) are referred to as Pakistani Muslims. Their spoken language is Punjabi-Mirpur, which is similar to Sikhs who speak Punjabi. Muslims who originate from Gujarat (in India) tend to speak Gujarati or Kutch dialect. Certain groups of Hindus that live in Gujarat also speak the same dialect. Muslims from other parts of India may speak Urdu. There is also wide use of Arabic among Muslims who have their origins in countries such as Saudi Arabia. Muslims also originate from China and other parts of the world where the host language is spoken fluently. In the opening case study the daughters of Mr Mohammed could not speak fluent Sylheti even though their father could. This illustrates how generational differences impact on the extent that the individual is fluent within ones own non-English mother tongue.

There are overarching rules that Muslims are required to abide by, although they will differ between individuals. Firstly, practising female Muslims will be veiled. Secondly, practising male Muslims tend to have a beard. Thirdly, all Muslims adhere to the main principles in Islam as religious education is compulsory for all Muslim children under the age of sixteen. Here the *Qur'an* (the holy book) and the main principles of Islam are taught. Praying five times a day is important for practicing Muslims, especially on the holy day, Friday. On holy day practising Muslim men are required to attend the mosque at midday to pray. A nurse can accommodate practising Muslim patients by making them aware that prayer rooms and adequate washing facilities are available. In the opening case study this was not made clear to Mr Mohammed, which heightened his anxiety and desire to leave the hospital. Muslims do not eat pork, and will only eat Halal meat (where the animal has been slaughtered according to Islamic law). In the absence of Halal meat, Jewish Kosher meat may suffice, or in the absence of either, a vegetarian meal.

Muslims also fast twice a year, referred to as **Ramadan**, which lasts for a month at a time. During this time Muslims can eat only at dusk and dawn. It is important for a nurse to be aware of Ramadan, so that they can discuss this in relation to treatment. The general rule is that all Muslims have to fast, unless a woman is pregnant or the individual has a particular condition where fasting will be detrimental to their health.

Think about this

Imagine that Mr Mohammed was in hospital during the fasting period of Ramadan. How would you tailor the consultation accordingly, when advising him on diet change and medication?

Health beliefs

It is important to take health beliefs of patients into consideration as they influence their health behaviours (see Chapter 15). Health beliefs may also determine medical outcomes such as adherence to medication (see Chapter 16). Addressing the different health beliefs that patients hold indicates that a nurse is culturally competent. In addition the nurse is promoting **holistic care** as the individual is understood in light of their previous experience and perceptions. This was not seen in the opening case study where the nurse helped and provided information to Mr Mohammed from the biomedical standpoint alone. There was no attempt by the nurse to consider Mr Mohammed's other possible health beliefs. It should be remembered that even though patients are receiving care from the NHS, which fully embraces the biomedical perspective, they may not agree with such a perspective when interpreting their symptoms. This was the case for Mr Mohammed who held a health belief influenced by the **personalistic systems** viewpoint. This overarching health belief model attributes the cause of illness to supernatural forces.

If a patient holds another health belief model, a nurse advocating the biomedical viewpoint alone may result in the patient not fully committing themselves to the medical advice. Even worse, as in the case of Mr Mohammed, the patient could appear to agree with medical advice but not adhere to the treatment and recommendations once discharged. This can have significant consequences; particularly as the patient could be readmitted to hospital with more severe symptoms than he or she initially presented (refer to Chapter 16).

The Nursing and Midwifery Council's (2004) Code of Conduct encourages practitioners to embrace holistic care. The NHS agenda for 2008 entitled 'Patient-led NHS' (Department of Health, 2005) endorses this further by highlighting the patient's viewpoint as important. This in turn emphasises the consideration of patient health beliefs as being an important contributor when carrying out individualised patient-led care. Spector (1996) acknowledges that the needs of patients who hold differing health beliefs from the mainstream health care provider, are the most difficult. However, finding 'a way of caring for the client that matches the client's perception of the health problem and its treatment is important' (Spector, 1996, p. 4).

The need to understand health beliefs other than the biomedical model has become more important because of the changing nature of patient problems that have to be addressed. Today's patient is living longer than ever before (Helman, 2001). As a result, diseases of today cannot be cured by a quick fix. Instead, chronic illnesses need to be addressed from a cooperative approach, as well as the patient becoming a co-healer. Thus Helman (2001) advocates 'a deeper understanding of the patient's needs, health beliefs and realities of everyday life' (p. 67). Below is a brief consideration of the main overarching belief systems that can be held by patients.

Biomedical health beliefs

In order for a nurse to understand differing health beliefs, it is important to remember that nurses are trained within the biomedical perspective.

Think about this

Think about health beliefs and health sayings you held before commencing on the pre-registration nursing course. Compare those previous beliefs with current health beliefs. Are they different? The chances are that as individuals progress through the nursing course their beliefs will be influenced by the biomedical approach.

The biomedical model is based on the principle that germs, genes and chemicals may contribute in different ways to the causes of disorders. Subsequent treatments are usually also based on physical interventions, e.g. medicines and surgery (Curtis, 2000). Even though the nurse in the opening case study was providing the appropriate advice, treatment and care to Mr Mohammed, she failed to acknowledge that he could have perceived his ill-health from a different perspective. From the biomedical perspective, the emphasis is on the individual to maintain good health and manage their illness to the best of their ability (Helman, 1994; Jackson, 1993). In Mr Mohammed's case, there was an emphasis on dietary changes and the cessation of smoking, which are based on the biomedical perspective.

Personalistic systems

According to Holland and Hogg (2001, p. 19), within personalisitic belief systems there are three main causes of illness:

- supernatural forces (e.g. God);
- non-humans (e.g. ghosts, ancestors or evil spirits);
- human beings, witches or sorcerers.

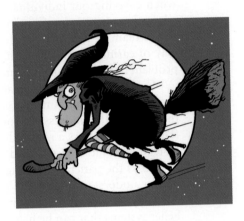

In the opening case study, Mr Mohammed believed that his illness stemmed not from physiological changes, but from supernatural forces. Within the personalistic system there is the belief that individuals are not in control of their own health, but instead are victims of supernatural forces (Jackson, 1993). Witchcraft and sorcery can have an influence on many people's belief systems both outside and within the United Kingdom. In this case, Mr Mohammed was adamant that someone had cast a spell. Today, this practice is an official religion within certain parts of Africa, famously referred to as voodoo. Another commonly held belief that stems from the personalistic systems is that of the evil eye. This is a belief system where it is believed that that someone who is jealous will cast their evil eye, which brings with it ill-health and loss of money.

Patients who have a belief system attached to any element of the personalistic system may see the cause of their illness in a different light to the biomedical perspective. Usual cures are to visit a supernatural healer, in order to 'undo' spells that have been cast. This could be seen in the case of Mr Mohammed, who wanted to seek solace by receiving the advice of a supernatural healer.

The influences of personalistic systems can be seen in every country around the world. However, the personalistic system is very much dominant within certain parts of Africa, the Caribbean, India, Dominican Republic, Central and South America, Middle East and Europe. During the Middle Ages in the United Kingdom, witchcraft was a commonly held belief. Influences of such beliefs may still be around today. At the same time, not every person will reside their beliefs within personalistic systems, even if their birthplace has been from the above-mentioned countries. For example, Mr Mohammed's two daughters did not accept Mr Mohammed seeking advice from a spiritual healer as the best option.

Naturalistic systems

Naturalistic systems, which largely have their ancient origins within China and India, equate illness to an imbalance of elements within the body, such as excess heat or cold. This system is most popularly referred to as holistic medicine/system. The Chinese medical system is based on the naturalistic systems. The famous yin (cold) and yang (hot) and chi (see picture), which represent force or energy, need to be in constant balance. A person seeking help within this system will seek out a traditional practitioner, who will attempt to restore the balance with the use of acupuncture, foods, herbs, exercise and dietary restrictions (Holland and Hogg, 2001). Sometimes coins are also used to treat the patient (Gervais and Jovchelovitch, 1998; Jones, 1994; Schott and Henley, 1996).

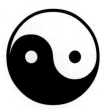

The naturalistic systems feature very much within post-natal care practices. According to Pillsbury (1984) this is because women are vulnerable to illness, as it is believed that the body has become depleted of heat. For the heat to be restored the woman is confined to the home for a specified period and will eat only food that will achieve this aim. Cold foods such as raw vegetables are forbidden. Naturalistic systems are not exclusive to the Chinese culture. Postnatal care and confinement in the home for new mothers are preserved by many other cultures. Muslim women, for example, are confined to the home for 40 days and Sikh women for 35 days (again, this can differ). It is important for the nurse to take such factors into account when arranging postnatal follow-up appointments. If appropriate explanation is given regarding why such appointments are necessary within a certain space of time, most new mothers will comply. Many elements of the naturalistic systems are observed across many cultural groups and countries.

Another example of naturalistic systems is **Ayurvedic** medicine, which has its roots in ancient India 3000–5000 years ago (Gerson, 2006). Again there is emphasis on the body restoring or maintaining a balance within the four elements of fire, water, earth and wind, which are referred to as **humors.** When a person is ill, Ayurvedic practitioners interpret this as an imbalance among the humors. Diet and herbal medication are placed in high stead for treatment and restoring balance. This perspective does not reside with every individual who is Asian or Indian or who has their origins within the Indian subcontinent. At the same time, this perspective, along with its sister perspective of Chinese medicine (which is largely herbal-based), is very much in vogue and can be seen on many high streets in Western countries. Hence, those individuals who are not Asian or Indian may adhere to the Chinese or Ayurvedic medical perspectives as well.

Think about this

Did you know that in America and the United Kingdom there are Ayurvedic colleges? These have been open since the 1970s or even earlier, but have come into the spotlight because of the recent trend in alternative care practices. In turn it is possible that any patient, irrespective of their ethnic origin, can have their health beliefs influenced by Ayurvedic medicine.

Kleinman's three sectors of health care

Kleinman is a researcher who has explored differing health beliefs in relation to health care practice for many years and has categorised the many health beliefs under three overarching sectors of health care: the popular sector, folk sector and the professional medicine sector.

The first sector of health care that Kleinman (1980) refers to is the **popular sector.** This sector consists of: 'lay, non-professional, non-specialist advice and help without any payment and consultation of folk healers or medical practitioners that are involved' (Helman, 2001, p. 51). As a result of the widespread use of the Internet, this sector has become the one that is most frequently used by patients. This has direct implications for the nurse who is caring for the patient. There are many concerns surrounding Internet use, the first one being that the lay individual may not seek out the originator of the source. What is more concerning is that some individuals are seeking solace in certain sites that actually promote ill states of health, but are written in a manner that appears to be seeking to make the individual better. The classic and most cited examples are those of the pro-anorexia and pro-bulimia websites.

Another influential aspect of the popular sector is that of the media, which heavily influences the health beliefs of individuals. For example, the many recent news reports of breast cancer drug treatments have resulted in women being pro-active in seeking 'more effective treatment'. Clearly this may be helpful. However, individuals may watch documentaries of an individual enduring the same illness as them and reject the biomedical perspective, just because the sufferer in the documentary did. This could result in the individual not undertaking or adhering completely to the treatment being provided, which potentially has dangerous implications for their heath.

Advice from family and friends is also embraced by the popular sector. This is more so when the advice being provided is from a current or recent sufferer of the same illness, or similar state of health. Acknowledging that patients may seek advice from family and friends and more importantly heed such advice, should be taken into account by the nurse.

The second sector that Kleinman (1980) presents is that of the **folk sector.** This is a sector regularly seen in developing and non-Western countries. This sector tends to include healers who cure illnesses with the use of herbal medicine, prayer and, in certain countries, spells. It is good practice for a nurse to be aware that a patient could be seeking help from a healer or even a clairvoyant while at the same time be seeking health advice from health practitioners within the NHS. It is important for the practitioner to ask about and discuss the possible treatments they may be receiving outside the biomedical perspective. Discussing this in an open manner will ensure that if a patient cannot carry on seeing a healer (because of adverse effects to medication), then once justification is given, the patient will hopefully oblige. In the case study above, Mr Mohammed placed all his faith in the spiritual healer. Had the nurse acknowledged this, she could have explained how important the biomedical treatment would be in preventing another heart attack.

The final sector is the **professional medicine sector** that nurses work within. People employed within this sector offer care and work within the guidance of the Nursing and Midwifery Council code of conduct. Procedures are followed on the basis of seeing a patient and interpreting their symptoms according to the biomedical approach, as opposed to spiritual causative factors, for example. This sector also includes holistic care and complementary health practices, e.g. acupuncture for back pain.

Think about this

In the opening case study which of the two sectors of health care clashed? How could the nurse have communicated with the patient differently so that there would have been a negotiation between the two sectors?

How to communicate effectively

The above section provides an insight into the differing health beliefs and practices that patients could possibly be influenced by. It is clear that not everyone within the same ethnic minority group, religion or even generational group will hold the same beliefs and carry out the same practices. Instead, there is enormous diversity within groups. This can include educational variables, social support, where the patient has lived and where they live today, experience of previous illness from others, their own experience; the list carries on. Hence, it is incorrect to assume that a patient holds a certain belief system because of the ethnic or religious group they are affiliated to (see Chapter 4 for a section on stereotyping).

Think about this

An example of a stereotype is that when you say 'university student' two of the most common associations would be: beans on toast and heavy alcohol consumption. In reality, there is enormous variation to this stereotypical association.

This is exactly the same for the above religions, sectors and health beliefs. Individuals may reside within a particular faith, sector of health or health belief, but each individual will vary as to how they will live their day-to-day lives. The opening case study illustrated the differences that can exist, firstly with the nurse assuming that there were similarities with Indian subcontinent languages, and secondly the assumption that because Mr Mohammed and his daughters were related that they could all speak the same language fluently.

In order to provide the best possible care, the nurse should communicate with each patient so that no assumptions are made about their beliefs and practices. This should result in both the nurse and patient being happy with the treatment and advice. The following is a step-by-step guide for nurses on how to communicate with patients who have different health beliefs so that they do not feel alienated or offended.

Step one

The nurse is to acknowledge that the patient's ill health will be interpreted and treated from the biomedical perspective. Even though the biomedical perspective will be the overriding one when treating the patient, the nurse should ensure that, when he/she is communicating with the patient, the biomedical perspective is not put across as being superior to other belief systems. This is referred to as **ethnocentrism** where an individual believes that one's culture or beliefs are superior to others (Dosani, 2003), which can result in the patient feeling alienated. The case study highlighted how it is possible for the nurse to build a mental wall between him/herself and the patient, so that the patient will not confide in the nurse.

Step two

In the case study the nurse should have explored the possibility of the patient holding health beliefs that differ from the biomedical perspective. A patient will often deny having different health beliefs when asked directly. At the same time not discussing the subject may mean that the patient will not mention their differing health belief. They may believe that it is not worthy of discussion if the practitioner did not acknowledge its existence. It is better to ask questions that are less direct in order to elicit what health belief and perspective the patient is interpreting in their current health state.

Jackson (1993) proposes the following questions that are helpful when attempting to gain an understanding about the patient's health beliefs:

- What do you think caused your problem?
- Why do you think it started when it did?
- What do you think your sickness does to you?
- How does it work?
- How severe is your sickness?
- Will it have a long or short course?
- What kind of treatment should you receive?
- What are the most important results you hope to receive from this treatment?
- What are the chief problems your sickness has caused you?
- What do you fear most about your sickness?

The above questions should be used carefully, and the following points are useful when incorporating the above questions in a consultation. Firstly, only one or two questions should be used per consultation. Secondly, it takes a while before the nurse can employ these with confidence. The key to these questions is to elicit and explore the patient's health beliefs without alienating them or allowing them to give a yes or no answer that would prevent further exploration.

Step three

Other practical ways to find out about patients' health beliefs and practices are listed by Mares *et al.* (1985):

- Avoid trying to change the traditional practices of people because they do not fit in with the expectations of the health service institutions.
- Any proposal for practical action should be made as far as possible with representatives of the community. It is pertinent to find out what changes, if any, members of the community might like to see.
- It may be useful to undertake a detailed exploration of the health beliefs and practices of the people you are with which relates to your area of practice.

Step four

Mares *et al.* (1985) also suggest the following useful tips:

- Find out about the health beliefs and practices of people in your area by reading the available literature and information. It may be useful to compare this with what people in the local community tell you.
- Establish the use of traditional healers and, if possible, meet them and discuss their approaches to care.
- Establish which illnesses are significant in the community and what people are most concerned about. Find out about people's beliefs in the causes of illness and effective prevention and cures.
- Find out which symptoms are regarded as serious. Make sure that your colleagues know that people may need reassurance about symptoms which health staff do not consider as serious.
- Give guidelines on symptoms that should be seen by a doctor.
- Try to build up a picture of the normal chain of referral within the community.
- Explain your role carefully and describe your relationship with other members of staff who may be involved in terms that patients can understand.
- Involve local people in education programmes, especially key members of the community.

Step five

The end result should be a negotiation of a care plan between the nurse and patient and what they are both happy with. This has been advocated by Jackson (1993), who has suggested the following steps in order to reach a negotiated care plan that is culturally sensitive to the patient's beliefs and values, as well as workable for the nurse within the biomedical framework.

- Explain the relevant points of biomedicine in simple and direct terms. This could comprise an explanation of the cause, signs and symptoms and likely treatment for this particular illness. Even though explanations could at first seem alien to the patient, they may be of value to them. Interpreters at this stage would be useful.

- Openly compare the patient's belief system with biomedicine. This is a good opportunity for the nurse to become aware of any discrepancies between the patient's and nurse's belief systems. Jackson (1993) suggests that this is a useful exercise, as it will enable the nurse to predict any potential problems when the health practitioner is becoming familiar with the patient's culture.

Step six

Several transcultural health care models exist, which can act as a framework for nurses to work within, when helping a patient who may hold a different health belief from the biomedical perspective. The models in Table 9.2 can act as a framework to help when working with a patient who is from a different cultural background.

Table 9.2
Transcultural health care models

Model	Researcher
The sunrise model	Leininger (1995)
Theoretical models based on practice and education to guide nurses in this area of care	Gerrish and Papadopoulos (1999) and Le Var (1998)
Range of teaching and learning strategies for transcultural health care education and training	Gerrish (1997)
The CAPP model: allows nurses to develop cultural competence and awareness	Middlesex University (2001) Papadopoulous and Lees (2002)
The ACCESS model	Narayanasamy (1998, 1999)

This chapter will focus on the **ACCESS model** (Narayanasamy, 1999). The ACCESS model consists of the following stages that the nurse should follow, in order. This should ensure effective communication with a patient, and that information is gathered about their perception and explanation of their illness:

1. **A**ssessment: Focus on cultural aspects of client's lifestyle, health belief and health practices. The following questions could be used about a patient's health beliefs:
   - What do you think caused your diabetes?
   - Why do you think it happened when it did?
   - What effects will having diabetes have on you?
   - What kind of treatment do you think you should receive?
   - Do you believe diabetes can be serious? Why?
   - Do you think your illness will last over a long period of time?
   - What are some of your problems that your illness has caused?
   - Some persons forget to take daily medications/injections; does this happen to you?
   - What have you done to help you remember to take your pills?
   - What things about high blood pressure frighten or worry you?

2. Communication: Be aware of variations in verbal and non-verbal responses.
3. Cultural negotiation and compromise: Become more aware of aspects of other people's culture as well as understanding client's views and explaining their problems.
4. Establishing respect and rapport: A therapeutic relation that portrays genuine respect for client's cultural beliefs and values is required.
5. Sensitivity: Deliver diverse culturally sensitive care to culturally diverse groups.
6. Safety: Enable clients to derive a sense of cultural safety.

The ACCESS model is one of the most useful and workable framework types for the nurse communicating with patients in a multicultural setting. A survey carried out by Narayanasamy (2002) found that up to 90 per cent of pre- and post-registration nurses found the model to be useful when implementing transcultural care practice.

Another model that has helped nurses to identify and work in a culturally competent manner is the cultural competence model (Purnell and Paulanka, 1998). The model is based on 12 domains of culture, which are seen as necessary when assessing the ethno-cultural attributes of a patient (Purnell and Paulanka, 1998, p. 10):

● overview, inhabited localities and topography;
● communication;
● 'family roles and organisation;
● work-force issues;
● bicultural issues;
● high-risk health behaviours;
● nutrition;
● pregnancy and child-bearing practices;
● death rituals;
● spirituality;
● health care practice;
● health care practitioners.

Working with a translator/interpreter

Within every NHS setting there are translators who are available for nurses when the need arises. Translators vary across PCTs, to reflect the local communities. The use of translators and interpreters is necessary, as they perform a crucial role when the nurse is attempting to communicate with a patient who cannot speak or understand English.

Translators and interpreters play a central role within the services that the NHS provide for patients (Webb-Johnson, 1992). However, it does not mean all communication problems will be solved when a translator is utilised. In the opening case study the nurse booked a translator who was of a South Asian origin. The nurse made the assumption that the South Asian translator could translate the English language into any one of the South Asian languages. Mr Mohammed was a Bengali Muslim who spoke Sylheti, which the translator could not speak or understand. The nurse assumed that the translator could communicate with Mr Mohammed as she had done so with other

A translator working with a doctor and patient

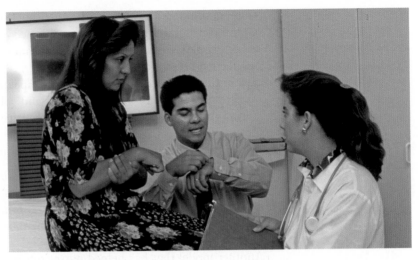

Tony Freeman/PhotoEdit

Muslim patients. As seen in the earlier sections, there is enormous diversity in relation to languages that are spoken by individuals who are Muslims.

Family members as translators

In this particular case study, Mr Mohammed's two daughters were asked to be translators for him and the nurse, as there were no other translators who could speak Sylheti. The use of family members as translators is warranted in situations where there is an emergency or when no other translator is available. However, there are certain factors that should be taken into consideration when family members or friends of the patient are utilised as translators.

Firstly, the nurse needs to be aware that the family translator may not disclose all the information; especially information that will evoke emotion in the patient. Hence, not all the information that the nurse needs to relay to the patient will be translated. Secondly, if there is no choice but to use a family member as a translator, the nurse may need to take into consideration confidential issues, as well as personal privacy issues. For example, for certain cultures having a son translate to his mother about her breast examination could evoke enormous embarrassment for both parties, which in turn could result in all the information not being fully relayed to the patient and back to the nurse. In the opening case study, certain parts of information, such as challenging their father's smoking behaviour, caused embarrassment for Mr Mohammed's daughter. In such circumstances the nurse needs to take into consideration the relationship between the patient and the translator. Where possible, ask the patient and translator individually if they will be happy for the family member to translate. However, professional translators should be used at all times if possible, especially in interactions that require the patient to disclose emotive or sensitive information.

The problems that untrained translators can bring in for the patient have been listed by Royal College of Nursing (1994), cited in Holland and Hogg (2001, p. 6), as:

- inaccurate translation, because of the inability to translate important ideas and words;
- bias and distortion, caused by inability to put aside personal bias;
- no confidentiality, the importance of confidentiality may not be recognised, and this may inhibit clients from being open in interview;
- not understanding their role – untrained interpreters may answer questions from staff without putting them to the clients, and may only relay part of the information to the client;
- no explanation of cultural differences – untrained interpreters may not be sensitive to differences in culture, values and expectations, and this limits their effectiveness;
- personal unsuitability – people brought in to interpret on an ad hoc basis may be the wrong sex or much older or younger than the client. Their backgrounds may be very different and they may even belong to a group antagonistic towards the client's own group.

How to work with a professional translator

When working with a professional translator, there are certain things that need to occur to ensure the most effective use of the service. First, it is vital to ensure that the patient and translator speak and understand the same language. This has been reiterated by researchers such as Henley and Schott (1999, p. 283) who state that the following features are essential for an effective translator:

- trained and experienced;
- fluent in both English and the patient's mother tongue;
- able to understand medical terminology and what the health professional is trying to achieve;
- someone both the health professional and the patient can trust.

The way a nurse makes use of a translator will determine their effectiveness. In the opening case study, the nurse spoke to and maintained eye contact with the translator. This is the most ineffective way to use a translator in a consultation. The most productive way is to talk to and maintain eye contact with the patient. This should result in all information being communicated between the patient and nurse (refer to Chapter 17 for further exploration of verbal and non-verbal communication).

The nurse should also be aware that medical terminology, as well as everyday words, might not translate or have a meaning in another language. By being aware of this and making sure that the patient understands the information being given should overcome this issue. It is important to discuss the use of medical terms with the translator. This has been illustrated with the work of Webb-Johnson (1992) who suggested that,

> Words are culturally loaded and have different meanings and concepts in different languages. Therefore the interpreter has to decode within the cultural context which is being expressed behind the words in order to communicate the full message to the professional. (Webb-Johnson, 1992, p. 86)

Think about this

Consider the following terms. Which terms are culturally loaded and would take extensive explanation by the interpreter when communicating with the patient?

- Blood
- Placebo
- Anaemia
- Abdominal pain
- Excessive pain

If an interpreter has been selected from the local community, the patient should be asked if they are happy to discuss personal and private issues. There could be a concern for the patient in regards to breeches of confidentiality or 'telling others' within the community about the patient's state of health.

Translators and interpreters are in constant demand. There will be times when a professional translator, or a family member performing the role of translator, will not be available. It has been found that in 46 per cent of emergency department cases involving patients with limited English proficiency no interpreter was used (Baker *et al.*, 1996).

Non-verbal communication

Nurses who work with patients who cannot speak fluent English will be heavily reliant on information that will be conveyed via non-verbal communication (refer to Chapter 17). Non-verbal communication can also vary across cultures. For example, when a patient talks and at the same time looks away when making a particular statement, it can be interpreted as a sign of lying or not feeling comfortable with what they have stated (also refer to Chapters 3 and 4). This is referred to as **incongruent** behaviour. However, members of certain ethnic minority groups will look away as a sign of respect for the nurse. Also, not maintaining eye contact is seen as a sign of modesty for females from particular cultural areas.

There are also variations in the way that individuals express themselves. For certain cultural groups, excessive hand gesturing and a higher-pitched tone of voice is a sign of sincerity. This can often be misinterpreted as aggression.

Conclusion

The United Kingdom has a population that is rich in diverse cultures. These cultures change with new influxes of immigrants. They are also dynamic as a result of changes in education, the environment and influences from peers and the media. The nurse's role involves caring and communicating with patients. Patients, nurses and the organisation (e.g. primary care trust, hospital) all have their own cultures which impact on the dynamics of the patient–nurse relationship. A nurse who is aware of such influences and accommodates for them is a nurse who is culturally competent and aware.

Being aware of differing health beliefs other than the biomedical model is becoming more accepted within health care practices than ever before. This can be seen with complementary practices and medicines becoming commonplace within, rather than hidden from, hospitals. This is also mirrored in consultations, which have also become open forums in which differing health beliefs and practices can be discussed. The most important contributor to a nurse being culturally competent and aware is to acknowledge that enormous diversity exists within cultural groups. Being culturally competent does not necessarily mean an awareness of the ethnicity of a patient but instead an appreciation of the many factors that result in the unique health experiences of each individual patient.

Summary

- Culture is dynamic and forever changing (Andrew and Boyle, 1995). Other researchers, such as Henley (1993) have echoed the dynamic nature of culture, and stated that culture changes in response to new situations and pressure. Because of the dynamic nature and culture and the enormous diversity within cultural groups, it is very easy to stereotype patients or not give them the appropriate care according to their own cultural needs.

- De Santis (1994) states that there are three cultures that interact when the patient is in hospital: organisational culture, patient culture and nursing culture.

- The biomedical perspective is the health model in which both the patient receives care and the nurse is trained in. The fact that patients receive care from a health care institution that is in the main based on the biomedical perspective does not mean that the patient's health beliefs are wholly biomedical. Other health beliefs that a patient can hold stem from personalistic systems where supernatural forces are identified as the main cause of illness; popular sectors where media, friends, family and the Internet impact on health beliefs and naturalist systems where illness is identified as being caused by an imbalance with the main elements of the body.

- There are many cultural framework models that a nurse can work with as a guide, when delivering culturally competent care. One of these is the ACCESS model (Narayansamy, 1999). The six stages of ACCESS are Assessment, Communication, Cultural negotiation, Extra respect, Sensitivity and Safety.

- When communicating with a patient who may hold a different religious or health belief, it is important to use questions that are open rather than closed. Jackson (1993) has advocated several open questions that can be used to explore the health beliefs of the patient in an open manner.

- Ethnocentrism is where an individual believes that their health belief or perspective is superior to any other. This should be avoided from the perspective of the nurse when listening to patient's health belief, irrespective of how strange or different they may be.

- When using a professional translator it is important to maintain eye contact and carry on talking to the patient, rather than the translator.

- A nurse who has to use family or friends as interpreters should be cautious as they may not relay all the information you want translated.

- Non-verbal communication has enormous variances when looking at it from a cultural perspective. Variations exist to the general rules of non-verbal communication.

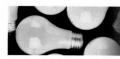

Check your understanding

- There is enormous diversity within cultural groups. Discuss variables that contribute to diversity.

- De Santis (1994) highlights three interacting cultures that are evident when caring for a patient. What are these? Describe and discuss their possible influences on the outcome of a care plan.

- Describe and distinguish between the three sectors of health that Kleinman (1980) describes.

- What is ethnocentrism? How can this negatively impact on the care of your patient? How can this negatively impact on the care that the nurse provides.

- Jackson (1993) has provided several questions, which can help the nurse when exploring the patient's health beliefs. Reiterate four of the questions in relation to Mr Mohammed, when attempting to explore his supernatural health beliefs.

- Describe each stage of the ACCESS model.

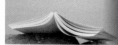

Further reading

Clegg, D.J. (2001) Cultural sensitivity: a practical approach to improving services. *Nursing Standard,* **15** (33).

Cowan, D.T. and Norman, I. (2006) Cultural competence in nursing: new meanings. *Journal of Transcultural Nursing,* **17** (1), 82–88.

Gibbs, K.A. (2005) Teaching student nurses to be culturally safe: can it be done? *Journal of Transcultural Nursing,* **16** (4), 356–360.

Hill, J. (2006) Management of diabetes in South Asian communities in the UK. *Nursing Standard,* **20** (25), 57–64.

Leishman, J. (2004) Perspectives of cultural competence in health care. *Nursing Standard,* **19** (11).

Lovering, S. (2006) Cultural attitudes and beliefs about pain. *Journal of Transcultural Nursing,* **17** (4).

McGee, P. (2002) Nursing with dignity. *Nursing Times,* **98** (9), 33.

Narayanasamy, A. (2003) Transcultural nursing: how do nurses respond to cultural needs? *British Journal of Nursing,* **12** (3), 185–194.

Royal College of Nursing (1994) Black and ethnic minority clients: meeting needs. *RCN Nursing Update,* **7**, 3–13.

Shen, Z. (2004) Cultural competence models in nursing: a selected annotated bibliography. *Journal of Transcultural Nursing,* **15** (4).

Weblinks

Melting Resource	http://www.wolfson.tvu.ac.uk/maryseacole/melting	A site aimed principally at nursing students to help them learn about transcultural issues in care.
Making Practice Based Learning Work: Bournemouth University	http://www.practicebasedlearning.org/resources/diversity/ethnicity.htm	This site been put together by Bournemouth University's health department which acts as a links to over 30 websites that are related to culture and communication within health.
Transcultural C.A.R.E. Associates	http://www.transculturalcare.net	Run by Dr Josie Campinha-Bacote, which provides regular updates of her theory on cultural competence.
National Library for Health	http://www.nelh.library.uk/	Gateway for electronic resources relating to a variety of conditions and clinical settings, and provides useful links to other similar sites.
London College of Traditional Chinese Medicine	http://www.lcta.com	
Cross Cultural Health Care program: NWRC	http://www.xculture.org/NWRCwelcome.php	Information ranging from cultural competent practice to working with patients from diverse cultures.
Transcultural Nursing Society	http://www.tcns.org/	Useful information related to transcultural nursing issues.
Research Centre for Transcultural Studies in Health: Middlesex University	http://www.mdx.ac.uk/www/rctsh/homepage.htm	Extensive links and information, updated on a regular basis.

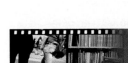

Media example

Bend it Like Beckham A funny portrayal of how first- and second-generation Asians living in the United Kingdom differ in the way they live their day-to-day lives in accordance with their faith, in a dynamic and changing environment.

Chapter 10

Working with older adults

Learning outcomes

When you have read through this chapter you should understand:

- How the acknowledgement of individual differences within the 'older adult group' can result in effective nursing care.
- How various internal and external factors being specific to the elderly patient can confound the communication process between the nurse and the older patient.
- How the principles within gerontology nursing are useful when working with an older patient.
- How preconceived perceptions, stereotyping of the older patient and ageism can result in care being hindered.
- How dementia and Alzheimer's can impact on the type of care and communication that the nurse provides.
- How dignity can be maintained for the elderly patient.

Case study

Delia Jones is a 72-year-old woman who lives alone. She is very independent and does not like to rely on others. In the past couple of years, Delia's GP has become gradually concerned about Delia living alone, as her mental and physical well-being have declined. In particular her Alzheimer's and visual impairment have become worse. The GP's concern for Delia has been further exacerbated by the number of falls that Delia has had. These falls have resulted in various bone fractures.

Delia herself is also aware that over the past couple of years both her daily confusion and visual deterioration have become more frequent. At the same time she wants to ensure that she does not consent to an environment that will mean dependency on others. This belief has been strengthened by the reactions of some of her children who in the past have been reluctant to take care of her when she needed help.

Recently, Delia had forgotten that she had placed a meal under the grill. It was only when she smelled burning that she realised her mistake and walked quickly into the kitchen. During this walk, she hit her leg on a table and fell. A neighbour who could see the small fire from the kitchen window called for help from the fire services and the paramedics. The paramedics decided to admit Delia into hospital as she had broken her right arm and appeared to be highly confused and tearful.

During Delia's stay in hospital the consultant noted that the patient's mood began to lift in the specialist ward that cared for Alzheimer's patients. Delia enjoyed her stay in hospital and found it comforting to know that the nurses and other health care staff understood her needs. After a couple of days Delia had to be moved to another ward. It was during her stay in this particular ward that Delia's mood began to deteriorate. Delia felt that the nurses on this ward did not understand her needs and only attended to her essential physical needs. During such interactions Delia felt that the nurses communicated with her in a patronising way and did not allow her to do anything for herself. She felt that she was talked over and not given the opportunity to express herself. She was further angered by how the nurses referred to her by her first name without asking. She also felt the nurses thought that she moaned about her pain.

Delia could not wait until she could be discharged from hospital. The way she had been treated further confirmed to Delia that she did not want to move into a nursing home. One late evening when resting, Delia overheard a conversation between her eldest son and the sister on the ward. The sister was urging Delia's son to think about a nursing home. The thought of a nursing home frightened Delia so she decided to walk out of hospital by herself. Delia only got to the top of the corridor where she was stopped by the nurse and was taken back, only to be talked to like a child and called 'silly'. Three months later and Delia is living alone but she receives an enormous amount of help from external authorities, agencies and family. She has not had any accidents and is very happy to still be independent. She is grateful to her GP, who made her family understand that she did not want to live in an environment that would stop her being independent.

Why is this relevant to nursing practice?

Nurses working in and around geriatric nursing need to be familiar with the issues surrounding the care of the elderly. Health care practitioners, especially nurses, are currently faced with working with a growing ageing population. The 2001 Census estimated that 11 million (11 125 000) older people (those aged 60 years and over) would be living within the United Kingdom during 2004 (Population Trends, 2005) with the following breakdown:

- 9 280 000 in England
- 968 000 in Scotland

- 602 000 in Wales
- 275 000 in Northern Ireland

The elderly population within the United Kingdom has been projected to increase further in the future. '11.4 million of people who are over the pensionable age in 2006 to 12.2 million in 2011, and will rise to over 13.9 million by 2026, reaching over 15.3 million in 2031' (National Statistics Press Release, 2005, cited in Age Concern: 2006a).

With the projected increase, the NHS will be registering elderly patients more than ever before. Hence, familiarity within the area of the care of the elderly is warranted, as the elderly population are and will continue to be the most frequent users of the NHS.

For example, Delia had also been admitted into hospital earlier that year with a similar accident, resulting in a hip fracture. In addition to this, Delia is also a regular user of the NHS as an outpatient in relation to her Alzheimer's. She is also a frequent visitor to the diabetes and asthma clinics. Elderly patients with several illnesses are likely to access the NHS more frequently than their younger counterparts, which has been mirrored in recent and predicted statistics: 'In 2003, in a three-month period, 24 per cent of those aged 75 and over had attended the casualty or out-patient department of a hospital compared with 14 per cent of people of all ages' (Department of Health, 2006, cited in Age Concern, 2006a).

The probability of treating a patient who is elderly and staying longer in hospital (apart from paediatric branch) is high. 'In 2003, of those admitted to hospital in the previous 12 months, the average stay was 8 nights. However, those aged 75 and over spent on average, 14 nights' (Department of Health, 2006, cited in Age Concern, 2006a).

The longer stay for the elderly in hospital could in part be explained by the increased probability of chronic illnesses with the ageing process. For example, 'In 2003, 60 per cent of people aged 65–74 and 64 per cent of people aged 75 and over in the General Household Sample reported a longstanding illness. Of those aged between 65 and 74, 37 per cent and, of those aged 75 and over, 44 per cent said that they had a long term limiting illness' (GHS, cited in Age Concern, 2006a).

The chances of becoming ill, enduring a long-standing chronic illness or having an accident increase among the elderly. Again this increases the probability of the elderly patient utilising NHS resources. Delia was not only a patient with a hip fracture but also endured other chronic illnesses such as Alzheimer's, asthma, a hearing impairment and diabetes.

The Alzheimer's Society estimates that there are currently over 750 000 people in the United Kingdom with dementia, of whom only 18 000 are aged under 65 (Alzheimer's Society, 2006, cited in Age Concern, 2006a). When caring for the elderly, different needs arise because of the possible multiple losses that are associated with illness. In the case study above, the two nurses did not communicate with Delia appropriately. They should have taken into account that being forgetful could have been a feature of her Alzheimer's.

The exploration of illnesses and disabilities, as well as the limited functioning that older age can bring, are important to consider if nurses are to deliver appropriate care to the elderly patient. **Gerontological nursing** refers to the knowledge, as well as the type of care a nurse should deliver to meet the needs of an elderly patient. This chapter will examine certain **chronic illnesses** that the elderly are more likely to encounter, such as **Alzheimer's disease**.

Even if a nurse is not working on a geriatric ward, the chances are that they will still encounter many elderly patients, who will require different types of skills and care. For example, in the case study above, Delia was admitted to the hospital because of a broken arm. The nurses on the second ward who were caring for Delia were not specialists within geriatric nursing or Alzheimer's. As a result they were not aware of how the patient's pre-existing illnesses were having an impact on her current physical and mental well-being. A basic knowledge of gerontological nursing is a necessity for any nurse, irrespective of what branch that you are specialising within.

In the case study above, the nurses on the second ward were clearly not communicating effectively with Delia. Lack of understanding can result in appropriate care not being given (Bush, 2003). Coverage of material within this chapter will raise awareness of the certain types of illnesses that the elderly patient is more likely to encounter, and the appropriate care and communication that is required.

In the case study above, the nurses on the second ward may not have known that they communicated to the patient in an ineffective way. There are many plausible explanations, including a lack of familiarity within gerontological nursing, a lack of contact with the elderly and the limited use of the nurse's **self-awareness**. Encompassing self-awareness, especially within the area of gerontological nursing, is useful when exploring your own attitudes and perceptions of the elderly, especially those that could be negative in nature and lead to stereotyping. An ageism survey was carried out by Age Concern, in conjunction with the University of Kent entitled 'How Ageist is Britain?' (Age Concern, 2006a). In this piece of work, out of the 1843 people interviewed about their perceptions of the elderly, it was found that one in three of the respondents said that the over 70s are viewed as incompetent and incapable (Age Concern, How Ageist is Britain?, 2006a, p. 3).

Negative attitudes and stereotypes about the elderly are referred to as **ageism**, which will be considered within this chapter. Consideration of the potential impact that negative attitudes can have on the care you provide for the elderly patient will be explored. In the above case study, the nurses on the second ward held a stereotype of the elderly being unable to do anything independently. This negative connotation left Delia feeling frustrated, helpless and wanting to go home. **Communication** and the area of **neglect** will be considered within this chapter. The exploration of **stereotypes** of the elderly as well as treating the elderly patient with respect and **dignity** will also be explored.

Defining 'the elderly', and its implications for communication and care

Think about this

Think about the definition of 'the elderly' and 'old'. What actually designates an individual being classified as 'old' or referred to as 'the elderly'? Is there a particular age that assigns a distinction between the transition from middle-age to 'elderly', or are such distinctions marked by how the individual physically and mentally feels and functions?

Within the United Kingdom the ages of 60 for a woman and 65 for a man mark the time when society allows an individual to retire from the world of work. Most commonly referred to as 'pensioners' or 'the elderly', these individuals also have access to free prescriptions and other health care services, irrespective of their state of health. Can everyone of a pensionable age be referred to as the elderly? There is a problem when attaching the same label to everyone who is retired and thereafter referring to *all* as 'the elderly'. There are many problems that can arise from such labels. Firstly, there has been an increase of life expectancy in recent decades. Take a look at Table 10.1, which demonstrates the increase in life expectancy over the years.

Life expectancy has increased vastly, which means that 'pensioners' are living for a longer period of time, even after they have 'retired'. As a result, to group all of the elderly (aged 60 or 65 and above) as being the same, results in stereotyping, especially as this period can span 50 years, from the age of 60 years all the way to as much as 110 years of age.

Imagine all individuals from birth up until 50 years of age being grouped together under one label. How many mistakes in terms of communication, stereotyping and assumptions would we make? Any categorisation of chronological age obscures the physiological, psychological and social diversity of older people (Bowling *et al.* 2005). This in turn obscures their unique and different health needs. This has implications as to the lack of individualised care that is provided to elderly patients.

	Year	65–74 years (%)	75–84 years (%)	Over 85 years (%)
Table 10.1 The increase in life expectancy: growth of UK elderly population as a percentage of total UK population	1948	7.2	2.9	0.4
	1951	7.3	3.1	0.4
	1956	7.4	3.4	0.6
	1961	7.5	3.6	0.7
	1966	78	37	0.7
	1971	85	39	0.9
	1976	9.1	4.2	1.0
	1981	9.2	4.7	1.1
	1986	8.8	5.3	1.3
	1991	8.8	5.4	1.5
	1996	8.6	5.3	1.8
	2001	8.2	5.5	2.0
	2006	8.2	5.5	2.0
	2011	8.9	5.5	2.2
	2016	10.2	5.7	2.3
	2021	10.4	6.3	2.5
	2026	10.6	7.3	2.7
	2031	12.0	7.6	3.1
	2036	12.5	7.9	3.7

Source: Population Trends (2000).

According to Suzman and Riley (1985) 'people over 65' can be divided into at least three stages:

- The young-old (65–75 or 80)
- The old-old (75 or 80 to about 90)
- The very-old or oldest old (those aged over 85–90 and over).

The above distinction enables the practitioner to assess and care for individuals according to their particular health needs, which are reflective of the chronological development stage that they reside within. This also enables the nurse to be aware of illnesses and impairments that are more likely to influence individuals at each particular stage, and hence tailor their communication and care plan in consideration of these possible influences.

Think about this

Patient Delia is a 72-year-old woman who resides within the 'young-old' stage. What particular deficiencies, if any, is Delia most likely to encounter that the nurse should be aware of? Was the communication between the nurses and Delia adequate, in relation to possible assumed sensory deprivation of a young-old person? Did the nurses communicate with the patient as a 'young-old' patient, or as an 'old-old' patient?

The nurses on the second ward clearly treated Delia as 'an old-old' person. This was displayed by speaking loudly, as well as talking over and not caring for Delia as an active patient. As a result, she felt patronised, humiliated and that she was 'talked down to'. This is what can happen when the over-65 age group are grouped together, without any individual variability taken into consideration.

On many variables, such as mental and physical performance the young-old resemble the middle-aged, as opposed to the old-old age group (Schaie and Willis, 1996). Riley and Riley (1994) and Shneidman (1989) have provided evidence of the 70s being a rewarding and active period of life for those who are bright and well educated. The blurred distinction between middle-age and young-old have been further enhanced with the emphasis in society being that of an age-integrated one. As a result, once an individual has reached their 60s, they do not like to be classed as being in the same 'older' age group as a 90+-year-old. This is demonstrated by the photo overleaf of the vast differences within the categorisation of the 'older' group, where individuals like Barbara Windsor are fully active and not dependent on others around them.

Government policy

Older people are the main users of health care services because of the increased probability of illness with the advancement of age. Services have not always addressed these population needs adequately (Department of Health, 2001b). Nurses need to be aware of policy development, as this has a direct impact on the elderly patients that you will be caring for. Nurses also have an important part to play in shaping future policy. This will impact on the framework that nurses will be working within when caring for the elderly (Webster, 2002).

I don't class myself as older than the rest!

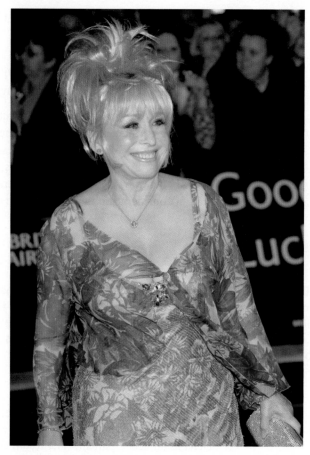

Allstar Picture Library/Alamy

One main factor that differentiates a nurse caring for an elderly patient, rather than a younger or middle-aged person is the multiplicity of age-related physical, psychological and social needs (Webster, 2002) that the elderly patient may have. Take, for example, Delia in the opening case study. She was admitted to hospital because of a broken arm. However, she also suffers from Alzheimer's disease, asthma and diabetes and has a slight visual impairment. This particular patient will require specialist care to cater for the needs that arise from her pre-existing state of health, as well as her present ill-health. At the same time, the patient is clearly an independent woman who does not want to be totally reliant on the nurses and carers around her.

Government policy has taken such factors into account, as reflected within documentation stating that older people should have their *individual* needs acknowledged and that living longer is something to celebrate (Department of Health, 2001b). The **National Service Framework** (Department of Health, 2001b) has working targets. It aims to:

- tackle age discrimination, to make it a thing of the past and ensure older people are treated with respect and dignity;
- ensure older people are supported by newly integrated services with a well-coordinated, coherent and cohesive approach to assessing individual needs and circumstances and for providing services for them;
- promote the health and well-being of older people through coordinated health and social care services.

Enhancing privacy, dignity and respect for the elderly patient

Delia overheard the nurse and her son discussing nursing homes. Delia felt that she had no privacy or control over her life and felt vulnerable as a result. She also felt that at times her dignity was compromised when going to the toilet and having a shower, as it was assumed that Delia was totally dependent.

Invasion of space, dignity and lack of respect, have been highlighted in many studies. For example, Calnan *et al.* (2003) cited a European Union funded study carried out in 2002, which asked elderly patients what they saw as important when receiving care within the hospital setting. The results of the study highlighted 'dignity' as important. The following list was concluded from the study, which looked at what was meant by lack of dignity and other aspects of care that were a problem for elderly patients:

- lack of thought given to helping people with their personal appearance;
- the attachment of labels to older people such as 'bed-blockers' or 'geriatrics';
- exposing a patient's nakedness to strangers or to other patients when using a hoist;
- not asking the person how he or she would like to be addressed;
- mixed sex wards;
- lack of thought being given to the gender of the carer;
- mixing tablets into food.

When working towards maintaining dignity and respect for the elderly patient, there are a number of different principles that researchers and nurse consultants highlight, all of which have psychological underpinnings such as person-centred care, unconditional positive regard and empathy (refer to Chapter 3). Calnan *et al.* (2005) carried out a study whereby employers within the NHS were asked what 'dignity' meant. Table 10.2 lists the findings. Nurses should find these useful, as these variables are drawn from professional experience when working with the elderly.

Ensuring that the elderly are provided with dignified care has a positive impact on their treatment, social outcomes, and health and well-being (Ranzijn *et al.*, 1998; Tadd *et al.*, 2002; Walsh and Kowanko, 2002). In the case study, Delia was not given respect or treated as an independent

Table 10.2
What is 'dignity'?

Identity	Rights	Autonomy
Respect	Choice	Independence
Self-respect	Equality	Control
Self-esteem	Consent	
Exposure	Confidentiality	
Inclusion	Innate dignity	
Communication		
Personal appearance		
Treat as an individual		
Privacy		
Emotional care		

Think about this

Think about the opening case study in this chapter. Which of the concepts of dignity in the table above were, or were not, taken into account when interacting and caring for the patient? How could the nurses have provided dignified care?

individual. In addition, her dignity was compromised, resulting in her wanting to go home. Her self-worth could have been negatively affected because of this experience.

Raising awareness

Even though a nurse may not be a specialist within geriatric care, it is likely that they will care for many elderly patients. It is acknowledged that nurses can not be specialists in every impairment and illness that elderly patients may have. This was seen in the case study, whereby the nurses did not acknowledge Delia's pre-existing state of health, aside from her broken arm. The patient's state of health and their stay in hospital can be vastly improved by acknowledging existing impairments and their impact on the patient. Had the nurses on the second ward acknowledged that Delia not only had the pain of her broken arm to cope with but also her pre-existing illnesses, the nurses could have tailored their care and communication accordingly. This section will provide a few examples of illness and impairments that tend to be age-related and the associated losses that come with them.

Alzheimer's/dementia

Think about this

Delia had the diagnosis of Alzheimer's disease five years ago. What possible impact will this have on her physical and mental well-being if it is not taken into account when providing care for her?

It is estimated that 700 000 people in the United Kingdom have dementia. The incidence of dementia increases with age and is thought to double every five to six years after the age of 65. In comparison, there are about 18 500 people under the age of 65 with dementia in the United Kingdom (Burgess *et al.*, 2006). Dementia is signified by a decline in memory and thinking, present for six months or more, and to a degree, sufficient to impair functioning in daily living (WHO, 1993).

One of the main characteristics of dementia is cognitive impairment. Nurses should be aware that dementia care is no longer seen as a collection of deficits where there is no hope for a patient. Instead, nurses should involve the patient as actively as possible, as well as utilising their strengths and abilities (Burgess *et al.*, 2006). The quality of life can be improved with adequate communication and individual care for the patient. This can be further enhanced when nurses co-operative with specialist dementia nurses, who can provide help. In the above case study, the nurses on the second ward needed to change their perception of dementia to a more positive one, rather than making Delia feel helpless and useless. Adapting communication so that it is slower and simpler will put a dementia patient at ease. This will also make the patient feel comfortable when responding at their own pace.

Attitudes of nurses in the way they view dementia is vital, as they influence how the patient feels and the satisfaction they have with the care that they have received (see Chapter 16). The nurses in the case study had a stereotypical view of the elderly as the inability to function and dependence on people around them.

An elderly person with dementia will naturally be more dependent on others because of the psychological, social and behavioural disturbances that accompany this disease. Dementia can result in the disruption of daily activities (Roper *et al.*, 1983). This can result in having to be dependent to some degree on others for particular daily activities (Bush, 2003). At the same time this does not mean that they are dependent for every daily task. For example, Delia could still go to the toilet and move herself freely. A nurse who acknowledges that an individual can become angry and frustrated because of their dependency, will be more empathetic and understanding of the patient (refer to Chapter 3). At the same time, a nurse needs to be aware that dependency may not be a necessity for every daily task.

Another issue that arises out of the opening case study is that the non-specialist nurses took into account only the broken arm when caring for Delia. Her other impairments were ignored. Elderly patients are more likely to be treated for their 'present illness', while their pre-existing illnesses are ignored. For example, Hellzen *et al.* (2003) found that although they also had dementia, long-term schizophrenia patients were treated as schizophrenic patients only.

The nurse should aim to involve the patient in conversation about themselves, rather than just talking about their present illness. The **person-focused approach** is dominant here. One of the aims is to maintain personhood in the face of failing mental powers (Kitwood, 1997). Dewing and Blackburn (1999) define maintaining personhood as: love, attachment, inclusion, comfort, identity and occupation (see Chapter 3).

Bush (2003) cites the work of Cheston and Bender (2000), which endorses that the focus should be on the person with dementia (not his or her diseased brain), on the person's emotions and understanding (not memory losses) and on the person within the context of marriage or family, and within a wider society.

According to Bush (2003), these can be attained with core values that stem from the humanistic approach:

- **Congruence:** what the nurse verbally states is also displayed via the non-verbal channel or in actions, which portray genuineness.
- **Unconditional positive regard:** caring for an elderly patient without any conditions or constraints on the relationship. For example, the illness or impairment or even pre-conceived ideas about ageing should not bias the nurse's perception and care they will provide (apart from the needs that arise from illnesses).
- **Empathic understanding:** is where the nurse attempts to understand how the elderly patient, feels, thinks and perceives their symptoms as well as the environment around them.

Communicating with an elderly dementia patient

Validation therapy, developed by Feil (1992), has techniques that are useful for nurses who are caring and communicating with elderly dementia patients. Validation therapy is the process of communicating with a disorientated older person by validating and respecting the person's feelings, in whatever context is real to that person at that time, even though it may not be connected with the present reality.

Prouty (1990) put forward a number of principles to help nurses when caring for elderly patients with any kind of impairment. Van Werde and Morton (1999) reviewed these principles and aligned these with specific techniques which are known as **pre-therapy** (Bush, 2003). Below are the techniques put forward as reflective points which can aid a nurse when communicating and caring for elderly patients with one or more impairments.

- *Situational reflections*: Used to strengthen contact with the world, and relate to facts, situation, people, environment and events.
- *Facial reflections*: The nurse states the emotion that is apparent in the client's facial expression.
- *Word-for-word reflections*: Coherent communication or meaningful sounds are repeated by the nurse in an attempt to support communicative contact.
- *Body reflections*: The nurse mirrors the posture or movements of the patient or reflects them via verbal description.

According to Iliffe and Drennan (2001), concentrating on effective communication with a patient who has dementia is the key to both understanding and resolving behaviour disturbances. Had the nurses simplified information and been empathetic to Delia's slow cognitive functioning, they would have realised that they were not communicating or providing care that was individualised to her circumstances. Underlying all these approaches is the emphasis on enhancing the quality of life for the elderly patient, by keeping them actively involved.

Cognitive impairments

The opening case study clearly exemplified the frustration and anxiety Delia felt as a result of people not understanding her dementia. There are a number of losses which are associated with **cognitive impairments**. Hall (1988) divides these into four:

- *Intellectual loss*: Loss of memory, loss of sense of time and loss of expressive and receptive language abilities.
- *Affective/personality loss*: Loss of affect, antisocial behaviour and paranoia.
- *Planning loss*: Loss of ability to plan activities and functional loss.
- *Low stress threshold*: Decreased ability to tolerate stress.

By reflecting on these four principles when caring for patients, communication can be tailored accordingly. For example, in the case study above, if the nurses had acknowledged the low stress threshold that she had, resulting from her previous illnesses, they would have understood the possibility of dysfunctional behaviour. Instead, the nurses ignored Delia and felt that she did not respond appropriately when they spoke to her.

The following six principles have been listed by Hall (1994) as maximising associated negative behaviour, such as Delia's agitation and 'shouting out':

- fatigue;
- changes in caregiver routine or environment;
- overwhelming, inappropriate, misleading or inadequate stimulus levels;
- internal or external demand that exceeds functional capacity;
- affective responses to perception of losses; and
- physical stressors such as pain, discomfort, infections or medications.

Rantz and McShane (1995) when looking at nursing home staff experience working with chronically confused patients, found four categories of effective nursing intervention: interpreting reality (encourage family members to bring in a photo album), maintaining normality, meeting basic needs (allowing a daily walk outside with supervision) and managing behaviour disturbances (identifying early warning signs for events that trigger an impending behaviour disturbance and redirecting the elderly patient, by calmly walking him or her away from the situation).

Think about this

In light of the study carried out by Rantz and McShane (1995), had the nurses met three or four of the principles when communicating with Delia, would she still have become agitated and attempted to escape?

Pain

Research has shown that pain has been poorly controlled in hospitals (e.g. Carr, 1990; Kuhn *et al.*, 1990; Marks and Sachar, 1973; Melzack *et al.*, 1987; Seers, 1987; Sriwatanakul *et al.*, 1983). A few studies have documented this specifically within elderly patients (e.g. Closs *et al.*, 1993). It is useful for nurses to consider how elderly patients manage pain compared with their younger counterparts. Closs (1994) highlights specific areas of concern, when looking at the management of pain among the elderly. Firstly the elderly may perceive and/or report pain differently from younger patients. This may be due to cultural differences and physical and psychological changes as a result of ageing. Secondly, cognitive impairment and dementia present barriers to pain assessment. Thirdly, patients may be at risk of over- or under-treatment because of age-related changes in response to analgesic drugs. Nurses may under-medicate due to the dangerous side effects of the drugs (Closs, 1994). Paying very close attention to these potential barriers can result in pain control medication being prescribed that is more appropriate.

The following psychological techniques highlighted by Closs (1994) are also useful when attempting to control pain, in addition to medication:

- *Distraction* – visual concentration with rhythmic massage and breathing techniques (although nurses should teach these techniques when the patient has minimum pain; McCaffey, 1983). Prayer and other more general techniques are also a useful form of distraction from the experience of pain.

- *Relaxation* – evidence shows that those who have mastered deep relaxation techniques are generally able to better cope with pain (Diamond and Coniam, 1991). One example is concentrating on relaxation on one part of the body (Latham, 1988). Yoga and meditation are two approaches that help individuals to relax and have recently gained enormous popularity among many elderly people worldwide (see picture).

The following 10 principles have been cited by Closs (1994), which have resulted from the work of Ferrell (1991), in relation to pain management for elderly people:

- Always ask elderly patients about pain.
- Accept the patient's word about pain and its intensity.
- Never underestimate the potential effects of chronic pain on a patient's overall condition and quality of life.
- Be consistent in the assessment of pain. An accurate diagnosis will lead to the most effective treatment.
- Treat pain to facilitate diagnostic procedures. Don't wait for diagnosis to relieve suffering.
- Use a combined approach of drug and non-drug strategies where possible.
- Mobilise patients physically and psychosocially; involve patients in their therapy.
- Use analgesic drugs correctly. Start doses low and increase slowly. Achieve adequate doses and anticipate side effects.
- Anticipate and attend to anxiety and depression.
- Reassess responses to treatment. Alter therapy to maximise functional status and quality of life.

In the case study, Delia was thought by the nurses to be constantly 'moaning'. The nurses labelled her as an awkward patient and that was typical of an elderly patient who moaned constantly. Had they asked Delia why she was 'moaning', they would have realised that she did not want to be a nuisance, but was dealing with her intense pain by moaning and humming. As far as

Yoga is an example of a form of relaxation which has gained popularity worldwide, especially among the elderly who have found this both to slow down the ageing process as well as manage pain more effectively.

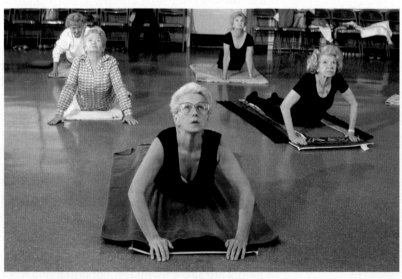

Mark Richards/PhotoEdit

Delia was concerned, she was not made aware that she could have asked the nurses to increase the pain relief drip.

Age stereotyping and ageism

Think about this

This section overlaps with Chapter 4. In the case study did the nurses stereotype and have ageist attitudes, which resulted in poor care for Delia? Discuss what being 'ageist' and 'age stereotyping' mean.

Stereotyping can be defined as a 'set of beliefs about the characteristics of the members of a social group' (Ashmore and Del Boca, 1981). More specifically, **age stereotyping**, generalised beliefs and judgements about ageing, old age and older people (Kruse and Schmitt, 2006).

We all are prone to **stereotype**. This is more so when we have not had day-to-day experience and contact with the particular group/individual we are stereotyping. Fill in the following questionnaire from Schaie and Willis (1996), which looks at the perceptions and myths, as well as facts about older people. For each statement decide if you think it is true or false. Once you have answered this questionnaire, think about the following question with a partner: 'are we all capable of stereotyping the elderly at one time or another'?

There was a stereotype within the case study where the nurses assumed that Delia was totally dependent because of her age. According to cognitive theories of stereotyping (see Chapter 5), we hold prototypes, which represent information for particular groups. This can have a negative impact, as we tend to go out and confirm what we have a misconception of, or negative connotation about. For example, the nurses in the opening case study perceived Delia as old, passive and unable to do much for herself. As a result, they did not give her a chance to be active within her own care, or even have a two-way conversation. Instead, the nurses cared for Delia so that she was passive in every respect.

This also had the possibility of Delia behaving in a way that was expected of her by nurses. This is referred to as **self-fulfilling prophecy**, whereby an individual begins to behave in a way that they are expected to behave. Slater (1995) exemplified this in the light of dependency:

> If you expect older people to be dependent, and consequently treat them as if they are dependent, and encourage them to respond as if they were dependent, eventually they may indeed become more dependent. Low expectations will necessarily lead to under-achievement (Slater, 1995, p. 17).

This has also been demonstrated with the words that you use and their effect on the patient's mental well-being as well.

Commonly held beliefs about ageing

1. Most people over 65 are financially insecure

2. Most people over 75 are in nursing homes or other institutions

3. Rarely does someone over the age of 65 produce a great work of art, science or scholarship

4. Ageing parents often reverse roles with their adult children, becoming childishly dependent on them

5. Remarriages among old people are generally unsuccessful

6. The shock of retirement often results in deteriorating physical and mental health

7. Women don't enjoy sex much after menopause

8. Old people are not very interested in sex

9. Most child molesters and exhibitionists are old men

10. Impotence is usually psychological, except in old men, where it is more or less inevitable

11. Men are more interested in sex than women

12. Rape is the result of intense sexual needs of some men

13. People tend to become more conservative and inflexible in old age

14. Old people are harder to motivate than young people

15. Old people get rattled more easily

16. Old people should stay active to keep their spirits up

17. Old people prefer to reduce the number of their activities and friendships

18. Old dogs can't learn new tricks

19. A failing memory is the worst intellectual problem in old age

20. In old age, memories of the distant past are clear and vivid, but memories for recent events are fuzzy

21. With all their intellectual deficits, old people don't benefit much from education

22. Intelligence peaks around the age of 20 or 30 and then declines steadily

23. With age comes wisdom

24. Those who are most able in their youth decline the fastest in old age

25. Women live longer than men because they don't work as hard

26. Soon people will live to 150 or 200

27. There are certain groups of people in South America and Russia who live to extraordinarily old ages

28. Elderly patients do not respond well to surgery

29. After 65, the majority of people are unhealthy

30. It is possible to 'worry oneself sick'

31. Hard work never killed anybody

32. Most old people become senile sooner or later

33. Senile old people cannot be helped by psychotherapy

34. Women are more susceptible to mental disorders than men

35. Unmarried people are more susceptible to mental disorders than married people

36. Most people who are faced with their imminent death try to deny it

(Answers at the end of the chapter.)

Source: Schaie, K., Warner, Willis, Sherry L., *Adult Development and Aging*, 5th Edition, © 2002, Pgs. 16-17. Reprinted by permission of Pearson Education, Inc., Upper Saddle River, NJ

How to avoid stereotyping

Stereotyping is something that we all do in order to make sense of the world. However, in professional practice there are certain 'raising awareness' exercises (like the one above) that a nurse can take part in. These will aid reflection on practice and prevent the use of ageing stereotypes. Firstly, filling in questionnaires like the one above can dispel many myths held about the elderly. Secondly, acknowledging the impact stereotyping and using ageist remarks can have on the patient's physical and mental well-being. Thirdly, acknowledging the impact of self-fulfilling prophecy and hence moving out of the mindset that the elderly are passive in their health care and instead facilitate the patient to be active within their care, irrespective of how frail they may be.

Literature that has looked at health promotion within the elderly has emphasised the perception of the elderly as being active, rather than passive, recipients of care. In the case study above, the nurses were reinforcing the view that Delia was not capable of doing anything for herself.

'Taking previous illnesses and impairments into account enhances a positive hospital experience for the elderly'. How do I achieve these as a nurse?

In the opening case study, Delia clearly did not have a positive hospital experience. The non-specialist nurses concentrated on the present health problem and did not address the other pre-existing illnesses. According to Odell and Holbrook (2006) the care that should be provided for older people requires special expertise, for the following reasons:

- Physiological ageing alters the presentation of disease and effects of medication.
- Incidence of depression, dementia and delirium become increasingly common.
- Pre-existing conditions can make self-care more difficult.
- Social support for successful discharge requires complex organisational skills.

Emotional support is also important, as the elderly can be more dependent on individuals around them (McCormack, 2001). By taking these into consideration, a nurse can provide more effective care to meet the needs of the elderly patient.

Neglecting the needs of the elderly and the potential for elder abuse

Elder abuse has been documented widely in research. It is a potential cause for concern because of the vulnerability that increases with advancing age and illness.

Elder abuse has been defined as: 'Single or repeated act, or lack of appropriate action, occurring within a relationship where there is an element of trust, which causes harm or distress to an elder person' (Action on Elder Abuse, 1995). The possibility of abuse occurring within hospitals can be due to a lack of understanding among staff, inadequate management structures, low staff morale or inadequate training (Hudson, 1992). Nursing students can begin to prepare to avoid such situations as the one in the opening case study by being aware of the potential for abuse.

Since 1999, the Nursing and Midwifery Council (then referred to as UKCC) (UKCC, 1999) put elder abuse high on its agenda and ever since has had working targets, so that staff and patients are both equally supported. The areas that the Nursing and Midwifery Council has focused on for both pre- and post-training for nurses are as follows:

- staff attitudes;
- supervision;
- resources;
- policies and procedures;
- staff support and management;
- education and professional development.

When there is a shortage of staff, it is very easy to ignore individual needs. This can sometimes result in neglect. Hence, it is important for nurses to be aware of the basic needs of elderly patients that need to be met, even on a busy ward.

Communication with the elderly patient

Communication with patients has been recognised as one of the most important aspects of nursing elderly people (Armstrong-Esther *et al.*, 1989; Hockey, 1976; Van Cott, 1993). According to Wilkinson (1991), effective communication does not just depend on the use of the right communication skills. Instead, Caris-Verhallen *et al.* (1999a) have identified and written a paper exploring three groups of variables that are important in determining the nurse–patient communication:

- nurse (provider) variables;
- patient variables; and
- situational variables, such as the ward setting (Caris-Verhallen *et al.*, 1997).

(See Chapters 9 and 17.) It is important for nurses to explore these three variables and be aware that they have an impact on nurse–patient communication.

Think about this

In relation to the three variables mentioned above, which of these contributed to Delia feeling frustrated?

Provider (nurse) variables

In the above section, attitudes in relation to ageism and their influence on the type of care provided to the elderly patient were explored. Research has suggested that the same impact can be seen with how the nurse communicates, and their attitudes and preconceptions about the elderly. For example, studies have found that those nurses who had a favourable attitude towards elderly people were also more likely to have attached value to conversations. In comparison, nurses who had a less favourable attitude placed higher importance on the delivery of physical and hygienic care only (Armstrong-Esther et al., 1989).

Job satisfaction and how it impacts on the care that is provided has also been explored. Kramer and Kerkstra (1991) showed that nurses with high levels of intrinsic job motivation and satisfaction with colleagues were more sensitive to elderly patients' needs than nurses with lower levels of job satisfaction. Caris-Verhallen et al. (1999a) also highlighted a link between educational and training levels and their impact on the communication process between the nurse and the patient. Caris-Verhallen et al. (1999a) highlight the study by Davies (1992) who found that although trained and untrained staff used broadly the same range of verbal strategies, trained staff used proportionately more of those strategies that promoted patients' dignity, self-respect, choice and independence. Unqualified nurses were less sensitive to underlying meaning in verbal communication of elderly clients.

In their own study, Caris-Verhallen et al. (1999b) found that more highly educated nurses showed more task-related communication and employed less small talk and banter with their patients. A negative association was found with level of education and the nurses' non-verbal communication, especially eye-contact and head nodding. The researchers found that highly educated nurses were often engaged with technical nursing care, during which they nodded less, because their gaze was directed to the task.

The above variables are important to consider when raising awareness. Communication is very important within the area of geriatric care because of the possible sensory difficulties the patient may have, resulting in communication barriers (Greene et al., 1994). The agenda of the elderly may also be different from that of their younger counterparts because of differences in values and expectations (LeMay and Redfern, 1987). In the case study above, Delia had a preference to be referred to as 'Mrs Jones' rather than 'Delia'. Referring to the latter by younger individuals was perceived as a lack of respect by Delia. In instances such as these, it is always best to ask the patient what their preferences are in relation to names, as every elderly patient will have their own preference.

The previous focus of the Department of Health and nurse training on 'patient-centred' as well as 'patient-led' care will also seem very new to many elderly patients, who are used to the practitioner 'telling the patient' what to do. As a result the elderly are less likely to challenge the authority of health care providers, become less involved in decision-making and avoid discussing psychosocial issues (Greene et al., 1994). A concerted effort needs to be made with the elderly in reassuring them that active participation is encouraged within the nurse–patient relationship.

Patient variables

In the opening case study, the nurses did not interact with Delia, even though they carried out their routine daily tasks with her. A study carried out by Armstrong-Esther and Browne (1986) found that nurses interacted significantly less with confused elderly patients than with their other elderly patients with no impairments. Even though no comparison was seen in the opening case study it was clear that interaction with Delia was kept to a bare minimum by the non-specialist nurses.

Situational variables

Having many demands placed on nursing staff can result in communication and care not being as efficient and effective as it should be.

Caris-Verhallen *et al.* (1999a) highlighted a few studies that exemplify the link between time pressure and care provided. They cited a study carried out by Gibb and O'Brien (1990) who reported that nurses who were responsible for the ward during morning care and were time-pressurised were brief and task-related in interaction with their patients. They used mostly closed rather than open questions, and did not negotiate about the care delivered. Other studies have highlighted that time pressure does not always necessitate lack or ineffective communication with the elderly patient. Wilkinson (1991), for example, compared nurses on six different wards in a general hospital and found that the ward where the best communication took place was a busy one.

As a result of the contradictory findings on time pressure and its impact on the communication process, Caris-Verhallen *et al.* (1999b) refer to the studies carried out by both Salmon (1993) and Turner (1993), which found that on wards where special activity programmes were arranged, there was a positive influence on the amount of nurse–patient interaction. The special activity programmes consisted of a particular time that the nurse and the elderly patient spent together, which was unrelated to any task the nurse had to perform.

Communication with the elderly: what is the right balance?

Research has highlighted that within caring, there are two aspects: **instrumental** and **affective** (Caris-Verhallen *et al.*, 1997). Instrumental aspects of care address the need for information, clarification and physical care. Patients also have emotional needs, such as reassurance, concern and understanding, which are referred to as affective (Engel, 1988).

Think about this

In the opening case study what aspect of care did the nurses on the two wards focus on – instrumental or affective? Discuss situations within the hospital where it may not be possible to provide affective care. How should the nurses have cared for Delia?

Bottorff and Morse (1994) have categorised behaviours into four categories:

- 'Doing', focused on tasks excluding the patient. The object of these tasks is to get the job done. There is rarely any communication with the patient or very brief task-related communication.
- 'Doing with' refers to tasks are focused equally on patient and the task. The object is to involve the patient and there is two-way discussion about care, patient needs and instructions.
- 'Doing for' refers to tasks focused on the patient, where the patient is given the opportunity to direct his/her own care. There is communication about care or social talk.
- 'Doing more' refers to establishing a relation and its focus on the patient as a person. The nurse wants to understand patient experience of illness and treatment. The dialogue is intensive, with emotionally supportive statements by the nurse.

A mixture of these is usually warranted within every context. However, the balance is dependent on the end goal. When working with the elderly, as in the case study above, it is clear that routine procedures had to be carried out: 'doing tasks'. At the same time, 'doing more' needed to have been incorporated when Delia needed emotional support. In addition, a supportive role was needed for her pre-existing illnesses and her pain.

Other researchers have voiced communication as being important, especially within a supportive emotional role for the elderly. Communication is important with patients like Delia, who may have a sensory impairment. Effective communication can be made difficult and hence should be concentrated on more, because of the possible generation gap which results in differing values and beliefs (LeMay and Redfern, 1987). This was portrayed in the above case study, when the patient was referred to as 'Delia'. However, the patient was not asked her preference as to what she would liked to have been called. Delia saw this as a sign of disrespect, as she would have liked those that are younger and did not know her to call her 'Mrs Jones'.

Non-verbal behaviour

Delia is a person who clearly likes her independence and enjoys living by herself. However, this is now becoming a problem with her increasing sensory impairment, worsening symptoms of dementia and increasing immobility, which has resulted in frequent visits to hospitals after falls. Her husband passed away 15 years ago. She has her extended family that tends to visit her every other weekend. In comparison to an individual who is fully mobile and functioning around the house, Delia has seen a decline in the amount of physical contact that she has.

Interaction results in support, comfort, love and affection, needs that all individuals have (Moore and Gilbert, 1995), especially the elderly. Comfort and empathy are components of affective care, which are conveyed both verbally and non-verbally. Researchers tend to emphasise the essentials of non-verbal communication when conveying such components (Bensing *et al.*, 1995; Roter and Hall, 1992).

In the case study Delia has a slight visual impairment. The nurses in the case study did not touch Delia in any supportive manner. Instead, touch was seen only when routine tasks were carried out. For patients that have sensory impairments, non-verbal communication is even more important, when attempting to interact with the patient. Caris-Verhallen *et al.* (1999b) have emphasised the importance of non-verbal communication with the elderly patient, especially those who have a hearing or visual impairment, as touch can form an important part of the caring relationship. Table 10.3 is largely collated from the material presented in the paper by Caris-Verhallen *et al.* (1999b), who reviewed studies that looked at the types of non-verbal communication that are important when working with the elderly patient population.

Think about this

Look at Table 10.3 and consider which of these the nurses could have used when communicating with Delia, so that she was less likely to become frustrated.

The picture below demonstrates how the nurse's non-verbal communication, such as smiling and touch, can convey understanding of what the patient has said, as well as the nurse taking time out to listen to the patient.

A nurse uses non-verbal communication

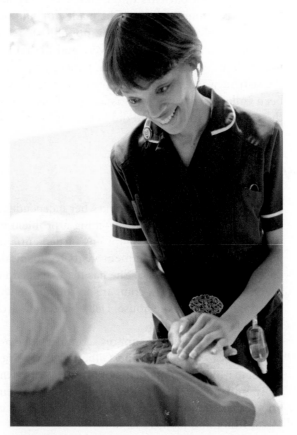

Bubbles Photolibrary/Alamy

Table 10.3
Non-verbal communication

Type of non-verbal communication	Description	Example
Eye gaze behaviour	Signal for readiness to initiate interaction with others (Eibl-Eibesfeldt, 1971, 1972; Von Cranach, 1971). Moderate or high levels of eye contact convey a sense of interest, looking away while a patient is talking is a sign of disinterest, detachment and dislike (Heintzman *et al.*, 1993).	Need to maintain eye contact to convey empathy to the elderly patient.
Affirmative head nodding	Schabracq (1987) three functions • regulation of the interaction, especially changes in turn taking, • support of spoken language, • comment upon the interaction concerning the rapport and the content of communication. Encourage client to tell their story. Conveyance of friendliness and concern (Heintzman *et al.* 1993)	Nurses could have used affirmative head nodding to reassure Delia that they understood her pain.
Smiling	Most important if want to establish rapport with patient (Schabracq, 1987; Heintzman *et al.*, 1993). Signifies warmth, sympathy and good humour (Reece and Whitman, 1962).	Smiling by the nurses could have put Delia at ease.
Body positioning	Indicates listening, attending and being involved (Von Cranach, 1971; Gross, 1990). Interest and leaning forward conveys awareness and immediacy (Schabracq, 1987) and attention (Rosenfield, 1978). Stimulates the other person to carry on talking (Reece and Whitman, 1962; Caris-Verhallen *et al.*, 1997).	Nurses could have 'leaned in' when Delia was talking, so that she felt that the nurses were attending to her as a person rather than just a routine task being carried out on 'another patient'.
Touch	Conveys affection, care and comfort (McCann and McKenna, 1993). Moore and Gilbert (1995) found that elderly patients experienced more immediacy and affection from nurses who used expressive touch than those nurses who did not. Hollinger (1986) found a relationship between nurse's touch and verbal responses by the elderly patient.	Touching Delia's hand when she fell or even when she was in pain would have indicated that the nurses were sympathetic and understanding.

Feeding and nutritional problems among the elderly

As a result of her illnesses, Delia has recently experienced both visual and auditory deterioration. This has resulted in Delia not being able to function as effectively as she used to, which resulted in her fall. Any communication with Delia will have to take this into consideration so that further confusion does not occur for the patient.

Malnutrition and underfeeding among the elderly are also major causes for concern. Statistics suggest that four out of ten older people admitted to hospital have malnutrition on arrival (European Nutrition for Health Alliance, 2005). The concern is that six out of ten older people are at risk of becoming malnourished, or their situation worsening in hospital (European Nutrition for Health, 2005). This has been raised by Age Concern who have stated that:

> One of the most frequent issues raised with Age Concern by the relatives of older people who have been in hospital, is the lack of appropriate food and the absence of help with eating and drinking for people who are unable to manage for themselves (Age Concern, 2006b, p. 4).

This could have been the case for Delia, who was not adequately supported and/or helped with her food. Delia is typical of an elderly patient who has dementia. Typical patients are more prone to malnutrition, both on arrival, depending on their personal circumstances, as well as during their stay in hospital, if adequate support is not provided. This 'additional' support is much needed, rather than the patient being 'left to get on' with eating their food, particularly with statistics suggesting that up to 50 per cent of older people in general health hospitals have mental health needs (Department of Health, 2005b).

Think about this

In relation to the material you have just read regarding malnutrition among the elderly, do you think there could be a possibility that Delia could be malnourished?

Research has suggested that with illnesses such as dementia, the actual illness is characterised by a decline in all activities, including eating (Volicer *et al.*, 1987). Even when there is enormous affective care provided, the loss of ability to feed oneself is often accompanied by nutritional problems (Sandman *et al.*, 1987). What can nurses do so that such problems do not occur or become worse?

The **EdFED questionnaire** (Watson, 1994) has been used in studies such as Watson and Deary's (1997) study which explored feeding difficulties and nursing interventions in elderly patients with dementia. The questions that constitute the EdFED questionnaire can be useful for nurses when assessing and helping an elderly patient eat. The questionnaire consists of the following questions:

- Does the patient require close supervision while feeding?
- Does the patient require physical help with feeding?

- Is there spillage while feeding?
- Does the patient tend to leave food on the plate at the end of a meal?
- Does the patient ever refuse to eat?
- Does the patient turn his head away while being fed?
- Does the patient refuse to open his mouth?
- Does the patient spit out his food?
- Does the patient leave his mouth open allowing food to drop out?
- Does the patient refuse to swallow?
- Indicate the appropriate level of care for feeding required by patient: supportive-educative; partly compensatory, wholly compensatory.

Possible answers to questions a = never; b = sometimes; c = often.

According to Lennard-Jones (1992), doctors and nurses need to be educated to develop 'a habit of instinctively noting under-nourishment and a sensitivity to situations in which it might occur.'

Tierney (1996) has listed further questions a nurse may need to ask when attempting to identify malnutrition.

- Has food intake reduced recently?
- Are there physical difficulties with eating?
- Is the patient confused or depressed?
- Has there been diarrhoea or vomiting?
- Has the patient been able to shop and manage food preparation (or had help)?
- Has the patient (or family) noticed weight loss, e.g. by fit of clothes; if so, over what period?
- What does the patient regard as normal weight?

It is clear that the non-specialist nurses who were caring for Delia did not take any of these questions into account. As a result, they did not see the lack of eating as an issue.

The attitude of the nurse towards the elderly and feeding also needs to be taken into consideration. If the nurse does not consider eating a priority, then malnutrition can go undetected. Barnes (1990) explored nurses' feelings about feeding elderly, long-stay patients. Patients who were described as being fussy, difficult to feed and who 'just won't eat anything' provided little reward for the nurse. Nurses were rarely observed encouraging underweight patients to eat more (see Chapter 6).

Conclusion

People are living longer which means that there will be more patients aged over 60 who will be accessing health care. The ageing process brings with it a number of health concerns, along with deterioration in physical and mental well-being. As a result, irrespective of what area a nurse may specialise in, caring for an older patient will be likely (unless working in a children's hospital or ward). This brings many different needs and requirements that a nurse has to consider when caring for and communicating with an elderly patient. It is important to be mindful of the way particular illnesses and sensory decline that accompany ageing can impact on communication and understanding. At the same time, nurses also need to be aware that patients, irrespective of age, like to maintain independence and be communicated to as people within their own right.

These issues span across areas such as dignity and ensuring that the patient is functioning both physically and mentally within their capacity. Nurses need to encourage this rather than ignore it. It is very easy to address only physical needs but conversations, psychosocial issues and general interaction that do not act as a reminder of their age or ill-health are just as important to prevent further physical and mental decline. Gerontology nursing brings with it a reminder of the importance of caring for the unique needs that the elderly patient presents, as well as the facilitation and encouragement of present physical and mental functions to ensure a healthy older age.

Summary

- The census of 2001 suggested that there are 11 million older people living in the United Kingdom. These figures are set to increase to 13.9 million in 2026.

- The main users of the health service are the elderly. 24 per cent of those aged 75 years and over visited a casuality out-patients department in the last three months, compared with 14 per cent for the rest of the population.

- The group 'the elderly' has enormous variances in relation to the care that the elderly patient requires. Suzman and Riley (1985) have divided the elderly group into three: young-old (65-75/80 years), old-old (75/80-90 years) and very-old (85-90 and above).

- The Government has outlined working targets for the NHS and the elderly patient population. These have been set out in the National Service Framework (Department of Health, 2001b), which tackle the areas of age discrimination and promoting health and well-being for the elderly patient.

- Dignity within the elderly patient population, is a key area to consider. Calnan *et al.* (2005) identify three sub-groups: identity, rights and autonomy, as being central to the explanation of dignity.

- Much research has highlighted the importance of treating and caring for the elderly patient in a holistic manner. This requires that not only the present illness is taken care of, but that previous illnesses and impairments are also considered.

- Morton (1999) identifies three types of reflections that can be used when communicating with an elderly patient who may have a sensory impairment: facial reflection, situational reflection and bodily reflection.

- It has been established that pain is hard to assess, and in turn control, in the hospital setting, especially for the elderly patient. Potential barriers in the way that pain is expressed can arise because of cultural and generational differences.

- Ageism and stereotyping of the elderly are prevalent within society. Nurses can counteract these prejudices by reading around the area of gerontological nursing, as well as raising awareness.

- Slater (1995) highlights the issue of dependency within the elderly. There are certain illnesses and impairments whereby the individual is, to an extent, dependent on caring staff. The danger is that nurses can further encourage dependency with the self-fulfilling prophecy.

- A balance of care should be aimed for by nurses that includes both instrumental and affective care, even on a very busy ward.

- The EdFED Questionnaire (Watson, 1994) provides a way of establishing whether the patient is receiving adequate nutrition. This is useful when assessing elderly patients who may come into the hospital malnourished.

- A mixture of doing tasks, doing with, doing for and doing more when working with the elderly ensure that adequate care has been provided (dependent on the context the patient is receiving care within). (Bottorff and Morse, 1994).

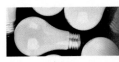

Check your understanding

- What are the three categories that the elderly group can be divided into, so that they are not all grouped together as just being 'the elderly'?

- An elderly patient being treated for their current ill-health state is in hospital. In order to provide appropriate care that meets the need of the individual patient, what else needs to be considered?

- When providing care for an elderly patient, it is important that both instrumental and affective care are provided. Define and distinguish the two types of care.

- What is a self-fulfilling prophecy? Explain how easy it is for the nurse to promote the self-fulfilling prophecy for the elderly patient when looking at the issues of dependency.

- Name three things that need to be taken into consideration by a nurse on a busy ward, so that the elderly patient's basic needs are not neglected.

- List five questions that a nurse can ask a patient to ensure that they are eating adequately.

- List four things that should be taken into consideration when assessing the elderly patient's current pain.

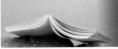

Further reading

Caris-Verhallen, W.M.CA., de Gruijter, I.M., Kerstra, A. and Bensing, J.M. (1999) Factors related to nurse communication with elderly people. *Journal of Advanced Nursing*, **30** (5), 1106–1117.

Copeman, J. (1999) *Nutritional Care for Older People: A Guide to Good Practice*. London: Age Concern.

Department of Health (2000) *No Secrets: Guidance on Developing and Implementing Multi-agency Policies and Procedures to Protect Vulnerable Adults from Abuse*. London: Department of Health.

Department of Health (2001) *National Service Framework For Older People*. London: Department of Health.

Heine, C. and Browning, C.J. (2004) The communication and psychosocial perceptions of older adults with sensory loss: a qualitative study. *Aging and Society*, 24, 113–130.

National Nursing, Midwifery and Health Visiting Report (2002) *Promoting Nutrition for Older Adult In-patients in NHS Hospitals in Scotland*. Edinburgh: Scottish Executive.

Weblinks

Age Concern	http://www.ageconcern.org.uk	Many research and statistical papers that have been put together on this website. 'Hungry to be heard: the scandal of malnourished older people in hospital', is included here.

| Department of Health | http://www.dh.gov.uk/ | Includes policy documents in relation to the elderly, including the National Service Framework document. |
| National Gerontological Nursing Association | http://www.ngna.org | Website providing information related to care of the elderly and dignity, with information on recent policy changes as well as helpful information for nurses. |

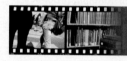

Media examples

Remember, produced by Arden T. Kayce. Cheryl, a victim of early-onset Alzheimer's disease, has become a burden and a source of frustration for her loving husband Jerry. Desperately needing a break from his caregiving duties, Jerry escapes out of the house. Cheryl, alone, loses her tenuous grasp on reality and floats in and out of her past memories. Jerry returns to find her reliving the happiest day of her life and his – their wedding.

The Royle Family A UK comedy that looks at dispelling the stereotypes of how older adults live their day-to-day life.

Answer sheet (see p. 272)

1. False
2. False
3. False
4. Partly true
5. False
6. False
7. False
8. False
9. False
10. Partly true
11. False
12. Partly true
13. Partly true
14. Partly true
15. Partly true
16. True
17. False
18. False

19. Partly true
20. Partly true
21. False
22. False
23. Partly true
24. False
25. False
26. False
27. False
28. False
29. Partly true
30. Partly true
31. False
32. False
33. Partly true
34. False
35. False
36. True

Chapter 11

Patient loss, bereavement and terminal illness

Learning outcomes

When you have read through this chapter you should understand:

- How the meaning and impact of loss change through the lifespan.

- How bereavement models can help the nurse to communicate adequately within the context of loss, anticipated loss and bereavement.

- Why nurses participate in nursing rituals that centre on bereavement.

- How the nurse can maintain a positive state of mind when helping patients and families through the experience of loss and grief.

- How the nurse can promote healthy grief work.

- How communication by the nurse can be carried out appropriately within the context of loss and bereavement.

- How patients' grief work is subject to cultural and religious rituals and experience of loss and bereavement.

Case study

Jim, his wife Rose and their three children are overjoyed at the news that Rose is expecting a baby. A couple of months into the pregnancy Rose has unexpectedly been taken into hospital with severe abdominal pains and bleeding. A few hours later and the couple have had their worst nightmare confirmed: Rose has had a miscarriage. They are both shocked by the news. The senior staff nurse can see that both Rose and Jim are finding it difficult to come to terms with the miscarriage and has decided to help the couple with their grief, so that coming to terms with the miscarriage will be easier for both of them.

The senior staff nurse introduces herself and expresses how sorry she is for the couple's loss. Rose looks back at the nurse with a blank expression while Jim states that they will be fine and that they can do nothing about it now.

Rose is kept in hospital for a couple of days until her health becomes more stable. During her stay, the senior staff nurse, as well as other nurses, encourage Rose to talk about her feelings. Rose does not reveal any of her emotions or feelings. Three days later Rose's physical health has improved, and she is prepared for discharge.

Knowing that Rose will be discharged, the nurse decides to talk to Jim; she is concerned that Rose has shown no emotion. The staff nurse explains to Jim that she is concerned about his wife's grieving process, as she has not spoken about her feelings. She hands Jim a leaflet that lists organisations that can further support Rose. Jim becomes tearful and the nurse reassures him that the grieving process will become easier over time. She further emphasises the positive things in life that they need to focus on, such as their three children, and compares their situation those of others who have miscarried and have no children. Jim thanks the nurse and begins to feel guilty about being upset.

Why is this relevant to nursing practice?

Death and loss are things that a nurse will have to deal with on a continual basis, irrespective of the particular branch of nursing they specialise in. Helping a patient to come to terms with their diagnosis, loss or multiple losses all require the patient to go through **grief work**. Grief work is an emotional process consisting of many emotional states. Working through grief is vital in order to reach acceptance of a changed physical state or status after a loss. When considering grief work, a common question that arises is, 'did the nurse help or hinder grief work?' This chapter will consider grief work, what entails grief work and grief work models. These are useful models for a nurse to be aware of as they will help him or her understand the patient's emotional state and communicate with the patient accordingly.

Individuals are living longer and are more likely to experience chronic, rather than acute, illnesses. As a result, a nurse will not only have to deal with the death of patients but will also have to deal with the mental and physical losses that occur throughout a patient's illness, while the patient is alive. In addition, the nurse will also be at the forefront of breaking bad news both to the patient and the patient's next of kin. Because nurses are involved in supporting patients and families of deceased patients, knowledge of the theory of bereavement is important. The supportive role of a nurse during bereavement is crucial. Exploration of this area is therefore warranted, as the nurse will have the potential to influence how the first steps of grief work are taken.

According to the World Health Organization, the need to offer family and significant others support, not only during the patient's terminal illness but also in bereavement, is significant and is the contemporary philosophy of palliative care (WHO, 1990). After the theory of grief work was developed by Kubler-Ross (1969), it became more acceptable for people to talk about death in an open manner. As a result, quality of life and the needs of the dying patient have been given the same importance as those of a patient who is not dying.

Even for nurses who are well-read around the area of palliative care, the prospect of caring for your first dying patient, breaking bad news for the first time or even carrying out a ritual such as the **last offices**, can be daunting. Research has shown that it is common among newly trained nurses to have feelings of inadequacy when it comes to the area of palliative care. De Araujo *et al.* (2004) found that, in the main, nurses felt that assisting terminally ill patients is a frustrating and sad activity. This is important, as nurses' attitudes towards death influence the type of care that they will administer to patients. Nurses also require additional emotional and psychological support. Within an area such as palliative care, many uncertainties are raised, as well as personal fears; previous experiences of loss may resurface for the patient as well as for the nurse. Having a ritual such as the last offices, as well as appropriate communication skills, will protect the nurse from becoming emotionally involved and affected in a loss situation. Communication and rituals within a loss situation will be looked at in this chapter.

Nurses may feel inexperienced or inadequate when communicating with a dying patient, which may have a negative influence on the care being provided, as well as resulting in feelings of failure for the nurse. Nurses may even question if this is the right career for them (Rooda *et al.*, 1999). Research has shown that feeling inadequate and not exploring the area of bereavement in great depth can result in the avoidance of those patients who need the most care; as a result, these patients have to wait longer for assistance compared with patients who are less seriously ill (LeShan, 1994). This chapter will enable you to begin to explore the area of bereavement, and discusses the 'dos' and 'don'ts' when caring for a dying patient or a patient who is experiencing loss. In addition, this chapter will also discuss your own attitudes and experiences towards loss and death. This chapter will hopefully equip the nurse with the confidence and communication skills to deal with 'the dying patient' and the patient who is experiencing or will be experiencing some kind of loss.

Think about this

Has the senior staff nurse in the opening case study facilitated healthy grief work for the couple? Could she have approached the situation better? What was wrong and right in her communication with Jim and Rose? What are the potential long-term implications for Jim and Rose's grieving?

Several **grief work models** have been put forward to explain the process of grief. A student nurse who has explored these grief work models can begin to understand the process that his or her patient will experience, and mirror their communication accordingly. This is a difficult area, especially for a training student nurse who may not have had experience with loss in a professional capacity. Many areas come to light in the case study. Firstly, both Rose and Jim have been hindered with their **grieving**. In such a case, **shock** is a common initial response, and features in the majority of models as the first stage of grief. The shock experienced by Rose for a couple of days resulted in the senior staff nurse being more proactive in her attempts to help the patient. Knowing when to be concerned for patients experiencing loss and responding appropriately do not only result from years of experience, but having the knowledge base of grief work models and appropriate communication, which this chapter will look at. The problem is that although grief models display the process of grief work, they do not necessarily clarify how a nurse should communicate with their patients. In addition, every situation is unique in its own right. The senior staff nurse in the opening case study compared other cases of miscarriage with that of Jim and Rose. Even though the nurse's intention was good, this did not facilitate **good grief**, simply because the family circumstances were unknown. What if the three children at home were from Rose's first marriage? What implications would there be had the unborn child been the first one that Rose and Jim had conceived together?

Communication and counselling skills are vital when helping patients and their families with loss. A student nurse who only has personal grief as experience can encounter problems when helping a patient through loss if they are not familiar with the basic skills and information that exist relating to helping patients deal with loss or anticipated loss. It will become clear that dealing with loss within a professional setting requires different communication skills to those used when comforting someone who has experienced loss within a personal context. What can be said in a personal setting to a family member, e.g. 'be grateful that at least you have three others at home', is not what you can say in professional practice. This is typical of the **sympathy versus empathy debate**. Nurse training emphasises the importance of **empathy**. However, this changes when it comes to loss and grief, as the different phases of the grieving process warrant both empathy and sympathy.

The last comment the nurse in the case study made, 'think about the three children at home, some do not even have them', resulted in Jim feeling guilty about grieving. The nurse facilitated **bad grief**. Psychology attempts to explain what happens when there is bad grief and or abnormal grieving. Making Jim feel guilty will result in a delay in the grieving process. The longer this is delayed, the more problems Jim and Rose will have later on when attempting to accept their loss. This area overlaps with the psychodynamic approach (see Chapter 4) as grief work models encompass **defence mechanisms**. In this case, Jim may use **denial** for a longer period of time because of the guilty feeling he felt during the initial stages of grieving. Facilitation of good grief work, as opposed to negative grief work, will be explored within this chapter.

Different phases across the lifespan result in different conceptions of, and reactions to, loss. The grief work models are based on an adult understanding of loss. Children, on the other hand, have a different understanding of loss, which changes rapidly with increasing age within childhood. Each of Jim's children may have reacted to the news of the loss differently. This chapter will focus on the phases of childhood and associated conceptions of loss. There is also diversity in how individuals understand and react to loss and bereavement. This chapter will help the nurse to become more aware of how cultural and religious influences impact on such an experience.

Death, loss, bereavement, grief and mourning

Death, bereavement, mourning and grief are terms that are used widely within any loss context. It is important to define these terms in order to acknowledge how they are distinct from one another, as well as their similarities.

Death is the irreversible cessation of life. This involves a complete change in the status of a living entity, which is signified by the death of the organism as a whole, preceded by the death of individual organs, cells and parts of cells. Death has been thought to occur when the vital functions cease, e.g. breathing and circulation (as evidenced by the beating of the heart). This view has been challenged, as medical advances have made it possible to sustain respiration and cardiac functioning through mechanical means. More recently the concept of brain death has gained acceptance. In this view, the irreversible loss of brain activity is the sign that death has occurred. This is the same throughout the world for every living being.

Bereavement has been defined as depriving someone of a beloved person through death. Bereavement is derived from the old English term *bereafian*, which means to have been deprived or robbed. In comparison to the term death, bereavement is an overarching term, which refers to the feelings and emotions one goes through during the period of loss.

Think about this

Think about a time when either yourself or someone you know had a car or their home broken into. What kind of feelings did you/they experience?

The feelings that you experienced may include fear, denial, anger and many more. Any of these feelings/emotions may feature within the bereavement process and are included within the bereavement models. Any type of loss that has been experienced – loss of a limb, loss of a job, loss of a pet, loss of a family member or friend – will result in emotions, reactions and feelings, which are all part of the same bereavement process.

During the process of bereavement, grief and mourning are experienced. The amount of time spent grieving and mourning depend on how attached the griever was to the deceased (e.g. day-to-day contact), and how much time was spent anticipating the loss. The terms below are therefore very much subjective.

Mourning is 'the process by which people adapt to a loss' (National Cancer Institute, 2005). Mourning is a signal of distress, which is influenced by religious rituals as well as societal rules that help with the process of coping during loss.

Nurses within the United Kingdom are trained within the biomedical model, which brings particular rituals and patterns within the hospital setting. Even though ethnic minorities adapt and adhere to rules within the hospital setting, there will be differing mourning patterns and rituals carried out by different cultural groups. These mourning patterns may seem alien to a nurse who has not come across them before, and which diverge from what he or she is familiar with. This will be looked at in greater detail within the section on culture.

Grief can be defined as feeling sadness and sorrow as a result of a loved one's death or loss, which can be one's own loss. This reaction to loss can be displayed physically, emotionally, cognitively and socially. Physical reactions include eating and sleeping problems. Mental reactions can include anxiety, sadness and despair. Social reactions include readjusting to life without the deceased, or readjusting to life after the loss of a limb or diagnosis of a chronic illness. The grieving process is dependent upon the relationship with the person, factors surrounding the loss (e.g. sudden or impending), as well as unresolved issues with the deceased.

All of these factors influence whether a person will go through a 'normal' or 'abnormal' grieving process. For example, death resulting from an accident increases the likelihood of there being an abnormal grieving pattern than a death resulting from a long terminal illness, where individuals have been told that their family member or friend will die. The opening case study is an example of sudden loss, which increases the likelihood of abnormal grieving.

Overlap and summary of the above terms

Even though the terms above have been looked at individually, in reality they overlap, as they are all interlinked. For example, *bereavement* involves the consideration of multiple *losses* experienced after the death of someone significant (Doka, 2000). *Grief* is the response to that/those loss(es) (Corr, 1992), and *mourning* the behavioural expression of grief (Wendell Moller, 1996), shaped by a given society or cultural group (Stroebe, 1998).

Children's understanding of loss

There are vast differences across childhood and adolescence in the understanding of loss. The understanding of loss changes rapidly throughout childhood as individuals experience cognitive and social changes that are reflected in how a child perceives, comprehends and thinks about loss and bereavement. It is useful for any nurse, regardless of specialism, to become familiar with this area as children may experience loss and have to be helped by nurses within many situations. In the opening case study Jim and his wife Rose had three children. Jim may have brought his children to the hospital when visiting Rose. This could have opened up the possibility for any of the nurses to sit with the children and talk about the loss; the nurses may also have talked to Jim, who may have taken the opportunity to ask the nurses on the ward for advice on how to communicate the recent loss to his three children.

Table 11.1 shows the different stages a child goes through, and the influence this has on dealing with any issue related to loss, grief, death and terminal illness. It demonstrates how differently children understand loss and death according to their particular age group. For example, a 3-year-old will confuse death with sleep, whereas a 9-year-old will understand that death is final and cannot be reversed. Children should not all be seen as having the same understanding of loss; how they need to be communicated with and helped differs. Table 11.1 should be taken only as a guide, not a prescriptive framework, suggesting that all children in a particular age group will have the same understanding of loss. The age groups, the transition to each age group and understanding of loss will become blurred as a result of experiences, peer influence, number of siblings, etc.

Three questions that children tend to ask in a loss context

According to the National Cancer Institute (2005), children's grief expresses three issues:

- *Did I cause the death?* As documented in Table 11.1, children have a belief system whereby they believe they have magical powers. This can cause enormous guilt. For example, a parent dies and the child remembers a time when their parent was disciplining them and said, 'You'll be the death of me'. As a result, children may attribute the cause of death to themselves.
- *Is it going to happen to me?* The death of another child can be especially difficult. If the child reasons that the death could have been prevented (by a parent or doctor), the child may think he or she could die.
- *Who is going to take care of me?* Since children depend on a parent or main caregiver, the death of a caregiver can result in the child asking 'who will care for me now?'.

Think about this

From the points highlighted above, as a nurse what issues would you take into consideration and how would you communicate with a chid that is grieving. Would you be honest? Direct? What kind of words would you use? Should children be involved? Below are some further areas that should be taken into consideration when communicating with a child who is grieving.

How can the child's grieving process be made easier?

Not talking about death will not help a child in any way. By using this approach, a child will feel guilty and grieve secretly without any adult input. Nurses can play a vital role here. The nurse should be open and honest when questions are asked (unless carers have made an explicit request not to do so). Each child should be given information that is simple and direct but if requested by the child, should contain as much detail as possible. Children

Age	Understanding of death	Behavioural/expression of grief	What can the nurse do when caring for a child who is grieving or is terminally ill?
Infants	Do not recognise death. Feelings of loss and separation are part of developing an awareness of death.	Separated from mother – sluggish, quiet and unresponsive to a smile or a coo. Physical changes – weight loss, less active, sleep less.	Awareness by nurse that even though the infant does not recognise death, they are still affected by the lack of presence of the significant other.
2–3 years	Confuse death with sleep. Begin to experience anxiety by 3.	Ask many questions, e.g. 'How does she eat?' Problems in eating, sleeping and bladder and bowel control. Fear of abandonment. Tantrums.	Death is associated with something that is mystical, magical and peaceful so make sure that your answers reflect this. Giving the child as much security as possible via non-verbal communication, e.g. comfort, attention, love, is crucial.
3–6 years	Still confuse death with sleep, i.e. is alive but only in a limited way. Death is temporary, not final. Dead person can come back to life.	Even though saw deceased buried still ask questions. Magical thinking – his or her thoughts may cause someone to die. Under 5 – trouble eating, sleeping and controlling bladder and bowel functions. Afraid of the dark.	Answer by acknowledging that the concept of death is something magic and peaceful, e.g. daddy is with the angels like you saw him in your dream, up until approximately age 5. From 5 and thereon, this begins the process of change to being associated with something that is scary and painful, hence afraid of the dark during the latter phases of this age group.
6–9 years	Curious about death. Death is thought of as a person or spirit (skeleton, ghost, bogeyman). Death is final and frightening. Death happens to others, it won't happen to me.	Ask specific questions. May have exaggerated fears. May have aggressive behaviours (especially boys). Some concerns about imaginary illnesses. May feel abandoned.	Communication here should take into account the child's comprehension of death, which has changed from something that is magical and painless to something that is painful and destructive. Even if a parent has protected the child from the subject of death, children will have an understanding from peers, education and the most influential – media.
9 years and older	Everyone will die. Death is final and cannot be changed. Even I will die.	Heightened emotions, such as guilt, anger, shame. Increased anxiety over own death. Mood swings. Fear of rejection, not wanting to be different from peers. Changes in eating habits. Sleeping problems. Regressive behaviours (loss of interest in outside activities). Impulsive behaviours. Feels guilty about being alive (especially related to death of a parent, sibling or peer).	Guilt is a predominant feeling when grieving at this stage. Encourage the child to talk as much as possible and work through the guilt. Closing up over a long period of time may result in referral to a counsellor. Peer support networks are highly beneficial here.

Source: partly adapted from National Cancer Institute.
http://www.cancer.gov/cancertopics/pdq/supportivecare/bereavement/Patient/allpages/

Table 11.1   Understanding death and loss across the different developmental ages in childhood

will also need to be reassured about their own insecurities, e.g. they will not die, or they did not have a part to play in the death of the deceased. Proper words should be used such as death, cancer, dying. Phrases such as 'he passed away', 'is sleeping' and 'we lost him' should be avoided, as the child will misunderstand what is happening.

Taking the above areas into consideration when communicating with a grieving child, as well as being direct and honest about the issue of death, will help a child mourn and take pressure off the parent(s) or caregiver. It can benefit their child/children to see the body of their deceased parent, as this will begin to confirm to the child that their parent will not be coming back. This is beneficial, as imagination is often far worse than reality (Byrne, 2005).

You should not underestimate the amount of experience a child has with death, for example the loss of a pet or even a favourite toy involve the grieving process. In these instances it may be slightly easier to explain death.

Communicating with a dying child

Problems can exist between the dying child and their family during the final stage of illness. It can often be difficult for the family to embrace the subject of death at all. On the other hand, the dying child may find it frustrating that the subject of death is not discussed. Nurses working within palliative and paediatric care need to be aware of the wishes of the dying child, who may not be able to talk to their family but instead may speak openly to the nurses around them. The nurse may be in a key position to communicate the needs of the dying child to the family and to encourage discussion and eventual healthy grief work for those left behind. Below is a case study by the researcher Kubler-Ross (2001), who illustrated this point in many of her case studies.

Research in focus

Elisabeth Kubler-Ross, E. (2001), *Living with Death and Dying.* New York: Touchstone Books; Simon and Schuster[1].

Case study

L. was a 13-year-old girl whose big dream in life was to be a teacher. She was hospitalised during the summer and was found to have an abdominal tumour. After surgery, the parents were reassured that everything malignant had been removed, and they were confident that their daughter's life was no longer in danger. Before school started L. developed new symptoms, and by September she began to deteriorate rapidly. It became clear that she was full of metastasis and that she would no longer be able to return to school. In spite of the pleas of her parents, her physician refused to put her on Brompton mixture for pain relief, and a search for a new physician who was willing to use the most effective oral pain management was in vain. She could no longer be transported to Chicago, where her previous treatment was given. It was at this point that I was consulted and started to see the young patient and her family in their home.

▶

The mother, an open, deeply religious and courageous woman, spent much time with her daughter and discussed frankly all issues that her child brought up. L. was in a comfortable bed in the living room so that she was able to participate passively with the family activities. Her father, a quiet man, did not speak much about the illness or impending death but showed his love and affection in little extra attention and would often return from work with a bouquet of roses for his oldest daughter.

The siblings, ranging from six to ten, were brought together one day in the living room after school hours. I had a session with them in the absence of any adults. We used spontaneous drawings of children, a technique taught by Susan Bach, and they happily cooperated and explained the pictures. Their drawings clearly indicated their knowledge of their sister's serious illness, and we discussed her impending death without euphemisms. It was the six-year-old who had courage to bring up his problems, namely his inability to watch television, to bang doors, and to bring friends home after school. He felt intimidated by the adults, who started to tiptoe around the house, and wondered openly how long this ordeal might last. Together the children discussed the things they would like to share with their sister – all the things they would like to say to her prior to her death – and, needless to say, we encouraged doing so without delay.

After several difficult days – each one expected to be the last, L. simply lingered on. By now she had an enormously enlarged abdomen and her arms and legs were similar to the ones I had seen in the concentration camps. L. simply could not die. We brought her tapes of her favourite music; her mother sat many hours at her bedside and was quite open to answer whatever questions her daughter had. It seemed impossible to figure out what held this little girl to life.

During one of my house calls – and with the mother's permission and in her presence – I asked her straightforwardly, 'L., is there something that prevents you from letting go? You cannot die, and I cannot figure out what it is. Can you tell me?' With great relief L., confirmed this by saying, 'Yes, I cannot die because I cannot go to heaven.' I was shocked by this statement and asked her who in the world had told her this. She then related this that she was told too many times by 'my priest and the visiting sisters' and that 'no one goes to heaven unless they loved God more than anyone else in the world.' With her last physical strength, she leaned forward, put her fragile arms around my shoulders, and whispered apologetically, 'You see, I love my mommy and daddy more than anyone else in the world.'

My initial reaction was one of anger. Why do people whom 'represent God' use fear and guilt instead of representing Him as God of love and mercy? I also knew from past experiences that no one could help another person by demeaning another person's approach. This is the time when the use of parables or symbolic language is the only answer. The following dialogue took place:

'L., I will not get into a debate about who has the right answers about God. Let us talk about things we always shared. Let us take your school as an example and answer me one single question. Sometimes your teacher gives especially tough assignments to some students in class. Does she give this to her worst students, to just anyone in her class, or to only very few, especially chosen ones?' L.'s face lit up and she said very proudly, 'Oh, she gives this only to very few of us.' My response to her: 'Since God is also a teacher, do you think He has given you an easy assignment that He can just give to any child, or has he given you an especially difficult one?'

A very moving, nonverbal communication took place at this time. She leaned up for a moment and took a long, hard look at her own emaciated body, her protruding abdomen, her skinny arms and legs, and with the most extraordinarily pleased look she stared at me and exclaimed, 'It was no longer necessary for me to say, "And now what do you think He thinks of you?"'

The above case study illustrates the point of being honest, open and direct (with the permission of the parents). It illustrates the role in which a nurse can find him- or herself; the nurse can both facilitate the discussion of loss and begin the process of healthy grief work.

Bereavement models/theoretical perspectives

Think about this

What emotional and physical states are experienced when an individual is grieving? Do individuals differ in what they experience? Does the grieving process encompass a particular order? Does grief have any purpose?

A number of models attempt to highlight the different stages that are involved within grief. The overall aim of the grief models is to demonstrate what is involved when grieving, known as grief work. These models emphasise that all individuals will experience particular emotional and physical states but will vary as to the amount of time that is spent at each stage. All models emphasise the need to experience these stages in order to reach acceptance. Grief work models are applicable in the main to adults but can also be applied to the grief process that children will go through before reaching acceptance. Grief work is described as 'an effortful process that we must go through entailing confrontation of the reality of loss and gradual acceptance of the world without the loved one' (Stroebe, 1998).

Parkes's (1972, 1986) four-stage model describes the phases of bereavement and, in turn, grief work that one faces (Table 11.2). An individual has to work through the stages of grief in order to reach acceptance. Nurses can apply this model to terminally ill patients when helping them to reach an end goal of acceptance of their illness. Patients who have been diagnosed with a terminal illness will go through exactly the same grieving process as someone who has lost a loved one. Parkes's model is easy to apply when attempting to understand what a patient is experiencing, but nurses should not expect each patient to experience each stage and the accompanying reaction in order (Greenstreet, 2005). In reality the grieving patient may miss a stage or move back rather than forward through the stages. Also, there seems to be an emphasis on grieving not being normal until a resolution has been reached in the find stage (Costello, 1995). This can have a negative impact on the care the nurse is providing. Try to place more emphasis on the individual making the most of each stage. This provides a base from which the nurse can work from and with when helping and communicating with the patient.

Another example of a stage-like model is Kubler-Ross's (1969) five-stage bereavement model, as shown overleaf. This model has provided a framework for caregivers and nurses working with individuals experiencing loss.

Table 11.2
Parkes's four-stage model of grief work

Name of phase	Reactions, emotions in each phase
Phase One	Initial reaction: shock, numbness or disbelief
Phase Two	Pangs of grief, searching, anger, guilt, sadness and fear
Phase Three	Despair
Phase Four	Acceptance/adjustment. Gaining a new identity

Source: Parkes (1986)

Kubler-Ross was one of the first researchers to study patients and their families from the diagnosis of a terminal illness up until death; she analysed the experiences and mental states of both the dying patient and the family around them. It was only after Kubler-Ross's research that more emphasis was given to palliative care and the importance of quality of life for a dying patient. This pioneering work resulted in death and terminal illness no longer being a taboo subject and thus changed nursing/palliative care forever.

Kubler-Ross's five-stage (DABDA) model

The **five-stage (DABDA) model** has the following stages.

Denial and isolation

During this stage there is constant denial of the new status of a patient. Typical reactions could be: 'It can't be me, you must have the results mixed up', or 'my daughter is not dead, she is perfectly healthy' (see also Chapter 4). In the case study, one explanation why Rose had a blank expression could have been because she may have denied the miscarriage and hence was oblivious to the emotional reactions around her. During this stage, the nurse should make it obvious to the patient that they are there if the patient would like to talk. In the case study, the senior staff nurse did do this by encouraging Rose to talk a number of times. The senior staff nurse also noticed that Rose did not cry or talk about the miscarriage; this was noted and Jim was encouraged to refer to the support that existed for couples who have miscarried.

Anger

In this stage the griever will be angry, and possibly displaying anger towards close family and health practitioners. Typical reactions include 'because of you [the nurse], I can't go home and pick my children up from school' or 'it's okay for you, you can go home at the end of the day'. Also, there is a shift from 'no it can't be me, it must be a mistake', to 'oh yes it is me, it was not a mistake'. It is useful for a nurse to be familiar with this stage, as any outburst of anger towards the nurse or other loved ones around the patient are part of the grieving process and should be acknowledged as such.

Bargaining

During this stage it is not uncommon for patients to seek help from alternative care practices outside the biomedical approach. At this stage, people who are enduring a terminal illness and looking for a cure or 'a bit more time' will pay any price for this. It is not uncommon for patients who have never been religious to pray, e.g. 'if I pray will you grant me another extra couple of days?' The problem is that even when the couple of extra days are granted, they are never enough, as the patient will always want more.

Depression

In the fourth stage the individual will undergo the process of 'letting go' of anger. This is replaced by feelings of intense loss. This time is very much a quiet, dark and reflective time. Feelings during this stage can be similar to those of an individual who is experiencing depression. The dying patient does not want reassurance from a nurse, but at the same time does not want to be ignored. During this time the family members of the dying patient begin the five-stage model, so are in denial that the family member is going to die. They may even become angry at the patient for 'giving up'. The dying patient would like people around them to be quiet, and this is where nurses can make a difference; all they want is someone to be present, who does not question and is not angry. There will be questions the patient will ask and they need to be answered honestly. The patient may also like the nurse to anticipate questions, since unasked questions can be the most important ones.

Acceptance

During this stage the individual is neither depressed nor angry. They have worked through feelings of loss and have found some peace. During this stage, the patient has let go of the world around them. Family members on the other hand are very angry or questioning why the patient is at peace when they still want to change the status of the patient. The patient, however, is ready to move on.

Analysis of Kubler-Ross's model

This is one of the most easily applicable grief work models and the one most frequently referred to by nurses. However, it is an outdated model, which reads in a very prescriptive manner, i.e. this is what you should do, or what grieving looks like. In reality grieving does not occur in stages and there are enormous individual variations. For example, it is not uncommon for patients and grieving families to oscillate between stages, e.g. depression then anger then back to depression. What you need to be aware of is when a patient resides in one stage for a long time, additional support from a counsellor may be needed. Do not work or push a patient to the next stage. There will be more therapeutic benefits if you work with the patient's reactions, rather than against them. Taking something positive out of particular reaction and building on that for increased self-esteem; enable the patient to be proactive in a situation in which they are helpless. In the opening case study the senior staff nurse was very passive in her approach with Rose, even though she monitored her physical well-being. The nurse could have approached a conversation with Rose by emphasising how her physical health was progressing, or how caring her husband is. This would also have built up trust between the nurse and Rose which would have increased the likelihood of Rose confiding in the senior staff nurse.

Communication

How a patient is helped through their grieving process is determined by the communication that takes place between the nurse and the patient. This can be difficult for newly qualified nurses who have not had much experience with end-of-life or loss situations. It can also prove to be challenging in areas such as cancer care where sensitive end-of-life topics will be at the forefront of care (Curtis *et al.*, 2001)

The following information is a brief guide for nurses who need to establish what they can and cannot say when helping a grieving person. Firstly, the nurse will need to distinguish between what can be said within a personal and a professional loss context when attempting to help an individual. There are many reasons for this. Firstly, the way you would communicate and sympathise with a family member is different from how you would communicate with patients and their family members in practice. Take for example the senior staff nurse in the opening case study. In an attempt to make Jim feel better, the senior staff nurse stated 'at least you have three lovely children'. Even though this statement could be used within a personal loss context, in practice, using such a statement could have negative implications. Jim felt guilty about feeling sad and emotional after this statement was made by the nurse. Nurses are in a key position to facilitate grief work that will be healthy and result in the patient reaching acceptance.

In addition to this, excellent communication skills are needed (refer to Chapter 17). Some of these skills will be required more than others. *Empathy* will have to be used interchangeably with sympathy. The prevailing rule is that within the loss context, empathy is required when helping a patient to move through the grief work model. Sympathy will also be required: for example, touch can make the dying patient aware that you are with them. Empathy and how to use it as a communication skill is looked at in Chapter 3. Tables 11.3 and 11.4 give suggestions related to what a nurse can and cannot do when communicating with the grieving patient or family members.

Table 11.3
What the nurse can say or do when communicating within the context of loss.

Do show genuine caring and concern – remember if it is genuine it is fine (refer to Chapter 3).

Do be available to listen or help when needed at any time – saying this to the patient will put them at ease, as they will know that even though you are busy, you are still thinking of them. Also they know that you are not avoiding them and that they can call upon you if need be (refer to Chapter 4).

Do say you are sorry about the pain and/or what happened – as long as it is genuine, it is fine and is often a good starting point for a conversation. Do not rush from one patient to another and start with 'I'm sorry'. You need to take a couple of minutes out before you can begin a conversation like this so that your non-verbal communication shows that you would like to spend time with the patient and that you are relaxed.

Do allow them to express as much unhappiness and feeling as they want – this is fine as this will give them a release and reduce anxiety. This is part of grief work and helps the patient work towards the end goal of acceptance. Also remember that patients may not be able to talk to family members, as there may be conditions on their relationships, e.g. as a dying parent they may not be able to show their children how really upset they are. Your relationship has no conditions, so you are not judging the patient in any way and do not want any return from the patient (refer to Chapter 3). As a result, the patient will be able to express themselves freely.

Do encourage patients – if a dying patient is still capable of doing things for themselves, e.g. able to sit up by themselves, then allow them to do so. This will result in the patient feeling that they are not totally dependent on nurses and are still able to perform a function, which will enhance their self-esteem and mood (refer to Chapter 6).

Do allow them to talk about loss as much and often as they want – this should be encouraged as it is all part of grief work and is healthy. Changing the subject will stop the patient/family beginning and/or completing their grief work (refer to Chapter 4).

Do talk about special enduring qualities of what they have lost – it is fine to highlight positive parts of the person's personality to the family, as this would be what the family remember as well.

Do reassure the family that the staff did everything possible – reassurance is the most important thing that can be carried out by a nurse when talking to the family of the deceased. Families who have been reassured by staff can go home and begin the grieving process in a healthy way. However, those families who are not reassured are more likely to be angry and question whether the staff did everything possible to help the patient.

Breaking bad news

Within a loss context, the nurse may have to accompany the consultant when breaking bad news. In the opening case study, the senior staff nurse may have accompanied the consultant when it was confirmed to Jim that Rose had miscarried. 'Breaking bad news is an experience that can be recalled for a long time by both the recipient and the bearer of the bad news' (Finlay and Dallimore, 1991). There are models put forward which can be used by the nurse as a reference when out on placement. This will help the nurse to gain confidence when having to break bad news.

The possibility of patient confusion needs to be considered when delivering bad news. Greenfield *et al.* (1985) questioned 100 women who were diagnosed with breast cancer. It was found that there was substantial misunderstanding of prognostic and survival information, with 73 per cent not understanding the term 'median' survival when a practitioner used it. Using information that is simplistic and employing counselling skills that enable you to facilitate patient questions will enable the clarification of any possible misunderstandings that occur.

Table 11.4
What the nurse cannot say or do when communicating within the context of loss

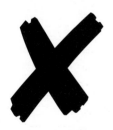

Don't let your own helplessness keep you from reaching out – there may be certain losses that nurses encounter within professional practice that mirror a personal loss of their own. In this case, the nurse will need to be self-aware and reflect on their feelings and interactions with the patient (refer to Chapter 6). Through reflection, the nurse will reveal if they have been avoiding the patient, talking about their personal experiences to make the patient feel better or feeling emotional. The next step will be to speak to a mentor who will be able to help.

Don't avoid them, as this is uncomfortable – as a nurse you are very busy dealing with several tasks and patients at once. If you have not made yourself known to a patient or wait until they ask you to come over, it could be clear to the patient you are avoiding them. Eventually you will have to interact with the patient and this will be uncomfortable for you. More to the point, a patient who is terminally ill will get straight to the point and tell you. Remember a patient in bed is picking up on your verbal and non-verbal behaviour more than you can, because you are so busy.

Don't say you know how they feel – even though you have dealt with that particular loss many times or have been through the experience within your personal life, never use this as an example of how you or others have dealt with their losses. Every situation is different and the patient should be treated as having their own unique experience.

Don't say you ought to be feeling better now – never use the bereavement models to suggest how the patient should be feeling, or the particular stage of the grieving process they should be in. Every situation is unique. You may need to think of referral systems when a patient is fixated in one stage for too long.

▶

Table 11.4 Continued

Don't tell them what they should be feeling - leave this to the consultant. Again, the models should be used as a rough guide only, rather than a clear guideline. Work with their feelings and build upon positive aspects, rather than working against or overriding feelings, which will only have a negative therapeutic effect.

Don't change the subject each time the patient mentions or relates to their loss - avoidance could result in the patient not disclosing their feelings.

Don't find positive things to say - when talking to the family, do not try to find positive things to say about the patient or deceased if there was nothing positive that you could recall. Remember that the family knew the patient/deceased a lot longer than you did. Finding positive things that were not there will result in the family questioning how truthful your profession is and lead to other negative doubts, such as did you do everything possible to help the deceased?

Don't make comments that suggest the loss is their fault - this will only facilitate guilt, which results in a bad grieving process rather than healthy grieving. All judgements need to be left behind.

Another issue that has been highlighted by studies is detecting distress. One qualitative study looked at five oncologists, out of whom only one was able to reliably assess patients' distress resulting from bad news (Greenfield *et al.*, 1985). This brings into focus the importance of acknowledging patient distress and anxiety (refer to Chapters 4 and 13). Nurses are prone to enduring stress both before and after breaking bad news. This can result in the nurse not paying full attention to the patient or the family. Acknowledging that nurses can experience stress during such interactions and being more self-aware will help the nurse to pay full attention to the patient and the family.

There are two main areas that practitioners fall short on when delivering bad news: willingness to talk about dying and the ability to give bad news. Both have central importance (Curtis *et al.*, 2001). Curtis found that problems arose as a result of discussing bad news at a time and place not appropriate for a serious conversation, being blunt, giving a sense of no hope and failing to maintain a balance between sensitivity and honesty. Referred to as **ABCDE'S delivery of bad news**, the guidelines below are designed to help health practitioners such as nurses break bad news in the most effective and sensitive way:

1. *Advanced preparation*
   - What does the patient know/understand already?
   - Arrange for the presence of a support person and appropriate family members
   - Arrange a time and place where you will be undisturbed
   - Prepare yourself emotionally
   - Decide on which words and phrases to use – write a script

2. *Build a therapeutic environment/relationship*
   - Arrange a private, quiet place without interruption
   - Provide adequate seating for all
   - Sit close enough to touch if appropriate
   - Reassure about pain, suffering and abandonment

3. *Communicate well*
   - Be direct – 'I am sorry, I have bad news for you'
   - Do not use euphemisms, jargon and acronyms

- Use the words 'cancer', 'AIDS', 'death' as appropriate
- Allow for silence
- Use touch appropriately

4. *Deal with patient and family reactions*
   - Assess patient or family reactions: physiological responses, cognitive coping strategies, and affective responses
   - Listen actively, explore, have empathy

5. *Encourage and validate emotions, evaluate the news*
   - Address further needs: what are the patient's immediate and near-term plans?
   - Make appropriate referrals for more support
   - Explore what the news means to the patient
   - Express your own feelings

Source: Western Journal of Medicine (1999) **171**(4), 260-263, adapted and reproduced with permission from the BMJ Publishing Group

Think about this

How could the senior staff nurse in the opening case study have used these stages when communicating with both Jim and Rose? Could any of these strategies have been further used when caring for Rose and talking to Jim?

Cultural diversity

Cultural influences impact on how individuals react to loss. Having a basic awareness of the different cultural practices that exist and their impact on how individuals mourn or carry out rituals for the dying patient or the deceased, will enable the nurse to be more understanding at a difficult time both for the dying patient and the grieving family. The sections below introduce religious beliefs and how they influence cultural practices within a loss situation (refer to Chapter 9).

Judaism

According to the traditional Jewish faith, followers would do anything to preserve life, as it is believed that life is a special gift from God. This underlying belief is extended to health professionals such as nurses and doctors, who are perceived to be 'God sent' and are thus expected to have healing powers. Because of this underlying belief and perception of health professionals, the nurse should never say that the end is imminent (Neuberger, 1994b).

'Accepting' death for the Jewish community is difficult. Up until the actual time of death, they expect the dying patient to continue to eat and drink. Within palliative care, facilitating 'good death' is alien to traditional Jewish thinking. Being aware of this and sensitive to such issues is a necessity.

When a person dies it is customary for psalms to be recited. The dying person is not allowed to be left alone during the final stages, as it is believed that by leaving the dying person alone, death will occur more quickly. In addition, keeping the dying patient comfortable is essential; removing pillows and cushions is believed to hasten death. This has implications for pressure area care and other nursing procedures that involve moving the patient. Explanation of medical procedures for the dying patient is accepted and welcomed.

When a person dies, the body should be left alone for ten minutes. A feather is placed on the dead person to ensure that there is no breathing and that death has occurred which is important before any organs can be removed. Burial should take place within 24 hours and is only delayed by Sabbath. Traditionally, one of the children of the deceased should close the eyes of the dead patient.

To signal the beginning of bereavement, large quantities of earth are thrown on the coffin, using spades. This is then followed by seven days of mourning (*shiva*), with prayers at home every evening. The next phase is 30 days of lesser mourning (*sholushn*), with prayers at the synagogue.

Care should be taken to make sure that Jews are permitted to follow their rituals by providing an environment which is understanding and allows the Jewish family to grieve. If certain rituals cannot be carried out, explain why – this provides justification for the bereaved family.

Islam

According to those following the Muslim faith, a religious requirement is to bury the deceased as quickly as possible. Burial within Muslim countries would be within 3–4 days of death (Gatrad and Sheikh, 2002). There will be many people, who may come from all over the world, to pay their last respects; not doing so would be offensive to the family who are beginning to grieve. According to Gatrad and Sheikh (2002), Muslim communities are closely knit. From their own personal experiences, 200–300 people visiting the home of the deceased would not be unusual.

The nurse should acknowledge that a Muslim patient who is dying can have large numbers of family and friends to visit because of the quick burial thereafter. It is clear that some families will have to bring children because they cannot find a babysitter. Accommodating this, and where possible, moving the patient into another room, would be ideal. If a room is not available and other patients are being disturbed, politely asking the main family to request that relatives be as quiet as possible would be fine. It would be offensive to the family to allow only small numbers of people to visit, since not everyone would be able to pay their last respects. The first few days of bereavement until the person is buried will be a time where eating and drinking should not be fully taken advantage of.

Gatrad and Sheikh (2002) have highlighted several other points of best practice for the nurse dealing with Muslim patients after death:

- After death, the face of a Muslim patient, young or old, should be turned towards Mecca. Mecca is located on the west side of Saudi Arabia, and hence lies in a direction roughly south-east to the United Kingdom.
- The feet of the deceased should not be allowed to face Mecca.

- Relatives should be notified immediately, as burial should take place within hours.
- The death certificate should be issued promptly.
- A post-mortem should only be requested if absolutely necessary.
- A person of the same sex as the deceased should usually be in close proximity to the body.
- A bereavement officer/Muslim chaplain who can communicate in the appropriate language should be available.

Greeks

To signify mourning and bereavement, it is common practice for Greeks to wail. However, this varies depending on the individual's education, religious faith and cultural standards. Historically, in Greece mourning and wailing have been considered as an obligation to the dead.

Hinduism

A priest will tie a sacred thread around the neck and wrist of a dying person as a blessing (Rees, 1997). These, as well as jewellery and other religious objects, should not be removed from the body.

After death, the family usually wash the body at home or within close proximity. If death occurs in the hospital and relatives are not available, the nursing staff may wash the body, but should obtain permission first. Staff should wear disposable gloves and the body should be wrapped in a plain sheet without any religious emblem (Nyatanga, 2005). The priest may sprinkle holy water from the River Ganges over the dying person's body, and also place a Tulsi leaf in the patient's mouth (Nyatanga, 2005).

Sikhism

Baptised Sikhs will incorporate the following, referred to as the five Ks, as part of their dress code: *kesh*, uncut hair; *kanga*, wooden comb worn in the hair; *kara*, steel silver wristband; *kirpan*, short sword worn across the body; *kacha*, shorts worn underneath clothing.

Under no circumstances should the five Ks be removed from the dying patient unless there is a valid reason, which will need to be explained to the family. Only baptised Sikhs will wear the five Ks, irrespective of sex and age. Other Sikhs are born into the Sikh religious following but are not baptised, so will not live their daily lives according to the religion, e.g. they will not wear the five Ks, but could adhere to certain aspects of their religion. For example, Sikhs also believe in reading from their holy book, *Guru Granth Sahib* to the dying patient, irrespective of being baptised or not. This is to keep peace and ensure that a peaceful death will occur with the spiritual guidance of the *Guru Granth Sahib*. A request may also be made to keep the *Guru Granth Sahib*, or a mini version of the religious scripture by the bedside of the dying patient. If this is the case, the holy book can be touched by a nurse only if they have washed their hands. Sikhs value a peaceful expression on the face of the deceased, as the face will be displayed to those paying their last respects. The body should be covered in a plain white sheet with no religious emblem. Sikhs are always cremated, except stillbirths, where a burial may be a possibility (Nyatanga, 2005).

Buddhism

Buddhist groups will differ with regard to care of the dying. The most important consideration across all Buddhist groups is the state of mind at time of death. A Buddhist will want to die with a 'clear mind', free from sedation, as this has an effect on the nature of rebirth. Clinical experience suggests that most Buddhists are reluctant to take analgesics, especially opioids (Nyatanga, 2005). If the patient cannot talk, then the nurse should ask the next of kin if analgesics can be administered. If so, everything must be documented, as well as any alternatives, e.g. acupuncture, that have been offered.

Buddhists believe in peace and quiet, which are imperative at death as this influences the nature of rebirth. Meditation and chanting may be seen as a way of calming and relaxing the mind and body.

Christianity

There are cultural differences in the way Christians in different countries view death (Neuberger, 1994b). For example, Roman Catholics and Protestants in Ireland actually celebrate death, whereas their counterparts in Britain tend not to (Neuberger, 1994b). Death in Britain is still viewed as a taboo subject, perhaps because of the uncertainty and fear that is associated with death (Nyatanga, 2005).

It is clear that there is diversity within religious groups as a result of generational, educational and regional differences. You will not be able to learn about every practice performed by every religious group when death approaches. However, being familiar with some of the practices common to the religious group and then asking questions to family members or community link workers, will enable each dying patient and family to have their own individual needs met. A nurse who reads the extract above and assumes that every person within that particular religious group carries out the same practices will not meet the unique needs that each dying patient requires. Chapter 9 further considers religious groups and practices.

What do dying patients require?

The first thing that a nurse needs to take into consideration is that a dying patient who can see their surroundings is aware of non-verbal communication around them. The dying patient will notice if a nurse avoids them, rushes around or talks quickly and leaves. Personal issues may resurface when dealing with a patient who is in a similar situation to one that the nurse may have experienced before. This may contribute to the nurse avoiding the patient. The nurse may need to explore this with a senior staff member or seek some counselling.

Dying patients are fully aware of the time pressures and constraints that face nurses, however. Taking a couple of minutes out before breaking bad news or sitting down with a dying patient will enable the nurse to gather their thoughts. This will facilitate congruence in your verbal and non-verbal communication when talking to the dying patient, and give the impression that you want to be there. The following points are also useful for consideration when working with a dying patient and his or her family.

Reassurance

During their final stage of illness, a dying patient does not want reassurance. During this stage, sympathy is more appropriate. A dying patient will need the nurse just to accept them for who they are (unconditional positive regard), rather than having constraints placed on their relationship, e.g. still having to be a husband/wife/parent.

Touch

Touch signifies personal caring to a dying patient. Calling a dying patient by the first name also signifies personal caring. A dying patient will appreciate touch to make them aware that the nurse is with them.

Questions

Dying patients do not have much time to 'pussyfoot' around issues and situations. As a result issues about their illness need to be addressed. These need to be explored with the patient in an open and honest way. It is clear that dying patients understand that there are unasked questions; they prefer nurses to anticipate, as it is these questions that are often the most important ones.

Eye contact

Maintaining eye contact is vital, as this will signify to the dying patient that you are honest in what you are saying and genuine with the care that you are providing. Most importantly, this will show that you are comfortable with the dying patient and still accept them as a living human being. Sitting down can further enhance comfort, especially if the nurse is at eye level with the patient. This demonstrates that you have time for the patient and that you are comfortable with them. In comparison, standing over the patient can seem rushed and inappropriate.

What do a patient's family require?

The family of the dying patient or family members who have experienced loss, will also need questions and anxieties addressed. Communicating and forming interpersonal relationships with families can cause anxiety for nurses (Garcia *et al.*, 2000). Research has shown that nurses feel inexperienced in communicating with families about end-of-life issues. Families also reported dissatisfaction and distress if a nurse was uncaring in their delivery of bad news or made careless remarks (Contro *et al.*, 2004) as well as providing no reassurance to family members. Below are communication issues that should be considered when communicating with family members. Breaking bad news and communicating with the grieving family in the best way possible is important as this will determine if the nurse has facilitated the beginning of a good or bad grieving process. Honesty and reassurance are two key areas that should be addressed with family and friends within the loss context.

Honesty

The most important thing that a nurse can do with a family is to be honest with them. Being dishonest or highlighting a personality attribute of the deceased to a family member that is untrue will only raise questions about the honesty of the nurse and how they cared for the dying patient. The family may like to hear the last words of the dying patient, and a nurse can highlight positive attributes of the deceased patient that are true.

Reassurance

Reassurance should be verbally stated to the family, as this is important when dealing with grieving family and friends. Stating to the family that 'we did everything possible that we could do while the patient was in our care' will begin the process of facilitating good grief for the grieving family. The senior staff nurse in the opening case study failed to do this when she was communicating with Jim. If reassurance is not offered, family and friends may question whether the nurse did everything possible. This pattern of thinking will result in the increased probability of bad grieving.

Nurses coping

Nurses need to ensure that they are coping well during the time they care for a patient, as well as after a death has occurred. **Self-awareness** (refer to Chapter 6) is one way for the nurse to monitor their own emotions and feelings. The following points can also help a nurse:

- Do not use your own experiences to help a patient; this will result in your having to take baggage home, reliving experiences or feeling emotional outside work. Also there will be a danger of making the patient's experience insignificant.
- Early on in the grieving process, i.e, early stages of a terminal diagnosis, empathy and counselling skills are vital in order for your patient to grieve healthily as well as allowing you to keep an emotional distance.
- Do not emotionally invest everything in one patient; this may be an easy mistake to make as a newly trained nurse. From experience you will realise that doing this results in the patient becoming dependent on you. Not distancing yourself and having a patient emotionally dependent on you will affect the care you are providing for others.

- If there is a personal experience or first death on placement, and you are finding it difficult to talk to a mentor or senior staff nurse, you will need to explore your feelings with another professional; this will enable you to carry on caring for other dying patients in a healthy manner. If you do not get help via resources at work, then see a counsellor, especially if there is a grieving experience you have never spoken about but which resurfaces.
- Through experience there will be coping strategies that you will eventually develop, which will enable you to deal with dying patients in the best way possible. For example, one strategy that has been popular among many health professionals is mental imagery. Follow the steps below (refer to Chapter 13).

1. After a shift, when getting ready to go home, do not rush out.
2. Take a couple of minutes to first clear your mind and begin to breathe deeply from the stomach.
3. Sense the heavy weight on your shoulders and the physical strain on your body and convert these to mental and physical baggage (actual bags as if you are going on holiday), and leave them in the hospital.
4. As you begin to get changed start mentally unloading a couple of the bags.
5. As you are walking out, carry on dropping the bags, mentally visualising this as you go along.
6. Your final bag should be dropped outside the hospital exit door.
7. Always remember you can pick them up again when you arrive at work the next day.

Last offices

When a patient has died, a nurse will be required to prepare the body to be taken away and for the close family to spend some time with the deceased. This is a necessary part of a nurse's job which is referred to as 'the last offices'. A procedure manual entitled *Last Offices* (found in every PCT) provides details of the current care practices to be performed by nurses after the patient has been pronounced dead. Below are a few questions that help to explain the procedure. It may not seem obvious at first but the last offices is also a chance of the nurse to have closure, which is especially important if they were in continual contact with the deceased when they were alive.

- *What is the aim of 'the last offices'?*
  - To prepare the deceased for the mortuary, respecting their cultural beliefs.
  - To comply with legislation, in particular where the death of a patient requires the involvement of a Procurator Fiscal.
  - To minimise any risk of cross-infection to relative, health care worker or persons who may need to handle the deceased.

- *Where are the last offices carried out?* At the bedside where the dignity and privacy of the deceased is maintained.
- *Why do I as a student nurse participate in the last offices?* As part of placement you may observe the last offices being carried out, or you may be involved in the procedure with another nurse. Nursing students may find

this difficult at first, especially if they have not encountered death within a professional setting. It is important for you to acknowledge that the reason why you may be asked to participate in this ritual is because this will be an opportunity to find closure, especially if you cared for the deceased over a large part of your placement.

Research has found using effective coping strategies in practice is beneficial for nurses when working with dying patients. Yan and McIlfatrick (2001) suggest that coping strategies and stressors associated with caring for the dying patient must be addressed within health education, so that better care of the dying patient is facilitated.

Conclusion

Irrespective of which branch the nurse specialises in, helping and caring for those experiencing loss will form a necessary part of their role. This chapter should help the nurse understand the stages of grief work that different types of patients and their families will experience. Having a knowledge base of grief work models as well as the appropriate communication that is required, will result in the nurse effectively facilitating the patient and family through the beginning stages of grief work that will be healthy and non-problematical. More importantly, the nurse will also understand how they themselves will need to be self-aware regarding their emotions and reactions in such situations, so that the quality of care they offer will not be affected.

Summary

- According to the World Health Organization, the need to offer family and significant others support during the patient's terminal illness and in bereavement is significant, and is the contemporary philosophy of palliative care (Sepúlveda, 1990).

- Death is objective and occurs when the vital functions cease – breathing and circulation (evidenced by the cessation of the beating of the heart).

- Bereavement is an overarching term that involves the consideration of multiple losses experienced after the death of someone significant (Doka, 2000).

- The experience of the grieving process is dependent on the beliefs of the particular individual grieving; grief is therefore subjective (Corr, 1982; Stroebe, 1998; Wendell Moller, 1996).

- Within childhood the perception and understanding of loss differs vastly. Nurses need to be aware of this and not stereotype all children as having the same understanding of loss.

- 'Proper' words need to be used with children: for example, 'is dead' rather than 'has passed away'.

- Grief work models are important theoretical tools, which need to be acknowledged as part of the communication with a dying patient.

- Parkes', (1972, 1986) four-stage grief work model encompasses the following: initial reaction (shock), pangs of grief, despair and acceptance/adjustment.

- Kubler-Ross's (1969) DABDA, stage-like model is the most popular model used by nurses. The acronym stands for the following stages in the grief work model: denial and isolation, anger, bargaining, depression and acceptance.

- A necessary job for nurses is to prepare the dead body for the mortuary, which is known as 'the last offices'. Every institution in the United Kingdom has a set procedure referred to as the *Last Offices*, which needs to be followed.

- Reassurance is the most important thing a nurse can give to the grieving family who did not see their family member die.

- Much emphasis in nursing practice is on the importance of 'empathy'. However, in relation to loss and grief, sympathy is also vital at certain stages of the illness mostly via non-verbal communication.

- When breaking bad news, it is important to be straightforward; give the most basic information, be sensitive and value hope.

- The ABCDE of breaking bad news is an important tool for nurses. The abbreviation stands for: **a**dvance preparation, **b**uild a therapeutic relationship, **c**ommunicate well, **d**eal with patient and family reactions, **e**ncourage and validate emotions.

- Cultural groups have different ways of dealing with death. The nurse needs to take into consideration that you should not stereotype every person from the same cultural group, but instead look at each person individually. The *Last Offices* need to be consulted when there are religious requirements.

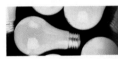

Check your understanding

1. List similarities and dissimilarities between the terms loss, grief, bereavement and death.

2. What does DABDA stand for in the grief work model provided by Kubler-Ross? Explain what happens to the patient at each of these stages.

3. List three 'do's' and three 'don'ts' when dealing with a terminally ill or dying patient.

4. Define the terms empathy and sympathy. When should a nurse use them during a patient's illness?

5. List each stage of the ABCDE of breaking bad news.

6. Explain the last offices in relation to the requirements of a Sikh patient and a Greek patient.

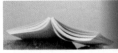

Further reading

Contro, N.A., Larson, J., Scofield, S., Sourkes, B. and Cohen, H. (2004) Hospital staff and family perspectives regarding quality of paediatric palliative care. *Paediatrics*, **114** (5), 1248-1252.

Faulkner, A. (1998) ABC of palliative care: Communication with patients, families and other professionals. *British Medical Journal*, 316, 130-132.

Greenstreet, W. (2004) Why nurses need to understand the principles of bereavement theory. *British Journal of Nursing*, **13** (10), 590-593.

Maguire, P. (2005) Breaking bad news: talking about death and dying. *Medicine*, **33** (2), 29-31.

Weblinks

Cruse	http://www.crusebereavementcare.org.uk/	National charity set up to offer free and confidential help to bereaved people. Booklets are also available from Cruse that look at coping with grief.
The Child Bereavement Website	http://www.childbereavement.org.uk/	Provides information on understanding bereavement, and sections dedicated to bereaved families, young people and one for professionals.
Macmillan Cancer Support	http://www.macmillan.org.uk/About_Us/ Specialist_healthcare/Specialist_Healthcare.aspx	Website that provides information about Macmillan health professionals' and nurses' work. Illustrated with case studies and a link to a learning zone.
The National Council for Palliative Care	http://www.ncpc.org.uk/	National Council for Palliative Care website which has an online library and publications as well as recent policies influencing palliative health care.

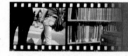

Media example

Death Becomes Her, a film starring Bruce Willis. A comedy that looks at mortality and how a preference is finally made to grow old gracefully, even though a chance to live forever has been given.

Part 3
Health psychology

Chapter 12

Risky behaviours: smoking, alcohol, diet and exercise

Learning outcomes

When you have read through this chapter you should understand:

- The health effects of smoking, alcohol, diet and lack of exercise.
- Why people smoke, drink alcohol to excess, eat poorly and do not exercise.
- What the nurse can do to improve the health behaviours of their clients/patients.
- What psychology can offer the nurse to help explain why people smoke and how to best improve health.

Case study

Colin Butt is a 60-year-old builder who is currently working in his own business but is looking forward to retiring shortly. He has worked continuously since he started his apprenticeship when he was 15 years old, and he is very proud of his achievements. He is still married to Nicki, the woman he met when he was 16 years old. He has two grown-up children and three grandchildren he adores. He loves to play football in the back garden with his grandchildren but is finding himself getting breathless frequently and thus not being able to enjoy playing with them as much as he would like. His grandson – Billie – worships his grandfather. However, Colin has noticed that Billie has started acting like him, plays 'smoking cigarettes', is refusing to eat anything other than chips and certainly isn't eating his portions of fruit and vegetables every day. Colin has had Type II diabetes for a number of years but it has recently become more poorly controlled. He drinks alcohol and eats typical 'builder's meals': a traditional fry-up in the morning, a sandwich or a pie at lunchtime with a couple of pints and a large evening meal with his family later. Colin likes a couple of pints at lunchtime as he thinks it is good to get together with his colleagues but his major drinking is at the weekend when he goes out with his friends and his wife down the local club. Here, Colin can drink nearly 15 pints during an evening while he enjoys the relaxing and social environment in the pub. Colin has smoked cigarettes since he was a teenager. He used to smoke heavily but has recently cut down to about 15 cigarettes a day. He suffers from early peripheral vascular disease and has a mild degree of lower limb neuropathy. He has been attending the clinic for routine care and monitoring. In order to prevent development of the more negative consequences of his condition it is essential for Colin to stop smoking and improve his diet.

Colin knows that he has to stop smoking but he has been doing it for over 40 years and feels he cannot stop. He is also aware that this behaviour and his diet are poor and are adversely affecting his health. However, he does not think he can change either of these. He sees you in the clinic and you realise that his health is severely compromised by his behaviour and he must change it or suffer serious consequences. How would you go about this?

Why is this relevant to nursing practice?

Over 30 years ago, Belloc and Breslow (1972) reported the impact on mortality of seven different behaviours (so-called **behavioural immunogens**, those behaviours that can protect health):

- sleeping seven or eight hours a night;
- not smoking;
- consuming no more than two alcoholic drinks per day;
- getting regular exercise;
- not eating between meals;
- eating breakfast;
- being no more than 10 per cent overweight.

This study followed up over 7000 healthy adults for over 15 years. The results of the study indicated that there were benefits of completing these types of behaviour and that these benefits were cumulative. The more an individual engaged in the behaviours, the more likely they were to live to an older age (Figure 12.1). At the 15-year follow-up, fewer than 4 per cent of those who were engaged in all seven types of activities had died, compared with 7–13 per cent of those who performed fewer that four of these activities. Also of note

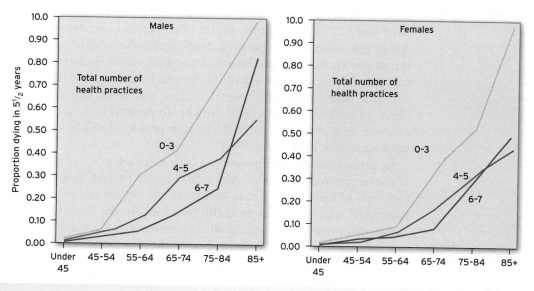

Figure 12.1 Effect of behaviour on health.

Source: Belloc and Breslow (1972)

was that the benefits of performing these activities were not simply additive but multiplicative: not smoking and moderate levels of drinking conferred more than twice the benefit of engaging in only one of these behaviours.

Think about this

How many of these behavioural immunogens do you and your colleagues engage in? What impact will this have on your life expectancy?

Colin is not a picture of health and he has several risky behaviours: smoking, alcohol consumption and a poor diet, and engages in few of those behaviours listed by Belloc and Breslow. What can the nurse do about these problems – how can they be improved and his health protected? This will be the focus of this chapter. Rather than try to deal with each of the 'Alameda seven' (i.e. the seven behaviours as recorded in Alameda as the behaviours listed above are known, the chapter will focus on the three major areas of behaviour: smoking, drinking and eating. Smoking is considered to be the single most preventable source of mortality and morbidity in the United Kingdom today. Doll and Hill (1952) were the first to link smoking and cancer and this has been followed by numerous reports highlighting the link between poor health and smoking. In the United Kingdom it is suggested that some 120 000 people die as a result of their smoking habit (440 000 in the United States). Deaths caused by smoking are higher than the number of deaths caused by road traffic accidents (3500), other accidents (8500), poisoning and overdose (900), alcoholic liver disease (5000), suicide (4000) and HIV infection (250). Almost half of all regular smokers will be killed by their habit. A man who smokes cuts short his life by 13.2 years and a woman by 14.5 years.

Most people know about this – it is over 50 years since the classic study (Doll and Hill, 1952) and the health effects of smoking are well known by almost the entire adult population. Smoking has been linked to heart disease, throat cancer, stomach and bowel cancer, lung cancer, leukaemia, peripheral vascular disease, premature and low weight babies, bronchitis, emphysema, sinusitis, peptic ulcers and dental hygiene problems, and can worsen the effects of asthma and infections. So why do people like Colin smoke? What can you, as a practising nurse, do to help people like Colin either not start smoking or quit the behaviour?

In terms of alcohol the picture is a little more complicated since low levels of consumption are not associated with ill-health (in fact, in some instances, a low level of consumption may be beneficial) but excessive consumption is associated with a number of health problems. In the short term, excessive consumption may be associated with an increase in the number of accidents (e.g. when driving, at work and at home), the amount of violence (either as a perpetrator or a victim), and an increase in the number of unwanted pregnancies, HIV or other sexually transmitted diseases. If there is regular heavy drinking then death may occur from liver cirrhosis and acute pancreatitis, neurological damage, increase in the risk from coronary heart disease and certain cancers, exacerbation of any psychological or social problems and a potential loss of employment and reduced career prospects. Over the past 30 years, annual alcohol consumption by the average British adult has increased considerably (Pirmohamed *et al.*, 2000); and, currently, 1 in 4 men and 1 in 10 women are believed to be drinking in a 'hazardous' or even 'harmful' manner, that is >21 and >14 units a week respectively (Paton, 1994; Pirmohamed *et al.*, 2000). Certainly, Colin's alcohol intake is not good, and he is damaging his health by drinking to excess, especially his binge drinking. But, again, why does he do this and what can be done about it?

Colin's diet is also poor and he is currently overweight. Despite having a physically demanding job, his poor diet and excess drinking mean that he is currently several stones over his ideal weight. Obesity can lead to a myriad of health problems: heart problems, Type II diabetes, hypertension, stroke and some cancers. A study (Rayner and Scarborough, 2005) estimated that food-related ill-health accounts for about 10 per cent of morbidity and mortality in the United Kingdom. The researchers concluded that the cost to the health service of dealing with poor dietary habits was significantly higher than the estimate for the annual cost of smoking, which is around £1.5 billion. They estimated that food accounts for costs of £6 billion a year.

It can be seen, therefore, that the key behaviours of smoking, drinking alcohol and diet can impact considerably on health. Indeed, Mokdad *et al.* (2004) suggest that these behaviours account for about half of all deaths in the United Kingdom. These behaviours will form the central themes of this chapter.

Smoking

Despite the health effects of smoking being known for over 40 years some 12 million individuals still smoke in the United Kingdom: 28 per cent of men and 24 per cent of women. These figures have shown a decrease in recent years – for example in the 1970s the comparable figures were 51 per cent of men and 41 per cent of women smoking. Although the number of people smoking has decreased considerably this is mainly due to the established smoker giving up: the number of young people starting to smoke remains, broadly, the same (ASH, 2007).

As we have seen in other chapters (see Chapter 8) the prevalence of smoking is not the same in different groups – about a third of those in the manual groups smoke compared with less than 20 per cent of the professional and managerial groups. Similarly, smoking is the highest in the 20–24 year age group (about 36 per cent) and the lowest in the over 65 years (about 15 per cent). This reflects the fact that many former smokers will have quit and also that about a quarter of smokers die before reaching retirement age (ASH, 2007).

Why do people start to smoke?

When exploring why people like Colin smoke, a distinction has to be made between why people become a smoker, and why they maintain the habit once they have started. One of the major reasons for starting to smoke is social pressure from peers or older siblings to experiment with tobacco. Early studies suggest that those who experiment with just four cigarettes become regular smokers (Salber *et al.*, 1963). Obviously this means that the prevention of smoking should begin early – in schools – and target young people before they have experimented with smoking.

The behavioural perspective (see Chapter 2) has been applied by researchers attempting to explain the initiation of cigarette smoking among adolescents (Akers, 1977). In short the behavioural perspective suggests that the smoking behaviour is learned according to the key learning processes of classical conditioning, operant conditioning, observational learning and cognitive processes (see Table 12.1 for explanation of how individual elements can be applied to smoking).

The social learning perspective suggests that the major influence on adolescents' cigarette smoking is a behaviour learned by modelling and social reinforcement. The most consistent and powerful predictor is whether their friends smoke (Dusenbery *et al.*, 1992; Urberg *et al.*, 1990). The other signifi-

	Concept	Rules	Example
Table 12.1 Key learning processes applied to smoking	Classical conditioning	Behaviours acquired through associative learning	Having a cup of coffee and a cigarette equals relaxation
	Operant conditioning	Behaviour is likely to increase if it is positively reinforced by the presence of a positive event, or negatively reinforced by the absence or removal of a negative event	Smoking is positively reinforced by social acceptance
	Observational learning	Behaviours are learned by observing others	Parents or friends smoking
	Cognitive factors	Other factors such as coping mechanisms or self-image may contribute	Belief that smoking looks 'cool'

cant influence is family; adolescents are more likely to smoke cigarettes if their parents smoke (Bricker *et al.*, 2005b; Huver *et al.*, 2006) or their siblings (e.g. Brandon and Brandon, 2005). For example, Bauman *et al.* (1990) found that lifetime parental smoking was strongly correlated with adolescent smoking. However, as adolescents develop, parents generally become less influential than peers (Valente *et al.*, 2005) and often the media (e.g. Gutschoven and Van den Bulck, 2005).

When we explore the reasons for people continuing to smoke we find that there are many different explanations. However, these can be broadly broken down into biological, social and psychological: conveniently the biopsychosocial model!

Biological explanations

The biological model suggests that smoking is a result of individuals becoming physically dependent on nicotine and the chemical substances found in cigarettes. When a person smokes a cigarette, nicotine enters the lungs and from there goes into the blood where it is carried to the brain. Here it leads to the release of various chemicals that activate the nervous system: heart rate and blood pressure increase and the body becomes aroused and alert. Once the person has stopped smoking the levels of nicotine reduce as do the 'positive' effects of smoking. From this, a model of nicotine regulation can be proposed: smokers continue to smoke in order to avoid withdrawal symptoms (Schachter, 1977). However, we do find people who stop smoking for a number of years (and hence all of the nicotine has disappeared from their bodies) but then start smoking again. We also find people – known as 'chippers' – who smoke a few cigarettes a day for a number of years but don't increase the amount they smoke (hence they don't show tolerance). Because of these issues it is recognised that the biological theories are not the complete picture – there must be other social and psychological factors involved.

Social factors

As we have seen, social factors are key to the initiation of smoking: parents, siblings and peers all have a part to play in the development of smoking. Although the relative importance of these various groups has been debated, all have agreed that they do have a role. Smoking is a social activity for many but this can differ from individual to individual and from cigarette to cigarette. Thus, for somebody at work smoking a cigarette may provide an opportunity to escape from the drudgery of the workplace and have a break. In contrast, in the pub the sharing of a cigarette was a means of strengthening social bonds with friends. For low-income mothers, smoking was used as a means of having a break after a certain number of activities or tasks or as a means of coping when something went wrong (Bottorff *et al.*, 2000; Graham, 1987; Irwin *et al.*, 2005).

Psychological factors

In terms of psychological factors a range of variables have been implicated. A number of models as explored in Chapter 15 have been used as predictors of smoking. Models of health behaviour, such as the health belief model, the protection motivation theory, the theory of reasoned action and the health action process approach, have been used to examine the cognitive factors that contribute to smoking initiation.

Research has also indicated that teenagers underestimate the health risk of smoking (Slovic, 2000) and they also believe that they will quit before they do themselves serious damage (Arnett, 2000). Hence, they smoke in spite of knowing the health damage effects of smoking – they know of them, they just don't think it will impact upon them. Furthermore, health is defined in terms of fitness and beauty (Murray and Jarrett, 1985; see also Chapter 1) and smoking is not thought to harm these features.

Think about this

On the basis of this, how would you design a health promotion campaign to prevent smoking behaviours in adolescents?

Stopping smoking

It has been suggested, of course, that getting people to stop smoking should be the cornerstone of every health care professional's advice to patients and clients. However, although it undoubtedly has benefits, quitting can be fraught with difficulties. People may get irritable, depressed, anxious and restless and will crave tobacco. In light of these factors a range of pharmacological treatments have been developed to help relieve them. For example, there are sprays, chewing gum, patches and inhalers, all of which can work to help people stop smoking (Cummings and Hyland, 2005). However, there must also be a psychological element to cessation or there will be no cessation. For example, at its most basic there must be a motivation to give up smoking.

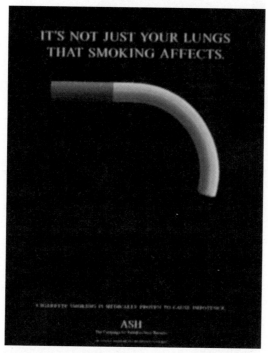

Image courtesy of The Advertising Archives

Transtheoretical model of change (TTM)/stages of change

However, the most influential psychological model that has been used in smoking cessation has been the 'transtheoretical model of change' or 'stages of change' (TTM; DiClemente and Prochaska, 1982). The model suggests that change proceeds through the stages summarised in Figure 12.2 and Table 12.2. Importantly, relapse can occur at any stage, and can mean that the individual goes back to the very first stage – it is not a linear model of simple progression from one stage to another where relapse means that you simply revert to the previous stage: you can revert to *any* previous stage.

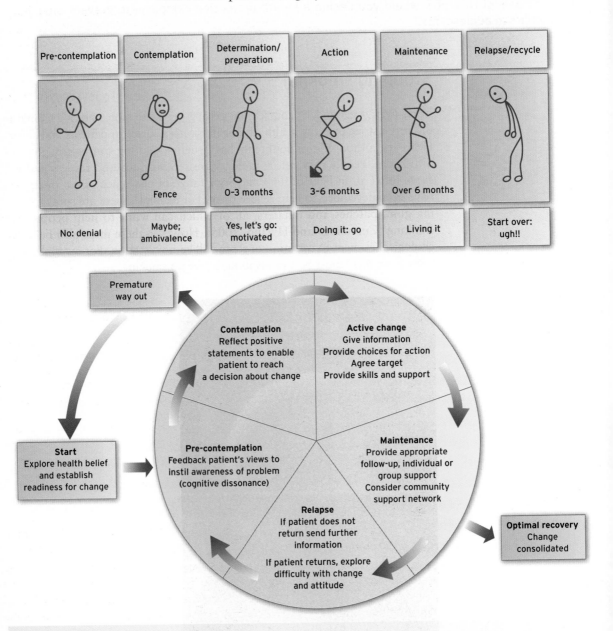

Figure 12.2 Model of stages of change model.

Table 12.2
Stages in the transtheoretical model of change

Stage	Definition	Description
Pre-contemplation	No intention of change	The person changing the behaviour has not been considered: the person may not realise that change is possible or that it might be of interest to them.
Contemplation	Intention to change	Something happens to prompt the person to start thinking about change – perhaps hearing that someone has made changes or something else has changed, resulting in the need for further change.
Preparation	Intention to change soon and plans of action have been made	Person prepares to undertake the desired change – requires gathering information, finding out how to achieve the change, ascertaining skills necessary, deciding when change should take place – may include talking with others to see how they feel about the likely change, considering impact change will have and who will be affected.
Action	Making changes	People make changes, acting on previous decisions, experience, information, new skills, and motivations for making the change.
Maintenance	Working to maintain behaviour and prevent relapse	Practice required for the new behaviour to be consistently maintained, incorporated into the repertoire of behaviours available to a person at any one time.

How can we use the stages of change model in the promotion of health and to assist individuals to quit smoking? The model is important because it allows us to identify where individuals are in their behaviour and then develop interventions – including computer and media based – founded on this information (e.g. Cobb *et al.*, 2005; Etter, 2005). For example, an individual smokes and has no intention of giving up – the thought had never crossed their minds. If this was the case then the intervention that we have to develop will be different from that for the individual who is preparing to give up. In the first example in the case where an individual has not considered quitting smoking then our obligation should be to try to get this into the person's thought processes. We want to try to get the individual to consider giving up smoking – we want to shift them from the pre-contemplation stage to the contemplation stage. So how can we do that? The most common method is a simple consciousness raising exercise: increasing information about the problem and how it can affect the individual concerned. So at this stage it would simply be a case of getting them to realise that smoking is health damaging and it can affect them individually, and then spelling out the individual health problems that they are either facing or could be facing because of their behaviour.

Velicer *et al*. (1993) have developed self-help interventions, based on the TTM, designed as substitutes for skilled smoking cessation counselling. These courses achieved quit rates equivalent to those achieved using smoking cessation counselling and nicotine replacement therapy (NRT). The intervention included a stage-based manual, which gives a detailed description of where individuals are in the stopping process, and provides exercises that engage the appropriate processes of change to move forward. This was supplemented by an expert system letter. Hence, the theoretical basis underlying the intervention appeared to be of benefit to quitting smoking.

Think about this

Talk to a smoker about their behaviour and discover what stage they could be considered to be at. How could they be prompted to move from one stage to another? Or maintained in their non-smoking stage?

Nurses and smoking

There are important consequences if nurses smoke: for themselves, their colleagues and their patients. In terms of their colleagues, nurses who smoke can create workplace problems that may need to be addressed (Sarna *et al*., 2005). Sarna and her fellow researchers reported that nurses who smoke:

● take more breaks;
● spend less time with patients;
● are less committed to their profession because they need to smoke during their shift.

The study found that some nurses structured their work day around such breaks because of their powerful addiction to nicotine. Smoking among nurses was described as an integral part of their work routine, affecting management of patient care and timing of breaks. The perception that smokers take more and longer breaks, and were less available for patient care, was an important theme in discussions with both smokers and former smokers, and clearly created conflict in the work environment. Such perceptions – imagined or accurate – create dissension, resulting in what one nurse in the study characterised as 'a war between the smokers and the non-smokers'. Also, those professionals that smoke often felt unwilling or uncomfortable devising, implementing or participating in stop smoking interventions with their patients, assuming that they were not good role models. In response to this, nurses often tried to cover their smoking behaviour from their patients and families by using such behaviours as regular teeth-brushing, washing their hands, sucking mints and applying scents to hide the smell of smoke. Furthermore, they feared the stigma of being a 'nurse that smoked' along with guilt when their 'secret' smoking is discovered by patients or family members.

How many nurses smoke?

Surely, being health care professionals, the level of smoking will be very low among nurses? A survey by McKenna *et al.* (2001) found that 25.8 per cent nurses were smokers, 19 per cent were ex-smokers and 55.2 per cent were non-smokers. This level of smoking was similar to that of the population from which the sample was drawn and in line with results from other studies (e.g. Nagle *et al.*, 1999). Of course, this is to be expected: nurses are part of the general population and their behaviour should simply reflect that from that population. Conversely, however, the nurse should be a role model in promoting health.

Since all health care professionals have a responsibility to promote health and to encourage all of their patients and clients to stop health-damaging behaviours and engage in health-protecting behaviours then we should try to ensure that all nurses quit smoking and are in a position to provide stop smoking advice. As those nurses who are smokers do not feel comfortable about providing stopping smoking advice, there is an obvious need to try to reduce the level of smoking by nurses. This is particularly important in certain specialities.

Nurses and smoking cessation

Smoking cessation after **myocardial infarction** is associated with a 50 per cent reduction in mortality after three to five years (Wilson *et al.*, 2000). Similarly, smoking cessation is associated with improvements in lung function in those with chronic obstructive pulmonary disease (COPD): improving lung function (Scanlon *et al.*, 2000) and reducing hospitalisation (Godtfredsen *et al.*, 2002). It is thus of key importance that nurses are involved in the smoking cessation process. Smoking cessation programmes with these patient groups have shown promise both in hospital and in the community. Systematic reviews (e.g. France *et al.*, 2001; Munafo *et al.*, 2001) show that smoking cessation interventions in hospital with long term follow-up (minimum of one month) after discharge are effective. But what is the role of the nurse in smoking cessation programmes? If the 280 000 nurses working within the UK health care system were each to help two people quit smoking per year, then the number of smokers in the United Kingdom would halve in the next decade.

Quist-Paulsen and Gallefoss (2003) reported a study that examined the success of a nurse-led smoking cessation programme on the smoking cessation rates of coronary heart disease (CHD) patients at 12 months follow-up. The results of the study were promising and indicated that 50 per cent in the intervention group stopped smoking compared with 37 per cent of the control group. The nurse-led intervention was minimal and consisted of the nurse providing a specially written booklet on how best to stop smoking and then following up by contacting the patients after discharge from hospital.

The booklet contained information on the benefits of quitting smoking – illustrating the differences in mortality between those who continued to smoke and those who did not. The booklet also contained information on how to prevent relapse, how to stop smoking for those that had not stopped or who had relapsed. Also contained was how to identify and cope with high-risk situations for relapse, with action plans.

Alcohol abuse

Not only does Colin smoke but he also drinks. Overall, he drinks over 40 pints of alcohol a week – well over the 21 units he is allowed! But surely Colin knows about alcohol abuse and the number of units that are in the alcohol that he is drinking? Most people do, indeed, know about the units associated with most drinks. For example, in a survey 83 per cent of people said that they had heard of measuring alcohol consumption in units (ONS, 2004). This knowledge had increased for both men and women between 1998 and 2004. In 1997, just under half (49 per cent) of men knew that a unit of beer is half a pint and this had increased to 59 per cent in 2004. Similarly, the proportion of women who drank wine who knew that a unit of wine is a glass had increased from 51 per cent in 1998 to two-thirds (66 per cent) in 2004.

Safe drinking limit

Sensible drinking limits (see box) have historically been quoted in units of alcohol, with limits set for weekly consumption: 21 units per week for men, 14 for women (although these figures are under review). So it is likely that Colin has heard of units and knows that he is over his weekly allowance. He knows that it is harmful to his health, so why exactly does Colin drink?

Think about this

How many units of alcohol did you consume in the past week? If you drink alcohol, why do you do so? What benefits does it bring to you – what sort of explanation does this lead to for people drinking and for problem drinking?

What are units?

The Department of Health advises that men should not drink more than three or four units of alcohol per day, and women should drink no more than two or three units. These daily benchmarks apply whether you drink every day, once or twice a week, or occasionally.

What is a unit of alcohol?

- A unit of alcohol is 10 ml of pure alcohol. Counting units of alcohol can help us to keep track of the amount we're drinking. The list below shows the number of units of alcohol in common drinks:
- A pint of ordinary strength lager (Carling Black Label, Fosters) – two units
- A pint of strong lager (Stella Artois, Kronenbourg 1664) – three units
- A pint of bitter (John Smith's, Boddingtons) – two units
- A pint of ordinary strength cider (Dry Blackthorn, Strongbow) – two units
- A 175 ml glass of red or white wine – around two units
- A pub measure of spirits – one unit
- An alcopop (e.g. Smirnoff Ice, Bacardi Breezer, WKD, Reef) – around one and a half units

Why do people drink alcohol?

A simple question to answer, you may think – and indeed it is, at one level! Drinking is a popular leisure activity primarily for its effects on the central nervous system (CNS): Colin drinks because it relaxes him after a hard day at work and allows him to socialise with his friends. The level of CNS relaxation varies with the amount of alcohol drunk. At the outset, the depressant effect on the CNS initially causes people to be less inhibited and have more fun. However, judgement and attention will also be affected. Consequently, government advise not to drink before driving or undertaking mechanical and professional tasks. Larger amounts of alcohol will cause other effects and could impede speech, other senses, increase sedation and interfere with temperature control mechanisms.

Problem drinking

There are three main theories of **problem drinking**: genetic theories, disease theories and learning theories.

Genetic theories

These suggest that certain people have a genetic predisposition to alcoholism and that some people are 'born alcoholics' (Ciccocioppo and Hyytia, 2006; Goldman *et al.*, 2005; Kreek *et al.*, 2005). Obviously even if people do have a genetic predisposition to alcoholism that does not mean they will necessarily develop into alcoholics: the general influence of the environment over genes has to be taken into account. This has obvious attractions (and detractions to others) to some as it suggests that people can evade social responsibility for creating or failing to solve social problems (Rose *et al.*, 1990).

Disease theories

These theories suggest that there is an 'at-risk' individual who has a predisposition to become an alcoholic once he or she starts to drink. A predisposition does not necessarily mean a genetic predisposition – it could be a psychological or physiological predisposition. A major implication of this approach is that treatment must emphasise the permanent nature of the alcoholic's problem and that the disease can be arrested only by lifelong abstinence. This approach is the approach adopted by Alcoholics Anonymous (AA). Despite a great deal of research there is no reliable empirical evidence for a psychological predisposition (Vaillant, 1983). Furthermore, there is now evidence that, rather than having to give up alcohol altogether, some alcoholics can be taught to return to controlled social drinking (e.g. Rosenberg, 1993).

Learning models

According to this approach, alcoholism is a way of drinking alcohol that has been learned either through conditioning (classical or operant) or through observational learning (Schuckit *et al.*, 2006). In particular, operant conditioning suggests that alcoholics receive rewards (e.g. positive feelings) which make the response (drinking alcohol) more likely. Of particular importance is the gradient of reinforcement: reinforcement that occurs rapidly after the response is much more effective in producing learning than delayed reinforcement. Hence, the reduction in anxiety and bonhomie following drinking alcohol is a stronger reinforcer than the negative reinforcement (hangover, health impairments, etc.) that occur much later. Social learning theories propose that patterns of drinking by parents are observed by children who may then imitate them in later life (Zucker and Wong, 2005). In adolescence, the drinking behaviour of favoured older peers may also be imitated, akin to the discussion presented previously concerning smoking.

Think about this

If people 'learn' to be problem drinkers, how can they 'un-learn' their problem drinking? What can the nurse do to help?

Other factors

Personality factors, such as impulsiveness and sensation-seeking, may predispose certain individuals to alcoholism (e.g. Elkins *et al.*, 2006; Kashdan *et al.*, 2005). Aggression and antisocial behaviour in boys may promote alcoholism later in life. Furthermore, in some individuals other psychological disorders (such as a depressive disorder or an anxiety disorder) may lead to alcohol problems. This is particularly the case in those with social anxiety disorder. Once the abnormal drinking behaviour has become established, alcohol may be used to cope with increasingly varied situations: boredom, depression, anxiety and frustration, as well as celebrations and interpersonal conflict.

Consequences of alcohol abuse

The consequences of alcohol abuse in the UK represent an enormous drain on the economy (Prime Minister's Strategy Unit, 2003), and are an ever-increasing burden on the health services (Pirmohamed *et al.*, 2000), costing an estimated £1.6 billion per year. Patients attending hospital with alcohol-related problems fall into two broad categories: (i) those with less severe drinking problems who may be amenable to brief interventions (Heather, 1996, 2002); and (ii) patients with features of alcohol dependence, requiring detoxification and ongoing treatment. Obviously appropriate management of both types of patient is required and nurses play a key role in both these aspects of alcohol abuse.

It is estimated that between 2 and 40 per cent of all those attending accident and emergency (A&E) departments are related to alcohol. As a consequence of these A&E admissions a significant proportion (5 per cent of all admissions) of those will end up being admitted to the hospital (with the majority for just one day) (Pirmohamed *et al.*, 2000).

Alcohol is, of course, one of the most significant factors in accidents. Accidents such as those that happen at home, at work or in unintentional drowning, fire injuries and road-traffic accidents (RTAs) are increased in those who drink. Furthermore, driving under the influence of alcohol impedes performance and both reduces the driving capability and increases risk-taking behaviour (Petridou *et al.*, 1998) with approximately 5 per cent of all RTA casualties involving illegal alcohol levels.

Psychological and psychiatric problems are also related to prolonged alcohol misuse. However, it is of course difficult to disentangle which came first: the alcohol problem or the psychological problem. For example, of all suicides in England and Wales, 15–25 per cent are associated with alcohol misuse, and almost 40 per cent of men and 8 per cent of women who attempt suicide are chronic problem drinkers (Morgan and Ritson, 1998).

Approximately 2–3 per cent of all A&E attendances are related to violent assaults and for at least half of these cases there is a causal relationship with alcohol misuse. This could be for either the perpetrator or the victim (Brismar and Bergman, 1998).

Incidence

Alcoholism is a growing problem in the United Kingdom, as is problem drinking (ONS, 2004). How we actually define these terms is rather difficult (see box). Just under a quarter of men (23 per cent) and a lower proportion of women (6 per cent) in England report drinking more than the recommended weekly limit. The rate of alcohol dependence associated with excessive drinking and complications is less (about 7 per cent of men and 2 per cent of women).

What is problem drinking?

Alcoholism is an imprecise term and the following terms are more accurate:

- *Alcohol abuse*: Consumption is likely to cause physical or mental damage in the future and may already be causing damage.
- *Alcohol-related problems*: Physical, psychological or social problems brought about through the use of alcohol.
- *Alcohol dependence*: Strong physiological and psychological desire to drink alcohol which takes precedence over all other activities. A withdrawal state or relief drinking may be experienced.

▶

As people often tend to hide their drinking, identification is often by screening. Many drinkers believe that an increased tolerance to the effects of alcohol means that they can 'handle drinking'. There are a number of questionnaires to detect abnormal drinking (e.g. Aertgeerts *et al.*, 2001) and one such is the CAGE (Ewing, 1984). A positive answer to two or more of the following screening questionnaire (CAGE) is highly suggestive of problem drinking:

- Have you ever thought you ought to **Cut** down on your drinking?
- Have people **Annoyed** you by criticising your drinking?
- Have you ever felt **Guilty** about your drinking?
- Have you ever had a drink first thing in the morning (**Eye-opener**) to steady your nerves or get rid of a hangover?

Consequences of alcoholism and problem drinking

Individuals who continue to drink heavily are likely to die about 15 years earlier than the general population, with the main causes being heart disease, cancer, accidents and suicide (Room *et al.*, 2005). General health may be impeded and chronic conditions may result such as alcoholic hepatitis, cirrhosis, gastritis, peptic ulcer, oesophagitis and oesophageal, acute and chronic pancreatic and carcinoma of the mouth, tongue, larynx, pharynx and oesophagus. Furthermore, cardiovascular problems are a relatively common complication of problem drinking – with hypertension, cardiovascular accidents and cardiomyopathy being potential consequences. Since the CNS is affected by alcohol (in a positive manner, as some would see it, as relaxation is a consequence) then it is apparent that there may be serious disorders resulting from excessive alcohol intake. Indeed, this is the case with disorders of the nervous system including **Wernicke-Korsakoff syndrome**, cognitive impairment and alcoholic dementia (Room *et al.*, 2005). Finally, it should be remembered that excessive alcohol can lead to reproductive problems including loss of libido and reduced sexual activity among heavy drinkers. About a third of children born to women drinking 15 units a day develop foetal alcohol syndrome (Eriksson, 2007).

Psychological symptoms include depressive symptoms (up to 70 per cent of heavy drinkers) and about 30 per cent have a secondary affective disorder. Up to 15 per cent of alcoholics end their lives by suicide and more than a third of individuals who commit non-fatal deliberate self-harm have alcohol in their blood.

Clinical treatment of alcohol problems

Initially following on from the disease concept it was believed that the only cure for alcoholism was complete abstinence. However, in time, it was felt that severely dependent alcoholics could be taught to drink moderately. Several factors seem to be important in predicting which problem drinkers may succeed at controlled drinking rather than complete abstinence. Individuals who have the best prospects are relatively young, married, employed and have a relatively brief history of alcohol abuse. Controlled drinking does not seem to be an effective method for chronic alcoholics who are severely dependent. Once severe dependence has occurred, the alcoholic no longer has the option of returning to social drinking – complete abstinence still appears to be the preferred goal for most patients that need clinical treatment.

A number of different therapies have been suggested as effective interventions for people with problem drinking. Although the nurse may be involved in all of these, there are some that may be more applicable to practise.

Aversion therapies

These therapies reduce a person's desire for alcohol by pairing an aversive experience with alcohol (whether this be sight, smell or taste). If successful, these alcohol stimuli should then elicit the unpleasant experiences and clients should acquire a conditioned aversion to alcohol (Thatcher and Clarke, 2006). Examples of aversion include electrical aversion therapy which pairs alcohol cues with electrical shocks until a conditioned response (anxiety) develops in response to these alcohol cues. Anxiety should then trigger alcohol avoidance. In chemical aversion therapy patients who have been given a vomiting-inducing drug are then administered alcohol a few minutes before vomiting occurs. Finally in verbal aversion therapy the noxious stimulus consists of aversive imagery which is repeatedly paired with alcohol-related imagery. The initial procedure involves pairing drinking stimuli with vivid imagination of nausea or other uncomfortable consequences of drinking. At a later phase, non-drinking alternatives, such as pouring out the drink or leaving the drinking setting, will be added. Results of empirical evaluations have been somewhat more encouraging for chemical and verbal aversion than for electrical aversion therapy.

Operant conditioning

This involves the individual's environment being managed so that positive consequences follow desired behaviour and either negative or neutral consequences follow undesirable behaviour (Thatcher and Clarke, 2006). Crucial to the planning of therapeutic strategies based on contingency management is the identification of reinforcers that maintain drinking behaviour as well as the rewards that may be manipulated to modify the drinking. Partners are essential to these therapies and hence they have to be included in designing therapy. Thus partners of alcohol abusers have to be taught basic principles of behaviour modification.

Self-management procedures

These accept that individuals can arrange their own reinforcement contingencies (see Chapter 1) in order to make certain behaviour more likely. For example, they can reward themselves for doing something which is unpleasant or punish themselves for transgressing predetermined rules. Hester and Miller (1995) suggests the following components of a self-management programme:

1. Setting limits on the number of drinks per day.
2. Self-monitoring of alcohol consumption.
3. Changing the rate of drinking.
4. Setting up a reward system for achievement of goals.
5. Learning which antecedents result in over-drinking and which in moderation.
6. Practising refusing drinks.
7. Learning coping skills as an alternative to drinking.
8. Learning to avoid relapse back into heavy drinking.

The Alcoholics Anonymous (AA) programme

This treatment involves the self-help groups run by ex-alcoholics using the 12 steps (see box) aiming to maintain lifelong abstinence. Kownacki and Shadish (1999) report on a study of the effectiveness of AA. Following a review of the literature, the authors state that 'the present results lend at least some weak support to AA-based inpatient treatment, although so few randomised studies of such treatment exist that the results are preliminary at best.' Moos and Moos (2006), however, report that regular attendance at AA meetings resulted in a better outcome at 16-year follow-up. Results more clearly support some components of AA, including the use of recovered alcoholics as counsellors, and training in specific AA procedures such as the 12-step programme and the 'honest inventory'. The authors also state that from their results 'it is probably a bad idea to coerce individuals to attend conventional AA meetings' as 'coercion apparently yields significantly worse results than treatment alternatives and non-significantly worse than doing nothing at all'.

Twelve steps of Alcoholics Anonymous

1. We admitted we were powerless over alcohol – that our lives had become unmanageable.
2. Came to believe that a Power greater than ourselves could restore us to sanity.
3. Made a decision to turn our will and our lives over to the care of God as we understood Him.
4. Made a searching and fearless moral inventory of ourselves.
5. Admitted to God, to ourselves, and to another human being the exact nature of our wrongs.
6. Were entirely ready to have God remove all these defects of character.
7. Humbly asked Him to remove our shortcomings.
8. Made a list of all persons we had harmed, and became willing to make amends to them all.
9. Made direct amends to such people wherever possible, except when to do so would injure them or others.
10. Continued to take personal inventory and when we were wrong promptly admitted it.
11. Sought through prayer and meditation to improve our conscious contact with God, as we understood Him, praying only for knowledge of His will for us and the power to carry that out.
12. Having had a spiritual awakening as the result of these Steps, we tried to carry this message to alcoholics, and to practise these principles in all our affairs.

Motivation enhancement therapy

This approach relies on the therapist trying to create a warm, empathic relationship with the client and uses a gentle and indirect approach in order to elicit, rather than impose, an increase in motivation to change behaviour, improve self-esteem and develop the feelings of self-efficacy for putting changes into practice. Further effective therapeutic techniques include social skills training, not least those needed to abstain or drink moderately in situations where others are drinking heavily, and training in psychological strategies designed to prevent a full-blown relapse from occurring after a single occasion of relapse. Heather (2001) suggested that motivation enhancement therapy proved effective, although it consisted of only 4 as against 12 sessions over a 12-week period (compared with the usual 12 in other forms of treatment). This finding applied equally across clients with problems of relatively high and low degrees of severity.

Nurse interventions: evidence for effectiveness

To date, the majority of screening and brief intervention research has focused on GP-led interventions (Freemantle *et al.*, 1993), although some studies included nurses in a supporting role (Fleming *et al.*, 1997; Kristenson *et al.*, 1983; Ockene *et al.*, 1999; Persson and Magnusson, 1989). Indirect evidence of the efficacy of nurse delivery of screening and brief intervention was reported in a World Health Organization (WHO) multi-centre study involving 10 countries (Babor and Grant, 1992).

In addition to brief treatments, there has been a great deal of recent interest in opportunistic interventions by GPs, nurses and other professionals to individuals who have come to seek their advice for other reasons. These were first introduced to encourage smoking cessation and their success led to similar studies of advice to cut down on drinking. The impressive evidence comes from a WHO study (Babor and Grant, 1992) in which 1655 heavy drinkers in 10 countries were given one of: (a) an assessment only of the individual's alcohol problems (control group); (b) assessment plus five minutes interview with a health worker who advised them to cut down; (c) assessment, advice and 15 minutes counselling on a habit-breaking plan; or (d) assessment, advice and extended counselling consisting of at least three further sessions. Men in all three intervention groups performed equally well, cutting down 25 per cent more than the control group. In the case of women, all four groups showed equally reduced consumption so that, for them, the mere fact having been assessed was sufficient to motivate them to cut down.

These findings have considerable significance for public policy. The cost effectiveness of brief interventions for those requesting help and very brief opportunistic interventions for those who do not request help appears to be relatively high and interventions offer health care systems excellent value for money. It should, however, be emphasised that they have been designed for individuals with relatively low levels of alcohol dependence and problems, rather than for those with severe dependence.

There is growing evidence to support the effectiveness of screening and brief alcohol intervention. Studies that have investigated the effectiveness of nurse-led screening and brief intervention approaches for problem drinkers in hospital settings have reported that a single session from a specialist nurse alcohol counsellor resulted in significantly better outcomes than routine medical care for male problem drinkers (Chick *et al.*, 1985); and that three increasing levels of nurse-administered screening and brief intervention resulted in an overall reduction in alcohol consumption for the sample as a whole (Watson, 1999).

School-based studies have reported significant reductions in quantity of alcohol use and intention to drink by US urban high-school youths who received screening and brief intervention from registered nurses compared with controls (Werch *et al.*, 1996, 1999, 2003). Some studies have reported that in primary health care settings, screening and extended counselling by primary health care nurses is more effective in reducing patients' alcohol consumption than screening and brief intervention (Israel *et al.*, 1996; Woollard *et al.*, 1995).

Research has shown that many nurses hold negative attitudes towards engaging in alcohol-intervention work (Gerace *et al.*, 1995), worry about losing rapport with patients if they discuss sensitive issues such as alcohol consumption (Lock *et al.*, 2002), are pessimistic about successful treatment outcomes (Rassool, 1993; Rowland and Maynard, 1989) and feel ill-equipped to care for people with an alcohol problem (Brown *et al.*, 1997; Owens *et al.*, 2000). However, with experience, seniority, education and training, this negative view can be modified (Brown *et al.*, 1997; Gerace *et al.*, 1995; Ockene *et al.*, 1997; Rassool, 1993).

One study, which sought to examine patients' views on the most appropriate professional to deliver preventive advice in primary health care, found that patients viewed the nurse- and GP-delivered interventions as equal (Eggleston *et al.*, 1995). Another study found that young women in particular preferred to speak with the nurse about alcohol issues rather than the GP (Lock, 2004). In this study it was felt by some participants that nurses would have more time to discuss alcohol issues than a GP, and that they were easy to talk to, approachable and understanding, yet persuasive.

Think about this

What opportunities are there going to be for you to promote sensible drinking? How and what should you do to encourage this?

Research in focus

Chang, G., McNamara, T.K., Orav, E.J., Koby, D., Lavigne, A., Ludman, B., Vincitorio, V.A. and Wilkins-Haug, L. (2005) Brief intervention for prenatal alcohol use: a randomised trial. *Obstetrics and Gynaecology*, **105**, 991–998.

Background

One of the leading preventable causes of birth defects is maternal prenatal alcohol use. Such alcohol use can lead to birth defects, mental retardation and neurodevelopmental disorders. Despite the widespread evidence that alcohol use can affect foetal development, pregnant women continue to drink (approximate 13 per cent of women drink, and 6 per cent drink frequently). Total abstinence during pregnancy is the aim for women and it is therefore important that there is early identification and modification of prenatal alcohol use. The T-ACE (Tolerance, Annoyed, Cut down, Eye-Opener) is a validated screening instrument for prenatal alcohol use that may help with early identification. The purpose of this randomised trial was to test the effectiveness of a brief intervention that was enhanced by including the partner of the woman. The hypothesis was that those randomised to the group with brief intervention with a partner would have a greater decline in antenatal alcohol consumption.

Method

Participants: Potential participants completed a series of questionnaires including the T-ACE attending a range of obstetric practices. The T-ACE asked four questions. T: How may drinks does it take to get you high (scored 2 if more than 2 drinks required)? A: Have people ever annoyed you by criticising your drinking? C: Have you ever felt you ought to cut down on your drinking? E: Have you ever had a drink first thing in the morning to steady your nerves or get rid of a hangover? Participants were recruited if they scored 2 or more on these questions. The second criterion for inclusion was being at risk for prenatal alcohol use, which was defined as any alcohol consumption during the three months before the study enrolment while pregnant. Finally participants had to be less than 28 weeks pregnant, intention to carry pregnancy to term and agree to the study terms.

Intervention: The intervention lasted less than 25 minutes and included four elements: (i) basic knowledge about a healthy pregnancy; (ii) the participant was asked to describe her prenatal drinking and goals during pregnancy along with the reasons why – participants were told that total abstinence was the ideal; (iii) the participant was asked to identify situations where they might be tempted to drink alcohol and identify some alternative behaviours; and (iv) a summary of the intervention was then provided to the participants.

Results

A total of 152 participants were recruited to the control group, along with 152 to the intervention group. At the outset, more than 80 per cent of women were drinking and nearly 30 per cent had two or more drinks at a time. Both the control group and the intervention group reduced their drinking behaviour at follow-up. However, the main finding was that the brief intervention for pre-natal intervention was more effective than the control group. Furthermore, the effects of the brief intervention were enhanced when a support partner participated.

Implications

A brief screening, assessment and intervention with partner can result in reduced antenatal alcohol use and minimise foetal risk.

Diet

What about Colin's diet? He eats fried food and very few fruit and vegetables – the only vegetables he has that are not fried are the 'two veg' he has with his Sunday lunch. How can we help him improve his diet and, just as importantly, help his grandson start to eat sensibly?

The consequences of a poor diet

Around 30 per cent of all cancer deaths can be attributed to smoking cigarettes, but around 35 per cent can be attributable, in some part, to a poor diet. A diet involving significant intake of high-fat foods, high levels of salt and low levels of fibre appears to be particularly implicated (Key *et al.*, 2007). In additional to cancer, excessive fat intake has been implicated in disease and death from several serious illnesses, including coronary heart disease. CHD arises because the fat molecules from food are excessive in some cases, the circulating levels become high and plaques (fatty layers) are laid down on the artery wall causing them to thicken (**atherosclerosis**) and restrict blood flow to the heart. Reduced fat intake is therefore a target of health interventions, not solely because of its effect on body weight but because of its link with CHD. Studies have indicated that a 10 per cent reduction in blood cholesterol is associated with a 54 per cent reduction in the incidence of CHD at 40 years of age (Navas-Nacher *et al.*, 2001).

Salt intake is also a target of preventative health measures, with high salt being implicated with high blood pressure (hypertension). A systematic review of the evidence suggested that reducing the salt reduction resulted in reduced **systolic** and **diastolic blood pressure** (Hooper *et al.*, 2002). Current guidelines suggest that 6 g per day for an adult and 5 g per day for a child should be treated as maximums. Colin's intake is considerably more than this and he obtains his salt not just from that added to his fried foods and vegetables but also in the pre-packed meals and pasties he frequently eats.

Obviously eating the right foods can prevent illness and promote health. For example, eating fruit and vegetables may offer protection against some forms of cancer (e.g. bowel). Block *et al.* (1992) suggested on the basis of 132/170 studies that there is evidence that fruit and vegetables offer a significant protection against cancer and other studies have indicated that it is also of benefit for stroke and heart disease (Ness and Powles, 1997; Ness *et al.*, 2002). Current recommendations are to eat five or more portions of fruit and vegetables a day; however, less that 20 per cent of boys and 15 per cent of girls aged 13–15 were found to be doing so (Bajekal *et al.*, 2003) and there is substantial evidence that adults are not following these recommendations either (Baker and Wardle, 2003; Wardle and Steptoe, 2003). So why don't people eat this amount of fruit and vegetables given that most people, it has been found, are aware of the guidelines? The simplest and most obvious answer is that it is down to the taste! Most adolescents report that they choose the food they do because it either 'tastes good' (67 per cent) or 'it fills me up' (43 per cent) rather than because it is healthy (22 per cent). Unfortunately, tasting good and being filling was associated with fatty foods such as biscuits, crisps and other snacks.

The choice of food stuffs is usually a result of parental behaviour – parents play a major role in setting down patterns of eating, food choices and leisure activities. Food preferences are generally learned through socialisation within the family, and in the case of Colin and Billie there could be trouble ahead – it appears as if Billie's eating habits have been influenced by inter-generational transmission of preferences and tastes.

The Food Dude Programme

The problem

Various interventions have tried to increase the intake of fruit and vegetables and one such programme is the Food Dude Programme. This has been developed by a group of psychologists at Bangor University in order to increase healthy eating habits in children using psychological techniques (including those described in this text – see Chapters 1 and 15). Previous approaches involved educating children about what they should and should not eat, i.e. basic information and education about what constitutes a 'healthy diet' in the hope that children would change their eating habits accordingly.

Food Dude Programme

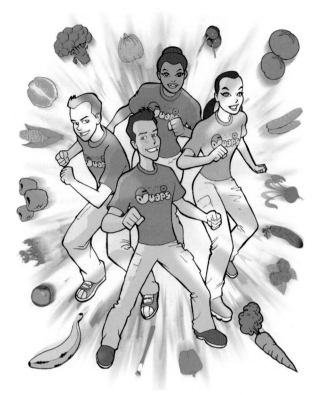

University of Bangor

What should and shouldn't be eaten

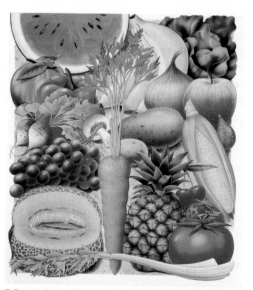

© Dan McGowan/Illustration Works/Corbis

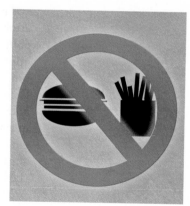

Christian Darkin/Science Photo library

Despite considerable efforts over a number of years, there is limited evidence to support this approach and research has indicated that children's eating habits have remained unaltered over the years of this intervention (Bajekal *et al.*, 2003; Department of Health, 1998; Gidding *et al.*, 2005). Clearly, even if children do know what they should be eating (and there are doubts whether this is the case), this does not necessarily translate into their actual dietary behaviour. The Food Dudes Programme was based on the sensible assumption that what was required was not simply information but providing help in changing to healthy behaviour on the basis of firm psychological principles.

The theoretical position is based primarily on research into learning and cognitive processes (see Chapter 1, or the previous discussion on smoking). When exploring food choice, it is suggested that once children are verbally adept (see Chapter 7) then they will begin to view food in a different light. Food is no longer seen as simply an object with sensual features (i.e. taste, appearance and smell) but will also be associated with other verbalisations that both the individual child along with significant others make. For example, a child may start to refuse vegetables if they hear a significant friend express a dislike of vegetables.

Admired friend: 'I hate vegetables', 'Vegetables are disgusting'

↓

Child adopts this view: vegetables are horrible

↓

Child views themselves as someone who does not like vegetables

↓

Parents view child as someone that does not like vegetables

↓

Parents' behaviour change

↓

Child's view reinforced

The Food Dude Healthy Eating Programme employs positive verbal associations with vegetables to help overcome potential problems associated with a child tasting fruit and vegetables, along with learning to like them. The approach adopted is to provide opportunities for children to see and hear others tasting fruit and see the positive reactions associated with this tasting. If children do see and hear others reacting positively and continuing to taste and experience the flavour and texture and that there are no negative consequences of eating these foodstuffs, then they will begin to see themselves as a child who 'eats' and 'likes' fruit and vegetables. A number of studies have shown that repeated tasting of a food enhances preference for that food (Lowe *et al.*, 2004; Tapper *et al.*, 2003).

The Food Dude Healthy Eating Programme brings together two variables already known to be powerful influences on human behaviour: **peer modelling** and **rewards**.

Peer modelling

Considerable research has indicated that peer modelling or observational learning (see Chapter 1) can have a significant impact on behaviour and this is particularly the case when:

- the models are perceived by the observer to be similar to him/her;
- the models are of similar age or slightly older than the observer;
- the model's behaviour is rewarded;
- the observer's imitation of the model is rewarded.

Sportacus promoting healthy eating and exercise in children

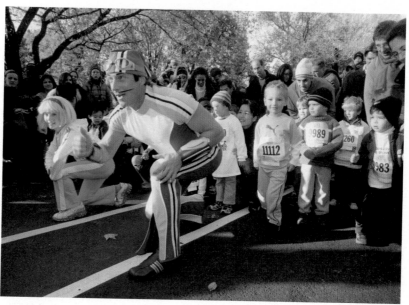

Getty Images

This is one of the methods that has been employed in the Food Dude Programme (Horne *et al.*, 2004), but has also been used in less academic settings (see picture).

Rewards

There is also a considerable literature base that supports the effectiveness of contingent rewards in altering behaviour (see Chapter 1). Rewards can be extremely effective in altering children's behaviour. The evidence indicates that if they are to be effective, rewards:

- are best presented in the context of 'real-life' settings;
- should be potent (i.e. they should be something that the children really want);
- should be delivered contingent upon performance of the desired behaviour (i.e. upon actual consumption of the targeted food but not otherwise);
- should be clearly specified as to what they are and how they can be earned (i.e. 'if you eat X, then you will get Y') in instructions given to children; and, most importantly,
- should be delivered in an appropriate context (i.e. that conveys not that they are compensations for low-value, disliked options, but rather that they are for behaviour that is high status and enjoyable.

Way forward

The Food Dude Healthy Eating Programme is specifically designed for 4–11-year-olds to encourage consumption of fruit and vegetables. The programme comprises two key elements:

- Video adventures featuring hero figures, called the 'Food Dudes', who like fruit and vegetables and provide effective social models for the children to imitate.

- Small rewards (e.g. stickers, notebooks, pencils) to provide an incentive for children to begin to taste the foods.

Two additional elements provide support for the programme:

- Food Dude letters – provide contact and information from the Food Dudes.
- Food Dude Homepack – includes a diary to record fruit and vegetable consumption at home, plus tips and advice on healthy eating.

The aim of the programme is to encourage children to *repeatedly* try fruits and vegetables so that they begin to enjoy the taste of the foods and eat them for this rather than for external rewards. In addition, they also come to think of themselves as healthy eaters who eat fruit and vegetables, ensuring that dietary changes last in the long term.

Effectiveness of the Food Dude Programme

Long-term effectiveness of the programme has been reported, with particular gains among children who ate less fruit and vegetables at the study outset (Horne *et al.*, 2004). The Food Dude Healthy Eating Programme research has indicated that both the quantity and range of healthy foodstuffs – fruit and vegetables – are increased following the intervention. Furthermore, these changes appear to be long lasting and generalise from the school (where the intervention typically happens) to the home life. Finally, it is also important to note that the greatest gains were made by those individuals who ate the least fruit and vegetables at the outset. Evidence presented by the Food Dudes research group (Tapper *et al.*, 2003) seems to support this contention (Table 12.3).

	School location	Increase in fruit consumption at lunchtime (%)	Increase in vegetable consumption at lunchtime (%)
Table 12.3 Results from the Food Dude Programme	Salford (Manchester)	154	300
	Brixton (London)	119	50
	Harwell (Oxford)	78	190
	Bangor (Wales)	43	54

Think about this

On the basis of the Food Dude Programme, how do you think an individual programme could be developed for Billie?

Conclusion

There are many behaviours that have an implication for health and illness. In particular, this chapter has focused on smoking, drinking alcohol and poor diet. These behaviours account for over 50 per cent of all deaths in the Western world and it is essential that the nurse understands why some people engage in these behaviours and how best to try to reduce them. Another key issue that can be gleaned from this chapter is that each of the behaviours can be conceptualised and treated in a similar manner. Hence, for example, it is possible to treat smoking in a similar way to that presented for alcoholism. Furthermore, the transtheoretical model can be applied to each of these behaviours and the potential of the stage-based interventions should be highlighted (e.g. John *et al.*, 2003, report on the use of TTM to encourage fruit and vegetable consumption).

Summary

- The benefits of a healthy lifestyle can add decades to an individual's life.

- Smoking is the single most preventable cause of illness in the United Kingdom.

- People start to smoke for a variety of reasons but for most it is a learned behaviour from family and friends.

- The transtheoretical model (TTM) of change suggests that quitters process through a series of six stages when they are quitting and that relapse can occur at any of these stages.

- The TTM can be used to design interventions based upon whatever stage individuals are at.

- Nurses can encourage people to stop smoking whenever they are in consultation with them.

- Most people know of the safe drinking limit, but many still drink above it.

- People drink alcohol for many reasons, although its impact on CNS is the major explanation!

- Alcohol abuse costs the country some £1.6 billion per annum.

- Treatments for alcohol abuse include aversion therapies, operant conditioning and self-management procedures. However, brief interventions by nurses or other health care practitioners can be as effective as more extensive interventions.

- A poor diet can lead to illness, including cancer and heart disease.

- Most people understand that eating five portions of fruit and vegetables will protect their health; however, many do not do this. This primarily because of socialisation: parents, peers and families are not encouraging healthy eating.

- Healthy eating can, however, be promoted by the use of various psychological techniques. In particular, the positive rewarding of tasting and eating healthy foods.

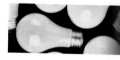

Check your understanding

1. What are the healthy amounts for (a) smoking; (b) alcohol; (c) fruit and vegetables?

2. What responsibilities does the nurse have in promoting healthy behaviours?

3. What can the nurse do in clinical practice to encourage clients and patients to quit smoking?

4. Devise a programme to encourage (a) children and (b) adults to eat a healthy diet.

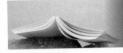

Further reading

Ladder, D. and Goddard, E. (2004) *Drinking: Adults' Behaviour and Knowledge in 2004,* Series OS no.26. ISBN 1 85774 589 2. London: HMSO.

Orford, J. (2001) *Excessive Appetites: A Psychological View of Addictions,* 2nd edn. Chichester: John Wiley.

Weblinks

Action on Smoking and Health (ASH)	http://www.ash.org.uk/	ASH is a campaigning public health charity working for a comprehensive societal response to tobacco aimed at achieving a sharp reduction and eventual elimination of the health problems caused by tobacco.
Society for Research into Nicotine and Tobacco	http://www.srnt.org/	The mission of the society is to stimulate the generation of new knowledge concerning nicotine in all its manifestations – from molecular to societal.
WHO resource on tobacco	http://www.who.int/tobacco/en/	Mortality and morbidity statistics for individual countries.
Smokefree	http://www.gosmokefree.co.uk/	The UK's online community for quitting smokers by quitting smokers.
Department of Health Tobacco page	http://www.dh.gov.uk/en/Publichealth/ Healthimprovement/Tobacco/index.htm	Provides a range of links on tobacco use and policy developments.
eBMJ collected resources on smoking	http://bmj.com/cgi/collection/smoking	Over 300 papers on smoking.
Institute of Alcohol Studies	http://www.ias.org.uk/	The Institute of Alcohol Studies (IAS) is an educational body with the basic aims of (1) increasing knowledge of alcohol and the social and health consequences of its misuse and (2) encouraging and supporting the adoption of effective measures for the management and prevention of alcohol-related problems. The Institute is financially independent of both government and the drinks industry and is supported by the Alliance House Foundation, a registered educational charity.
Department of Health alcohol misuse pages	http://www.dh.gov.uk/PolicyAndGuidance/ HealthAndSocialCareTopics/AlcoholMisuse/ AlcoholMisuseGeneralInformation/fs/en	The pages are intended primarily as a resource for a wide range of professionals and managers. Some of the information will also be of interest to parents, young people and students.

eBMJ collected resource on alcohol	http://bmj.com/cgi/collection/alcohol	Over 50 articles on alcohol use and abuse.
British Nutrition Foundation	http://www.nutrition.org.uk/home.asp?siteId=43&sectionId=s	The home page for the British Nutrition Foundation, which 'promotes the nutritional wellbeing of society through the impartial interpretation and effective dissemination of scientifically based nutritional knowledge and advice'.
Food Standards Agency	http://www.food.gov.uk/healthiereating/	The Food Standards Agency is an independent food safety watchdog set up by an Act of Parliament in 2000 to protect the public's health and consumer interests in relation to food.
Harvard School of Public Health: The Nutrition Source	http://www.hsph.harvard.edu/nutritionsource/	The Nutrition Source is designed to get you started on the path towards the healthiest diet possible.
Bandolier's Website on Healthy Living	http://www.jr2.ox.ac.uk/bandolier/booth/booths/hliving.html	These Healthy Living pages are developed from medical literature. Whenever possible, papers of the highest quality are reviewed, ideally systematic reviews or meta-analyses of epidemiological data as these are the most likely to give us trustworthy answers.
Treatment of Obesity	http://www.york.ac.uk/inst/crd/obesity.htm	A systematic review of the interventions for the prevention and treatment of obesity, and the maintenance of weight loss from the University of York's NHS Centre for Reviews and Dissemination.
wBMJ collected resource on obesity	http://bmj.com/cgi/collection/obesity	24 papers from the BMJ addressing obesity.
Healthy Eating	http://www.healthyeating.net/he_1.htm	A comprehensive site on healthy eating with links to other resources concerning diet, health and exercise.
The Nutrition Society	http://www.nutritionsociety.org/	Provides extensive nutrition information and diet, along with links to various other related sites.
British Dietetic Association	http://www.bda.uk.com/	Provides extensive nutrition information and diet, along with links to various other related sites.
Food Dudes	http://www.fooddudes.co.uk	This site is designed to provide information about the Healthy Eating Programme, and other Food Dude research conducted by the Bangor Food Research Unit at the School of Psychology, University of Wales Bangor.
Department of Health	www.doh.gov.uk/en/Publicationsandstatistics/Statistics/index.htm	DoH survey statistics

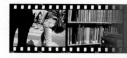

Media examples

Withnail and I All told, Withnail is shown drinking roughly $9\frac{1}{2}$ glasses of red wine, half a pint of cider, 1 shot of lighter fluid (vinegar or overproof rum are recommended substitutes), $2\frac{1}{2}$ shots of gin, 6 glasses of sherry, 13 glasses of whisky and half a pint of ale.

Arthur Perhaps the best known film about alcoholism.

Drunks The most comprehensive film made depicting the structure and dynamics of an AA meeting. With Richard Lewis and Faye Dunaway, the story describes a meeting from beginning to end during which time a program veteran bolts from the room, drinks during the evening, and then returns to AA.

Leaving Las Vegas with Nicolas Cage and Elizabeth Shue (Oscar winner). Important emphasis on the links of alcohol with depression and suicide and the intentional use of alcohol for ending one's life. No recovery.

Chapter 13

Stress and stress management

Learning outcomes

When you have read through this chapter you should understand:

- The definitions of stress.
- The various models of stress.
- The link between stress and ill-health.
- How people cope with stress.
- Social support and stress.
- Stress management techniques for both patients and nurses.
- Burnout and the practising nurse.

Case study

Joe Gallagher is a 40-year-old man who has worked in the Civil Service for all of his adult life. He was committed to his work and, despite having little opportunity to progress, had remained loyal and determined to his chosen career. His father had died many years ago, and other than his children his elderly mother was his only surviving relative for many years although she passed away three months ago. He married Mary when he was 18 years of age and they had twins – Delilah and Joseph Junior (JJ), now 8 years old. Joe's marriage deteriorated and six months ago the pair split up, with Joe moving into rented accommodation. Mary had subsequently filed for divorce and refused access to his two children. Currently, Joe is living alone and sees few people outside his work environment.

At work Joe, although dedicated, has recently been overlooked for promotion and has been told that he was 'next in line for redundancy' by his manager with whom he does not see eye to eye. Because of this he has been sidelined by his colleagues and has very little interaction with them at all.

Joe recently consulted his GP after a series of recurrent chest infections which cleared up with appropriate medication. Other than this Joe considers himself relatively healthy and rarely went to the doctors. He does tend to overeat, however, and took up smoking and drinking when his marriage broke up. He takes very little exercise and has few interests, although he does enjoy reading historical novels. Joe has recently been admitted to the accident and emergency unit after complaining of chest pains which appeared cardiac in nature. He was subsequently admitted to hospital where it was found that he had suffered a mild heart attack.

Why is this relevant to nursing practice?

Reviewing the case history, why do you think that Joe suffered from a heart attack? Consider all the factors in the case study that you think are relevant to the case – what about his relationships at work? What about the smoking and drinking? What about his chest infections? Obviously he has had some stresses in his life: his marriage has broken up and he has lost contact with his children. Furthermore, he has had trouble at work and is facing redundancy and possible money worries. On top of all this Joe appears to be losing his friends and family. He has lost his parents, and his wife and children no longer have any contact with him. In addition, his work colleagues have deserted him and it appears as if Joe has a particularly joyless existence. It is not surprising, therefore, that Joe has had a heart attack. This is the common view of **stress** and health: something stressful happens to an individual and, as a result, their health suffers.

Stress probably affects all of us, like Joe at some time in our lives, and for some it may be a relatively permanent state. There is a popular belief that stress can lead to illness – cancer, heart attacks and so on. A number of studies worldwide have found that heart attack patients report that their health problems were either initiated or compounded by stress. A considerable amount of time, money and effort have gone into investigating stress and how it can affect all areas of our lives, including our health status. Unfortunately, not all of the investigations have provided consistent results and there is some debate about the exact impact of stress. This is probably a result of some of the controversies that we will discuss in this chapter.

Stress is an everyday phenomenon and can impact on your everyday practice, either because the patients that you see will relate their health to their stress levels or may find the health care environment stressful, or because your work environment may be extremely stressful. Learning about stress and **stress management** strategies may be of benefit to both you and your patients. As we have seen with the case study, Joe has been under stress (as most people would define it) and has suffered the consequences (in terms of his heart attack). It is important that we explore the validity of the claim that stress can impact on health, and subsequently what the practising nurse can do about it. Furthermore, we also need to explore the stress in the workplace – how we can recognise it in ourselves and how we can best deal with it.

Definition of stress

Although many of us consider stress to be an element of everyday life, when you stop to consider it: what exactly is stress? Researchers have found it a difficult concept to define, and indeed, some even question whether stress exists. For example, Engel (1980) suggested that: 'Stress is neither a noun, nor a verb, nor an adjective. It is an escape from reality'. Since it is so poorly defined and misused, some have suggested that the term is no longer of any use and should be abandoned (e.g. Kasl, 1983; Kemeny, 2003; McEwen and Lasley, 2002). Indeed, Massé (2000) identified that members of the public associated 'stress' with approximately 2000 different terms and concepts.

But why is this the case? Surely, if you and your colleagues try to list all those activities or events that you would consider stressful then you would probably come up with a common list, for example, exams, going to the dentist, parachuting or giving a verbal presentation. However, even though there will be a great deal of commonality, there will probably be some activities that you could not agree on. For example most would consider giving a presentation to an audience stressful, however, some of you may consider it a 'thrill' or exciting rather than being a negative experience. (Does stress always have to be a negative experience?) What about going to the dentist? Again, most of us would consider that it is a stressful experience, yet others do not get stressed and some (a few admittedly!) actually enjoy the visit.

This is the first model of stress that we could investigate. This model suggests that stress is there on the 'outside'. It is something that happens to us and we can do little about it. However, as we will see it is rather difficult to say that something is definitely stressful just by listing the events.

What about those feelings that you get when you are stressed? Perhaps this could provide a better way of describing what stress is. Most of us could describe how they feel when they are under stress (for example, having an increased heart rate or butterflies in the stomach), but is this the case for all people? How would we know when people are under stress other than by asking them, or recording their physiological responses? Does this take us any further forward?

These are two of the three major definitions of stress and the third includes these elements as well. This model suggests that stress is an interaction between the event and the person (i.e. **interactional model**). That is how the person perceives the event is stress. So it takes into account the **stressor**, what a person thinks of the event, and their bodily reactions.

What is stressful for some is enjoyable for others.

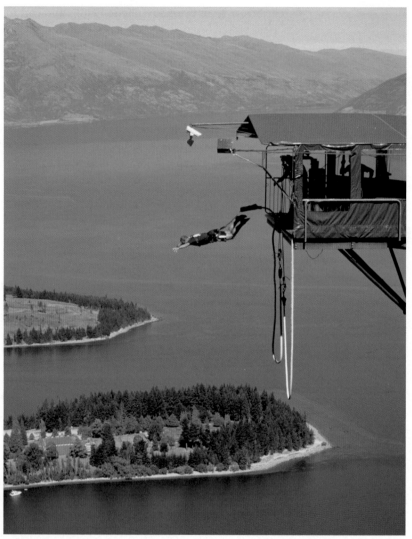

© Douglas Pearson/Corbis

As you can see from this brief description each of the models has some positive elements, but also has some problems that need to be reviewed. Each of the models will be explained in more detail in the next section, starting with the earliest chronologically.

Stress as a response

One of the earliest models of stress focused on the body's reaction to stress (Kemeny, 2003). This is the physiological **general adaptation syndrome (GAS)** identified by Selye (1956). If we try to recall how we feel when we consider ourselves under stress we will come up with a common set of responses: increased heart rate, increased blood pressure, increased respiration and so on. These are all part of the '**fight or flight**' syndrome which prepares the body for action and are mediated through the nervous and endocrine system (see Figure 13.1).

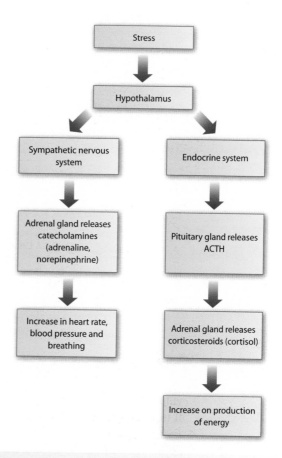

Figure 13.1 Model of the consequences of the GAS.

Previous research by Cannon (1929) suggested that when animals and humans perceive danger, these physiological systems are activated in preparation for the animal to 'fight or flight'. Obviously in the short term this prepares the animal or human for appropriate action (depending on the stressor) but in the long term it may be harmful. On the basis of the physiological reactions described in the 'fight or flight' response, Selye (1956) observed the reactions of animals to various stressful stimuli. He noticed that this reaction was the start of a series of reactions the body makes in response to stressors. On the basis of this he developed the GAS (Figure 13.2). The GAS has three distinct phases:

- *Alarm phase.* The function of this stage is to mobilise the body's resources so the body is ready to cope with the stressor. At this stage, the nature of the stressor is not important: there will be, according to Selye, an equivalent response to both psychological and physical stressors. This stage is like the fight or flight response in terms of mobilising the body's resources ready for action. However, in time the body's resources become depleted, leading to fatigue, and at this stage the second stage, the resistance phase, occurs.
- *Resistance phase.* In this stage the body tries to adapt to the stressor, physiological arousal declining although remaining higher than normal. The ability to resist new stressors is impaired, so that individuals become

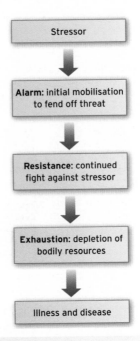

Figure 13.2 Model of the general adaptation syndrome (GAS).

vulnerable to health problems resulting from impaired immune functions. If this occurs for too long then the exhaustion phase is entered.

- *Exhaustion phase*. The true state of exhaustion occurs when the body's ability to respond is exhausted such that recovery and resistance are no longer possible. If stress continues then death may occur.

This three-phase explanation appealed because it describes people's experience of stress, and there is some evidence of the biological changes.

Implications

There are a number of criticisms of Selye's model:

- Stress is defined in terms of outcome. Hence, somebody could be considered as under stress only when a phase of the GAS was occurring.
- It does not allow for psychological activation. For example, you can become stressful just thinking about something happening.
- Individual differences are not accounted for, such as personality and previous experience.
- Selye's model can be viewed as describing the individual as passive and as responding automatically to the stressor.

Despite these criticisms the model still remains influential and most up-to-date models of stress have attempted to integrate some of the ideas from the GAS.

Think about this

Review the last time you were stressed. What bodily reactions occurred? How long did they last? Were you able to reduce these reactions by thinking about them?

Stress as a life event

In this definition, stress is defined as a particular event or set of circumstances in the environment. These are the stressors. If we look back at the case study we note that Joe had a number of 'life events', for example his divorce and his loss of job (Holmes and Rahe, 1967). It is these types of event that are considered negatively and can lead to stress and potentially illness. These sources of stress (the 'stressors') may take a number of different forms:

- *Chronic stressors*: for example, an illness, caring for somebody or living in poor surroundings.
- *Acute stressors*: for example, being admitted to hospital, going for a screening scan or taking an examination.
- *Daily hassles*: for example, trouble travelling to work, or mislaying a file.
- *Life events*: for example, getting married or divorced or losing a partner.

A popular notion was the view that stress was an event that happened to you. Holmes and Rahe (1967) suggested that stress was a consequence of the life events that an individual experienced: the greater the number, or the greater the magnitude of the individual event, the greater the extent of the stress. A key publication was the social readjustment rating scale (SRRS) of Holmes and Rahe (1967) (Table 13.1). This scale weighted each of a series of events on how stressful each was. The most stressful, as rated by the respondents, was the death of a spouse which scored 100, while marriage was rated 50, and Christmas 12. The scale consists of a number of everyday events which were rated on a scale of 1 to 100 which has been derived from a number of studies so represents an average level of stressfulness for each of the items.

However, many of the events listed in the SRRS are major life events and these happen, luckily, very rarely. Most of the stress that we suffer on a daily basis is not major events but minor events, or hassles. Recognising this, Kanner *et al.* (1981) designed the hassles scale which is designed to measure daily irritations (e.g. misplacing or losing things). This consists of 117 items, and the respondent indicates whether the event has occurred in the past month and then rates how severe each event was. In addition to this scale, the uplifts scale was developed, which is a list of 135 items (e.g. practising your hobby) that are likely to result in positive feelings.

Obviously in addition to these measures a number of specifically designed scales have been developed for specific populations. There are several, for example, for nurses, midwives and other health professionals. There is also one for students at university or college and some items drawn from this scale are provided (although it is American, it does highlight the issues that may be important). Table 13.2 provides a list of common events you may sometimes find unpleasant because they make you irritated, frustrated or anxious. The list was taken from the hassles assessment scale for students in college (Sarafino and Ewing, 1999).

Table 13.1
Examples drawn from the Social Readjustment Rating Scale

Death of a spouse	100
Divorce	73
Marital separation	65
Jail term	63
Death of family member	63
Personal injury/illness	53
Marriage	50
Fired	47
Marital reconciliation	45
Retirement	45
Change in health of family member	44
Pregnancy	40
Sex difficulties	39
Gain of new family member	39
Business readjustment	39
Change in financial state	38
Death of a close friend	37
Job change	36
Change in number of arguments with spouse	35
Mortgage/major loan	31
Foreclosure of loan	30
Change in work	29
Child leaving home	29
Trouble with in-laws	29
Outstanding personal achievement	28
Wife starts/stops work	26
School starts/ends	26
Change in living conditions	25
Trouble with boss	23
School/house move	20
Minor loan	17
Change in sleeping habits	16
Vacation	13
Christmas	12
Minor violations of the law	11

Source: Holmes and Rahe (1967)

Table 13.2 Common events that cause stress

Statement	Never or rarely (0)	Occasionally (1)	Often (2)	Very often (3)	Extremely often (4)
Annoying social behaviour of others (e.g. rude, inconsiderate, sexist/racist)					
Annoying behaviour of self (e.g. habits, temper)					
Appearance of self (e.g. noticing unattractive features, grooming)					
Accidents/clumsiness/mistakes of self (e.g. spilling beverage, tripping)					
Athletic activities of self (e.g. aspects of own performance, time demands)					
Bills/overspending: seeing evidence of					
Boredom (e.g. nothing to do, current activity uninteresting)					
Car problems (e.g. breaking down, repairs)					
Crowds/large social groups (e.g. at parties, while shopping)					
Dating (e.g. noticing lack of, uninteresting partner)					
Environment (e.g. noticing physical living or working conditions)					
Extracurricular groups (e.g. activities, responsibilities)					
Exams (e.g. preparing for, taking)					
Exercising (e.g. unpleasant routines, time to do)					
Facilities/resources unavailable (e.g. library materials, computers)					
Family: obligations or activities					
Family: relationship issues, annoyances					
Fears of physical safety (e.g. while walking alone, being on a plane or in a car)					
Fitness: noticing inadequate physical condition					
Food (e.g. unappealing or unhealthy meals)					

Source: Sarafino and Ewing (1999)

Table 13.2 Continued

Statement	Never or rarely (0)	Occasionally (1)	Often (2)	Very often (3)	Extremely often (4)
Forgetting to do things (e.g. to tape TV show, send cards, do homework)					
Friends/peers: relationship issues, annoyances					
Future plans (e.g. career or marital decisions)					
Getting up early (e.g. for class or work)					
Girl/boyfriend relationship issues, annoyances					
Goals/tasks: not completing enough					
Grades (e.g. getting a low grade)					
Health/physical symptoms of self (e.g. flu, premenstural syndrome, allergies, headaches)					
Schoolwork (e.g. working on term papers, reading tedious/hard material, low motivation)					
Housing: finding/getting or moving					
Injustice: seeing examples or being a victim of					
Job: searching for or interviews					
Job/work issues (e.g. demands or annoying aspects of)					
Lateness of self (e.g. for appointment for class)					
Losing or misplacing things (e.g. keys, books)					
Medical/dental treatment (e.g. unpleasant, time demands)					
Money: noticing lack of					
New experiences or challenges: engaging in					
Noise of other people or animals					
Oral presentations/public speaking					
Parking problems (e.g., on campus, at work, at home)					
Privacy: noticing lack of					
Tutors (e.g., unfairness, demands of, unavailability)					

Think about this

Complete the questionnaire for the previous month. Indicate against each of the events how frequently each occurred and then total your score – the higher the score the greater the level of hassle. On the basis of the results, how stressed were you? Do you think this was an accurate reflection of how stressed you were? Or did you feel more/less stressed?

With all these questionnaire approaches the idea is the same – the level of stress an individual has experienced can be measured by simply totalling the number of stressful events that have occurred within a specified time frame. This type of assessment has proved useful since it allows for direct comparisons to be made among individuals. Furthermore, many studies have found an association between these stresses, their severity and the onset of illness.

Think about this

What sorts of stressors are there in your health care setting for both the patient and the nurse? How would you rank these? Are there any which are extremely stressful, and some that are less so?

Interactional approach

In order to overcome problems associated with the two earlier models, the interactional (or **transactional**) approach was devised. Lazarus and his co-workers during the late 1960s and early 1970s proposed this alternative model of stress that took into account psychological variables (e.g. Lazarus, 1966, Lazarus and Folkman, 1987; Lazaurus and Gal, 1975). Lazarus argued that stress involved a transaction between individuals and their external world, and that a stress response was elicited if an individual appraisal perceived a potentially stressful event as being stressful. This model was developed by Lazarus and Folkman (1984) where they suggested two forms of appraisal.

Primary appraisal is applied to the event to assess whether it poses a threat (i.e. is negative), is positive or is neutral. For example, developing a cold may be seen as positive (because you will not have to go to work or to university tomorrow), neutral (because you will be able to carry on with whatever you intended to do whether you had a cold or not) or negative (i.e. stressful, because you have an important meeting tomorrow and the cold will not help). If primary appraisal considers the situation to be threatening then the *secondary appraisal* comes into play and questions how well we are able to cope with the threat. Hence, secondary appraisal involves an individual evaluating their coping strategies. Can we cope with this stress, and if so how? If on the basis of these forms of appraisal we both consider the situation to be threatening and we lack the resources to cope effectively with it then we will experience some form of stress. This model is presented in Figure 13.3.

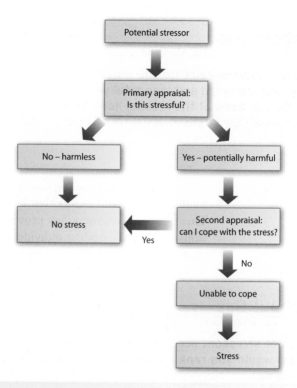

Figure 13.3 Transactional model of stress.

So how do people cope with stress? According to Lazarus and Folkman (1984) coping has two main functions: it can alter the problem causing the stress (i.e. problem-focused coping) or it can regulate the emotional response to the problem (i.e. emotional-focused coping).

Emotional-focused coping is aimed at regulating the emotional response to the stressful situation and this can be through either **behavioural coping** or **cognitive coping** methods. For example, dealing with the stress of exams by drinking alcohol or taking part in sports would be examples of behavioural strategies. It is not about changing the situation but reducing the amount of distress associated with the situation. Cognitive methods would include attempting to reinterpret the situation: 'there are worse things in life than exams', 'I have an opportunity to show how good I am' and so on.

Problem-focused coping is aimed at reducing the demands of the stressful situation or expanding resources to deal with it: for example, dropping out of university because of the stress of exams or devising a new schedule for studying (and sticking to it).

A number of different coping mechanisms have been described that lie in these broad categories (Folkman and Lazarus, 1988) and some of these are presented in Table 13.3.

Think about this

Using the table of coping strategies, how would you advise a person to cope with an injection?

Table 13.3
Coping mechanisms

Problem-focused mechanism	Example
Planning: analysing the situation to arrive at solutions to correct the problem	'I knew what had to be done so I doubled my efforts to make things work' or 'I made a plan of action and followed it'
Confrontative: assertive action taken	'I stood my ground and fought for what I wanted'
Social support	Gets practical support from friends
Emotional-focused	
Social support	Gets emotional support from friends
Distancing: detaching from the situation	'I made light of the situation and refused to get too serious about it' or 'I went on as if nothing had happened'
Escape-avoidance: thinking wishfully about the situation	'I wished that the situation would go away or somehow be over with' or 'I hoped a miracle would happen'
Self-control: modulate own feelings	'I tried to keep my feelings to myself' or 'I kept others from knowing how bad things were'
Accepting responsibility: acknowledging own role in the problem while trying to put them right	'I criticised myself' or 'I made a promise to myself that things would be different next time'
Positive reappraisal: creating a positive meaning from the situation	'I changed or grew as a person in a good way' or 'I came out of the experience better than I went in'

Source: Folkman and Lazarus (1988)

It should also be pointed out that coping differs in its success ratings for different people – what one person uses may not be suitable for another. It also has to be highlighted that some coping methods (e.g. drinking large amount of alcohol) may be useful for reducing stress, but increases other problems! Furthermore, individuals may engage in more than one coping strategy, indeed a combination of both emotional and problem-based coping strategies may be a necessity in some chronic long-term conditions (Aldwin and Park, 2004).

Think about this

Think about a recent stressful experience. How did you manage to cope with it? Did you use a range of methods, or just one or two? Which one worked best for you, or did you have to use many to get through?

Implications of the interactional model

There are a number of implications and problems with this model. The major problem is that by focusing on the perceptual world it is unclear what a stressful event is (Hobfoll, 1989). For example, people may be able to cope with a certain pressure because they are good at coping: are they under stress? On the other hand, some may find that the same event, perceived in the same way, is stressful since they do not have the resources to cope with it. How do you measure stress, therefore? It is always up to the individual and is therefore subjective.

However, the model has three important implications. Firstly, no event can be characterised as stressful (or unstressful) per se. Any situation can be appraised by one individual as stressful but not by another. Thus, some may appraise going to the dentist (or having an operation) as being stressful. Others will appraise it as unstressful. By the same token it is also important to recognise that something that we may take as an everyday occurrence may be stressful for others. We therefore have to consider this when dealing with patients, clients and members of the general public on a daily basis. Something we view as mundane and routine may be considered stressful and worrying.

Secondly, since the model is based on an individual's thought processes (i.e. **cognitive appraisal**) then it is susceptible to changes in mood, health and other mental states. An individual may interpret the same event in different ways depending on the way they are feeling. Hence, an individual may consider going to the dentist as stressful at the end of a tiring hard week, but consider it less stressful if they are fully relaxed and are motivated to get their teeth fixed.

Thirdly, a stressful response may be experienced irrespective of whether the situation is recalled, experienced or simply imagined. Hence, imagining going to the dentist can be considered by some just as stressful as actually going.

Think about this

What daily activities are you involved in that you consider routine and (almost) boring that you think others would consider stressful? How do you think you could best reduce the stress on others?

Stress and physical health

There are a number of potential indicators of stress and these may be broadly categorised in psychological and physiological (see Table 13.4). Obviously the psychological facstors can lead to poor mental health and, in chronic cases, poor physical health (Yehuda and McEwen, 2004).

There is widespread acceptance that stress does cause ill-health and this notion has been agreed upon for a number of years. For example, in an 1884 leader article in the *British Medical Journal* it was suggested that at funerals: 'The depression of spirits under which the chief mourners labour at the melancholy occasions peculiarly predisposes them to some of the worst effects of chill.' The author was suggesting that stress (i.e. the death of a loved one) led to a disease (in this case a cold or cough). However, not all have agreed, and some (e.g. Jones and Bright, 2001) have argued that the link between stress and physical illness is unproved. However, a number of illnesses have been linked to stress and continue to do so by both the general public and health care professionals alike (Clark, 2003; Lundberg, 2006).

	Psychological	Physiological
Table 13.4 **Indicators of stress**	Unease	Persistently elevated blood pressure (leading to clinical hypertension)
	Apprehension	
	Sadness	Indigestion
	Depression	Constipation or diarrhoea
	Pessimism	Weight gain or loss
	Listlessness	CHD
	Lack of self-esteem	Gastric problems
	Negative attitudes	Menstrual problems
	Short temper	
	Fatigue	
	Poor sleep	
	Increased smoking	
	Increased alcohol	

Surveys have indicated that stress and related conditions form a massive group of work-related ill-health conditions (HSE, 2005, Jones *et al.*, 2006). It is estimated that work-related stress, depression and anxiety affect over half a million people in Great Britain with an estimated 12.8 million lost working days due to these work-related conditions in 2003/4. This means that, on average, almost a month per year is lost per affected case and makes stress the largest contributor to the overall estimated annual days lost from work-related ill-health (HSE, 2006).

Evidence also suggests that most of those reporting work-related heart disease (some 66 000 people) ascribed its cause to work stress. These reports have mainly concerned the mental health effects of stress. However, there is also suggestions, and in some cases evidence, of a link between stress and physical illness (e.g. Cohen, 2005; Lundberg, 2006). This has come from a number of sources, and stress has been implicated in a number of different conditions. These include heart disease (Clark, 2003), cancer, HIV/AIDs and other infectious disorders (Langley *et al.*, 2006). It may be worthwhile to explore each of these conditions in turn to explore how the evidence stacks up: does stress cause illness?

Coronary heart disease (CHD)

Coronary heart disease is the physical condition for which there is the most comprehensive evidence for a link with stress (Bunker *et al.*, 2003; SIGN, 2007) and one that most members of the general public, including those that have had a heart attack, believe there to be a link (Clark, 2003). These results have some relevance – it is suggested that **psychosocial** variables have a risk similar in size to biological risk factors (hypertension and dyslipaemia), with each increasing the risk three- or four-fold (Bunker *et al.*, 2003). MacLeod *et al.* (2002) also report a strong and substantial relationship between self-reported stress and self-reported symptoms of CHD, and with admission to hospital for psychiatric disorders. There was also a relationship between stress and admission to hospital for various conditions associated with cardiovascular disease. However, the interpretation by these authors was that there was a tendency among those who were stressed to report more symptoms rather than to actually experience them, as objective measures of ill-health did not appear to correlate with self-reported stress. Nonetheless, the evidence does suggest that there is a link between stress and CHD: the greater the stress, the greater the chance of experiencing a heart attack.

Think about this

Looking back at Joe, what sort of stress could have caused his heart attack?

Breast cancer

Early studies were equivocal, and there are still arguments over the relationship between stress and breast cancer onset. Some have argued that there is a relationship between life events and the onset of breast cancer, although others suggest that the studies are flawed. In a large cohort study of 10 808 Finnish women, Lillberg *et al.* (2003) **prospectively** investigated the relationship between stressful life events and risk of breast cancer. In this way life events were recorded over a five year period and were linked to the subsequent development of breast cancer. The results indicated that life events, particularly divorce/separation and death of a close relative, were linked to the onset of the cancer. So again, although there is some academic debate about the quality of the studies conducted, there does appear to be a link between the onset of breast cancer and stressful events.

HIV/AIDS

There is some evidence that stress can lead to a progression of HIV/AIDS (Antoni *et al.*, 2000; Leserman, 2003). One such study was reported by Evans *et al.* (1997). This was one of the first studies to highlight the relationship between stressful life events and the progression of HIV in 93 HIV-positive gay men. Their findings suggested that the more severe the life stress experienced, the greater the risk of early HIV disease progression. For example, they reported that the risk of disease progression was doubled for every incident of severe stress in the preceding six month period. There is considerable interest in exploring the relationship between stress and HIV progression for a number of reasons: it can help elucidate the concept of '**psychoneuroimmunology**' and it obviously has considerable clinical relevance. Reviews of the literature (e.g. Leserman, 2003) suggest that there is substantial evidence linking stressful events and HIV disease progression.

Infectious disease

Obviously stress does not cause infectious diseases. However, it can reduce the body's defences against viruses by impairing the immune response. Cohen *et al.* (1993) used the cold virus in their study and found that emotional distress and high levels of stressful life events increased the risk of developing an infection and in the expression of the disease clinically. In a later study, Cohen *et al.* (1998) reported that those who had experienced stress of a long duration, primarily as a function of unemployment or family conflict, exhibited a substantially greater risk of developing a cold. They also reported that participants with low numbers of social ties were four times more likely to develop a cold than those with a higher number of ties (see Cohen, 2005, for a review of the impact of psychosocial variables on infectious disorders).

Other physical conditions

A number of other conditions, for example MS, rheumatoid arthritis, Type I (insulin-dependent) diabetes, systemic lupus erythemastosus, bronchial asthma and irritable bowel syndrome, have been investigated. However, for most of these conditions the evidence is equivocal. Although the role of stress in the primary aetiological process is limited, the stronger evidence suggests that the stress process can aggravate the severity of these disorders and is involved in the exacerbation of these disorders (Yehuda and McEwan, 2004).

Think about this

How does this information help you as the nurse? What does it mean for you as a professional?

How does stress affect health?

All of these studies indicate that there does appear to be a relationship between stress and health status in a number of different conditions. However, it is worth considering how stress actually affects health. There are a number of routes through which stress can influence health. Physiological reactions to stress play a part (see box); however, two are routes are also worthy of further investigation: through the immune system (psychoneuroimmunology); and through changes in behaviour.

Physiology of stress

The way stress affects health has been related to three different physiological pathways: the nervous; the hormonal and the immune systems.

The nervous system

The nervous system, which includes the central nervous system (CNS - brain and spinal cord) as well as the peripheral nervous system (all other neurons), controls the body's reaction to stress. ▶

The peripheral nervous system is divided into both somatic nervous system (responsible for movement and senses) and the autonomic nervous system (ANS) which serves the involuntary muscles and internal organs. There are two branches to the ANS: the sympathetic division, which deals with bodily excitation and the expenditure of energy, and the parasympathetic division, which is concerned with reducing bodily activity and restoring energy.

From this brief description it should be possible to see how the concept of Cannon's fight or flight can be interpreted in light of this physiological reaction, especially the sympathetic division of the ANS. Hence, when an individual is under stress the sympathetic division of the ANS **innervates** the adrenal medulla (part of the adrenal gland) and this results in the release of two chemicals, known as catecholamines: adrenaline (sometimes called epinephrine) and noradrenaline (or norepinephrine). These two neurotransmitters mobilise the body's resources, preparing it for fight or flight; for example, increasing the cardiovascular activity (heart rate, stroke volume and force of contraction), shifting the flow of blood to the muscles rather than digestion or the skin, widening the airways, speeding the rate of breathing and increasing the volume of air intake into the lungs, and many other such reactions. All of these bodily reactions are seeking to prepare the body for either fight or flight. These can be mapped onto the reactions of stress as highlighted in the table.

Physiological reaction	Potential symptom
Increase in heart rate	Rapid or irregular heartbeats
Increase in respiration rate	Hyperventilation or some form of asthma
Adrenaline released	Increase in heart rate
Noradrenaline released	Raised blood pressure
Muscle tightening	Tension headache, tense muscles, insomnia, fatigue, loss of concentration
Change in blood flow/circulation stomachs,	High blood pressure, cold hands, upset migraine, pre-ulcerous/ulcerous conditions, increased colitis, constipation, and sexual dysfunction
Senses heightened	Emotional irritability, poor impulse control, reduced communication abilities
Increased perspiration	Dehydration
Imbalance in hormone	Frequent infections, auto-immune disease
Saliva consistency change	Dry mouth

The repeated occurrence of these responses is one way in which stress can impact on health. For example, the repeated cardiovascular activation could lead to permanent damage to the arteries and veins and thereby cause elevated blood pressure.

Hormonal system

The hormonal (or endocrine) system consists of a number of glands throughout the body which secrete hormones in times of stress, although at a much slower rate than the neurotransmitters described above. For this reason they are mainly associated with chronic stressors (rather than the acute stressors that influence the nervous system). The hormones are carried in the bloodstream to various parts of the body where they act on the target organ (either directly or indirectly). These hormonal reactions are much slower to act than the neurotransmitters but also have a longer-lasting effect.

One major hormonal pathway through which stress exerts its effects is the adrenocorticotrophic hormone (ACTH). The anterior pituitary produces ACTH when it is stimulated by the **hypothalamus**. ACTH is released into the bloodstream and acts upon the outer area of the adrenal gland, causing it to produce a group of hormones – the corticosteroids. These regulate the blood pressure and hence this demonstrates one mechanism whereby the hormonal transmitted stress can exert a negative effect.

Immune system

The immune system protects us from infection and illness and consists of a series of coordinated responses to protect the body by defending it against invasion by antigens. Immune reactions involve two main types of response. In the first the immunity involves the action of a special white blood cell called the T cell, which kills invading micro-organisms. In the second, special chemicals known as antibodies or immunoglobulins are released into the bloodstream which attach themselves to the antigen and destroy it. A third type of cell involved in the immune response is known as a phagocyte, which envelops and devours foreign substances.

Psychoneuroimmunology (PNI)

The term **psychoneuroimmunology** was first coined by Ader (1981; see Ader *et al.*, 2001) and involves the study of the interactions between behaviour, neural and endocrine function and the immune process. The first evidence that appeared to link stress and the immune system came from the studies of bereaved spouses with reports that bereaved spouses have a weaker immune system than those in continuing relationships. This finding was extended by Kiecolt-Glaser *et al.* (1987) who found that a sample of women who had recently divorced or separated had a lower lymphocyte response than a control group and that hostile marital environments had a weaker immune system (Kiecolt-Glaser *et al.*, 2005) and those that had a positive marital environment had a better immune response (Heffner *et al.*, 2004). This means that those who got divorced had a weaker immune system than those that had not. Women who were more attached to the marriage showed the greatest response than those that showed less positive memories of the marriage. Similar findings were reported for men who had been separated or divorced.

Other stressful situations have been explored. It is important to note that this stress can be at either the acute level or the chronic level. In terms of chronic stress, for example, Kiecolt-Glaser and Glaser (1992) found immune suppression in carers of Alzheimer's patients. Carers for people with a dementing illness had a poorer immune system and hence were more prone to disease – a result confirmed in a longitudinal follow-up study (Kiecolt-Glaser *et al.*, 2003).

Workman and La Via (1987) explored the immune system in students undertaking an exam (an acute stressor) and noted a weakening in the immune system from a baseline prior to the exam, to during the exam and then after the exam. The studies have also found that the whole immune system appears to be affected, and this appeared to be the case even when behavioural factors such as lack of sleep, diet and drug use were controlled for. Hence, this study, among others, suggests that those students undertaking exams had a poor immune response and hence they were at a greater risk of developing infectious disorders. This is a finding that has been replicated on numerous occasions (e.g. Marazziti *et al.*, 2007; Weekes *et al.*, 2006). Overall, exams can be bad for your health since stress is bad for your immune system (Glaser and Kiecolt-Glaser, 2005).

Change in behaviour

When a person is under stress they tend to indulge in coping strategies in order to reduce the stress (as we have seen before with the transactional model of stress). Some of these coping strategies may be successful in reducing an individual's stress but may, ironically, result in an increased health risk: for example, smoking, drinking excessive alcohol and deteriorations in diet or exercise regimes.

Think about this

Think about the last time you were under exam stress. Did you change your behaviour? Did it become healthier or unhealthier? Did you, for example, smoke more, drink more or eat the wrong things?

Smoking

Research suggests a link between stress and smoking behaviour in terms of smoking initiation, relapse and the amount smoked. Carey *et al.* (1993) reported that people who experience high levels of stress are more likely to start smoking again after a period of abstinence than those who experience less stress. Other studies have reported that higher levels of stress were associated with smoking more cigarettes. This association was also found in one large survey of over 6000 Scottish men and women which showed that higher levels of perceived stress were linked to smoking more (Heslop *et al.*, 2001).

Alcohol

Many people have suggested that work stress may promote alcohol use. The **tension reduction theory** suggests that people drink alcohol because of its tension-reducing properties (Cappell, 1987). This theory is supported by evidence of a relationship between negative mood and drinking behaviour, which suggests that people are more likely to drink when they are depressed or anxious. Furthermore, in an interesting epidemiological study Boscarino *et al.* (2006) reported on an increased alcohol intake in those with greater exposure to the stressors of the World Trade Center attack on 11 September 2001.

Eating

There is an appreciation that stress leads to over-eating – people talk about 'comfort eating' or 'comfort food'. However, although the evidence does suggest that there is a link between stress and diet, it may not be as simple as the common-sense prediction. Greeno and Wing (1994) propose two hypotheses concerning the link between stress and eating. First, that stress increases eating generally and, secondly, that stress causes changes in eating in vulnerable groups of individuals (the individual difference model). It is the latter hypothesis that has the most support. For example, Michaud *et al.* (1990) reported that exam stress was related to an increase in eating in girls but not boys. However, in contrast, Conner *et al.* (1999) reported that those with greater daily hassles had greater levels of eating irrespective of gender or any other factor. In summary the evidence is contradictory. Stone and Brownell (1994) called this 'the stress eating paradox' since sometimes stress causes over-eating, while on other occasions stress causes under-eating. However, most of these studies were conducted in lab settings with an induced stressor (for example, a loud bang or a maths test). In a more thorough, large-scale survey, Cartwright *et al.* (2003) found that there was some evidence to support the idea of comfort eating. The report found that those under stress were more likely to eat fatty foods than fruit and vegetables and more likely to snack unhealthily. Furthermore the authors report: '... a dose–response relationships such that as stress increased, the likelihood of unhealthy dietary practice also increased'.

Exercise

Research has indicated that stress may reduce exercise (e.g. Heslop *et al.*, 2001) whereas stress management which focuses on increasing exercise has been shown to result in some improvements in coronary health.

Accidents

Research suggests that individuals who experience high levels of stress show a greater tendency to perform behaviours that increase their chances of becoming injured (HSE, 2006). Furthermore, some research indicates that the greater the stress, the greater the level of accidents at work and in the car.

Think about this

How does Joe's behaviour change because of the stress? How would you suggest he alters his behaviour to cope with the stress?

Mediators of the stress–health relationship

Social support

Social support is usually defined as the existence of people on whom we can rely, people who let us know that they care about, value and love us and the support they provide for us (Sarason *et al.*, 1983). There is a distinction between existence of social relationships and the functions provided by these. So the structure would be 'how many friends, colleagues, family relationships' you have. The functional aspect would refer to what these do. In essence you can have lots of friends but not interact with them and this may not be very useful. Social support can come from a variety of different sources and a variety of types of support (Cohen, L. *et al.*, 2000); for example, spouses, relatives, friends, neighbours, co-workers, superiors. But it can also come from professional sources and this can help reduce stress. The type and amount of social support an individual receives depends upon their social network but also on various demographic factors: their age, sex, culture, socio-economic status and so on.

Generally, social support comes in one of five types:

- *Appraisal support*: The person is encouraged to evaluate their own health through information and they are then able to put the stressors in context.
- *Emotional support*: A 'shoulder to cry on' is the traditional descriptor for this form of social support. It is being loved for, cared, protected, listened to and so on.
- *Esteem support*: Is a feeling that you are valued, or held in esteem, by others. If you feel that you are a competent and skilful person you are more likely to be able to cope with the stressors.
- *Information support*: Is support in the form of information or knowledge which can assist the person in doing the right thing to look after themselves – providing feedback on how well they are doing, for example.
- *Instrumental support*: Is practical support – people will help you. They will give you a lift to the clinic, or look after the children so you can have some time to yourself, for example.

Social support can play an important part in reducing the effects of stress and we will explore this in detail later. In a seminal study, Berkman and Syme (1979) published their results linking social support to mortality. Subsequent studies have confirmed reliable links between social support and better physical health (see reviews by Berkman *et al.*, 2000; Uchino, 2004). Studies have suggested that those with low levels of social support have higher mortality rates – from cardiovascular disease (e.g. Brummett *et al.*, 2001; Frasure-Smith *et al.*, 2000) or from cancer (e.g. Hibbard and Pope, 1993) and infectious diseases (e.g. Lee and Rotheram-Borus, 2001).

Think about this

How could you use social support in a health care setting? Think of a number of examples of how health care could be less stressful with the presence of some form of support.

How does social support protect health?

It has been suggested that social support can protect against the negative effects of stress. There are two main views as to why this may be the case. The first, the *main effect hypothesis*, suggests that social support is beneficial

Pregnancy and social support

A number of more recent studies have also indicated that social support during pregnancy can improve the health of the baby. For example Feldman *et al.* (2000) report that the greater the social support (from a variety of sources – baby's father, family and other functional support), the better the outcome in terms of infant birth weight. Women who had better support from a range of sources had higher birth weight infants. It could be that having greater social support may improve birth weight by enhancing positive health behaviour and promoting healthier lifestyles in pregnant women; for example improved nutrition, reduced smoking and substance misuse. Furthermore, women who perceive that more support is available during pregnancy may also seek health-related information and receive prenatal care earlier in their pregnancy. However, although the findings from this study suggest that support interventions may be an effective approach to reducing rates of low birth weight, findings from interventions studies have been equivocal, although they do tend to indicate a lower likelihood of Caesarean sections.

Support interventions to attempt to increase social support for the women have to involve more than is currently on offer. Hence rather than simply the provision of informational and emotional support by nurse, social worker or lay educator several times over the course of a pregnancy there need to be multiple forms of support and support from multiple sources of social support. Thus interventions may be needed to improve a woman's social networks.

A number of studies have been undertaken to investigate this. The classic example is that of Sosa *et al.* (1980) who found that the addition of a birthing companion lead to an easier birth that required less medication. Hodnett (2002) reports on a systematic review on the role of care-giver support for women during labour. This study suggested that the continuous presence of a support person resulted in a number of positive outcomes. For example, there was a reduced need for pain relief medication, operative vaginal delivery, Caesarean section, reduced length of labour and a more positive view of the labour.

In terms of health states, Arnetz *et al.* (1987) explored the immune function in a group of women (*n* = 25) who were either employed or unemployed. The unemployed group were split into two groups: in one group the individuals simply received standard economic benefits only, in the other they received the benefits and a psychosocial support programme. The results indicated that the group that received the psychosocial support showed better immune functioning than the subjects who received benefits only. It seems that social support improved immune functioning and thereby health.

per se to health and it is the absence of social support that is stressful. This suggests the more social support you have, the better. This is because large social networks provide people with regular positive experiences both in terms of emotional as well as physical support. Hence, social support promotes healthier behaviours such as exercise, eating healthily and not smoking as well as greater adherence to medical regimes.

The other major theory – the **buffering hypothesis** – of social support is that it buffers the individual against the stressor. As the name suggests this explanation suggests that the presence of social support acts as a buffer against the stress being experienced. The 'buffer' protects the individual against powerful stressors but has little effect when the stressors are weak. Rather than protect a person all the time against the minor hassles and stresses of everyday life, the buffer acts on the stressors when it is needed most. For example, when a person with considerable social support has a diagnosis of an illness then they *appraise* it as less stressful because they know people to whom they can turn. In contrast, those with lower social support might be unable to turn to anyone (Cohen, S., *et al.*, 2000).

Other variables that may mediate the stress-health link

Stress and control

The link between stress and control – defined as the extent to which a person feels they are able to change their own circumstances – has been studied extensively in the workplace. Broadly, the results suggest that the more control you have in a work situation, the less stressful it is. Obviously, there comes a point where you have more control but also considerable responsibility and this can be stressful as well.

Think about this

How much control do you have over your current working/study life? Are there any areas you would like more control? If you had more control, how do you think it would affect your stress levels?

Stress and hardiness

Kobasa (1979) put forward this concept which describes a set of **traits** which can protect a person from the effects of stress, and includes control as a factor. A 'hardy' person copes well with stress and is somebody who has a high sense of personal control, a person who is committed to things, and a person who likes challenges and sees them as a good thing in life.

Stress and personality

For some people, personality variables are simply a way of behaving. They represent the way a person reacts to stress – their behavioural response. One personality variable that has received much attention is the so-called Type A personality type. Type A Behaviour Pattern (TABP) can be defined as: 'an overt pattern of behaviour which is elicited from susceptible individuals in an appropriately challenging environment'. TABP was first noted by two cardiologists from the United States who noted a common type of behaviour in their patients (Friedman and Rosenman, 1974). This behaviour included:

- job involvement;
- excessive hard driving behaviour;
- impatience;
- time urgency;
- competitiveness;
- aggressiveness;
- hostility.

In a series of studies, a relationship between Type A personality and CHD was established. However, more recently the evidence has been questioned and the key factor suggested as being hostility (Kjelsberg *et al.*, 1997; Miller *et al.*, 1996).

There have been attempts at establishing a link between personality types and other illnesses – most particularly cancer – but these have largely met with limited success (e.g. Dean and Surtees, 1989; Greer *et al.*, 1979; Schapiro *et al.*, 2001).

Stress and hostility

Initially a component of the Type A classification system, hostility has been linked to the development of CHD. In particular researchers have suggested that hostility is not only an important risk factor for the development of heart disease but also as a trigger for a heart attack (Miller *et al.*, 1996).

Stress management

Obviously, since stress can cause ill-health, a number of methods – '**stress management techniques**' – have been devised to try to reduce stress. Stress management can be defined as the application of methods in psychology to reduce the impact of stress. There are a whole host of different methods for stress management and each of these can be explored in turn.

You should have noticed that the underlying concepts of all the stress management techniques is that they can be related to the interactional model of stress.

Obviously, the first method of reducing stress is to remove the stressor! We could take away or modify the demands or exposure to potential stressful conditions. Hence, if the person gets 'stressed out' whenever there an injection is required then the person could simply avoid having the injection. Obviously, this is easier with certain stressors than others. People can usually avoid the stressor of parachuting from an aeroplane, whereas going to hospital or having an injection may be unavoidable. However, in other areas, for example initiatives in the workplace such as job redesign, management of conflict or changes in working practices (Daniels, 2006), stressors can bring about positive change in levels of stress by altering the stressor.

Primary appraisal

If the person cannot avoid the stressor then perhaps attempting to get the person to reappraise the situation may prove beneficial. Hence, rather than seeing the dentist as a stressor, get the person to see the visit in more positive light – this will improve my teeth, my smile, remove my pain and so on. Obviously, this can take some time and may need professional assistance. This approach underlies many cognitive behavioural interventions and assertiveness training.

Coping strategies

One of the major psychological approaches to stress management is cognitive-behavioural and this is best developed in the **stress-inoculation-training (SIT) method** (Meichenbaum and Cameron, 1983). This is a self-instructional method for teaching individuals to cope with stress and are basically concerned with developing the individual's competence to adapt to stressful events. In this way, the individual can alleviate his or her stress and achieve personal goals.

The SIT approach involves three basic phases:

- *Cognitive preparation*: The person learns the nature of stress and how people react to it. For example 'Under what circumstances do you experience stress?', 'What do you do to reduce your stress?'
- *Skill acquisition*: The person learns behavioural and cognitive skills to use in emotion-focused and problem-focused coping. Some of these skills are general ones that all individuals would learn such as relaxation, cognitive redefinition while other skills may be specific to the individual (e.g. communication skills).
- *Application practice*: This involves the transfer of the learned material into practice. A variety of stressors are introduced into the sessions which are then generalised to other situations.

Another form of coping strategy enhancement comes in the provision of additional psychological resources. For example, providing more structured forms of practical support or by providing additional forms of social support.

The stress reaction

Finally, stress management can address stress responses directly through **relaxation** training, **biofeedback** and **meditation** techniques. The basic premise of relaxation for stress is that it is the opposite of arousal – so relaxing should be a good way to reduce stress. A number of methods have been used to induce relaxation. The most frequently mentioned in psychological terms is **progressive muscle relaxation (PMR)**. PMR originated from the work of Jocobsen in the 1920s and 1930s. Jocobsen (1938) proposed that the main mechanism influencing relaxation lies with the patient's ability to tell the difference between tension and relaxation. PMR involves the successive tensing and relaxing of various muscle groups.

For each of the muscle groups the therapist asks the client to tense them as tightly as possible and then relax them, and asks the client to note the difference. The client sits in a quiet relaxing room and the therapist takes the client through the following procedure:

- hands;
- forearms;
- upper arms;
- eyes;
- neck;
- forehead, and so on.

At the end of the session the client should be in a relaxed state and asked to focus on this and how it differs from the tense state. Research has indicated that PMR is extremely effective in reducing stress.

PMR can be extended to **autogenic muscle relaxation (AMR)**. In this the client is first taught how to relax following the PMR procedures. The relaxed state is then associated with a word, such as 'relax'. Hence, when the client is in a relaxed state, they say to themselves 'relax, relax, relax'. After a while, they associate the relaxed state with the word and can simply get into a relaxed state by saying the word at any time or in any place. This can then be successfully applied to other situations in which the client may feel under stress.

Think about this

How could you use some of these stress management programmes in your day-to-day practice? Is there anything that you would suggest to Joe to ease his stress?

Success of stress management programmes

Research has indicated that stress management programmes can result in reduced stress (obviously!) and generally provide better mental health than either sham or no treatment options. The more interesting question is whether these programmes can result in better physical health by reducing stress. The assumption is that, as we have seen, if stress either causes or exacerbates the illness condition then providing stress management should both reduce stress and help ameliorate the condition. Although there are a number of research reports in this area investigating a wide range of illnesses (e.g. asthma, Nickel *et al.*, 2006; and prostate cancer, Penedo *et al.*, 2006), studies have mainly concentrated on the following main disorders.

Hypertension and CHD

Johnson (1992) reported 25 published papers on stress management in hypertension. In these studies 823 patients had been studied who had received stress management and 578 patients who had acted as controls. The average reduction in blood pressure was 8.8 mm Hg (mercury), compared with 3.15 mm Hg for the control treatment (these figures are measures of blood pressure). It is clear from the studies that blood pressure can be reduced considerably with the use of stress management programmes. The long-term effects of stress management appear to be good with follow-up studies indicating a reduction at six months. But, what does this mean in practice? Does this have an impact on any illness? It is a relatively small reduction and may mean little in practice. Overall, the evidence (Williams *et al.*, 2004) suggests that: 'structured interventions to reduce stress (stress management, meditation, yoga, cognitive therapies, breathing exercises and biofeedback) have been shown to result in short term reductions in BP'.

Immune function

Kiecolt-Glaser *et al.* (1985) split a group of elderly patients into three groups; relaxation training, social contact or no social contact. The relaxation group showed the greatest improvement in immune functioning with the other two groups showing no change. However, at one month follow-up there was no significant difference between the three groups. That is, there had been no substantial improvements over time. McGregor and colleagues (2004) explored immune function in women with cancer. They found that a psychological intervention to reduce stress resulted in improved immune function. This improvement was noted both immediately after the programme and three months later when the group was followed up.

HIV

Hall and O'Grady (1991) in a sample of subjects who were HIV-positive used imagery and relaxation programmes in an attempt to improve their stress management of subjects. The results suggested that those who had undergone the stress management programme were more relaxed and, more importantly, had improved the immune status of the subjects. Antoni *et al.* (2002) reported on HIV-positive men participating in a 10 week cognitive behaviour stress management intervention programme. They reported that the men showed greater signs of immune system improvement over a 6–12 month follow-up than did control subjects. Since HIV-infected persons are at heightened risk for significant physiological consequences from chronic stress and depressed mood, they suggest that cognitive behaviour stress management might influence immune status by reducing tension and by altering maladaptive appraisals of stressful events.

Think about this

How would you treat Joe Gallagher on the basis of the stress management techniques outlined? How would you help with his chronic and acute stressors?

Stress and health care practice

Chronic workplace stress and the related concept of '**burnout**' are widely recognised phenomena in health care workers. There is considerable literature on stress and burnout in both qualified and student nurses. The Nursing Stress Scale (Gray-Toft and Anderson, 1981) has been used extensively to investigate stress and its relationship to clinical areas, job satisfaction and well-being. Other professionals such as physiotherapists, occupational therapists and podiatrists have also been studied. All studies have indicated that there are considerable levels of stress in health care and the need to address this has been recognised by the UK Government. Furthermore, there is evidence that workplace stress is having a greater impact on today's workforce than with previous generations. Obviously this could mean that there is additional intensity of stress from some potential stressors, or that there are more stressors.

Nursing provides a series of potential stressors and French *et al.* (2000) have identified nine areas of workplace stressors that might impact on nurses:

- conflict with physicians;
- inadequate preparation;
- problems with peers;
- problems with supervisor;
- discrimination;

- workload;
- uncertainty concerning treatment;
- dealing with death and dying patients;
- patients and their families.

The outcomes of stress may be severe. Ultimately, stress may lead to psychological and physiological distress, low job satisfaction and burnout. Burnout is described as a syndrome consisting of three dimensions: emotional exhaustion, depersonalisation (development of cold attitude) and personal accomplishment (loss of ability to value one's personal achievements). This can ultimately lead to high sickness absence, high staff turnover and problems for both clients/patients and the remaining staff workforce.

Obviously, some of these sources of stress need to address working and structural conditions in order to ameliorate any problems. However, there is little stress management training available to nurses and 'the need for the NHS to provide further stress management training is evident' (McVicar, 2003). A number of studies have investigated the effectiveness of stress management interventions for nurses, and these have ranged from personal relaxation techniques to increasing social support-based programmes. Although these have had a variable level of success, what is essential is that individual practitioners recognise what stress is, how it can affect individuals – themselves included – and the need to address the problem. Since stress is a transaction between the person and the environment, stress management techniques are best devised on an individual basis. However, the forms of stress management interventions can be at one of three levels: the individual level (e.g. stress education and monitoring, relaxation/meditation, cognitive coping strategies, assertiveness training, time management, counselling); individual/organisational interface (e.g. relationships at work, person–environment fit, role issues, participation and autonomy); and the organisational level (e.g. organisational structure, working conditions, selection and placement, training and development).

Think about this

What do you do when you are under stress? How can you deal with the stress of working clinically? Are there any elements in your workplace over which you can exert additional control? Or have you developed your own coping style?

Research in focus

Evers, K.E., Prochaska, J.O., Johnson, J.L., Mauriello, L.M., Padula, J.A. and Prochaska, J.M. (2006) A randomised clinical trial of a population and transtheoretical model based stress management intervention. *Health Psychology*, (4)**25**, 521–529.

Background
Stress is a considerable health concern for a large proportion of the population. Surveys have consistently indicated that stress is a major problem for the population and can have significant impact not just on the individual but on society as a whole. Stress can result in wide-ranging health effects and consequent impact on the workforce and economic productivity. Hence, a number of stress management techniques have been developed and introduced. This study recruited a national sample and devised an intervention based on a theoretical model – the transtheoretical model [TTM: see Chapter 12) that was tailored to the individual stages with the aim of producing long-term improvements in the effective management of stress.

Method
Participants: A national sample of over 1000 adults was proactively recruited for the study. The sample consisted of those adults who had a history of stress-related symptoms (identified as those with a history of purchasing over-the-counter products for symptoms related to stress). Two-thirds were female, and the ages ranged between 18 and 91 years (with a mean of 55 years). Almost three-quarters of the sample completed all questionnaires across the 18 month study period and hence there were 778 individuals in the final sample.

The sample was categorised (according to their response on a questionnaire) to a particular stage of change [see Chapter 12] for stress management: pre-contemplation (not considering stress management in the next six months), contemplation (intending to start stress management in the next six months) and preparation (intending to begin stress management in the next 30 days).

Measures: Participants completed questionnaires on the (both healthy and unhealthy) behaviours they used to manage their own stress along with a questionnaire on the perceived stress and coping methods. They also completed a depression questionnaire.

Intervention: Two groups were formed – a control group and a treatment group. The intervention was based on TTM and consisted of stage-matched feedback. Hence, participants received feedback about their use of stress-management behaviours and how best to implement stress management strategies (particularly for those in the preparation stage).

Results
Those in the treatment group were more likely to move into the action phase compared with those in the control group. Over 60 per cent of individuals in the treatment group who completed the study began practising effective stress management by the six month reporting period which was maintained at the 18 month follow-up. Furthermore, the results also indicated that participants in the treatment intervention group had reduced depression scores.

Implications
The results of the study indicate that a mail-delivered individualised TTM-tailored intervention aimed at increasing effective stress management on a population basis was effective. Of those that completed the study, over 60 per cent had changed their behaviour and were using appropriate stress management strategies (compared with 40 per cent of the control sample). Hence, a computerised public health intervention can help those at risk from stress related mental health problems.

Summary

- Stress is a difficult concept to define, even though it is a feature of all our everyday lives.

- Stress can be defined as coming from the inside (GAS), from the outside (life events) and as an interaction between the two (transactional model).

- Coping with stress can take one of two broad forms: problem focused or emotion focused.

- Stress has been implicated in mental health and in certain physical illness such as coronary heart disease, cancer and some infectious disorders.

- Stress can influence health through a number of routes, although through the immune system and because of changes in behaviour are two of the most investigated.

- There are several mediators of the stress–health link. For example, social support, control, hardiness, personality types and hostility have all been suggested as impacting on the stress–health link.

- Social support can prove effective in promoting health and reducing the consequences of stress.

- Stress management techniques include teaching improved coping techniques, increasing social support and promoting relaxation techniques.

- Workplace stress can lead to considerable problems for both individuals and organisations.

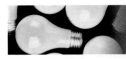

Check your understanding

1. Explore the explanations of stress. Which one offers the most comprehensive view of stress in practice?

2. What stressors face the individual being admitted to hospital? How can you help reduce the stress experienced by that individual?

3. What is the role for social support in pregnancy?

4. Does stress affect health and, if so, how?

5. How can stress be managed by the nurse?

6. How can stress be reduced in your workplace?

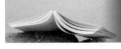

Further reading

Bartlett, D. (1998) *Stress: Perspectives and Processes*. Buckingham: Open University Press.

Weblinks

American Institute of Stress	http://www.stress.org/	Dedicated to advancing understanding of: the role of stress in health and illness; the nature and importance of mind-body relationships and the potential for self-healing.
International Stress Management Association	http://www.isma.org.uk/	The ISMA exists to promote sound knowledge and best practice in the prevention and reduction of human stress. It sets professional standards for the benefit of individuals and organisations using the services of its members.
UK National Work-Stress Network	http://www.workstress.net/	This site is intended to help raise the profile of work-related stress, its causes and how we can move towards eliminating it.
Guide to Psychology Practice	http://www.guidetopsychology.com/ stress_menu.htm	A common-sense approach to the management of frequent psychological problems.
Centre for Stress Management	http://www.managingstress.com/	The Centre for Stress Management is an international training centre and consultancy which runs modular courses in stress management, stress counselling, psychotherapy and coaching suitable for professionals wishing to gain more knowledge and skills practice in these subjects.
Health and Safety Executive leaflets on stress	http://www.hse.gov.uk/pubns/stresspk.htm	As it says on the tin!
HSE stress site	http://www.hse.gov.uk/stress/	These pages explain what HSE is doing to address the issue of stress at work, and provide access to a range of information, resources and further points of contact.
Stress – virtual library	http://www.dialogical.net/stress/index.html	The Stress Virtual Library keeps track of online information as part of the World Wide Web Virtual Library. Sites are inspected and evaluated for their adequacy as information sources before they are linked from here.

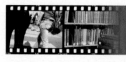

Media examples

Casualty/Holby City These popular BBC programmes demonstrate every week the stresses and strains of working in a high-pressure clinical environment.

Saving Private Ryan The opening sequence eloquently and shockingly demonstrate the reactions to hideous stress.

Chapter 14

The psychology of pain

Learning outcomes

When you have read through this chapter you should understand:

- The various definitions of pain.
- Historical definitions of pain.
- Inadequacies of the early definitions of pain.
- The gate control theory of pain.
- The different types of pain: chronic and acute pain.
- How to assess pain.
- How to manage pain by using medication and other medical methods.
- Behavioural methods for managing pain behaviours.
- Cognitive methods for alleviating pain.
- Multi-modal methods for treating pain.

Case study

Mrs Andrea Heskey is a 45-year-old woman who is married with two teenage children. Previously, Mrs Heskey was a senior administrative officer with the local council. However, 18 months ago she was involved in a minor car accident which has resulted in her suffering lower back pain. This bad back pain had continued despite all other symptoms now being resolved. Mrs Heskey had been signed off sick from her employment initially but had eventually been forced to resign. She was now receiving benefits in order to support her period without employment. A recent medical assessment had not revealed any significant anatomical or physiological abnormality but had revealed significant anxiety and depression. Mrs Heskey maintained both of these psychological ailments were a consequence of the bad back and her inability to work any further. At the medical assessment additional home support was provided: she now had a wheelchair, a stair lift and a bath hoist. Her husband, Eddie, had taken time off work in order to look after his wife and subsequently lost his job. The only relief that Eddie got was two nights a week when the two teenage children 'sat' with their mother while he played five-a-side soccer with his local pub team. However, he was considering (at his wife's request) giving this up in order that he could remain at home at all times to support his wife.

Mrs Heskey reported that she was in considerable pain and was on an increased dose of painkillers – the dose had been increased steadily over the previous 18 months and the medical staff caring for her considered there was a danger of her becoming dependent on the painkillers. However, Mrs Heskey stated that she was unable to sleep and survive throughout the day without these painkillers. As a consequence, the drugs remained at a high level. During the day Mrs Heskey spent most of her time in the wheelchair watching television, but now and again she did attempt to work in her garden – although after a few steps Eddie usually had to support his wife and help her back to the chair where she took some considerable time to recover.

Mrs Heskey had been requested to attend a pain clinic, which she did because 'she had tried everything else'. She lasted only a day and felt that the therapists did not understand the pain and suffering that she was experiencing. She felt that she needed effective drugs and possibly surgery.

Looking at Mrs Heskey's case – she is clearly reporting pain and is confined to a wheelchair, but there is no medical evidence of any damage of underlying structure. What does this mean: is she in pain or not? Do you think that there could be a psychological component to her experiences of pain? If so what methods could be introduced to help Mrs Heskey reduce her pain? Similarly, what about Eddie and the two children – are they helping Mrs Heskey deal with her pain or are they hindering her recovery?

Why is this relevant to nursing practice?

Pain will happen to all of us – although this is an unpleasant thought, it is a reality that at some stage of our life we will be in considerable pain. It may be related to an injury – an acute pain – or it may be more long term, such a chronic illness. Despite being unpleasant, it must be remembered that pain has a vital survival value as it serves to warn us we are in danger and should escape the situation. Consequently, it is vital to our continued existence. Those animals or humans that are born without the ability to experience pain do not live for very long.

Pain is one of the most common reasons for people to seek health care assistance. For example, over 80 per cent of the population will experience disturbing lower back pain problems at some time during their life. Similarly, some 30–40 per cent of the population will have experienced a tension headache in the previous year. Not only does this have serious consequences for the individual but also has an impact on society – the costs in terms of lost employment time, benefits and visits to health care practitioners are considerable. Furthermore, many people will experience pain when they enter the health care system and the treatment they receive may actually cause more pain in the short term. Obviously, for the nurse there is the requirement to minimise and reduce pain throughout treatment using a range of methods.

How can pain be described and how does it occur? What about the different forms of pain, for example, the difference between acute and chronic pain? If we can answer these questions then this should give us some insight into how pain can be treated and managed. What role does psychology have in ameliorating pain, and how can this be used in practice? These questions will be addressed during this chapter.

What is pain?

Pain can vary from a mild headache, through to a sharp pain as you receive an injection, to a severe stabbing pain following a major surgical intervention or accident. The International Association for the Study of Pain (IASP) defines pain as 'an unpleasant sensory and emotional experience associated with actual or potential tissue damage, or described in terms of such damage' (IASP, 1979). Although there are many different forms of pain it is worth outlining forms of pain that can be distinguished.

Think about this

What sort of pain have you come across in your own life? How can you categorise it – in terms of time, the severity and so on?

Acute pain is pain that occurs in the short term. This pain is generally the result of tissue damage or disease – a cut, bruise or broken bone, for example. This type of pain usually improves over time as the damage heals and lasts usually less than 6 months. When pain persists and becomes chronic, patients begin to perceive its nature differently. As the pain persists they see it as a permanent part of their lives. **Chronic pain** is difficult to define: it has been defined as pain that lasts more than 6 weeks, or 6 months, or 12 months! Although there is no generally agreed definition it is generally accepted that it is pain that does not go away after a minimum of 6 months. Lower back pain, headaches and the pain associated with cancer or arthritis are all examples of this form of pain.

This is an important area for psychology for a number of reasons. Firstly, there may be no sign of injury, or the pain reported may be disproportionate to the injury (think about the case of Mrs Heskey). Although an unclear area, it does suggest that there is more to pain than mere physical injury. Furthermore, psychology has played its primary role in the treatment of chronic pain, although moves towards the treatment of acute pain are now occurring.

Sub-categories of chronic pain include *recurrent acute pain* caused by benign conditions that is sometimes intense and sometimes disappears (e.g.

migraines). In contrast, *intractable-benign pain* is pain that is persistent and never really goes away (e.g. lower back pain). *Progressive pain* is pain that is both continuous and one that worsens over time (e.g. arthritis or cancer).

It is important to realise that pain is not merely a physiological response – psychological factors have an important role to play in all parts of pain. The IASP states that pain is never experienced in a **socio-cultural vacuum**: 'Psychological factors are always present, whether or not they are acknowledged by patients or therapists. They can be ignored, although their effect on pain may be powerful, or they can be systematically managed in such a way as to maximise pain relief' (IASP, 1992).

Think about this

Do you have chronic pain? A simple questionnaire is give in Table 14.1. Check through the questionnaire, and if you answer 'yes' to more than five questions then you probably have some form of chronic pain that can be helped by the methods discussed later in this chapter.

Table 14.1 Chronic pain questionnaire	**Question**
	1. Have you been experiencing strong pain three or more days a week for more than a month?
	2. Do you take painkillers four or more days a week?
	3. Do you often take painkillers to prevent pain before it begins?
	4. Has your pain been getting worse?
	5. Have you cancelled or avoided making social plans in the past month because you thought your pain would interfere with them?
	6. Do you ever drink alcohol to relieve your pain or the stress it produces?
	7. Have you seen more than three doctors about your pain?
	8. Are you afraid of performing physical activities, feeling they could elicit or aggravate your pain condition?
	9. Has you pain caused you to feel depressed and helpless for more than a couple of weeks or so?
	10. Do family or friends either seem annoyed by your pain or often ask how your pain is doing?

How to assess pain

In order to ease pain it is important to know how the patient/client feels. For example, with Mrs Heskey we would like to know where the pain is, what it feels like, how long it has occurred and how effective treatment has been and so on. We could then determine her readiness for treatment; to prioritise the type of intervention; to quantify how disruptiveness the problem has been to Mrs Heskey and her family; and then to assess the nature and impact of the patient's **implicit pain theory**. On this basis we could develop an appropriate intervention for Mrs Heskey.

There are a number of strategies that have been suggested that can help the health care professional measure pain. Depending on why, who and for how long you want to review will influence the selection of method.

Self-report measures

The most obvious method of measuring somebody's pain is simply to ask them! There are a number of methods, from the unstructured interview to the more formally structured rating scale. The **interview** discussions can focus on such items as the history of the pain, where the pain is, what it feels like and when it tends to occur, how strong the pain is, what treatments have been tried and what have/have not worked, emotional adjustment and the social context of the pain.

In terms of **self-report questionnaires** the simplest form is a **visual analogue scale** (VAS) with people simply marking a point on the scale which best describes their pain. For example, in its most simplest form a VAS would be from 'no pain' at one end of a 100 millimetre line to the 'worse pain possible' at the other. A variation on these is the verbal rating scale where people describe their pain by choosing a word or phrase from several that are given (see examples below). These scales can be used to measure how someone estimates their pain in general and how this changes over time, either with or without treatment. However, this scale only measures one form of pain – the intensity. Thus they only describe one element of the pain experience.

These are examples of a VAS:

No pain	0	1	2	3	4	5	6	7	8	9	10	Worst pain possible

No pain	_____	Worst pain possible

This is an example of a verbal rating scale:

No pain	Some pain	Considerable pain	Worst pain possible

Melzack (one of the key names in the psychology of pain) recognised the multi-dimensional nature of pain and suggested that these simple measures were not comprehensive enough. On the basis of this observation and some intensive research, the McGill pain questionnaire (MPQ; Melzack, 1975) was developed. There are two major elements to this questionnaire – the verbal descriptive scale consists of 102 pain descriptors which are sorted into groups describing different aspects of pain. These are classified into three major groups of words (example in Table 14.2): **sensory**, **affective** (emotional-motivational) and **evaluative**. The other component of the questionnaires is concerned with indicators of localisation, questions about medication and previous pain, change in pain over time, and a verbal rating scale of present pain intensity (PPI).

Table 14.2
Pain descriptors

Sensory	Affective	Evaluative
Flickering	Punishing	Annoying
Quivering	Gruelling	Troublesome
Pulsing	Cruel	Miserable
Throbbing	Vicious	Intense
Beating	Killing	Unbearable
Pounding		

The MPQ is the most well-known and widely used pain questionnaire and has many strengths as an instrument for assessing both acute and chronic pain. People in acute pain tend to score higher on the sensory descriptors while those in chronic pain score more highly on the emotional words. It has also been noted that people suffering from the same sort of conditions choose the same pattern of words. For example, those with a toothache are more

SHORT FORM McGILL PAIN QUESTIONNAIRE and PAIN DIAGRAM
(Reproduced with permission of author © Dr. Ron Melzack, for publication and distribution)

Date: _____
Name: _____

Check the column to indicate the level of your pain for each
word, or leave blank if it does not apply to you. —

	Mild	Moderate	Severe
1 Throbbing	—	—	—
2 Shooting	—	—	—
3 Stabbing	—	—	—
4 Sharp	—	—	—
5 Cramping	—	—	—
6 Gnawing	—	—	—
7 Hot-burning	—	—	—
8 Aching	—	—	—
9 Heavy	—	—	—
10 Tender	—	—	—
11 Splitting	—	—	—
12 Tiring-Exhausting	—	—	—
13 Sickening	—	—	—
14 Fearful	—	—	—
15 Cruel-Punishing	—	—	—

Mark or comment on the above figure
where you have had pain or problems.

Indicate on this line how bad your pain is – at the left end of the line means no pain at all, at right
end means worst pain possible.

No pain —————————————————————————— Worst possible pain

| S | /33 | A | /12 | VAS | /10 |

Figure 14.1 Short form of the McGill pain questionnaire.

Source: Melzack (1975)

likely to choose throbbing whereas those with arthritis are more likely to select punishing. However, the main limitation of the questionnaire is that the full version requires a fairly strong vocabulary (e.g. 'lancinating') and individuals are required to make fine distinctions between groups of words (e.g. 'beating' and 'pounding').

Behavioural measures

These assess the behaviours associated with pain – either counting them or observing how they change over time. For example, physical symptoms (e.g. limping or rubbing), verbal expressions (e.g. groaning or sighing) and facial expressions (e.g. grimacing or frowning). These measures are generally useful and can be used in either everyday situations or structured clinical sessions.

Physiological measures

Researchers have used putative physiological measurements of pain. For example, **electromyography (EMG)** can be used to measure muscle tension in patients with headaches and lower back pain. However, most research using these measures has failed to demonstrate a consistent relationship between these physiological measures and the experience of pain.

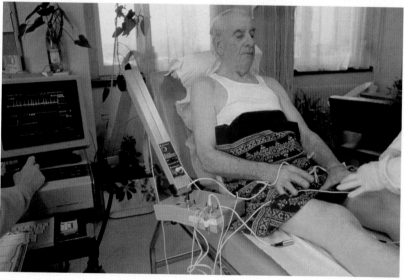

BSIP Laurent/Science Photo Library

Assessing children's pain

As mentioned, the assessment of pain using the MPQ requires strong verbal skills – something that can be missing from young children. In order to address this issue special forms of assessment methods are required. For example, pre-verbal children have to be assessed through observational methods (e.g. facial expressions, crying), older children can be assessed through picture-based pain scales (e.g. Figure 14.2).

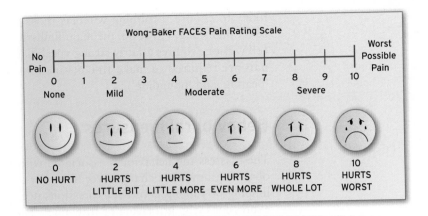

Figure 14.2 Example of the picture scale.

Source: Hockenberry, M.J., Wilson, D., Winkelstein, M.L.: *Wong's Essentials of Pediatric Nursing*, ed. 7, St. Louis, 2005, p. 1259. Used with permission. © Mosby

Think about this

How would you assess pain in these cases: a 6-month-old undergoing orthopaedic treatment, a 33-year-old man with chronic lower back pain, an 18-year-old woman undergoing dental treatment, an 88-year-old dementing adult and Mrs Heskey's case.

Concepts of pain

The first explanation of pain was provided by Descartes (1644) who (Melzack and Wall, 1973, p. 126): 'conceived of the pain system as a straight through channel from the skin to the brain'. That is, there was an injury in one particular bodily area and the hurt or damage in this area was transferred through the nervous system to the brain which experienced the pain. A development of this was the **specificity theory** developed by Von Frey in 1894 who assumed that there were specific sensory receptors responsible for the transmission of sensation, warmth and pain. All of these models have a series of underlying principles:

● Damage to the body causes the sensation of pain.
● Psychological reactions are a consequence of the pain.
● No psychological variables are associated with modifying the pain.
● Pain is an automatic response to injury.
● Pain has a single cause.
● There were only two forms of pain – organic ('real' pain when an injury was visible) or psychogenic ('all in the patient's mind').

If these models were correct then it should be relatively easy to treat pain by interfering with activity in pain pathways. Simple variations on this model are still around today: the linear-biomedical model. There are practitioners and treatments based on this thinking (that the pain is simply connected to the tissue damage experienced); this underlies the surgical treatment of pain explored later.

Think about this

Think about this simple biomedical model: what sort of evidence would suggest that this is an inadequate explanation? Think about the last time you experienced pain: what sort of things made it better or worse? Were any of these things non-physical actions and activities?

Problems with earlier models

These simple **linear models** (from injury through to the experience of pain) were very popular until the twentieth century, when it became increasingly recognised that there were many lines of evidence to suggest that a more complex model may be necessary. Firstly, it was noted that treatments for acute injury (e.g. medication) were not particularly useful for treating more long-lasting, chronic pain. Secondly, there was evidence that pain is not simply a direct response to a given stimulus – there were observations that different individuals with the same amount of tissue damage reported experiencing different levels of pain and required different levels of pain relief. A classic study that reported on this phenomenon is that of Beecher (1959). He

Soldiers in the Second World War

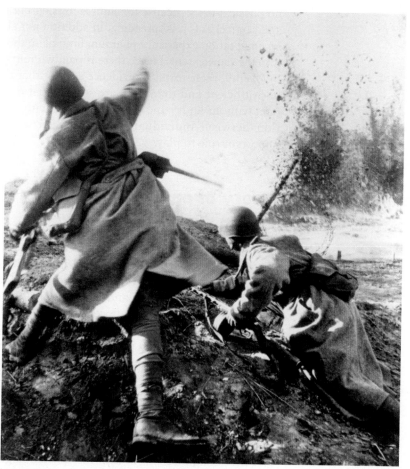

© Dmitri Baltermants/The Dmitri Baltermants Collection/Corbis

compared the pain experiences of civilians and soldiers during the Second World War. He found that similar levels of tissue damage needed greater levels of painkillers in civilians compared with soldiers. Only one in three required painkillers in the soldier group, whereas in the civilian group four out of five required medication. Beecher suggested that the meaning of the situation was affecting the pain. The soldiers' pain was offset by the fact that they had escaped death on the battlefield and were on their way home from the battle, whereas the civilian's pain had singularly negative connotations. This suggests that pain in itself is not simply a consequence of excited nerve impulses, but that psychological factors can play a part.

Think about this

Think about the work of Beecher. Have you come across this type of behaviour in clinical work – how a person's pain alters depending on the situation they are in? How do you think you could use this work to improve the experience of pain patients?

Another form of evidence is that of **phantom limbs** where there are no nerve transmissions, but there is pain. People who have lost limbs through amputation often have severe pain in the missing limbs. Phantom limb pain has no physical basis because the limb is missing but the pain can feel excruciating and can feel as if it is spreading. In addition not all those who have experienced an amputation experience phantom limb pain; those who do, do not experience it to the same extent. Hence there is pain without physical activation.

Overall, these forms of evidence suggest that the linear-biomedical model is not sufficient and that there are some variations among individuals: there is pain without injury and there is no pain with injury. Since there is this variation between individuals then it is perhaps psychology which has an important role to play.

The gate control theory of pain

In order to overcome some of the problems identified, Melzack (a psychologist) and Wall (an anatomist) published a new theory of pain: 'the gate control theory' (Melzack and Wall, 1965). It combined both a biomedical element and a psychological element. It described a role for both physiological causes and interventions and psychological causes and interventions. The simple description of the gate control theory is that pain is a consequence of pain messages. These pain messages travel through a gate: if the gate is open then more pain messages get through and hence more pain is experienced. On the other hand, if the gate is closed then fewer pain messages get through and so less pain is experienced.

The central idea of gate control theory is the presence of **neural mechanisms** in the spinal cord which can somehow close a gate, and so prevent pain messages from travelling to the brain (obviously this gate can also be opened and therefore allow the message to travel to the brain). The theory proposes that the gating mechanism is in the **substantia gelatinosa** of the dorsal horns, which are part of the grey matter of the spinal cord (Figure 14.3).

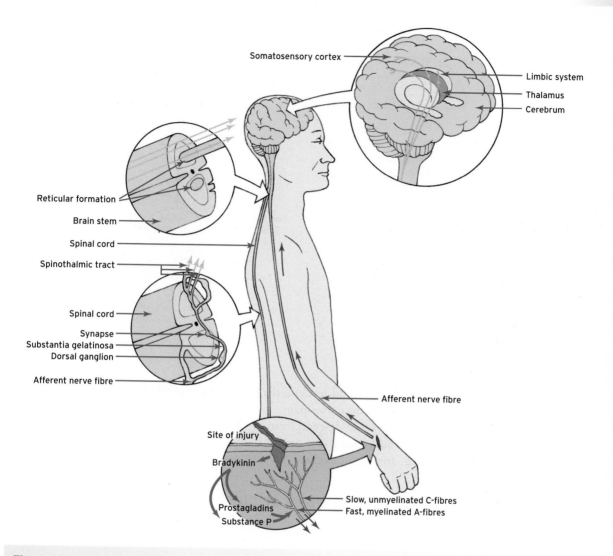

Figure 14.3 Anatomy of the gate control theory of pain.

Source: www.wildirismedicaleducation.com

In the model (Figure 14.4) you can note that signals from the injury enter the gating mechanism (substantia gelatinosa) of the spinal cord from pain fibres (A-delta and C fibres). After these signals pass through the gating mechanism they activate transmission cells which send impulses to the brain. When the signals reach a critical level the person perceives pain: the greater the output beyond this level, the greater the pain intensity. When the pain signals enter the spinal cord and the gate is open the transmission cells send impulses freely. But if the gate is closed then the output of the transmission cells is inhibited. The following factors close or open the gate:

- The amount of activity in the pain fibre: the greater the injury the active the pain fibres, the more open the gate.
- The amount of activity in other peripheral fibres: some small fibres, A-beta fibres, carry information about harmless stimuli (e.g. touching or rubbing

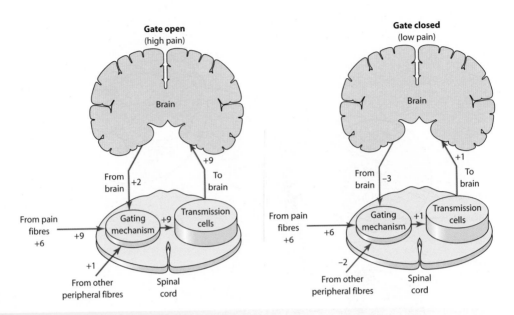

Figure 14.4 Gate control theory model of pain.

Source: Sarafino (2005)

of the skin) tend to close the gate. Hence, gentle massage or applying heat to muscles decreases pain.

- Messages that descend from the brain: impulses from neurons in the brain-stem and cortex can open or close the gate. The effects of some of these (e.g. anxiety or excitement) may open or close the gate.

What factors open or close the gate?

Emotional factors

Factors that open the gate (i.e. make the pain worse):

- Anxiety: the more anxious a person is the worse the pain experienced.
- Worry: the less worried a person the less pain they experience.
- Tension: the greater the tension the greater the pain.
- Depression: the greater the pain the greater the depression, and the greater the depression the greater the pain.

Factors that close the gate (i.e. reduce the pain):

- Happiness: If you are happy then there is likely to be less pain.
- Optimism: the more optimistic you are the less likely the pain.
- Relaxation: if a person is more relaxed and rested then they are likely to experience less pain.

Cognitive and behavioural factors

Factors that opens the gate (i.e. make the pain worse):

- Focusing on the pain: if you focus in on the pain then there is likely to be an increase in the pain experienced.

- Boredom: little involvement in life's activities and the greater the pain (think about how this links to Mrs Heskey).

Factors that close the gate (i.e. reduce the pain):

- Concentration and distraction: if a person is distracted or concentrates on another activity then the pain is likely to be less.
- Involvement and interest in life activities: if the person is bored with life, or has little involvement with other activities other than focus on the pain then they will experience greater pain. Hence there is a need to develop interest in life's activities.
- Reactions of others: the way others react can influence pain. (Again, think about how Eddie and the children are impacting on Mrs Heskey's pain – are they making it better or worse?)

Physical factors

Factors that open the gate (i.e. make the pain worse):

- Extent and type of injury: a relatively obvious one – the greater the extent of injury, the more likely the gate is to be open to let the pain messages through.
- Inappropriate activity level: the lower the activity, the greater the pain experienced.

Factors that close the gate (i.e. reduces the pain):

- Medication: certain forms of medication will lead to a decrease in pain.
- Counter-stimulation (e.g. heat or massage): with certain types of pain (muscle strain for example) some form of heat or massage will help reduce the pain.

Think about this

Consider how these factors can be used in the management of pain. How can you use these factors to open or close the gate in order to reduce pain? Think about a recent experience in clinic: using a technique other than a medical one, how could you have suggested reducing the pain the individual was suffering?

Problems with the gate control theory

The gate control theory has been a great advancement over the previous models of pain and has stimulated a great deal of research since its initial description. Most, although not all, of these studies have offered support for the proposals. However, there are several problems with the model. Firstly, although a great deal of investigation has centred on the search for the neural mechanism of the 'gate', there has been little advance. Secondly, the input is still physiological rather than psychological. Hence, although the input from the injury is mediated by psychological factors, the model still assumes an organic basis for pain processes and is still based around a simple stimulus response process. Finally, although the gate control theory attempts to integrate mind and body it still sees them as separate processes. However, this being said, the gate control theory has 'been the most influential and important current theory of pain perception' (Weisenberg, 1977, p. 1012).

Management of pain

The management of acute pain and chronic pain are, obviously, different. However, they share many common elements in the form of approaches that may be useful. Hence in this section each of these types of approach will be explored and how it can be applied to both acute and chronic pain. The benefits and problems for the nurse and patient for each of these approaches will also be outlined. However, with all of these approaches it is important to remember that as Kanner (1986, p. 2113) notes: 'There is no single answer to pain' and that **multi-modal methods** may be required.

Methods of pain management

The most obvious method of pain management is by *pharmacological interventions*. These are most useful in reducing acute pain in the short term and can be extremely effective. There are many forms of drugs that can be taken to reduce acute pain. Analgesics (such as aspirin and ibuprofen) reduce fever and inflammation by interfering with the transmission of pain signals. Narcotics (e.g. codeine and morphine) work by inhibiting the transmission of pain signals and can be very effective at reducing severe pain. Local anaesthetics (e.g. for tooth pain or for an epidural) work by blocking the nerve cells in a small region from generating impulses.

Although effective drug treatments are available, not all patients receive appropriate pain relief 'resulting in the needless suffering of countless millions of patients' (IASP, 1992, p. 3). Indeed, there is often the tendency to prescribe drugs without consideration of the pain being experienced by the individual – rather on the basis of what pain the person is *thought* or *expected* to be in. This may result in many patients remaining in pain. A survey of over 3000 individuals discharged from hospital showed that some 87 per cent reported moderate or severe pain on leaving hospital (Bruster *et al.*, 1994). In children the picture is the same: Karling *et al.* (2002) reported that almost three-quarters of those children discharged were in pain and that a quarter of these were experiencing moderate or severe pain.

The prescribing of pain medication may also be influenced by the expectations of the health care professional of the patient. For example, it is suggested that men are viewed as 'tough' or 'macho' and hence are often prescribed less medication than a woman, irrespective of the individual's rating of pain. Similarly, those cultures that express their emotions more openly than others may have higher levels of medication than their counterparts, irrespective of the amount of pain that the individual may be in (Zborowski, 1952).

For example, Green *et al.* (2003) report on a number of pain differences in ethnic groups. For example, African-American patients were less likely to seek treatment for chest pain, to receive less anti-ischaemic therapy for chest pain, and to use less analgesic medication post-operatively than White

Americans. Marked ethnic differences in response to acute post-operative following limb fracture pain have also be found with White Americans having more pain medication than either African-Americans or Hispanics.

Think about this

What implications does the study of Zborowski (1952) and subsequent reports have for your professional practice? What warnings does it suggest for those trying to reduce pain in patients from different cultures?

Although medication for pain may be useful in the short term, it can lead to problems in the long term. The first problem may be that medication may not be sufficient in itself to manage and control pain since there may be more psychological explanations for the pain or the psychological factors may be more important than the physiological ones for treating the pain. There are a number of other problems that may arise in certain cases when an individual is prescribed drugs for chronic pain. Firstly, **tolerance** to the drug may occur, as may **dependence** (both physical and psychological). This may result in others – whether these be the patient's family, friends or health care practitioner – viewing the patient as 'addicted' to medication or 'weak'. Obviously, if this is expressed frequently and forcibly then the patient may also begin to see themselves as being 'weak' and a 'failure'. With this may come lower self-esteem, a lack of hope and demoralisation and resulting psychological problems. As predicted by the gate control theory these factors may open the gate and this may result in increased pain which, in a vicious cycle, results in an increase in the prescribing of pain medication.

Although these events can occur in some people some of the time, it does not mean that all of those with chronic pain should immediately be weaned off their medication! Far from it. For example, it is generally agreed that those with pain as a result of terminal cancer should have effective drug management. However, the undesirable side-effects of some medication, the possibility of tolerance and dependence and the lack of effect of some medication in isolation suggest that drug control of chronic pain will prove difficult in a large number of cases. Hence, other methods of controlling chronic pain are required.

Surgical methods

If the pain becomes severe or persistent enough then a surgical approach to pain management may be suggested. The thinking behind this technique is relatively straightforward: if the pain pathway to the brain is broken then the pain message cannot get through. Hence the surgery involves the division of nerve pathways, either by severing or destroying them, that reduce the perception of pain. This technique is most commonly used in those with chronic low back pain (mainly in the United States).

The technique is not particularly successful, however, and there may be limited benefits. Indeed, there may be some negative consequences: numbness, pins and needles and even paralysis in the region involved in the surgery. Furthermore, since pain messages can travel to the brain via different routes the pain may return in a month or two after the surgery.

Transcutaneous electrical nerve stimulation (TENS)

TENS involves stimulating the skin area over the site of the pain, using an electrical stimulator, and thereby replacing the pain messages with a tingling sensation. This form of pain management is reported to be effective in some form of chronic conditions: phantom limb pain, labour and pain following surgery in some individuals. However, despite being extensively used, the effectiveness of TENS is not firmly established (Khadilkar *et al.*, 2005) and the success rating in a range of studies has been mixed. The major methodological problem has been the lack of sufficient numbers and placebo-control groups in the studies.

Biofeedback

Biofeedback involves the monitoring of physiological data (e.g. heart rate, muscle activity, brain wave patterns and skin response) which are then presented to the patient, who attempts to control and change these biological variables. For example, a patient's muscle group is wired to an EMG machine and the results of the muscle tension presented to the patient. The patient is then shown how the muscle tension can be increased or decreased, by either tensing their muscles or relaxing. By providing feedback on how the biological variables respond, the patient over time learns how to control their physiological responses by changing thoughts or behaviour.

Biofeedback has been used in cases such as tension headaches, migraines and lower back pain. Vasudeva *et al.* (2003) reported that using biofeedback techniques in those with migraine headaches reduced their reports of pain, depression and anxiety. The biofeedback treatment involved the patients learning to control their cerebral blood flow velocity which was measured in

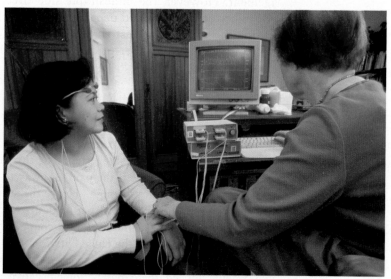

Michael Newman/PhotoEdit

the middle **cerebral artery** with a **transcranial Doppler** test. However, biofeedback can often be time consuming and expensive, especially as it is often considered nothing more than relaxation.

Relaxation is often a component of biofeedback so it is worth exploring this form of intervention for chronic pain. Most commonly, relaxation is used as a treatment for headache or migraine. The thinking behind these relaxation approaches to tension headache, for example, is relatively straightforward: tension headaches are assumed to result from persistent muscle contractions around the head, neck and shoulders and if this occurs, then relaxing these muscles should have the opposite effect – relaxed and pain free (there are, of course, other theories of headache development).

Since there appears to be a link between the tension and the pain then a suitable intervention would be **progressive muscle relaxation (PMR)** (see Chapter 13). In essence the PMR approach involves the tensing and relaxing of muscles to demonstrate to the patient the difference between the two and are taught how best to relax. They will also be taught to identify the signs of an onset of a pain episode so they can start to relax early to prevent the pain from increasing. It is not only the PMR method that can be used to relax and reduce the tension and hence the pain – there are a number of other forms of relaxation techniques.

Does relaxation work for various forms of pain? Yes, according to some reviews (e.g. Sarafino and Goehring, 2000), but not according to others (Carroll and Seers, 1998). However, the consensus appears to be that (as is often the case) the pain can be reduced by relaxation in certain people and as such should play a part in any multi-modal pain management programme. Whether they are effective as a stand-alone intervention is debatable.

Acupuncture

Although acupuncture may be useful in certain cases – dental surgery, lower back pain, headache pain – the evidence on its overall efficacy is equivocal and, ultimately, it is probably down to individual differences between patients. Manheimer *et al.* (2005) present a systematic review to suggest that acupuncture can reduce pain levels in individuals with lower back pain but the effects of the treatment were not as impressive when compared with other forms of more traditional treatment. Trinh *et al.* (2004) report another review that suggest that there is no evidence for the effectiveness of acupuncture in tennis elbow. Hence, overall, it is argued that the benefits may simply be a result of distraction rather than any underlying physiological or medical reason. This being said acupuncture can help some as part of an overall package of treatment.

Hypnotism

Hypnosis refers to an altered state of consciousness brought about by a trained therapist. There are anecdotal reports of hypnotised patients undergoing cardiac surgery, Caesarean sections and appendectomies with no medication. There are two main schools of thoughts about the effectiveness of it in the treatment of chronic pain: it works (e.g. Barber, 1998) or that it works merely as a placebo or that it is a relaxation technique (e.g. Spanos and Katsanis,

1989). Overall, however, the evidence is not substantial enough to be used in place of psychological or medical methods in the treatment of pain.

Take it easy

In this 'treatment' the patient is advised to take it easy with rest, and to avoid social, leisure and work activities. This can go on for a number of months and the patient will become more and more inactive. Ultimately, they avoid more and more activities and this can cause an increased focus on the pain since they no longer have any other activities on which to focus. Their lives tend to revolve around the pain and its treatment. As loss of rewards from the environment continues there is an increase in depression. Finally depression can lead to a greater increase in pain and a vicious downward spiral can develop.

Behaviour

Behavioural approaches to the treatment of pain were first applied by Fordyce *et al.* (1984). The behavioural approach argues that pain is a series of pain behaviours (or **operants**) and that pain can either be increased by reinforcing these pain behaviours (i.e. **positive reinforcement**) or by individuals avoiding an unpleasant or aversive situation (i.e. **negative reinforcement**). For example, it is argued that people in pain often receive certain benefits – attention seeking, comforting and sometimes even financial benefits. They also avoid unpleasant experiences – going to work or having to help out around the house may be examples.

In a behavioural approach the pain behaviours are noted – for example how often the patient makes an audible remark (e.g. moaning), expression (e.g. grimacing teeth), distorted posture or movement (e.g. limping), negative affect (e.g. depression) or avoidance of activity (e.g. not walking). The behavioural approach deals with these behaviours. Initially the patient is asked to do something small (e.g. walk a few paces) and this is reinforced by the health care practitioners and the family. In contrast to negative reinforcement the pain behaviours are left unrewarded. Hence, the grimaces are ignored and not reinforced by health care professionals. Important to the behavioural approach is the patient's family – it has been found that those with chronic pain are more likely to have 'caring' and 'over-supportive' families. Hence the patient's family are trained not to reinforce pain behaviours by not providing sympathy or reduction in domestic work. At the same time the pain medication is reduced and given on a time-based basis rather than on need as

Think about this

Think about the case of Mrs Heskey: how would you assess her pain behaviours? What sort of pain behaviours does she show? How are Eddie and her children reinforcing her pain behaviours? How could you try to reduce her pain behaviours by involving the rest of her family? What sort of difficulties do you think you would face?

expressed by the patient. Over time, this period is lengthened and/or the dosage reduced.

There is evidence to suggest that this behavioural approach can be quite effective for increasing activity levels, exercise tolerance and decreasing pain medication intake (Roelofs *et al.*, 2002) and this is especially true if the patient's family is involved and fully supportive of the programme. However, there are some problems with this approach. Firstly, the very basis of the behavioural intervention is not necessarily about the experience of pain, but rather improving the behavioural functioning of pain patients. Hence, detractors argue that the pain experienced is not reduced but only the outward manifestation of the pain. Roelofs *et al.* (2002) also suggest that the evidence shows there is no reduction in subjective measures of pain. Overall, therefore, patients still report the same amount of pain, but they did not show it. Furthermore, detractors of the behavioural approach argue that as soon as the intervention ends, the old pattern of inactivity and pain behaviour reappear. It should also be evident that this type of programme may not be suitable for all – certainly those with progressive chronic pain (e.g. cancer sufferers) would not benefit in the long term. Finally, although these types of approach can be effective in the long term they can be hard for the patient to complete and there is a large drop-out rate from programmes with this form of intervention. In certain cases this drop-out rate can be as much as one-third of all people on the programme.

Cognitive approach

Cognitive therapists stress that the way people think is important in their experience of pain. It is these thoughts that are the target for change in any cognitive programme. Often this approach is combined with a behavioural approach and is known as **cognitive behavioural therapy (CBT)**.

In terms of a person's cognitions, when we have an injection in hospital we may be thinking, 'This is going to hurt' or 'I'm scared of needles' or 'I am really anxious – I can hear my heart pounding'. All of these thoughts are more likely to increase the pain of the injection rather than reduce it since they focus the attention on the unpleasant aspects of the experience. Others having an injection may think to themselves 'I am going to be brave about this' or 'This is nothing, I have had worse' or 'Was that it?' and this may help reduce the amount of pain experienced. Obviously if somebody can help the patient reconceptualise their pain in a more positive light then the patient may be more likely to experience less pain. Cognitive therapy includes three elements:

- Patients are taught to reconceptualise their pain by emphasising how it can be controlled by thoughts, feelings and beliefs.
- Imagery and diversion techniques are important.
- The practice and consolidation of these techniques in general situations is assessed.

This script, taken from Holzman *et al.* (1986, pp. 45–46), highlights how the therapist helped the client examine the logic of her thought patterns and generate a list of ideas she believed that were incompatible with her irrational fears and hence reduce the amount of pain involved.

Therapist:	You know that all the tests have not shown anything: there is no brain tumour.
Patient:	Yes, I know they're not true but I cannot help it.
Therapist:	You don't think you have control over your thoughts.
Patient:	Yes, they come back to me.
Therapist:	Well, let's come back to the idea that your thoughts are automatic. First, let's break down your flood of negative thoughts and look at each part separately. Do you really think you have a tumour?
Patient:	I don't know. I guess not [pause] but it's hard not to worry about it. My head hurts so bad.
Therapist:	Yes, I know. So how do you convince yourself that you don't have a tumour or something else seriously wrong?
Patient:	Well, as you know I've been examined many times by the best neurologists around. They say I'm OK. Also, my pain never goes away and I've never had any other neurological problems. My only problem is the pain. But, it's hard to remember these facts when my pain is so awful.
Therapist:	It's much easier to be positive about your condition when you're not suffering. Nevertheless, rationally, you really are convinced that there's nothing seriously wrong.
Patient:	I guess so. If only I could remember that when my pain starts coming on.
Therapist:	So the goal of our work today could be to figure out a strategy to increase the likelihood that remembers the positive thoughts during a pain episode.
Patient:	Yes, that sounds good.
Therapist:	Let's start by generating a list of accurate statements about your pain. Then we can talk about ways you can cue yourself to remember the list when you begin to feel pain. You already mentioned a couple of beliefs about your pain: that is, that there's nothing seriously wrong, that the pain always goes away, and that, other than the pain, you feel pretty healthy. Can you think of other accurate and positive thoughts?

The cognitive (or cognitive-behavioural) approach can be used in both acute or chronic pain situations. There are a number of cognitive techniques that can be used when attempting to deal with pain (Table 14.3).

	Technique	Example
Table 14.3 Cognitive techniques	Distraction	This is a technique where the focus of attention is away from the painful experience. For example in dental surgery there is often a poster or hanging mobile from the ceiling as you sit in the chair receiving your filling. In a hospital setting asking a child to watch TV while they receive an injection might distract them from the experience. Furthermore, if they were asked to concentrate on the programme ('Describe what is happening') then they experience less pain. Getting the patient to sing a song or do multiplication tables are other techniques which may help distract the patient from the procedure.
	Imagery	If the patient is told to think about something pleasant then this may alleviate pain: for example, asking them to imagine lying on a beach with the waves gently lapping the shore and a summer breeze wafting through the palm trees (note the therapist is *guiding* the imagery). However, it does not have to be a gentle relaxing scene – some patients may wish to imagine they are watching a horse race or a football match. This form of technique is similar to the distraction technique, other than it is an imaginary event rather than a real event or object that is the distraction.
	Pain redefinition	The patient is asked to redefine their pain in more positive terms. As in the examples given above, 'I can handle this pain', or 'I can deal with this pain and I will be better after this'.

Morley *et al.* (1999) presented a systematic review of 25 trials of CBT for chronic pain (other than headache) in adults. They demonstrated that the treatment was more effective than alternative active treatment approaches (e.g. relaxation, exercise and education) or **waiting list controls**. Hence, CBT seems to be an effective way to reduce pain. Eccleston *et al.* (2002) reported similar conclusions for studies using CBT in children and adolescents.

Typical multi-modal programme

Psychological treatment

The psychological management of chronic pain is characterised by the use of a variety of techniques. This was best expressed by Keefe (1982): 'These programs share one common assumption: if chronic pain is complex, then a combination of treatment techniques is needed to successfully treat patients' (p. 903).

There are a number of approaches to pain management that may be useful for both acute and chronic pain. Acute pain can be dealt with successfully with both drug and psychological therapies in combination, with the emphasis on the former. For chronic pain it is worth repeating that 'if chronic pain is complex, then a combination of treatment techniques is needed to successfully treat patients' (Keefe, 1982, p. 903). This has been the basis of a typical multi-modal pain programme. The aims of a psychological pain management programme are generally considered to be

Typical distraction techniques for children

Distraction techniques, like the assessment, have to differ in children according to their developmental stage. According to Duff (2003) there are a number of rating scales/distraction techniques that can be used with children across variable age ranges and these are presented in the table.

Age	Pain measurement	Distraction technique
0-3 months	Biophysiological: heart rate, palm sweat	Oral glucose Rocking Dummy Blowing bubbles, singing
3-6 months	Observation: length of crying Parental reports	As above
6-18 months	Behavioural ratings (Neonatal Facial Action Coding System: N-FACS)	Action rhymes, kaleidoscopes, party blowers, touch, bubble blowing
18-24 months	As above	As above
24-36 months	As above	Simple cognitive strategies: counting, being read stories, music, drawing
36-60 months	Gross indications: 'no pain, little pain, lots of pain'. Can grossly mark on diagram where the pain is located	As above
5-7 years	Self-rating: accurately mark on body outline. Faces scale, pain ladders	Guided imagery Engagement in fantasy scenes
7-11 years	Visual analogue scales Likert scales	Listening to music Reading
11+ years	As above	As above

Source: Archives of Disease in Childhood, 2003, Vol. 88, 931–937, reproduced with permission from the BMJ Publishing Group

multi-faceted in nature. Firstly, it is important that the concept of pain management rather than cure is introduced to both the client and their family. In this way expectations are managed and the client is not expecting something that will be unfulfilled. Secondly, each person is encouraged to believe that they have control over their own situation – attempting to get the individual to consider that they have control over their own personal well-being rather than viewing it as a medical problem that must be 'treated' by a professional with no input from them. In this way it should be possible to enable and encourage each person to achieve control of their own situation. As part of any programme one of the key aims is to increase the participant's knowledge and understanding of factors that contribute to pain management (such as those outlined above) and to get the individual to use these in order to set goals for them and their family. If the programme is run as a group offering then it is likely that an environment that enables participants to gain support from group processes and sharing can be developed. Hence, rather than seeing the problem as individualistic, there is a possibility of learning from each of the group members and, thereby, promoting active questioning to clarify understanding and knowledge. The group is also useful in that it allows for the development of personal skills and the highlighting (and hopefully changing) of unhelpful habits which may be contributing to the pain. As part of the group process each member of the group will, hopefully, become more confident and improve their self-esteem. With the development of these personal attributes along with the development of skills and knowledge, it should ensure that each member of the group is fully equipped to continue to work independently at improving their pain management skills once the course has ended.

Although this provides an overview of the type of course programme it does not really provide any specific details. This is because many of the programmes can be tailored depending on the type of pain being experienced. For example, chronic pain will be treated differently from pain of a shorter duration. An example of the type of elements included in a programme for post-operative pain is included in Table 14.4. This method has been called the BASIC-ID (Lazarus, 1973) method and provides a useful mnemonic for remembering all the individual elements of such a programme.

Table 14.4
Programme for post-operative pain

B *Behavioural*: Do not reinforce pain behaviours (e.g. winces, complaints). Reinforce healthy behaviours (e.g. getting out of bed, behaving as normally as possible). It is important to involve the patient, the family and any support staff in these programmes to maximise success rates.

A *Affect*: Try to deal with any depression or emotional problems after the operation. As previously outlined, anxiety or depression can open the 'gate' and thereby increase the pain. Both conditions can be treated by psychological therapy and therefore intervening to assist with these psychological problems can also help to reduce the pain.

S *Sensation*: The area of pain sensation needs to be reduced or altered to a less painful feeling. This is really a component of imagery since the health care professional should try to get the patient to think of the pain in more positive ways (e.g. warmth) rather than a searing pain.

I *Imagery*: Try to get the patient to imagine positive thoughts and imagine good scenes (e.g. palm beaches, being fit and well). Again this may have to be guided imagery with the nurse or health care professional helping or guiding the patient through the imagined scene.

C *Cognitions*: The patient should think in a positive manner – the positives of the outcome of the operation rather than the pain itself. Rather than thinking 'This hurts' the patient should be taught to consider the pain to be 'worth it' or 'something I can handle for the good of my health'.

I *Interpersonal relationships*: Try to involve the family and friends of the patient in any programme. With their support progress is more likely.

D *Drugs*: The pain relief drugs should be reduced over time. In the initial instance the pain-relieving drugs should be provided but then offered on a time-based schedule rather than on demand (obviously there are exceptions!).

These elements are combined into programmes promoted across the country and combine medical, psychological and physiotherapy interventions. A typical programme from the United Kingdom would follow this sort of timetable:

Week 1	Introduction to the programme
	Introduction to exercise
	Stress and rehabilitation
Week 2	Pacing activity
	Seating
	Exercise session
	Deep muscle relaxation
Week 3	Goal setting
	Lifting
	Exercise and relaxation
Week 4	Pain pathways
	Gate control theory of pain
	Mid-course evaluation
Week 5	Thoughts and feelings
	Drugs and doctors
	Exercise session
	Self-hypnosis for pain
	Pain and sex
Week 6	Benefits of exercise
	Fitness
	Relatives session
	Self-hypnosis
Week 7	Pain behaviours and communication
	Exercise fitness circuit
Week 8	Beds and sleeping
	Autogenic relaxation
	Flare-up plans
	Evaluation

Outcomes of psychological interventions

Is there any evidence for the effectiveness of these programmes? To take one example, Dysvik *et al.* (2004) reported on the effectiveness of a multi-modal programme for the management of chronic pain. The authors recruited 76 patients, all of whom had chronic non-malignant pain (57 per cent had musculoskeletal pain, 16 per cent had headaches, 13 per cent had abdominal pain and the rest had other forms of chronic pain). The intervention was active and time-limited over an eight week period and included a multi-modal, CBT-based programme along with education and physical therapy. All participants were asked to evaluate their **quality of life** and their current pain intensity (using a VAS as previously described) at both the start of the programme and at the end of the intervention.

At the end of the intervention there was a significant improvement in mental health, vitality, social functioning, physical functioning and health transition. Furthermore, there was an improvement in pain intensity from 6.6 cm (on a 10 cm VAS) to 6.2 cm. However, although this was a statistically significant reduction, the clinical importance of this result is debatable and may be dependent on the characteristic of both the patient and the condition being treated.

Problems with pain programmes

Although these studies have reported a generally positive result (as in the example provided above from Dysvik *et al.*, 2004) there are a number of problems that have been raised when examining the evidence for the multi-component methods of pain management:

- Selectivity of patients: are patients typical of the pain patients? This study used a range of patients which means the group was **heterogeneous**. What conclusions can be drawn from the data on individual patients?
- Lack of **reinforcement** following programmes can mean behaviour becomes extinct. That is, once the patients leave the hospital the problems re-appear. The follow-up for this study was minimal: simply after the programme.
- It is difficult to identify the most efficient components of the programmes: they are all multi-faceted. Hence, why bother to provide all the interventions if it is just one component that is the effective one?
- The fluctuating nature of chronic disease is not taken into account: the pain could get better all by itself. Hence, the studies have to be carefully designed in order to prevent this occurring. In the example given, there was no control group so the patients may have improved because of time.
- Are patients simply trained to be more stoical? That is, they just suffer in silence more? This is certainly the case with behavioural interventions. The pain is not shown any more, but it still may be experienced.

Conclusion

Pain is a key concept for nursing as it is one of the most common occurrences in health care. Previously the view of pain was merely as a medical perspective, but there is now a recognition that there are considerable psychological factors involved in its experience. Consequently there are now numerous psychological approaches to the management of pain which can easily be incorporated, where necessary, into nursing care.

Research in focus

Haythornwaite, J.A., Lawrence, J.W., and Fauerbach, J.A. (2001) Brief cognitive interventions for burn patients. *Annals of Behavioural Medicine*, **23**(1), 42–49.

Background
When treating severe burns, regular changes in dressing and **debridement** of the affected area is required and this can cause severe pain despite treatment with medication (usually **opioid** medication). The use of psychological techniques to help reduce the experience of pain has been explored but the specific techniques that could be used have yet to be fully articulated. This study sought to explore whether particular psychological techniques (e.g. distraction or sensory focusing strategies) would help reduce pain and provide pain relief during burn dressing changes.

Method
Participants: The participants were 42 adult patients with burn wounds (32 men and 10 women) with an average age of 44 years that required hospitalisation due to severe burns. The percentage of the total body surface with a second or third degree burn ranged between 3 per cent and 65 per cent.

Intervention: Patients were split into one of three groups: (i) usual care with no additional psychological input; (ii) sensory focusing technique in which patients were instructed to focus their attention on their sensory experience during the dressing change; (iii) distraction techniques during which patients were given an extensive list of music to listen to and taught how to focus their attention on aspects of the music.

Measures: Patients with burns completed a series of questionnaires – a visual analogue scale for intensity of pain; a degree of pain relief due to the intervention (on an 11 point scale); level of satisfaction with their ability to control their pain; the coping with pain questionnaire which included a number of sub-scales: reinterpreting pain sensations, catastrophising and ignoring pain sensations; depression scale; and the total amount of analgesic medications.

Results
The results indicated that sensory focusing techniques increased ratings of pain relief and reduced patients' memories for pain during the procedure. Distraction did not show any beneficial effects. However, there was no reduction in pain ratings or improved patient satisfaction with either technique which was inconsistent with previous studies in this area. One suggested reason for the unclear results was the limited number of participants in the study.

Implications
Although there were some inconsistent results, the sensory focusing procedure showed 'some important benefits and deserves continued attention in future research' (p. 47). In particular, the technique resulted in a reduction in catastrophising thoughts which the authors considered important. This was essential, the authors claim, since catastrophising is an important predictor of pain experience in the acute setting of the burn treatment unit. It is suggested that sensory focusing techniques altered the cognitions associated with the pain experienced during the treatment whereas the distraction technique had no impact on the thoughts of the individual patient. Consequently, cognitive techniques can and should be used in those experiencing severe acute pain.

Summary

- Early models of pain were linear – there was a transmission of pain from the site of the injury to the brain and pain response.

- The gate control theory suggested a gate in the spinal cord which could be opened (to increase the pain) or closed (to decrease the pain).

- The gate control theory suggested a new conceptualisation of pain in which both psychological and physical factors could influence pain.

- Critics of the gate control theory suggest that no physiological basis has been uncovered, that the input is physical rather than psychological and that the mind and body are still seen as separate.

- Drug therapy for acute pain can be extremely effective. There needs to be, however, consistent review of the approach taken to ensure that maximum pain relief is achieved.

- There are a number of psychological methods for the management of chronic pain.

- Medical methods for treating chronic pain can result in a poor psychological outcome, and some approaches are not particularly successful.

- Psychological interventions have to be multi-modal involving Behavioural, Affect, Sensation, Imagery, Cognition Interpersonal relationship and Drug reduction (BASIC-ID).

- Behavioural approaches focus on pain behaviours and are useful, although the drop-out rate is high.

- Since low affect can increase pain, the improvement in affect can result in better pain management.

- Imagery techniques are also of use in pain management.

- The re-interpretation of pain sensation can be useful.

- Cognitive techniques aimed at altering illogical thinking can assist in the reduction of chronic pain.

- Relationships between patient and his/her family are of key importance in the behavioural management of pain.

- Drugs need to be reduced in order for more multi-modal programmes to be successful.

- Psychological interventions are successful in reducing reports of pain.

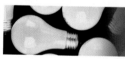

Check your understanding

1. How was pain conceptualised in the past, and how much is the gate control theory an advancement of previous models of pain?

2. How can psychological factors inherent in the health care system increase pain?

3. What psychological techniques can be used by the nurse to manage pain?

4. Consider each of the following cases and devise a programme for managing their pain: (i) a 12-month-old infant having regular injections; (ii) a teenager undergoing chemotherapy; (iii) Mrs Heskey; (iv) an individual with chronic headaches.

5. How useful is psychology in understanding and managing pain?

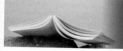

Further reading

Horn, S. and Munafo, M. (1997) *Pain. Theory, Research and Intervention.* Buckingham: Open University Press.

Weblinks

Systematic reviews on pain	http://www.jr2.ox.ac.uk/bandolier/painres/MApain.html	Bandolier list of all systematic reviews on pain (up until 1999).
University of Bath pain links	http://bath.ac.uk/pain-management	A thorough set of links from this recognised department.
Liverpool University Pain Research Institute	http://www.liv.ac.uk/pri/html/institute.html	The Pain Research Institute is part of the University of Liverpool, Department of Neurological Science. The Institute carries out research into the causes and treatment of chronic pain in humans.
International Association for the Study of Pain (IASP)	http://www.iasp-pain.org/	IASP is a non-profit professional organisation dedicated to furthering research on pain and improving the care of patients with pain.
The UK Pain Society	http://www.britishpainsociety.org/	The British Pain Society is the largest multidisciplinary professional organisation in the field of pain within the UK. Their membership comprises medical pain specialists, nurses, physiotherapists, scientists, psychologists, occupational therapists and other healthcare professionals actively engaged in the diagnosis and treatment of pain and in pain research for the benefit of patients.
The Oxford Pain Internet Site	http://www.jr2.ox.ac.uk/bandolier/booth/painpag/	This site is for anyone with a professional or personal interest in pain and analgesia. It is firmly based in the principles of evidence-based medicine and has pulled together systematic reviews with pain as an outcome.
Back pain guide	http://www.spine-health.com/topics/cd/pain/ chronic_pain_theories/chronic_pain_theory01.html	Provides a good, introductory overview on the models of pain.
	http://www.partnersagainstpain.com/	An excellent title!

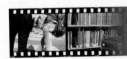

Media examples

Rambo and *Die Hard* Showing how despite physical injuries Sylvester Stallone and Bruce Willis still manage to get to the end of the film! These films demonstrate the importance of drive and psychological factors in mediating the painful consequences of a range of physical injuries suffered.

Chapter 15

Psychological models in health and health care

Learning outcomes

When you have read through this chapter you should understand:

- The role of psychological models in understanding the health and health behaviour of individual clients and patients.
- Locus of control (LoC) and how individuals can be classified into internal LoC, external LoC and powerful others LoC and what impact this has on behaviour.
- The health belief model (HBM) and how it can be used with individuals to improve health or health prevention.
- The theory of reasoned action (TRA)/theory of planned behaviour (TPB) and its relationship to health behaviours.
- The health action process approach (HAPA) and how it has been a development over other models.
- How to use psychological models in professional practice.

Case study

Elizabeth Dunn is 32 years old and is married to David. They have two children, a boy and a girl, under the age of 5 years. Both children are cared for by Elizabeth who has given up her job as a marketing consultant to care for her children. Her marriage to David is Elizabeth's second – she was previously married to Phil when she was much younger and has a 16-year-old daughter, Maxine, from this relationship. Maxine has some mental health problems (initially diagnosed as **schizophrenia**) but manages to cope well with these problems with the help of her local community psychiatric nurse (CPN). Maxine is starting to have sexual relationships with a number of 'boyfriends' and is considering setting up home independently. Elizabeth is worried that Maxine may end up becoming pregnant (as she did at the same age) and will potentially miss out on her schooling and future career plans. She is keen on encouraging Maxine and her boyfriends to use appropriate contraceptive methods in order to prevent unwanted pregnancies and practise safe sex.

Elizabeth is overweight – something she has been since she was pregnant with her second child. She also has asthma and arthritis in her knee. She is being encouraged to join a local gym in order to improve her heath and in particular decrease her weight. She has been attending the local Healthy Living Centre gym since January, when she joined as part of her New Year's resolution to lose weight and partly as some 'time to herself' – she either leaves the younger children in the crèche or with her elder daughter. However, although she started with good intentions – she initially attended three times per week – now she is attending rarely and puts this down to the problems of getting to the gym with her young children.

It is hoped that Elizabeth would follow a healthy eating plan and this would result in weight loss and health gains, enabling her to carry out everyday activities with considerably more energy, strength and vitality. If this occurred then her new healthier lifestyle would mean, as an asthma sufferer, that she would not need to use her inhaler as often, also because of her weight loss her knees would be much less painful.

There are a couple of key issues in this case study: why has Elizabeth started to take part in exercise, and how can we keep her there and improve her attendance at the gym? Also, what about Maxine: are there any concerns about her current lifestyle and the possibility of pregnancy? How can we prevent an unwanted pregnancy from occurring?

Psychological models have been at the vanguard into predicting and explaining heath behaviours – whether people engage in exercise, drink too much or eat the 'wrong' foods. The most frequently used models are those that are described as 'cognition models' or 'social cognition models' (the distinction will be outlined in more detail later). It is only recently, however, that there have been attempts at developing theory-based interventions – in the past the models were simply used as systematic attempts at predicting people's health behaviours. This chapter will explore these models and demonstrate how they can be used to predict behaviour and, ultimately, devise interventions on how best to improve behaviour. It will look at two particular heath behaviours to best demonstrate this: physical exercise and safe sex.

Why is this relevant to nursing practice?

All health care professionals should try to encourage positive health behaviours: we want people to exercise more, to eat healthily and to engage in safe sex, for example, so people can live long and healthy lives. By the same token, we want people to avoid health-damaging behaviour: promiscuous sexual activity for example, smoking or excessive alcohol intake. So we must know the best (or most appropriate) way of getting people to engage in such activity. Physical exercise is generally considered as an activity that is protective of health: it has been reported to reduce an individual's risk of developing cardiovascular disease, Type II diabetes and obesity (Knowler *et al.*, 2002; Kohl, 2001). Pate *et al.* (1995) concluded that 'cross sectional epidemiologic studies and controlled, experimental investigations have demonstrated that physically active adults, as contrasted with their sedentary counterparts, tend to develop and maintain higher levels of physical fitness' (p. 403).

Exercise has also been associated with psychological benefits in terms of elevated mood among both clinical and non-clinical populations (Mutrie and Choi, 2000). It is not simply that regular exercise brings about long-term benefits to mood as a result of improved body image or increased physical fitness. Limited frequency aerobic exercise has been found to be associated with reduced anxiety and improved self-esteem and general well-being (Biddle and Nigg, 2000). Indeed, Faulkner and Taylor (2006) report that 'we now have a convincing body of literature that supports the role of physical activity and exercise as strategies for promoting mental health'.

But why do some people exercise and others not? If we try to list all the reasons why people choose to exercise then we can come up with a variety of reasons for doing so:

- desire for physical fitness;
- desire to lose weight/change body shape and appearance;
- desire to maintain or enhance health status;
- desire to improve self-image and mood;
- as a means of **stress** reduction;
- as a social activity.

On the other hand, however, there are a number of people who do not exercise and they may cite a number of reasons for not exercising – it is not simply an absence of the desire for the goals listed above. Barriers commonly mentioned include:

- lack of time;
- cost;
- lack of access to appropriate facilities and equipment;
- embarrassment;
- lack of self-belief;
- lack of someone to go with/support.

Think about this

On the basis of this, suggest reasons why Elizabeth wants to exercise (i.e. the benefits) and what is preventing her from doing so (i.e. the costs). Now think about Maxine: what are the reasons for her using safe sex practices, and what are the potential costs involved? What other factors are important in Maxine's case?

What about sex – surely this is not a risky behaviour? Surely this is something that should be encouraged and enjoyed? Recently there has been a change in the way sex is viewed: previously it was regarded as a pleasurable activity but now (or really since the 1980s with the advent of the HIV campaigns) it is often seen as a risky activity. As a consequence, sex is now discussed in terms of health promotion, health education and self-protection. This shift has resulted in the psychological literature on sex as a risk both in terms of pregnancy avoidance and in the context of sexually transmitted disease (STD)/HIV preventative behaviour. But what sexual behaviours are people actually engaging in? Are people still involved in dangerous sexual activity despite the enormous monies put into 'safe-sex' campaigns?

The National Survey of Sexual Attitudes and Lifestyles (Wellings *et al.*, 1994) examined the sexual behaviour of over 18 000 men and women across Britain and produced considerable data on factors such as age of first intercourse, sexual behaviour and contraception use. The report indicates that for men and women aged 16–24 the most popular form of contraception was condom use. It was rather worrying however, that many young adults in this age group respondents reported using either no contraception at all, or potentially unreliable methods such as withdrawal or the safe period (Figure 15.1). In terms of safe sex, however, health care professionals should try and encourage condom use to prevent both STDs along with potentially unwanted pregnancies.

Other reports have investigated the views of both men and women. In general, men tend to report a number of negative **attitudes** towards condoms including reduction in spontaneity of behaviour or reduce sexual pleasure. Surveys of young women suggest they also hold these negative attitudes. However, they also tend to hold unrealistically optimistic estimates of personal risk of infection with STD or HIV (Bryan *et al.*, 1996, 1997). There are a number of other negative attitudes held by women that can potentially hinder condom use:

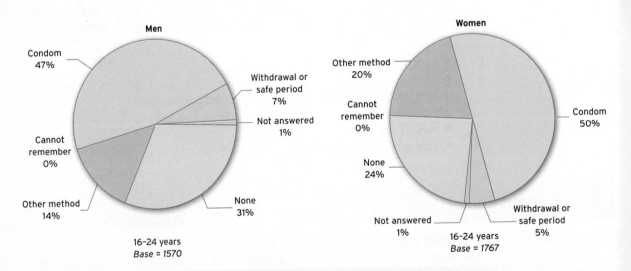

Figure 15.1 Forms of contraception used.

Source: Wellings *et al.,* 1994

- anticipated male objection to a female suggesting condom use (denial of their pleasure);
- difficulty/embarrassment in raising the issue of condom use with a male partner;
- worry that suggesting use to a potential partner implies that either themselves or their partner is HIV-positive or has another STD;
- lack of skill in condom use.

Think about this

Will Maxine and her partner use a condom the first time that they have sexual intercourse? What factors are preventing them from doing so?

Beliefs and attributions

Considerable research has been directed at attempting to predict health behaviour. Obviously if we could predict why people behave in a certain way then we could target our interventions more appropriately. It has been suggested that one of the major factors in explaining health behaviour are the health beliefs and **attributions** that people hold. For example, could we predict whether Maxine would use a condom or whether Elizabeth would exercise? What factors are involved in these decisions and how could we promote the health-increasing behaviours while reducing the potentially health-damaging behaviours? Leventhal *et al.* (1985) were some of the first authors to *describe* the factors that they suggested predicted health behaviour. These included:

- learning, modelling and social norms;
- genetics;
- anxiety, stress and other emotional factors;
- perceived symptoms such as pain, breathlessness and fatigue;
- beliefs of both the patient and the health care professional.

Ultimately, it was suggested that a combination of these factors could be used to predict and promote health-related behaviour. Most of this research has explored health beliefs of the patient, client, individual and has used this as an attempt to predict health behaviours. It is suggested that the beliefs and attributions people hold impact on their health behaviour – for example whether they diet, practise safe sex or take exercise. There is general agreement that health beliefs and attributions are important in explaining and predicting health behaviours and this will be the focus of this chapter. Approaches to health beliefs include **health locus of control**, unrealistic optimism and various psychological models which will all be featured and discussed in this chapter.

Health locus of control

Health locus of control (HLC) is based on the attributions people hold about their health. The concept of Locus of Control (LoC) was first noted by Rotter (1966) who suggested that people had either an internal LoC, where they placed responsibility for outcomes on themselves and considered that their action affected the outcomes, or an external LoC, where the outcomes were not controllable by them but was the responsibility for external factors such as luck, fate or others. Attributions have been explored in health in relation to locus of control. This was further developed by Wallston and Wallston (1982) who applied it to the health field. Specifically, they developed a measure of HLC. This measure categorised people into one of three types:

- **Internal:** If an individual regards their health as controllable by them (e.g. 'I am directly responsible for my health').
- **External:** If an individual believes their health is not controllable by them and in the hands of fate (e.g. 'whether I am well or not is a matter of luck').
- *Powerful others*: If an individual regards their heath as under control of powerful others (e.g. 'I can only do what my doctor tells me to do').

One important concept for the HLC is that it only becomes relevant if an individual values their health since an individual will only act on the valued outcomes (reflecting the **social learning theory** foundation of LoC; see Bandura, 1986, and Chapter 1). If individuals do not value their health, it is thought that they are unlikely to engage in health protective behaviour (even if they feel they have control over their health), because their health is not a high priority.

Think about this

Why would certain people not value their health? What is more valuable to some than their health? Think about Maxine: what would she consider to be most valuable to her at the moment?

It should be obvious that people with different types of LoC will act in a different manner. For example, it could reasonably be expected that those individuals with an internal HLC or a powerful others HLC are more likely to behave in a heath-protective manner than those with an external HLC. Of course, what action this takes may differ: those with a high internal LoC would be more likely to take their own action – for example starting an exercise programme at the gym. In contrast somebody with a powerful other HLC would be more likely to go to a local health clinic and get some diet advice. This type of person would be more likely to go and seek advice, direction and 'cures' from medical and health care practitioners. Those with external LoC would suggest it was not under their control but was due to other factors, such as fate, genetics or God's will.

Think about this

How could Elizabeth's behaviour differ depending on the different types of HLC? What type of HLC do you think (on the basis of the brief information contained in the case study) Elizabeth has? How would you record this?

The research into differences in HLC has revealed a rather understandable set of behaviours. For example, those with an internal HLC are more likely to engage in self-screening behaviours such as breast self-examination. In contrast those with an external HLC are more likely to engage in screening activity that involves a health care professional – for example obtaining a Pap smear.

Obviously, these types of study have been extremely useful in predicting the uptake of services and people's actual behaviours. However, what would be more useful would be if the HLC could be used to develop health messages – to encourage people into positive health behaviours. There are, fortunately, some studies like this around. For example, Wallston *et al.* (1976) reported that those with an internal HLC when matched with an appropriate programme and those with an external HLC when also matched with an appropriate programme lost more weight and were more satisfied with the outcome. Similarly, Quadrel and Lau (1989) reported that messages that were consistent with an individual's HLC was more likely to promote breast self-examination among women – this was particularly the case when follow-up messages/reminders were sent. Promoting the use of mammography was also reported to be enhanced by matching a woman's HLC with an appropriate message (Williams-Piehota *et al.*, 2004). Messages appropriately matched to women's HLC beliefs were, for the most part, more influential in promoting mammography than mismatched messages 6 and 12 months after the desired intervention.

On this basis, therefore, an appropriate intervention can be devised. When discussing, initially, a person's health behaviour, you can devise a programme on the basis of the individual's HLC. So, during the interview if you confirm that the person's HLC then you could devise appropriate follow-up or interventions match the recipient's HLC to yield an increase in health behaviours. Also, physicians, nurses or other health care professionals could take this psychological characteristic into account when presenting patients with information.

There are a number of studies that have explored the HLC and its relationship with health educating outcomes. For example, Shipley (1981) noted that those attending a smoking cessation clinic were more likely to have quit at six months follow-up if they had an internal LoC. More recently, Shaw *et al.* (2003) found that there was a relationship between LoC and recovery from fractured neck of femur (broken hip). In essence, the study reported that those with a more internal LoC had significantly better levels of independence 30 days post-surgery than those with either external or powerful others LoC. This finding was similar to those reported in other studies with individuals with wrist fractures and strokes (Partridge and Johnston, 1989). Furthermore, Stürmer *et al.* (2006), in a large-scale study ($n = 5114$), explored the relationship between a number of **psychosocial** variables and cardiovascular disease. They found a relationship between internal LoC and reduced risk for common chronic disease. They postulated that the relationship was mediated by health-related behaviour. Hence, those with an internal LoC had an impact on lifestyle factors such as smoking, alcohol consumption and dietary intake.

Obviously, these findings may have resonance for nursing practice. The results of these (and other) studies suggest that increases in perceived control in the rehabilitation process may improve and facilitate physical recovery or be protective of health. Since it is possible to promote perceptions of perceived control then it may be possible to enhance recovery by improving this psychological facet, or prevent illness by promoting internal control over health behaviours. Furthermore, this indicates a potential way of intervening to prevent people from either engaging in health-damaging behaviours or enhancing health-protective behaviours – by assessing their LoC and developing intervention strategies based on this.

Think about this

How can nurses promote perceived control? Think about the way you may act in practice with a range of different clients and patients.

Although the research on HLC does appear promising, the reviews have indicated that the relationship between protective health behaviours and HLC is only rather modest (Norman and Bennett, 1996). Consequently, research attention has turned to examining other issues and models.

How to assess HLC

The most frequently employed questionnaire for assessing HLC is that developed by Wallston *et al.* (1978) – the multi-dimensional health locus of control (MHLC) scale – hich provides a measure of three dimensions of health locus of control:

- *Internality*: Measuring the extent to which an individual believes the locus of control for health is internal.
- *Chance*: Measuring the belief in chance or external factors in determining health outcomes.
- *Powerful others*: Measuring the belief in the control over one's health of powerful others, particularly health care professionals.

The three subscales have six items each, and each method provides an indication of how strongly the individual believes in each dimension of control. The following are some examples.

Internal
- If I get sick, it is my own behaviour that determines how soon I get well again.
- I am in control of my health.
- When I get sick I am to blame.

Chance
- No matter what I do, if I am going to get sick, I will get sick.
- Most things that affect my health happen by accident.
- Luck plays a big part in determining how soon I will recover from an illness.

Powerful others
- Having regular contact with my doctor is the best way for me to avoid illness.
- Whenever I don't feel well, I should consult a medically trained professional.
- My family has a lot to do with my becoming sick or staying healthy.

Unrealistic optimism

Weinstein (1983, 1984) suggested that people often engage in risky or unhealthy behaviour due to what he termed 'unrealistic optimism'. This he defined as 'an inaccurate perception of risk and susceptibility' and noted that people engage in comparisons with others in their social circle or wider ('I do not smoke as much as my friend' or 'I am not as heavy as the bloke off the television') or ignore their own risk-taking behaviours ('I may drink to excess some times, but it is not that important') and may focus on their risk-reducing behaviour ('At least I don't inject drugs'). Weinstein *et al.* (2005) report on the unrealistic optimism of smokers – reporting that smokers underestimate their risk of lung cancer considerably relative to both other smokers and to non-smokers. Furthermore, they also demonstrate other misunderstandings of smoking risks (e.g. curability of lung cancer, exercise and vitamins undoing the effects of smoking). Weinstein (1987) suggested that there were four reasons underlying this unrealistic optimism, which suggested that perception of own risk was not a rational process:

- lack of personal experience with the problem;
- the belief that the problem is preventable by the individual action;
- the belief that if the problem has not yet appeared, it will not appear in the future;
- the belief that the problem is infrequent.

Weinstein *et al.* (2005) report on a survey of smokers' views on their tobacco intake. The results indicated that smokers engage in risk minimisation by convincing themselves that they are not as much at risk as other smokers. This recent study added to the considerable body of evidence that this was the case in a number of smoking populations (e.g. Sutton, 2002; Weinstein *et al.*, 2004). Consequently, the data highlight that smokers have an imperfect understanding of the risks of smoking, the difficulty in quitting, the number and strength of cigarettes they smoke. They believe that their risk is lower than the risks faced by other smokers. Therefore, the evidence is that smokers do not have adequate knowledge about smoking and its consequences. Hence, this means that smokers do need continual updating about their behaviour and the impact that it has on their own health.

Cognitive models of health behaviour

The factors discussed so far – attribution, locus of control and unrealistic optimism – along with various other psychological factors have been integrated into different models of health behaviour. These models are often called cognition or social cognition models and these will be the subject of the next section in this chapter. The earliest models were based on the belief that behaviours were a result of a rational weighing of the potential costs and benefits of that behaviour and that the behaviour is a result of rational information processing of these costs and benefits. (Have you spotted the potential problem?) Several models have been proposed as explanations for health behaviour and behaviour change.

The health belief model

The **health belief model** (HBM) was one of the first and best-known models (Becker, 1974; Rosenstock, 1974) developed in order to predict preventative health behaviours. It has also been used to describe the behavioural response to treatment in patients with both acute and chronic illnesses (Figure 15.2).

The HBM makes a series of predictions about behaviour and suggests that they are a result of a set of core beliefs. The original core beliefs are the individual's perception of:

- susceptibility to illness (e.g. 'my chances of getting HIV/AIDS are high');
- severity of the illness (e.g. 'HIV/AIDS is a serious illness');
- the costs involved in carrying out the behaviour (e.g. 'wearing a condom will reduce my/my partner's pleasure');
- the benefits involved in carrying out the behaviour (e.g. 'wearing a condom will prevent unwanted pregnancies');
- cues to action, which may be internal (e.g. some non-specific symptoms) or external (e.g. health education information/leaflets).

The model suggests that the likelihood of a behaviour occurring is related to these core beliefs. Consequently, the HBM can be used to predict whether a behaviour will occur or not. The original HBM has been updated and improved with 'health motivation' added to reflect an individual's readiness to be concerned about health matters (e.g. 'I am concerned that not wearing a condom might seriously damage my health'). More recently Becker and Rosenstock (1987) have also suggested that another factor should be added to the model–perceived control.

The HBM and preventative behaviour

For nurses, the HBM has been regarded, since its initial formulation, as a potentially helpful model to help clients assess and manage their illness

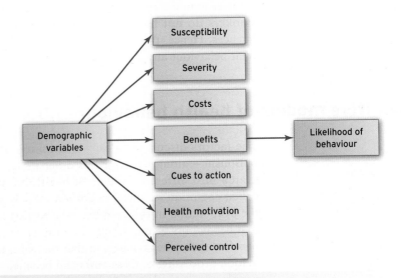

Figure 15.2 Health belief model.

Source: Ogden, J. (2004) *Health Psychology: A Textbook*, 3rd Edition, Open University Press. Reproduced with the kind permission of the Open University Press Publishing Company

prevention or prevent health problems. It has been used across a wide range of different practice areas by nurses, from breast cancer and osteoporosis to developing intervention/educational programmes. Furthermore, it has been shown that some people carry out a cost–benefit analysis when making decisions about seeking medical assistance in accident and emergency services (Walsh, 1995).

It has mainly been used, however, to describe why people attend screening services. For example, to help nurses understand some of the factors that influence whether women turn up for mammography screening (Holm *et al.*, 1999; Petro-Nustas, 2001; Yarbrough and Braden, 2001). One such study was reported by Jirojwong and MacLennan (2003) who explored the value of the HBM in predicting breast self-examination in a group of women. A total of 145 women took part in the study and completed a number of different questionnaires exploring the role of various components of the HBM in predicting whether Thai women undertook breast self-examination. It was reported that 'Perceived susceptibility to breast cancer, cues of triggers for screening, self-efficacy and the overall HBM are important factors influencing BSE' (p. 247) and that 'health professionals could use the important HBM factors: susceptibility to cancer, barriers to screening, cues or triggers for screening and self-efficacy, as a guide to encouraging BSE' (p. 248). Hence, if we explore the model with the various components then we can see how knowledge of the HBM can be employed to improve screening behaviours (Figure 15.3).

Implications for the planning of interventions

According to the HBM, if we can persuade people that they are susceptible to some diseases then we are more likely to convince them to engage in some form of preventative action. Furthermore, we also need to convince the person that developing that disease will have severe consequences and that if

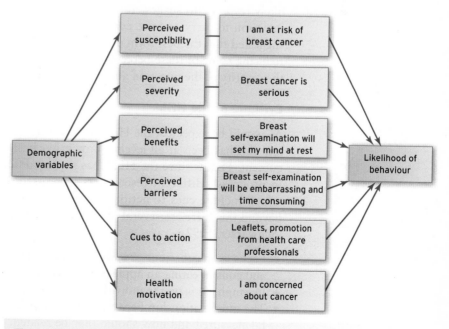

Figure 15.3 Use of HBM for breast self-examination.

Think about this

Using the following HBM factors indicate how they can be applied to the case of Maxine and condom use, or if Elizabeth had to take one of her younger children to A&E with a high temperature and rash:

- susceptibility to illness;
- severity of the illness;
- the costs involved in carrying out the behaviour;
- the benefits involved in carrying out the behaviour;
- cues to action.

they engage in the preventative action then they are less susceptible to the disease (or will reduce its consequences). Finally, we have to convince them that the costs of taking the action will be outweighed by the potential benefits of taking the desired action.

Whether this model is useful in promoting such positive behaviours has been explored in a number of different settings. Let us look at one such study, which relates to the case example previously presented: Abraham *et al.* (1992) reported on whether the HBM could be applied to condom use among teenagers in Scotland. This study reported on the relationship between the various components of the HMB and the intention to carry and use condoms. The study did report that there was a relationship between the various factors (e.g. perceived severity of HIV infection, perceived vulnerability to HIV infection and perceived effectiveness of condoms) and intention to use, although this relationship was modest at best. In contrast, perceived barriers to use (e.g. beliefs concerning pleasure reduction, awkwardness of use and partners' likely response to suggested use) were found to be much better predictors of intention to carry and use condoms. On the basis of these findings it can be suggested that the best form of intervention would be one that had a focus on reducing some of these perceived barriers rather than attempting to highlight the severity of the infection and condom effectiveness.

Critique of the HBM

As would be expected, the HBM has been subjected to considerable criticism and this has been at all levels – how it has been applied and its fundamental content. Firstly, since the HBM has several different versions (rather a work in progress!) different researchers have used different versions, not all of which include cues to action and health motivation. However, above and beyond this there are several other criticisms that can be applied to the model (Schwarzer, 1992):

- Focus is on conscious processing of information. (Do we weigh up the pros and cons of eating an apple or whether we clean our teeth in the morning?)
- Its emphasis is on the individual. (Do we act in a social vacuum?)
- The interrelationship between the different core beliefs – how should these be measured and how should they be related. (Is one more important than another, how can we measure them?)

- Absence of a role for emotional factors. (Do we change our behaviour dependent on how we feel?)
- Health beliefs are treated as static. (Do these remain the same throughout the process?)

With these criticisms in mind, however, a number of research studies have been conducted with the HBM and its value established in a number of different areas. For example, research has used aspects of this model to predict screening for hypertension, screening for cervical cancer, genetic screening, exercise behaviour, decreased alcohol use, changes in diet and smoking cessation. It obviously has a considerable part to play in both predicting behaviour and enhancing adaptive preventative behaviour.

The recognition that the HBM had several components that needed to be further developed, and some factors needed to be included, prompted researchers to refine this model: thus, the protection motivation theory (PMT) was developed.

The protection motivation theory (PMT)

The PMT was developed by Rogers (1975, 1983, 1985) who expanded the HBM to include additional factors (Figure 15.4). The PMT suggests that health behaviours can be predicted on the basis of four components:

- severity (e.g. 'heart disease is a serious illness');
- susceptibility (e.g. 'my chances of getting CHD are high');
- response effectiveness (e.g. 'doing some exercise would improve my health');
- self-efficacy (e.g. 'I am confident that I can engage in physical exercise').

These components predict behavioural intentions that are related (although somewhat tenuously) to behaviour. It should be noted that the last component of the sentence – the relationship between behavioural intent and actual behaviour has been the most difficult to conclude as there is only a weak relationship between these factors. Rogers (1985) also suggested a role for a fifth component, fear (e.g. an emotional response), in response to education or information. The PMT considers that severity, susceptibility and fear are part of the threat appraisal (external factors) and response effectiveness and self-efficacy as relating to coping (internal factors).

Using the PMT

When devising interventions based upon the PMT it is important that the assumptions underlying it are fully integrated into the intervention. For example, if self-efficacy for the given behaviour is low then this should be the first element to be targeted. There is no point in increasing the perceived risk of the condition if the individual has low self-efficacy as the individual will not feel able to engage in the protective action. When self-efficacy is low, however, that is, when individuals feel that they are unable to engage in a given action (e.g. dieting to lose weight), increases in vulnerability will probably not result in increments in intentions to behave in a certain manner. The intervention should merely be to provide information to increase self-efficacy.

In contrast, if the self-efficacy within the target population or individual is relatively high (that is, feeling ready and able to engage in the recommended health actions) then the provision of information should reflect this. In this

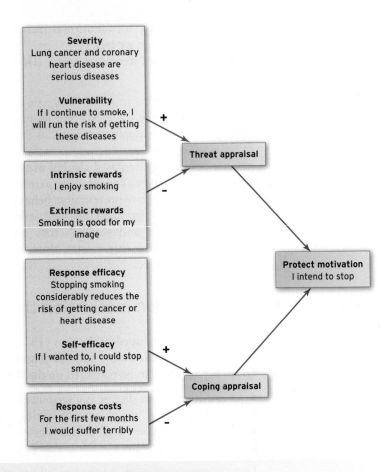

Figure 15.4 Protection motivation theory

Source: Stroebe, W. (2000) *Social Psychology and Health*, 2nd Edition, Open University Press. Reproduced with the kind permission of the Open University Press Publishing Company

case, information which increases the perceived vulnerability or severity should, as a consequence, increase protection motivation and thus intention to act. Basically, this suggests that if people feel able to engage in the desired health protective behaviour then increasing their own perceived risk will increase their intention to act, and as a consequence, they will be more likely to act.

If applied to enhancing physical exercise for Elizabeth, the PMT would make the following predictions:

- Information about the role of a lack of exercise in asthma and arthritis deterioration would increase fear, thereby increasing the behaviour.
- Increasing the *perceived severity* by increasing an individual's perceptions of how serious the arthritis was and therefore increase the likelihood of positive behaviour.
- Increase *perceived susceptibility* by increasing their belief that their health was likely to deteriorate – again this would mean an improvement in the pro-health behaviour.

If the individual also had positive *self-efficacy*, that is, they felt confident that they could increase their exercise and that the *response effectiveness* was positive (i.e. would have beneficial consequences), the behavioural intentions to change their behaviour would be high.

Houlding and Davidson (2003) used the PMT as a predictor of condom use in drug users. In a study of 72 injecting drug users, the study found that perceived vulnerability to infection from a regular partner and social norms were significant predictors of condom use. The results of the study suggested that to increase condom use then the perception of vulnerability needs to be increased, as does the view that condom use is the 'norm'.

Critique of the PMT

The PMT has been less widely criticised than the HBM; however, many of the criticisms of the HBM also relate to the PMT. For example, the PMT assumes that individuals are conscious information processors, and it does not include social and environmental factors.

Social cognition models

The two models thus far described have been further developed, and revised, in order to overcome some of the criticisms levelled against them. In particular, the models have been refined to include a role for the social context of the behaviour and not simply rely on the individual's **cognitions** or attitudes. Not surprisingly these models have been called 'social cognition models' (as opposed to 'cognition models'). Several models have been developed using this perspective and there are a couple that will be explored here: the **theory of planned behaviour** (derived from the **theory of reasoned action**) and the **health action process approach**.

Theory of reasoned action/theory of planned behaviour

The theory of reasoned action (TRA) was developed by social psychologists in the 1970s and has been used extensively to examine predictors of behaviours (Ajzen and Fishbein, 1970; Fishbein, 1967; Fishbein and Ajzen, 1975). The TRA was an important model as it was one of the first to place the individual within the social context. The first point to note about the TRA is that it predicts behavioural intent, which it assumed leads to behaviour – although this is far from an accepted reality as we have seen with the other models discussed so far. The TRA suggests that behavioural intention is a product of an individual's attitude towards performing the behaviour and of subjective norms. Each of these factors has further elements (Figure 15.5).

For example, a person's attitudes towards the behaviour will be a consequence of the likelihood of that behaviour being associated with positive outcome. Hence, Elizabeth's attitudes towards starting exercise is a function of the perceived likelihood with which physical exercise is associated with certain consequences such as being healthier and fitter and the evaluation of these perceived consequences. (Are they positive? Are they worth the effort?) Subjective norms make up the other element to the model and include two components: normative beliefs and motivation to comply.

Normative beliefs are the beliefs held by us about how people who are important to us expect us to behave. For example, Elizabeth might believe

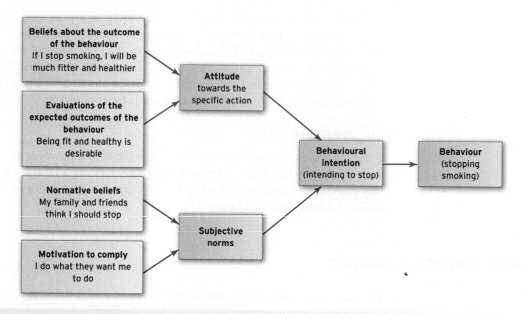

Figure 15.5 Theory of reasoned action.

Source: Stroebe, W. (2000) *Social Psychology and Health,* 2nd Edition, Open University Press. Reproduced with the kind permission of the Open University Press Publishing Company

that her husband, David, wants her to take up exercise so she can lose a bit of weight, or that he is worried that she is not as fit as she used to be. However, whether Elizabeth's intentions will alter depending on these subjective norms depends on her willingness to comply with it. Hence, subjective norms are a product of both normative beliefs and motivation to comply.

Theory of planned behaviour (TPB)

The TRA was developed by Ajzen and colleagues into the theory of planned behaviour (TPB; Ajzen, 1985, 1988) (Figure 15.6). The TPB suggests that behavioural intentions (i.e. to engage in a particular practice, to behave in a certain manner) are a consequence of a combination of several beliefs:

- *Attitudes towards a behaviour*: This comprises a positive or negative evaluation of a particular behaviour and beliefs about the outcome of the behaviour (e.g. 'exercising is fun and will improve my health').
- *Subjective norms*: These are composed of the perception of social norms and pressures to perform a behaviour and an evaluation of whether the individual is motivated to comply with this pressure (e.g. 'David is important to me and he will approve if I lose weight and I want his approval').
- *Perceived behavioural control*: This is an important component and suggests that the individual can carry out the particular behaviour considering both internal (e.g. skills, abilities and information, 'e.g. I can play squash and badminton and I know where to join a club') and external (e.g. 'I can make the Friday night when the badminton club have their sessions because I can get a babysitter'). Obviously both of these relate to previous experiences and behaviour.

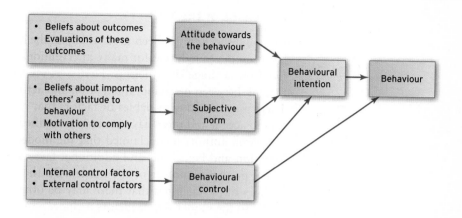

Figure 15.6 Theory of planned behaviour.

Source: Ogden, J. (2004) *Health Psychology: A Textbook*, 3rd Edition, Open University Press. Reproduced with the kind permission of the Open University Press Publishing Company

The TPB and preventative behaviour

Considerable research exists with the TPB in a number of different areas of preventative behaviour. For example, Armitage and Connor (2002) and Connor *et al.* (2002) found that the model predicted whether an individual intended to eat a healthy low-fat diet. Likewise, Hagger *et al.* (2001) reported that attitudes, perceived behavioural control were related to intention to engage in physical activity as reported by children, although there was no relationship with subjective norms.

The model has also been used to explore the uptake of a range of screening opportunities. Rutter (2000) reported that intention to attend a screening service was predicted by attitude, perceived behavioural control and subjective norm. However, it was also of note that only attitudes and subjective norms were related to uptake of screening.

The TPB and risk-reducing behaviour

The TPB has also been applied to risk-reducing behaviour: do people stop smoking, for example. Both Godin *et al.* (1992) and Norman *et al.* (1999) reported that the frequency of smoking behaviour could be explained primarily by low perceived behavioural control beliefs. It does appear as if the perceived behavioural control is an important element of the TPB.

Think about this

How would you use the TPB to increase the chances of Maxine's using a condom when she has sex with her partner? In particular, how would you increase perceived behavioural control?

Criticisms of the TPB

Although the TPB has been used widely in the health behaviour literature and has been the foundation for many interventions, it is worth noting that it suffers from a range of criticisms. Firstly, as indicated throughout this chapter, the link between behavioural intention and actual behaviour is not consistent. There must be other variables or factors that move an individual from intention to action and these have yet to be identified.

Several authors have claimed that the model accounts for the majority of intention and behaviour and additional factors would not lead to any additional predictive power of the model. On the other hand, however, several authors have suggested that there may be other factors that can add significantly to the model. These factors include:

- moral norms;
- anticipatory regret;
- self-identity;
- implementation intention.

Research in focus

Watson, P.W.B. and Myers, L.B. (2001) Which cognitive factors predict clinical glove use amongst nurses? *Psychology, Health and Medicine*, **6** (4), 399–409.

Background
Glove use aims to protect the user from blood/bodily fluid of patients suspected of carrying blood-borne viruses. Nurses may be exposed to such blood-borne viruses including HIV and various other pathogens including hepatitis. Professional recommendations are to minimise blood/body fluid contact and that appropriate barrier precautions (e.g. gloves) should be used where necessary. However, adherence to the recommended use is limited, with some reports suggesting that up to 40 per cent of practitioners were not wearing gloves when necessary (Adegboye *et al.*, 1997). The aim of this current study was to explore whether a modified theory of planned behaviour (TPB) was a good model for predicting self-report glove use.

Method
Participants: These were 103 registered nurses at a London teaching hospital with 25 per cent working in Accident and Emergency, with the remaining on various general medicine wards (e.g. renal, intensive care, paediatric, oncology).

Measures: Questionnaires were used to assess respondents' (i) intentions to use gloves on occasions where blood contact will occur; (ii) attitudes towards wearing gloves; (iii) subjective norms – whether the respondent felt under social pressure from colleagues; (iv) perceived behavioural control – whether the individual felt they could manage to wear gloves in all appropriate situations; (v) perceived barriers to wearing glove use – for example if it made the procedure more difficult; (vi) self-reported glove use – from always to never.

Results
A total of 43.7 per cent respondents reported that they always wore gloves in situations where contact with blood could occur (which obviously means that over 50 per cent did not). A multiple regression analysis was undertaken and the results indicated that intention to use gloves was the

most significant predictor, although perceived barriers (particularly availability of time) also made a large contribution. When looking at the variables that explained *intention* to use gloves, attitude to glove use, perceived behavioural control and barriers to use (particularly volume of blood) were highlighted as being important.

Implications

The TPB helped explain intention for glove use, which in itself was an important predictor of actual glove use behaviour. There were a number of important findings from this study. Firstly, attitude towards glove use was a fundamental factor in both intentions and actual behaviour. Secondly, specific barriers were significantly implicated in explaining both intentions and behaviour. The two major barriers identified were 'when expecting the amount of contact with blood to be minimal' and 'time pressure'. The latter suggests that nurses appear to be making decisions on circumstances they find themselves in, rather than making an appropriate risk-based decision. Finally, the report found that self-report glove use was low, with fewer than 50 per cent of nurses reporting always wearing gloves when contact with blood can occur. The authors suggest that the findings from the study have practical implications for the design of training programmes for nurses. These programmes should emphasise the risks associated with specific clinical procedures. Finally, the authors suggest that 'Innovative interventions based on prior theoretically driven investigations targeting attitudes, perception of risk and decision making need to be explored' if adherence to the safe practice of glove wearing is to be both maintained and improved.

The health action process approach (HAPA)

Schwarzer (1992) developed another model, the health action process approach (HAPA) on the basis of a thorough review of the literature. His review, and subsequent model development, suggested there was a need to include a temporal element into the understanding of beliefs and behaviours. Furthermore, the new model stressed the importance of self-efficacy as a determinant of both behavioural intentions and self-reports of behaviour. The HAPA, consequently, includes elements from all the previous models described and attempts to predict both behavioural intentions and, more importantly, actual behaviour (Figure 15.7).

Components of the HAPA

The HAPA model distinguishes between decision-making/motivational stage and an action/maintenance stage and has included both a temporal and process factor. It suggests that there is a two-stage process: individuals initially decide whether or not to carry out a behaviour (the motivation stage), and then make plans to initiate and maintain this behaviour (the action phase).

According to the HAPA, the motivation stage is made up of the following components:

- Self-efficacy (e.g. 'I am confident that I can get my partner to wear a condom when having sex').
- Outcome expectancies (e.g. 'using a condom will prevent unwanted pregnancies'), which has a subset of social outcome expectancies (e.g. 'my mum would not approve if I became pregnant').
- Threat appraisal, which is composed of beliefs about the severity of a condition and perceptions of individual vulnerability (e.g. 'Getting AIDs is serious and if I don't wear a condom I could catch it').

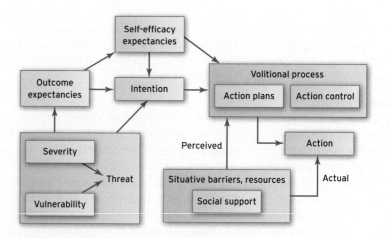

Figure 15.7 The health action process approach.

Source: Ogden, J. (2004) *Health Psychology: A Textbook,* 3rd Edition, Open University Press. Reproduced with the kind permission of the Open University Press Publishing Company

Ultimately, the end result (as with the other models) is an intention to act or behaviour in a certain way. Then, the action stage comes into play which includes cognitive, situational and behavioural factors. It is the combination of these factors that determines how the individual both starts and continues the behaviour. Hence:

- Cognitive factors: Composed of both action plans (e.g. 'If I start to have sex I will use a condom as I will remember the possible diseases I could catch') and action control (e.g. 'I can use a condom regularly and will always carry one'). This is really akin to the everyday concept of 'willpower'.
- Situational factors: Included in this are social support (e.g. 'friends tell me that carrying a condom is sensible') and the absence of situational barriers (e.g. not having a condom ready).

This model, it is argued, is an improvement over previous models inasmuch as it develops the link between intentions and actual behaviour. Furthermore, there is an explicit and implicit recognition of the importance of self-efficacy (Schwarzer, 1992).

Strategies for changing risk behaviour

So far in this chapter the various models that have been devised to predict people's behaviour have been outlined and explored and the value of these to nursing demonstrated. However, of course, one of the important areas for any health care professional is in altering an individual's maladaptive behaviour to positive health-promoting behaviour. This will be the focus of the final section of this chapter. In particular, the concept of **motivational interviewing** will be developed and discussed (Miller and Rollnick, 2002).

Motivational interviewing (MI) has as its goal the simple (some would say!) expectation that increasing an individual's motivation to consider change rather than showing them how to change should be the key step. If a person is not motivated to change then it is irrelevant if they know how to change. However, if a person is motivated to change then the interventions aimed at changing behaviour can begin.

MI is a technique based on cognitive-behavioural therapy which aims to enhance an individual's motivation to change health behaviour. The whole process aims to help the patient understand their thought processes and to identify how these help produce the inappropriate behaviour and how they can be changed to develop alternative, health-promoting, behaviours.

One of the foundations for MI is the **transtheoretical model** (stages of change: see Chapter 12) as developed by Prochaska and DiClemente (1982). Motivational strategies include eight components that are designed to increase the level of motivation the person has towards changing a specific behaviour. It is important to note that the motivation is specific to one behaviour, so being motivated to quit smoking does not simply transfer to being motivated to reduce alcohol consumption. The eight components are:

- giving advice (about specific behaviours to be changed);
- removing barriers (often about access to particular help);
- providing choice (making it clear that if they choose not to change, that is their right and it is their choice; the therapist is there to *encourage* but not *insist* on change);
- decreasing desirability (of the ambivalence towards change or the status quo);
- practising empathy;
- providing feedback (from a variety of perspectives – family, friends, health professionals – in order to give the patient a full picture of their current situation);
- clarifying goals (feedback should be compared with a standard (an ideal), and clarification of the ideal can provide the pathway to the goal);
- active helping (such as expressing caring or facilitating a referral, all of which convey a real interest in helping the person to change).

Creating the conditions for change

In order to create the conditions for changing behaviour, MI suggests that five basic principles are important:

- *Expressing empathy*: Empathy is fundamental to all cognitive therapies and this is about demonstrating an informed understanding of the person's predicament. This is obviously a skill and requires active listening and reflection. For example, 'I hear what you say about the problems about trying to stop smoking and how you use it to deal with stress'. This shows that the therapist understands, accepts and is interested in the person.
- *Avoiding argument*: Since MI is a challenging therapy then argument is unnecessary and counterproductive. The goal of MI is to encourage the patient to hear themselves why they want to change, rather than your own arguments.
- *Supporting self-efficacy*: It is important to encourage the individual to make positive statements that reflect self-efficacy so they reframe their thinking. The therapist's job is to ensure the patient statements counterbalance any negative view. If a patient says 'I have tried lots of times to quit smoking/lose weight' along with the implicit (or sometimes explicit) message that 'and I am a failure'. It is important to reframe this into a more positive reflection:

'you know what you need to change, you are motivated to change, and you are willing to keep trying under difficult circumstances'.

- *Rolling with resistance*: The aim here is not to argue but subtly challenge the thought processes underlying the behaviour. This can then change the patient's perspective of the situation. This can be done in a number of ways – asking for clarification or elaboration, helping the individual to see the incompatibility of their position and so on.
- *Developing discrepancy*: The individual needs to have goals to work towards and understand that their current circumstances have consequences and cannot continue. For example, not losing weight will have a health consequence – the knee joints will not improve, the breathlessness will continue.

How to do it

Miller and Rollnick (2002) suggest that there are eight steps of MI that allow the therapeutic process to work:

- *Establishing rapport*: The individual needs to learn to trust the therapist and this will take time. Ensure that the first sessions start and finish on time and the patient is clear about what has been covered and what is to come. The therapist's role is to create the conditions outlined above (develop discrepancy, support and encourage self-efficacy, give advice, provide feedback and clarify goals).
- *Setting the agenda*: The therapist and the patient must work together to ensure that there is a clear agenda. It is important not to attempt too much too soon, but to ensure that the agenda for change is carefully planned and any changes are prioritised. It is not worth attempting to quit smoking, reduce alcohol intake and increase exercise all at once – stages have to be prioritised.
- *Assessing readiness to change*: Level of motivation can be assessed in a variety of ways. At its most simple, asking the question, 'On a scale of 1 to 10 how keen are you to ...?' will provide some insight. This can be taken further – why a 3, rather than a 4 or a 5? This will also provide you with information about possible barriers, or support available.
- *Sharpening the focus*: As this stage suggests, the idea is to focus on precisely what the patient wants to change. Behaviours often comprise a series of complex different behaviours and it may not be possible to change all of them at once. At this stage, the most important stage and specific behaviour components can be identified. This is obviously sensible for a number of reasons, not least because it makes the task appear much more achievable.
- *Identifying ambivalence*: Obviously it is likely that the patient will disagree with, argue with or ignore a statement at some stage of the therapy. This is to be expected and probably indicates that the patient has reasons for and against change. This is a truism – if there are no problems then the behaviour will have changed.
- *Eliciting self-motivating statements*: The therapist should encourage the patient to phrase positively and to highlight successes. For example, rather than concentrating on the negatives, concentrate on the positives. Similarly, rather than the passive 'If only I could ...' change to 'I am keen to ...'
- *Handling resistance*: Again, this is to be expected and one way to deal with this is to use reflection. Expressing what you see and hear is important and it is useful to reflect back to the patient.

- *Shifting the focus*: If a patient talks about barriers then re-shift the focus. For example 'I can't give up smoking because of my wife' then this can be changed to focus on some of the beliefs that may underlie this – is it support from others that is lacking, is it the way a non-smoker is perceived?

Putting it all together: the case of STD

This chapter has now explored various models and motivational interviewing which can be used to help transform behaviour. This final section will explore how this can all be put together so the use of psychological models can be demonstrated.

If we refer back to Maxine, Elizabeth, her mother, is concerned about the possibility of her sexual promiscuity. This is for two reasons: her worries about becoming pregnant and because of the risk of STDs. The latter are a major cause of morbidity among adolescent girls, with an estimate of two-thirds of those acquiring a STD being less than 25 years of age. Evidence has suggested that although condom use has increased significantly over previous years (Ventura *et al.*, 1999), the majority of adolescent mothers still do not use them and are therefore putting themselves at risk from both STDs and the possibility of further pregnancy. A number of studies have indicated that there are a range of factors that influence condom use and these have indicated that the predictors derived from social-cognitive models are important (Jemmott and Jemmott, 2000). In consequence, it is important to develop safe sex interventions for women of this age and to use the variables from the social-cognitive methods outlined previously.

Such interventions, for this age group, require good, accurate information, that will capture the audience's attention and promote changes in both attitudes and behaviour. Shrier *et al.* (2001) explored whether an individual intervention based on various psychological models and implemented through motivational interviewing could improve condom use. The intervention began with a short video in which popular entertainers and sports figures discussed and dramatized condom names, buying condoms and negotiating condom use, and two female adolescents demonstrated condom use to their peers. Condom use was portrayed as normative behaviour.

In addition to this, a series of female health educators were employed and trained in various theories including being taught to use a standardised intervention manual that outlined key points to cover, activities to perform and the motivation strategies to employ. At the outset, participants were asked about how much they needed and wanted to change their sexual risk behaviour (on a so-called 'wheel of change'). The intervention ensured that the same information was provided to all participants but the educator tried to individualise the session based on the stage of change.

But what about Maxine's schizophrenia?

Maxine has schizophrenia, and this obviously will have some impact on the cognitive processes and how they can be dealt with. Hence, it could be argued that people with severe mental illness may have problems that could interfere with traditional motivational interviews. However, this does not mean that people with schizophrenia should be ignored and MI cannot be used. There are several strategies that can be used to prevent the possible attention and memory deficits, associated with schizophrenia, interfering with the various tasks associated with MI. Listing costs and benefits to individual actions can be especially helpful to persons with cognitive disabilities.

The type of schizophrenia that Maxine has and the individual elements associated with it (e.g. possibly anergia and disinterest) may prevent the usual reinforcers acting as a motivator for her. In this way, it is difficult to identify specific costs and benefits of any identified costs. Others with schizophrenia may show marked **anhedonia** which may make it difficult for them to list all the positive benefits (especially those concerning positive affect). It should be noted, however, that the motivational interview is only the first step and the goal might never be achieved by this method alone. There may be a need for additional support in order to achieve a specific goal. Hence, Maxine may need to have additional psychosocial interventions including skills training; cognitive therapies; supported employment, education and housing; and family education and support. The full range of psychosocial therapies is most effective, however, when it reflects the goals identified by the persons with **psychiatric disability**.

Conclusion

There are various models in health psychology that can be used to both predict an individual's health behaviours and how best to intervene to promote health behaviours and reduce inappropriate, health-damaging behaviours. These models have been developed over a number of years and have been refined in light of decades of research. This ultimately has led to theoretically derived interventions. These interventions at both a community and an individual level have proved useful and beneficial. It is likely that the nurse can use these models to improve the health care provided to their patients and clients. One such way of improving an individual's health behaviour is to employ motivational interviewing which has proved successful in changing and improving an individual's motivation to change.

Summary

- Considerable time, money and effort have been and continue to be spent on attempting to find variables that can predict why people behave in a certain manner and how these variables can be used to promote health protective behaviour.

- The health locus of control is an indication of whether they placed responsibility for their health on themselves, powerful others or external factors.

- HLC has been found to be related to predicting whether people will attend for health screening,

how likely they are to engage in such activities and how this can be facilitated.

- Many people engage in unhealthy behaviours because of unrealistic optimism – they believe they are 'immortal' and unlikely to suffer the consequences of the poor behaviour.

- The health belief model (HBM) was developed to predict which people would engage in health protecting behaviour.

- The HBM is based on susceptibility to illness, severity of illness, costs and benefits of carrying out the behaviour along with cues to action.

- The protection motivation theory (PMT) is another cognition model that attempts to predict behavioural intent. It suggests that health behaviours can be predicted on the basis of severity, susceptibility, response effectiveness, self-efficacy and fear.

- The theories of reasoned action/planned behaviour are social cognition models which are based on attitudes towards a behaviour, subjective norms and perceived behavioural control.

- The health action process approach (HAPA) is a two-stage model: the motivation stage and the action phase.

- The psychological models described can be used to both predict behaviour and also design intervention strategies to improve health behaviours.

- A particular method for developing behaviour is motivational interviewing which aims to increase an individual's motivation to alter their own behaviour.

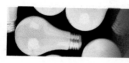

Check your understanding

1. How can a knowledge of an individual's health locus of control influence health education interventions?

2. Compare and contrast two social cognition models.

3. The value of social cognitive models in nursing has been seriously neglected. Discuss.

4. How can social cognition models be applied to an area of your professional practice?

5. Is the HAPA model a development over previous social cognition models?

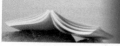

Further reading

Connor, M. and Norman, P. (eds) (1996) *Predicting Health Behaviour*. Buckingham: Open University Press.

Rutter, D. and Quine, L. (eds) (2002) *Changing Health Behaviour: Intervention and Research with Social Cognition Models*. Buckingham: Open University Press.

Weblinks

Ajzen Website on Theory of Planned Behaviour	http://www.people.umass.edu/aizen/	Personal website of Professor Ajzen which includes considerable information and publications on the theory of the planned behaviour.
Intute resource on health behaviours	http://intute.ac.uk/	Various resources available with links to reviewed sites.
Bridging the Intention-Behaviour Gap: Promoting compliance with medication for coronary heart disease	http://www.psyc.leeds.ac.uk/research/hlth/HealthPsyc/HealthBehaviours/index.htm	Report from research group at Leeds University, which contains some useful information (published October 2003).
Health Action Process Approach, HAPA	http://userpage.fu-berlin.de/~health/hapa.htm	Schwarzer's model described in all its glory.
	http://www.motivationalinterview.org/	A series of resources related to motivational interviewing.

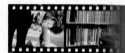

Media examples

Thirteen (2003) The value of subjective norms, attitudes and control factors are factors explored in this film. A naive adolescent girl is led down a path of sex, drugs and petty crime. Not surprisingly it isn't long before her new world and attitude finally take a toll on her, her family and friends.

25 Ways to Quit Smoking (1989) This is one of Bill Plympton's first films, and is a funny take on ways to quit smoking. The film focuses on 25 alternative methods to kick the habit, all of which have violent, bizarre and humorous results.

Chapter 16
Patient adherence to medical information and lifestyle change

Learning outcomes

When you have read this chapter you should understand:

- How the terms compliance, adherence and concordance are linked to patient outcome.
- How patient adherence is measured.
- What factors contribute to patients not adhering to medical advice and treatment.
- How patient satisfaction with a medical encounter impacts on adherence behaviour.
- How the nurse can tailor communication so that adherence behaviour is enhanced.
- How a nurse can improve adherence.

Case study

Mr Riaz is an 84-year-old man who has been diagnosed as having type II insulin-dependent diabetes. The consultant has referred him to the diabetes nurse who will help him to become familiar with the correct administration of the insulin injection. The patient also has a history of chronic asthma, high blood pressure and high cholesterol.

The nurse explains to the patient that the insulin needs to be injected twice a day and shows the patient how to use the injection correctly. Mr Riaz is also provided with information about the foods that should be avoided and what needs to be incorporated into his diet so that the diabetes can be managed appropriately. Mr Riaz is asked if he has understood everything and if he has any questions. The patient acknowledges to the nurse that he is satisfied with the information and has understood it well.

The following morning, Mr Riaz has his regular breakfast of sugary porridge. He then takes his insulin injection out of the box ready to be used. Mr Riaz then begins to think about his consultation with the diabetic nurse and remembers the dietary recommendations that were given. He then becomes confused as he remembers the nurse stating that he would need to change his diet so that high-fat foods and sugar were eliminated. As a result, Mr Riaz does not know if he should use the injection after having breakfast, which was high in sugar. He becomes highly anxious and begins to find the phone number for the diabetes nurse; however, he is unsuccessful in getting hold of her. Mr Riaz's daughter comes to visit him later on in the day to find him highly confused and agitated. He explains to his daughter that he cannot remember when he should and should not take his injection and recalls the nurse talking about other medication but cannot remember the exact details. In all the confusion Mr Riaz has forgotten to use his inhaler. As a result Mr Riaz has taken no medication during the day. His daughter gives him the inhaler and rings the diabetes clinic for clarification.

Why is this relevant to nursing practice?

It is crucial that nurses are familiar with adherence literature as it has a direct implication for their patients' future health. 'Good' **adherence** with drug treatment is an important factor in preventing readmission to hospital and improving health care (Rose, 1995). In the case study above, Mr Riaz became very confused and did not adhere to administering his insulin injection; as a result, he could have made his diabetes worse. If his confusion persists, he could end up being readmitted to hospital with more severe symptoms than he had initially. **Non-compliance** with prescribed treatments has implications for the health of the patient, the effective use of resources and the assessment of the clinical efficacy of treatments (Playle and Keeley, 1998).

The nurse is vital in facilitating the patient to adhere correctly to the medical advice and the medical regimen that has been set. The way the nurse provides information, as well as the communication process, is key in determining the extent to which the patient will adhere. In the above case study, the nurse was not **patient-centred**. As a result, the nurse did not gain an insight into the possible confusion that could have occurred. Research places a large part of the responsibility on practitioners for poor adherence among patients, largely because of inadequate communication and poor treatment planning (i.e. Rose, 1995). How to be patient-centred, as well as ways of providing information will be looked at within this chapter. Within this particular case study, had the diabetes nurse referred to the insulin injections by their colours, she could have ensured that Mr Riaz would be less confused about which injection to administer during different times of the day. Patients might not ask questions or mention certain aspects of their anxiety, as they will be afraid of appearing 'stupid' or think it is not worth mentioning.

The nurse should have taken more caution, as patients with chronic illnesses such as asthma, diabetes and any illness that lasts for more than three months tend to have higher non-adherence rates for treatment and lifestyle changes. For example, non-adherence rates of 50 per cent have been projected for illnesses that have to be managed over a long period of time (Haynes *et al.*, 1979). Within this case study, Mr Riaz was also confused with his morning breakfast and the injection. Adherence and the way information is communicated will be looked at in relation to both medication-taking and lifestyle change.

Mr Riaz is an elderly gentleman who is Muslim. Such factors are important as they determine how an individual prioritises health needs and treatment as well as the lifestyle that they are accustomed to. The nurse above did not take any of these factors into consideration, and should have done, as they will contribute to how more or less likely a patient is to adhere. With the notion of **holistic care**, demographic variables are important to consider during a consultation as they will indicate how the patient will follow advice outside the hospital: this will be explored in this chapter.

Another reason why nurses need to explore the area of adherence is because of the possible implications that can occur when the patient does not adhere to the medical advice or treatment that has been provided. These can range from deterioration of health, symptoms increasing to rehospitalisation and even compromising one's own life. This can be seen, for example, in HIV patients, whereby antiretroviral medications need to be taken 95 per cent of the time (Paterson *et al.*, 1999). Also with chronic illnesses such as diabetes not adhering correctly to medication can result in an increased vulnerability to eye disease, kidney disease, nerve damage and heart problems (Diabetes Insight, 2006). This has also been echoed within the mental health setting, where not adhering can result in an increase in rehospitalisation and a poorer outcome in people with psychotic disorders (Gabel and Piezcker, 1985; Helgason, 1990).

Up to 80 per cent of patients can be expected not to comply with their treatment at some time (Dunbar-Jacob *et al.*, 1995). These figures are mirrored in studies that have looked at several chronic illnesses, such as HIV (Wu, 2001), child and adult asthma (Rand, 1997), diabetes (Sadur *et al.*, 1999), hypertension (Berlowitz *et al.*, 1998), myocardial infarction (Horwitz *et al.*, 1990) and schizophrenia (Gabel and Piezcker, 1985; Helgason, 1990).

Think about this

The relationship between non-adherence and negative implications for health is a lot closer to home than you may think. Think back to the last time antiobitics were prescribed and you were instructed to take the full course. Even though you were instructed to take all your antibiotics, did you adhere to this advice, or did you stop taking them once the symptoms had disappeared? Stopping the medication too early or not taking the full prescription can result in the body being more likely to contract the illness again.

The World Health Organization (WHO) Report on Infectious Diseases for 2000 states that, 'not taking a full course of treatment, sharing medication with other people, or keeping part of the course for another occasion' (Davey *et al.*, 2002, p. 43) is a problem. This report brings to light how individuals may not adhere and how vast the problem is.

Defining the terms 'compliance', 'adherence' and 'concordance'

When referring to patient adherence, the terms '**compliance**' and 'adherence' are used interchangeably. Compliance was frequently used during the early stages of research, which investigated whether the patient followed their practitioner's instructions. Haynes *et al.* (1979) define compliance as, 'The extent to which the patient's behaviour (in terms of taking medication, following diets or other lifestyle changes) coincides with medical or health advice'. The term compliance implies that the patient will follow the nurses orders without any questions, is always in a less informed position and that a failure to comply is the fault of the patient (Donovan and Blake, 1992; National Asthma Council, 2003; Waitzkin, 1989). This term has been heavily criticised in nursing literature for its paternalistic view of the practitioner–patient relationship, in which the patient is perceived to be passive and expected to obey the clinician's orders (Snelgrove, 2006). Many nurses feel uneasy about the label, as it directs blame largely towards the patient (Russell *et al.*, 2003). For example, the term implies the patient is being deviant and labelled as non-compliant. In the case study above, Mr Riaz did not comply with the treatment advice that had been initially set as he became confused. The term compliance does not enable the nurse to distinguish between patients who have intentionally decided not to take medication (**intentional non-adherence**) and those such as Mr Riaz, who are confused and in turn have not adhered.

There is a small but growing body of nursing literature which argues that the dominant view of non-compliance fails to take sufficient account of the social context of patients' lives (Russell *et al.*, 2003). In the case of Mr Riaz, his background such as his lifestyle, demography and previous medical history, was not taken into account.

Nurse–patient consultations have changed as a result of health research, health education and government policies, from being heavily dominated by the practitioner, who instructs the patient 'what to do', to the consultation being 'patient-centred'. As a result, there is more emphasis on patients being encouraged to ask questions and the consultation focusing on the patient's individual needs. The term non-adherence has been used to reflect this shift and has almost replaced the term non-compliance, which had been given to the patient who does not take their medication as instructed or following the medical advice from the nurse. This move has been highlighted by Leventhal (1993), who states that:

> The conceptual shift from compliance to adherence represents an important first step in moving away from roles emphasising obedience to instructions toward models emphasising the independence, or self-regulatory activity of the patient.

According to the National Asthma Council (2003) adherence can be defined as 'A term that focuses more on patient commitment to the regimen. It is based on reasonable negotiations and more patient empowerment than compliance'. The term adherence moves away from the patient being a passive recipient of health care who should obey instructions from professionals (Gray *et al.*, 2002); this in turn attributes blame away from the patient. Take for example the case study above: had the term non-compliance been used to describe Mr Riaz not taking his insulin injection, the attributed blame would have been on him. On the other hand, the term adherence provides the scope to explore the communication process, which resulted in Mr Riaz not taking his injection. The term adherence is more reflective of the type of consultation that is now carried out between the nurse and the patient, where the patient is encouraged to have a more active role. Clearly in the case of Mr Riaz, this was not the case.

The term adherence has, however, also been criticised for still implying that the patient is, to an extent, passive within their care, and that the practitioner, e.g. the nurse has the dominant power weighting. As a result, more recently the term **concordance** has been used. Weiss and Britten (2003) describe con-concordance as 'The patient being an equal partner, supporting the ethos of shared decision-making between patient and health professional rather than more traditional paternalism'. This term is very much reflective and in line with the predicted ethos of the NHS, which is now working towards the new 'patient-led NHS' (Department of Health, 2005a). The term also enables the nurse to identify variables within the consultation that could have contributed to the patient not adhering to medical advice or treatment. At the same time the terms adherence and compliance have been and are still cited within health education material and research.

How common is non-compliance among the patients that I will be working with?

As suggested above, the general rate of non-adherence across illnesses has been 80 per cent (Dunbar-Jacob *et al.*, 1995). However, this figure will vary depending on what illness is being considered.

Think about this

Consider the following ill-health states:

- Flu
- Cold
- Depression
- Type II insulin-dependent diabetes
- HIV

To what extent will non-adherence vary? Are there any other factors that will determine the variation of non-adherence and or non-compliance figures?

Mental health

The average rate of non-compliance among schizophrenic patients has been estimated as being as high as 42 per cent by Cramer and Rosenheck (1998), who also found this rate to be similar for other mental disorders. Even though the study above exemplifies the consistency of adherence figures across mental illnesses, there also seems to be enormous variability across studies in the estimated rate of or compliance/non-compliance. For example, Quitkin *et al.* (1978) found the rate of non-compliance to be as low as 10 per cent among schizophrenic patients, whereas other studies suggest non-compliance to be as high as 73 per cent among this group. Gray *et al.* (2002) attributes such variances partly to the problems associated with the accuracy of measuring adherence and how adherence is defined.

Low adherence has not only been documented with schizophrenia alone. Bipolar disorder is another mental illness where low medical adherence is becoming a major clinical concern (McAllister-Williams, 2006). McAllister-Williams points out that there are implications for the patient, the most obvious being further deterioration in health, even though during the time of non-adherence the patient will be feeling very well or 'high'. Not taking medication as directed can also contribute to relapse in treatment overall.

The different factors and reasons for non-compliance vary depending on the mental illness that is being looked at. Nurses need to be familiar with the differing reasons why non-compliance occurs for specific mental health illnesses, so that these can be emphasised to the patient. For example, McAllister-Williams (2006) highlights the following four reasons why non-compliance occurs among bipolar disorder patients:

- Difficulty tolerating side effects of the medication.
- Dislike of medication controlling their mood or missing their highs.
- Wanting to stop treatment as soon as they feel well.
- Some see the need for drug treatment as symbolic of chronic illnesses.

These four factors need to be addressed before or during treatment so that each of these factors is managed well and, in turn, non-adherence is less likely to occur.

Paediatric

Studies have looked at the frequency of paediatric non-adherence across a range of chronic illnesses, such as diabetes, rheumatoid arthritis and cystic fibrosis. They have found that adherence levels at or below 50 per cent of prescribed dosages are common (Rapoff, 1999). Poor adherence rates have been commonly highlighted as a particular problem for children with asthma. For example, under-use of the inhaler steroids has been observed in a study, which suggested that the under-use could be seen for up to 55 per cent of the observation days (Coutts *et al.*, 1992). However adherence rates vary when looking at particular population demographics, such as ethnicity. For example, Vargas and Rand (1999) examined medication adherence among a sample of low-income African-American children with asthma aged 6–12 years, who reported using at least one inflammatory medication. Electronic monitoring over a two to three week period found that no single subject took the medications as prescribed for the full observation period.

Adult

Adherence problems with chronic illnesses in adults have been highlighted as a major problem. For example, in relation to HIV-positive patients, effective treatments are currently failing because of non-adherence and **drug-resistance** (Forgarty et al., 2002; Hellmann, 2001). Asim et al.'s (2007) study is one of many that have identified a link between lack of adherence among HIV patients and the increased likelihood of drug resistance and opportunities for viral breakthrough. In order to avoid these effects and keep the immune system as healthy as possible, HIV patients need to maintain an adherence rate of 95 per cent or more over many years.

In relation to other chronic illnesses such as diabetes, it has been found that individuals have to adhere to treatment as well as lifestyle and dietary change. As a result, adherence rates differ depending on the particular change that is being addressed (Glasgow et al., 1987; Kurtz, 1990). For example, research has shown better adherence rates for medication use than for lifestyle change (Anderson et al., 1993). In other studies, adherence rates of 65 per cent were reported for diet (Glasgow et al., 1987) but only 19 per cent for exercise (Anderson et al., 1993). In order to prevent non-adherence among diabetes patients, nurses need to spend more time concentrating on issues such as diet and exercise so that patients will not have a problem adhering to the recommended lifestyle changes.

Think about this

The diabetes nurse informed Mr Riaz that he was to avoid food that was high in sugar and/or fat. The nurse could have spent more time explaining the reasons behind such change, providing information that was tailored to his current lifestyle and explaining why people have problems adhering to long-term medication and lifestyle changes.

Individuals are more likely to have problems adhering to medical advice and treatment that have to be endured over a long period of time. Chronic illnesses, which are defined as illnesses that last three months or more, fall into this category. Diabetes, HIV and asthma are all examples of chronic illness as they have to be managed for the rest of the individual's life; as a result mistakes are more likely to be made. DiMatteo (1994) suggests that when looking at non-adherence in long-term illnesses, non-adherence figures can rise, on average, by 10 per cent.

Problems with adherence are also high for less serious states of ill-health such as flu. One early study revealed that only 12 per cent of patients who were prescribed penicillin for 10 days were still taking it by the tenth day, 50 per cent had stopped by the third day, 71 per cent by the sixth day and 82 per cent by the ninth day (Bergman and Werner, 1963). Patients who are provided with medication for a short period of time need to be informed that non-adherence is high and forewarned about the possible consequences of such. For example, nurses should emphasise that irrespective of symptoms disappearing, medication should be taken until the full course is completed as this will prevent reoccurrence within a short space of time.

As the above examples have demonstrated, non-adherence, non-compliance or non-concordance may vary depending on the type of illness, the number of changes that have to be made and if the illness is acute or chronic. This is before any consideration is given to the communication process between the nurse and patient, the demograpy of the patient or previous adherence behaviour. The next section will consider further explanations as to what contributes to adherence and non-adherence. Had the diabetes nurse been aware of the contributing factors that result in non-adherence, she would have explored Mr Riaz's confusion during the consultation. Once the nurse has understood the factors that contribute to non-adherence she can then think about factors that enhance adherence.

The nurse-patient relationship

The nurse–patient relationship is a contributing factor to the extent the patient will follow the advice and treatment regimen set. The following section will take a look at the different components of the nurse–patient consultation and how the communication process between the two can influence adherence.

Think about this

Before reading the section below, think about the consultation in the opening case study. Which components of the consultation resulted in the patient becoming confused and not adhering?

Patient satisfaction

One of the major contributing factors to adherence is **patient satisfaction**, which has been shown in a number of studies to increase the likelihood of medication and medical advice being followed. Phillip Ley (1981, 1989) developed the **cognitive hypothesis model of compliance**. According to this model, patient compliance can be predicted by:

- patient satisfaction with the process of the consultation;
- understanding of the information provided during the consultation; and
- the recall of this information.

Figure 16.1 exemplifies this further.

Numerous studies have highlighted the important role patient satisfaction has to play in influencing patients' adherence to medication and medical advice (Bartlett *et al.*, 1984; Bolus and Pitts, 1999; Falvo *et al.*, 1980; Francis *et al.*, 1969; Geersten *et al.*, 1973; Ley, 1990; Ley *et al.*, 1976; Smith *et al.*, 1986; Wartman *et al.*, 1983).

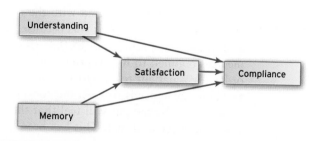

Figure 16.1 The cognitive hypothesis model of compliance.

Think about this

Which aspect(s) of the interaction between the nurse and patient will influence patient satisfaction? Once a nurse can establish which aspects of the nurse–patient interaction impact on patient satisfaction, these can be taken into consideration when communicating with patients so that problems with medical treatment, medication and advice are prevented.

It is as simple as a student completing their homework or an assignment! Think back to a time at school or college when an assessment or a piece of homework had to be completed. There would have been certain subjects that you would have given priority to. At the same time, there would have been subjects that you would have hated and given low priority to. Why was this? The answer is student satisfaction. The happier you were with the understanding of the subject, the more you liked the way your teacher/lecturer delivered the content and how well you were able to relate the subject to everyday life, resulted in you, the student, being satisfied. As a result, you were more likely to adhere to deadlines if you were satisfied with your learning experience! It is exactly the same for patient satisfaction and adherence.

Wolf *et al.* (1978) measured specific parts of a consultation, to determine what actually resulted in patient satisfaction. Wolf and his colleagues concluded that three parts of the consultation were perceived by patients to have been detrimental in influencing patient satisfaction: (a) the *cognitive* aspect – satisfaction with the amount and quality of the information provided by the doctor; (b) the *affective* aspect – the extent to which the patient feels that the doctor listens, understands and is interested; and (c) the *behavioural* aspect – the patient's evaluation of the doctor's competence in the consultation.

Think about this

To what extent was Mr Riaz satisfied with his consultation? What areas could have been improved?

Mr Riaz was not satisfied with the consultation that took place between himself and the nurse. This was because, firstly, he was not encouraged to ask any questions. In addition to this, the nurse did not attempt to relate the medical regimen to his everyday life. As a result, Mr Riaz was confused. In order for a patient to be satisfied with the cognitive aspect of the consultation, the nurse needs to keep the consultation as patient-centred as possible. As a result, the patient will feel that their anxieties and requests have been both addressed and met. This has been highlighted with studies that suggest that patients are more likely to be satisfied with their consultation if they perceive their requests to have been met (Like and Zyzanski, 1986, 1987). Patients are also more likely to feel satisfied if they feel that they have been understood. This was highlighted by researchers such as Zyzanski (1986, p. 335) who suggested that 'the understanding of the patient's perspective should be a core clinical task' as the patient's own perception and feelings of satisfaction may differ from that of the nurse. The nurse can ensure that the patient has had all their questions answered and any misunderstandings clarified by keeping the interaction as patient-centred as possible; this way the patient is more likely to understand the information provided to them.

Mr Riaz could have had a different explanation as to the origins of diabetes, which may have diverged from the biomedical perspective (refer to Chapter 9). Having two different explanations, such as one from a lay person and the other from a health practitioner will inevitably result in poor patient satisfaction, especially when the consultation is being dominated by the health practitioner's biomedical viewpoint (Bertakis, 1977). The diabetes nurse did not make any attempt to see if the patient had his own explanation or viewpoint regarding his insulin injection to manage his diabetes. Nurses need to be aware that patients may hold health beliefs regarding the origins, management, cure and treatment of an illness or state of ill-health, which may be different from the predominant biomedical viewpoint. Any potential clashes will need to be prevented so that patient satisfaction and, in turn, adherence will not be affected negatively. This can only be done by keeping the consultation as patient-centred as possible so that the patient will feel that their viewpoint has been taken into consideration (see Chapter 9 for more details).

Research has also highlighted the link between consultation style and patient satisfaction and adherence. Kenny (1995) exemplified the negative impact a physician-dominated approach can have on patient adherence. The study looked at patient satisfaction among ethnic minorities, specifically those from an Asian background. Kenny found that there was a strong association between the level of satisfaction and the degree to which patients felt their requests had been met in the consultation. The more they felt their needs had been met, the greater the satisfaction they reported. For example, 95.1 per cent of those reporting that their requests had been met expressed satisfaction with the consultation.

Patient satisfaction and being patient-centred

There have been numerous studies that have highlighted a positive link between being patient-centred and patient satisfaction (e.g. Little *et al.*, 2001). A positive association has also been found between patient-centredness, treatment adherence (Rao *et al.*, 2000) and decreased rates of malpractice claims (Levinson *et al.*, 1997).

Think about this

In the opening case study, the diabetes nurse dominated the consultation and was not patient-centred. What possible effect can this have on Mr Riaz, in relation to being satisfied and his non-adherence to the insulin injection?

But what does being patient-centred actually entail? Balint *et al.* (1970) have suggested that being patient-centred should involve the asking and receiving of questions and information which result in the patient understanding the health information and treatment being proposed. For example, the diabetes nurse could have asked Mr Riaz if he understood how diabetes is caused and how they would be treating it. This in turn would have allowed the nurse to clarify any confusion that he may have had, which is positive for adherence behaviour. So how could the diabetes nurse have been more patient-centred?

- The diabetes nurse should have asked questions to establish Mr Riaz's health beliefs and if these complemented or clashed with the biomedical approach (refer to Chapter 9).
- These could have followed in the format of, how do you think your illness began? What do you think is the best way forward, etc., (refer to Chapter 9).
- The diabetes nurse should have asked questions throughout the consultation (refer to Chapter 5).
- The diabetes nurse should have talked about the administration of the insulin injection in relation to other drug regimens.

If the diabetes nurse had met the above criteria throughout her consultation, not only would the consultation have been more patient-centred but, more importantly, Mr Riaz would not have been as confused about his medication and his diet.

Nurses need to be aware that every patient may not necessarily be happy with a consultation that is dominated by the person or patient-centred approach. In the case of Mr Riaz, a patient-centred approach was needed in order to establish his perception of the diagnosis and to ease any worries, confusion or anxiety he may have experienced. However he needed this only up to a certain point, as he also needed the nurse to dominate the information-giving part of the consultation.

The patient's preference in terms of the type of consultation is also important to patient satisfaction and adherence, as not every patient necessarily prefers a patient-centred approach. Lipton *et al.* (1998) observed the preferred interaction between the patient and the physician and concluded that the relationship varies, depending on the ethnic background of the patient. They concluded that patients who did not have health beliefs that stemmed from the biomedical approach, actually preferred a physician/nurse-dominated consultation. For example, Hall and Doran (1990) found no gender differences with patient satisfaction. However, those who are older and have less educational status are more likely to prefer a physician-dominated consultation.

Mr Riaz would have preferred the diabetes nurse to dominate the consultation because of the new diagnosis, but not to the extent that occurred; as a result the individual needs and concerns of Mr Riaz were ignored. For nurses a midway point needs to be found, where questions and anxieties are addressed as well as information being conveyed to the patient in the best way possible.

Swenson *et al.* (2004) have suggested a 'flexible' approach to patient-centredness when attempting to enhance patient satisfaction and adherence. They urged practitioners to use a flexible approach, whereby patients are encouraged to have a consultation within a patient-centred arena, but acknowledge that parts of the consultation and some patients require a core nurse-dominated approach.

Think about this

Using the flexible approach for each of the situations below, will a patient-centred, directive or mixed approach take predominance?

- Emergency surgery.
- Treatment explanation to a newly diagnosed diabetes patient such as Mr Riaz.
- Patient who is feeling unwell but does not know why.
- Patient who has not been adhering to the correct dosage of the asthma inhaler prescribed.
- Blood pressure reading.
- Administering drugs.

Table 16.1 is a physician assessment questionnaire (adapted from Swenson *et al.*, 2004) which assesses the extent to which patient-centredness is used by the practitioner. Use the questionnaire to establish the extent to which the diabetes nurse was patient-centred.

Communication

Cognitive factors: understanding

Mr Riaz was clearly confused when contemplating the administration of his insulin injection.

Think about this

How could the diabetes nurse have improved her information-giving, so that Mr Riaz would not have become confused when administering his insulin at home? The section below examines the role of information giving and the cognitive factors that influence patient recall.

Table 16.1 Physician assessment questionnaire

Patient-centred characteristics

	(Definitely yes)				*(Definitely not)*		
The doctor suggested a good plan for helping the patient	1	2	3	4	5		

	(Very strongly agree)					*(Very strongly disagree)*	
The doctor seemed narrow-minded	1	2	3	4	5	6	7
The doctor was interested in the patient as a person	1	2	3	4	5	6	7
The doctor gave the patient a chance to say what was on their mind	1	2	3	4	5	6	7
The doctor gave the patient his/her full attention	1	2	3	4	5	6	7

Other characteristics

The doctor took the patient's problems seriously	1	2	3	4	5	6	7
The doctor communicated in simple, clear language	1	2	3	4	5	6	7
The doctor seemed to know about the risks and benefits of alternative medicine	1	2	3	4	5	6	7
The doctor seemed indecisive	1	2	3	4	5	6	7

Global measurements

This is a doctor I would trust	1	2	3	4	5	6	7
I would recommend this doctor to my friends	1	2	3	4	5	6	7

Source: Swenson *et al.* (2004)

The hospital setting can be a highly anxious and distressing environment for a patient, which means they may find it difficult to absorb information (see Chapter 5). Take for example Mr Riaz, who has just been diagnosed with diabetes in the hospital environment. Even though the diabetes nurse may have assumed her instructions were simple and straightforward, this may have not been the case.

The guidelines in Table 16.2 will ensure that the information being given is provided in the best way possible and that the patient remembers what they have been told. The patient will therefore be less likely to forget or become confused and more likely to adhere. (See Chapter 5, which explores information-giving.)

Accuracy and recall of information can be further improved by:

- bearing in mind that patients tend to remember the first part of the message;
- stressing the importance of compliance;
- simplifying information given;
- using repetition;
- being specific;
- following up with additional interviews.

Table 16.2 Guidelines for providing information	**Guidelines when information-giving, to ensure adherence**	**Example: Mr Riaz and the diabetes nurse**
	Keep information as simple as possible	Diabetes nurse simplifying the diagnosis and medicine-taking instructions
	Most important instructions and information should be given at the beginning	Talking about the insulin injection at the beginning of the consultation
	Divide the consultation into several 'chunks', rather than one piece of information	Divide the consultation between information-giving, asking about the patient's lifestyle, talking about diet and instructions regarding the insulin injections
	Convert meaningless information to meaningful information	Explanation of terms such as insulin, diabetes
	Ensure the patient is listening	Making parts of the consultation patient-centred by asking questions

The more complex a regimen is, the more likely it is a patient will not fully adhere (Bender, 2002). In order to make treatment instructions as simple as possible, it is important for the nurse to provide instructions in light of the patient's current lifestyle, as well as the drugs they may be taking or the treatments they are currently involved in. In the case study above, had the diabetes nurse spoken about the insulin injection in relation to Mr Riaz's current diet and other medications, Mr Riaz would not have been as confused.

Oral and written information

There are different ways in which a nurse can provide treatment instructions, which can influence how likely a patient is to remember them. For example, the more oral and written information you can give a patient, the more likely you are to enhance their adherence (McDonald *et al.*, 2002). This is because information that is received by more than one sense is more likely to be registered within memory and retained for a longer period of time (see Chapter 5 for further elaboration).

How many times have you visited a doctor or any other medical practitioner and not been able to recall the instructions that they gave you? The answer is, usually, many times! Writing information down can help an individual remember. Think about Mr Riaz. If the nurse had written down instructions that reiterated what she had said, then Mr Riaz would have been more likely to have remembered what injection he should have taken in the morning.

Tailoring medication instructions to the patient's daily activities

A nurse should ensure that a complex treatment plan is prescribed and explained in light of what the patient does on a daily basis (McDonald *et al.*, 2002). In the opening case study, no attempt was made by the nurse to relate the insulin injections to Mr Riaz's day-to-day life. The diabetes nurse could have explained the timing of injections for each day by firstly asking Mr Riaz about his daily routine. It would then be possible to relate the timing of his injections to features of his routine, thus encouraging him not to become confused or forget what he was instructed to do. Taking into account both previous and current states of ill-health, as well as what the patient has come in for is also important, as previous adherence patterns with other medication can influence the patient's current motivation to adhere.

The research in focus box is an example of how pre-existing states of ill-health can influence the patient's current motivation to adhere.

The research in focus box demonstrates the importance of acknowledging the patient's previous treatments, illnesses and current day-to-day routine, so that the patient will be more likely to adhere and not get confused or forget treatment instructions like Mr Riaz. Research is favourable towards health practitioners being able to easily provide instructions in such a manner that has the benefit of the patient adhering correctly to medical instructions. For example, Seaton (2005) concluded from his findings that clinicians can quickly adjust a treatment regimen to fit a patient's lifestyle. When patients

Research in focus

DiMatteo, M.R., Lepper, H.S. and Croghan, T.W. (2000) Depression is a risk factor for non-compliance with medical treatment. *Archives of Internal Medicine*, **160**, 2101–2107.

Aim
Depression and anxiety are common in medical patients and are normally associated with decreased health care utilisation. The authors of this article carried out a review of studies aimed at finding correlations between patients' non-adherence to medical treatment and their levels of anxiety and depression.

Sample
The authors looked at 25 studies carried out between 1968 and 1998, 12 of these were about depression and 13 about anxiety.

Method
In order to qualify for this review, studies had to measure adherence, patient anxiety or depression and involve a control group who were not being treated for either of these disorders, but instead had been asked to follow a medical regime by a doctor who was not a psychiatrist.

Results
The studies examined by the authors showed that there seems to be no correlation between anxiety and non-adherence but a strong correlation between depression and non-adherence.

Conclusions
Compared with non-depressed patients, depressed patients are three times more likely to fail to adhere to a medical regime. The authors point out that it remains to be determined whether treating depression will result in improved patient adherence but that the recognition of depression as a risk factor for non-adherence has the potential to improve health care outcomes for some patients.

perceive their treatment and prescribed drug plan to be adjusted and related to their daily living, not only do they feel more confident that the proposed treatment is workable but also the chances of adherence success have been found to increase.

Adherence support tools can also be used to help a patient adhere. A calendar pill remainder box (see picture) is one example of an adherence support tool. Today such a tool is frequently used by patients like Mr Riaz who need to take several medications in a day. Even though an injection cannot be fitted into these, Mr Riaz could have been made aware of this tool so that less confusion would occur when taking his other pills as well as the injections. Pillboxes are sold in pharmacies and have been found to decrease the frequency of non-adherence (Poppa *et al.*, 2003; Simoni *et al.*, 2003).

Nurses are also encouraged to recommend calendar pill reminders, as practitioners can now prescribe them for groups of patients who could have potential problems with adherence. These include patients who tend to forget their medication times, elderly patients who live by themselves, patients who have an illness such as HIV where several medications have to be taken or, like Mr Riaz, patients who are required to take several medications because of having more than one illness. Nurses are also encouraged to demonstrate the use of pill calendar reminders to patients.

Calendar pillboxes are helpful for patients who forget to take their medication or have several medications to take daily. The calendar pillbox acts as a visual reminder.

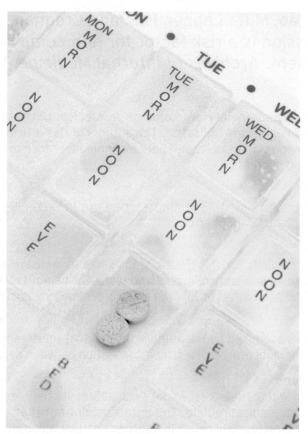

Geoffrey Kidd/Alamy

Health beliefs and patient adherence

Health beliefs (see Chapter 15) have an important role in determining if a patient will adhere or not. In the opening case study, Mr Riaz was clearly confused. However, because he was not asked the right questions, we were unable to grasp how Mr Riaz perceived his diagnosis (see Chapter 9).

'**Social cognition** is concerned with how individuals make sense of social situations' (Conner and Norman, 1996, p. 5). The **health belief model** (HBM) (Janz and Becker, 1984; Rosenstock, 1974) is one example of a social cognition model that has been applied to adherence behaviour in patients. This model suggests that the likelihood that someone will engage in a given health behaviour, e.g. adherence, is a result of the following four functions: perceived susceptibility, perceived severity, perceived benefits/barriers and cues to action (refer to Chapter 15).

According to the HBM, in weighing the pros and cons of taking preventative action such as medication, people arrive at a decision as to whether the perceived benefits (e.g. taking insulin injections) outweigh the perceived barriers or cost (e.g. taking time out to become familiar with self-administration of an injection).

The evidence for the HBM predicting compliance behaviour has been very strong. For example, a review has shown that the HBM has been able to distinguish between people who do and do not comply with medication. According to this model, individuals are more likely to adhere to medication if they believe that their health may become worse (e.g. susceptibility). In addition, another predictive element, which results in high adherence, is where the benefits of protective behaviour (e.g. taking medication to prevent serious side effects) outweigh the costs of taking the medication (e.g. time taken out to visit the surgery for repeat prescriptions). This model cannot be applied to Mr Riaz as he was simply confused with his medication instructions. This model brings in the notion of **intentional non-adherence** or non-compliance whereby an individual will willing decide not to take medication.

Self-regulatory model, illness perception and adherence behaviour

The **self-regulatory model** postulated by Leventhal and Cameron (1987) is more relevant when understanding adherence behaviour of patients. The model acts as a framework to examine why a patient, through their understanding of their illness, has resulted in their current adherence behaviour. According to this model, coping responses such as adherence behaviour, are heavily influenced by the patient's own beliefs or representations of the illness, which differ from person to person (Cameron and Leventhal, 2003). Table 16.3 displays the possible thought patterns that Mr Riaz could have experienced when making sense of his diagnosis of diabetes, and which the nurse should have acknowledged during the consultation.

According to Leventhal et al. (1980), how patients think about their illness can be structured around four (and, in a later model, five) cognitive dimensions. These are *illness identity*; which refers to the label one gives to a

Table 16.3 Possible thought patterns	**Mr Riaz making sense of the new diagnosis of diabetes**	**How the nurse could have acknowledged this during the consultation to ensure that Mr Riaz would adhere to his insulin injections**
	The diagnosis of diabetes will be able to be managed just like the flu - I will get better after a while.	Should have made Mr Riaz aware that diabetes is a chronic illness that will have to be managed for the rest of his life.
	What on earth does diabetes have to do with insulin?	Explain the link between the two.
	Just like my asthma, won't be that severe if I miss an injection - I will be fine. I have been so far.	Explain the consequences of not adhering.
	In my culture there is no such word as diabetes. They don't understand that Asians tend to have a diet that is high in fat.	Explain that his current diet will not have to change vastly. Small changes will be most beneficial.
	The pain of administering an injection, and I hate injections!	Reassure Mr Riaz and explain the type of discomfort that will be experienced. Also, recommend relaxation techniques.

disease and the symptoms that indicate it. *Causes and underlying pathology*: ideas about how one gets the disease. *Timeline*, beliefs about how long a disease takes to appear or last. *Consequences*, the expected effects and consequences of an illness and finally, *cure and controllability*, whereby assumptions are made about how one recovers and the extent to which this can be controlled by the patient or by external sources (Croyle and Jemmott, 1991). These five cognitive dimensions can help a nurse understand how the patient makes sense of their illness. As a result the nurse will be able to acknowledge these structures during the consultation when adherence to treatment may become a problem, i.e. when managing a chronic illness.

During this process, any kind of mismatch between the nurse and the patient can result in the patient not adhering or even accepting the illness. A nurse who is aware of the five cognitive dimensions can effectively tailor the communication and consultation around the patient's needs and weak spots. As a result, the patient will more likely adhere. Below is an example of Mr Riaz attempting to 'make sense' of his newly diagnosed insulin-dependent diabetes:

- *Illness identity* – 'the diabetes nurse says that I have diabetes, but I have no symptoms that suggest that I am diabetic'. The nurse will need to make Mr Riaz aware that diabetes does not necessarily present obvious symptoms straight away. The nurse will need to make him aware of what is happening in his body, as well as the symptoms that could emerge if he fails to comply with his medication.
- *Causes and underlying pathology* – what ideas does Mr Riaz have about the origins of his diabetes? The nurse will have to establish what Mr Riaz perceives the causative factors to be. If these are factious, the nurse will need to highlight this and present factual information, e.g. relevance of biological as well as psychosocial factors. There could be causative factors that do not reside within the biomedical or biopsychosocial model. For example, if Mr Riaz thought that his diabetes had stemmed from genetic

factors alone, he would have to be informed about other factors such as diet, lifestyle and the environment.

- *Timeline* – a commonly held coping mechanism is that newly diagnosed illnesses (especially those that the patient does not know much about) are viewed in the same way as previous illnesses. The nurse will have to highlight to Mr Riaz that this is a chronic illness, which he will have to manage for the rest of his life, unlike the common cold. Also very different from asthma and the use of inhalers.

- *Consequences* – the patient should be made aware of the consequences of not taking an insulin injection. In addition to this, the patient should be informed about the necessary lifestyle changes, particularly in relation to his diet and prioritising his insulin injection.

- *Cure and controllability* – the patient will need to know that diabetes cannot be cured and that the severity of the illness will depend on how it is managed. The nurse will need to highlight what Mr Riaz can do to manage his illness, e.g. change of diet and exercise, as well as acquaint him with all the social support networks that are available, e.g. walking for life groups.

Studies have found that working on each of these cognitive components with a patient can result in better adherence; this was documented in a study carried out by Griva *et al.* (2000). Researchers tested these dimensions by administering the **illness perception questionnaire** to 64 adolescents (15–25 years) with insulin-dependent diabetes mellitus (IDDM), who were outpatients at two affiliated hospitals in London. It was found that those patients who had a strong illness identity and a belief that there would be serious consequences associated with diabetes were more likely to correctly adhere to their diabetes treatment.

Beliefs about medication and adherence behaviour

The Royal Pharmaceutical Society of Great Britain (1997) has suggested that how individuals perceive and think about medication (**medication beliefs**) is important when considering treatment adherence and should be a priority for future research. Nurses should be aware of their patients' medication beliefs if they want to break the enormous barrier of non-adherence to medication. There has been a clear link outlined between medication beliefs and adherence behaviour. For example, Horne (1997, p. 32) has stated that

Decisions about taking medication are likely to be informed by beliefs about medication, as well as beliefs about the illness, which the medication is tended to prevent or cure, which would inevitably influence adherence behaviour.

According to Fallsberg (1991) there are three broad categories of lay beliefs concerning medication:

- Positive view of medication, which stems from the beneficial effects of taking medication.
- Negative view of medication, which derives from the perception and/or experience of the harmful effects of medication, e.g. poisonous, necessary evil.
- Dual nature of medication, which refers to beliefs about the potential harm as well as the benefits of medication.

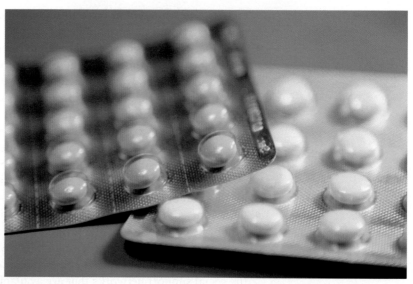

Peter Banos/Alamy

The second category can help to explain intentional non-adherence. For example, Fallsberg (1991) has cited that, within the remit of *negative views of medication,* fear of becoming addicted or too dependent are key reasons for intentional non-adherence. Mr Riaz may have perceived the insulin injections as 'another batch of medications' that would result in being addicted to them for the rest of his life. The diabetes nurse would need to rule out any misconceptions, so that non-adherence does not occur. Many of these misconceptions and negative views of medication are influenced by social systems around the patient, e.g. what other people say and the media.

Another example of this is the recent debate about the measles, mumps and rubella (MMR) vaccine for young babies. The media highlighted recent research on the link between MMR vaccines and autism. As a result, there were many mothers who did not adhere to the practitioner's requests to have their babies vaccinated. Instead, they adhered to what the media were stating.

A negative view of medication can also extend into altering the dosage of medication. For example Mr Riaz could have excused his behaviour by stating that missing one injection would not hurt as he did this with his inhalers. Conrad (1985) highlights another reason for intentional non-adherence; a fear self-reliance and addiction to medication. Patients could deal with this by changing their doses of medication so that they would be less likely to become addicted. Nurses need to make patients aware of the dangerous side effects of taking medications in this manner and state how these effects can potentially be more serious.

Think about this

Other than Mr Riaz being confused, what factors could have resulted in him having a negative view of medication?

One factor that could contribute to Mr Riaz holding a negative view about medications is the potential side effects. Nurses should make the patient aware that with chronic long-term illnesses such as diabetes, the negative consequences of not taking medication outweigh the long-term effects of the medication itself. Morgan and Watkins (1988) looked at hypertensive patients and found that it was common to find patients intentionally not adhering when taking their anti-hypertensive medication. The justification for this was that by stopping medication it would give the body a break.

Another possible explanation for Mr Riaz failing to adhere could be that he is comparing his negative view of the insulin injection with another model of health. For example, medication is more likely to be viewed in a negative manner with unnatural properties if it is compared with herbal remedies which are seen as 'safer'. A patient like Mr Riaz will need to have their awareness raised about herbal remedies, which can also contain unnatural properties and could have dangerous side effects when taken in conjunction with biomedical medicine.

Mr Riaz could have been faced with the dilemma of the necessity of the medication on one hand and the concern about the medication on the other. This necessity–concerns dilemma is strongly correlated with adherence behaviour (Horne and Weinman, 1999). Scores high on the necessity component result in higher adherence behaviour, while scores high on the concerns component result in lower adherence behaviour.

Mr Riaz's view of the harmful effects of his insulin injection may not necessarily have been about the injection itself. The negative view could stem from more general beliefs about medication having negative side effects (Horne *et al.*, 1999). The nurse needs to be aware that the patient could have been influenced by a general view of medication, which is usually linked to their unnatural chemical origins. Links to the adverse effects of medication (Horne *et al.*, 1999) and the link between harmful substances and the general overuse of them by practitioners (Horne *et al.*, 2001) can also result in non-adherence (Peters *et al.*, 2001).

Social support and adherence

Mr Riaz did not bring any family members or friends with him to the consultation. The likelihood of adherence, as a result of absent **social support** is therefore reduced. Numerous studies have suggested that social support enhances the likelihood of adherence. For example, Glasgow *et al.* (1989) suggested that greater levels of social support, particularly diabetes-related support from spouses and other family members, are associated with better adherence.

Social support has been found to serve many functions in patient adherence. One is that it serves to buffer the adverse effects of stress on diabetes management (Griffith *et al.*, 1990). In the case of Mr Riaz, it was clear from the outset that his chances of adherence were low, as there was no one with him who could correct his confusion by recalling parts of the previous consultation. However, his daughter, who arrived later, helped her father by clarifying his confusion.

For those patients, especially the elderly, who may not have family or friends living very close to them, the immediate social support network may be the nurse. The social support provided by nurse case managers has been shown to promote adherence of diabetic patients to diet, medications and weight loss (Sherbourne *et al.*, 1992). The nurse can provide many types of social support to the patient:

- *Informative*: Information regarding the illness or state of ill-health where literature could be provided as well as the nurse providing information.
- *Educational*: Providing instructions to the patient about medical interventions and treatment. Could also involve the first steps in providing instructions for treatment which the patient will have to practise thereafter, e.g. coping skills, relaxation skills.
- *Behavioural*: How to carry out a task or skill that the patient has been taught (then doing). For example, showing the patient how to administer an injection on a piece of fruit. Also, practising skills with the nurse, e.g. relaxation skills, deep breathing.
- *Emotional*: Providing emotional support where the nurse will listen to the patient and be there for them so that they can discharge their emotions.
- *Counsellor*: Even though nurses will not be professional counsellors (unless you have an accredited counselling qualification and can practise), they will still have to use elementary counselling skills: for example, by asking the patient to elaborate with the use of an open question (see Chapters 3 and 17).

The nurse in the above case study only provided brief instructional support, which is why Mr Riaz did not adhere. Depending on the type of ward and department you will be working in, there will be interactions whereby the nurse cannot fulfil every role. In circumstances such as these, highlighting to the patient the types of social support network within the local area would be very useful. However, there will be certain support networks that could also hinder the adherence behaviour of the patient: for example, friends who would encourage the patient not to take medication, or those who would encourage behaviour that could be detrimental to the management of their illness. The nurse will need to work with the patient to ensure that such networks are avoided when first managing or changing habits. For example, the diabetes nurse has advised Mr Riaz that he needs to lose weight. However, she should have worked with him in relation to the avoidance of triggers, e.g. rewarding himself with a pamper session rather than eating fatty foods (see Chapter 2). In this instance it would have been beneficial if the nurse had referred Mr Riaz to the dietician for additional support.

Putting it all together

The box gives an overall look at what a consultation should take into consideration where patient adherence is essential or when there are pre-existing issues with adherence behaviour. Further advice on information giving can be found in Chapter 5.

Fact Sheet: Helping the nurse to encourage the patient to adhere through communication

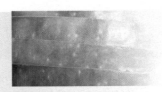

- Listen to the patient.
- Ask the patient to repeat what has to be done.
- Keep the prescription as simple as possible.
- Give clear instructions on the exact treatment regimen, preferably in writing.
- Make use of special remainder pill containers and calendars.
- Call the patient if an appointment is missed.
- Prescribe a self-care regimen in concert with the patient's daily schedule.
- Emphasise the importance of adherence at each visit.
- Gear the frequency of visits to adherence needs.
- Acknowledge the patient's efforts to adhere.
- Involve the patient's spouse or other partner.
- Whenever possible, provide patients with instructions and advice at the start of the information to be presented. When providing patients with instructions and advice, stress how important they are.
- Use short words and short sentences.
- Use explicit categorisation where possible (for example, divide information clearly into categories of aetiology, treatment or prognosis).
- Repeat things where feasible.

Conclusion

This chapter has demonstrated the many different factors that contribute to the adherence behaviour of patients. The chapter has shown that such factors determine if the patient decides intentionally or unintentionally not to adhere. The main factors that contribute to intentional non-adherence range from concerns about the side effects of medication and an individual's own explanation as to how the illness occurred, to not placing a high concern on one's own health. Unintentional non-adherence results from factors that stem from the consultation itself. These range from confusion and not understanding the health practitioner to being unable to follow treatment correctly because of confusion arising from pre-existing medical advice and instructions. A nurse who is familiar with the factors that contribute to adherence can address such factors during the consultation, thus increasing the likelihood that the patient will adhere correctly when medical advice or instructions have been given.

Summary

- Over time researchers have used differing terms to describe patient behaviour when advised by a practitioner to take medication or make significant changes to their lifestyle. Compliance refers to the patient following the practitioner's orders. Adherence implies that the patient follows the request with more negotiation. The most recent term is concordance. Concordance implies a complete power balance between the practitioner and the patient in which they both come to an agreement. Adherence has also been divided into intentional and non-intentional adherence.

- Rates of non-adherence vary, depending on the nature and duration of illness as well as the patient variables. There is a general consensus that on average there is an 80 per cent rate of non-adherence in general.

- According to Ley's (1989) cognitive hypothesis, compliance is predicted by three variables: The patient's overall satisfaction with the consultation, the patient's understanding of the information provided during the consultation and how well the patient can recall this information

- Wolf et al. (1978) highlighted three aspects that contribute to overall patient satisfaction: cognitive, affective and behavioural.

- There is link between patient-centredness and enhancing compliance. However, not every patient is satisfied with the patient-centred approach; instead, they may prefer a practitioner-dominated approach.

- The way information is communicated can have an impact on the way the patient recalls and understands the consultation. To ensure that information is communicated effectively it should be: simple, specific and tailored to the individual.

- Social cognition models (Conner and Norman, 1996) such as the health belief model (Rosenstock, 1974) can predict the adherence behaviour of patients. According to the health belief model adherence can be predicted by assessing an individual's beliefs concerning: susceptibility to illness, severity of illness, perceived benefits and barriers of performing the behaviour and cues to action

- The self-regulatory model predicts adherence behaviour of patients. The illness perception questionnaire, which is based on the self-regulatory model, identifies five dimensions that contribute to the self-regulation or the individual making sense of their illness: identity of illness, cause of illness, timeline of illness, consequences of illness and cure of illness, all of which predict adherence.

- Individual beliefs about medication are valuable in explaining adherence behaviour. The three categories that have been identified are: positive beliefs about medication, negative beliefs about medication and dual nature view of medication.

- Social support can have a positive influence on adherence behaviour. The nurse can provide many types of social support to the patient including: informative, educational, behavioural, emotional and counselling.

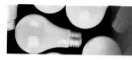

Check your understanding

- Define and distinguish the terms compliance, intentional adherence, non-intentional adherence and concordance.

- The rate of non-adherence varies depending on what particular illness you are looking at. Discuss how non-adherence varies between long- and short-term illnesses.

- Outline Ley's (1988) cognitive hypothesis model.

- Explain the five components that make up the self-regulatory (illness perception) model. How do these explain the adherence behaviour of patients?

- Describe three possible components when looking at beliefs about medication. How do they contribute to the adherence behaviour of a patient?

- Think about eight techniques that are important to incorporate into a consultation so that the patient understands and can recall information at ease.

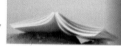

Further reading

Badger, F. and Nolan, P. (2006) Concordance with antidepressant medication in primary care. *Nursing Standard*, **20** (52), 35–40.

Beswick, A., Rees, K., West, R.R., Taylor, F.C., Burke, M., Griebsch, I., Taylor, R.S., Victory, J., Brown, J. and Ebrahim, S. (2005) Improving uptake and adherence in cardiac rehabilitation: literature review. *Journal of Advanced Nursing*, **49** (5), 538–555.

Caress, A.L. (2003) Giving information to patients. *Nursing Standard*, 17 (43), 47–54.

Delamater, A.M. (2006) Improving patient adherence. *Clinical Diabetes*, **24** (2), 71–77.

Enriquez, M., Lackey, N.R., Mary, C., O'Connor, M.D., David, S. and McKinsey, M.D. (2004) Successful adherence after multiple HIV treatment failures. *Journal of Advanced Nursing*, **45** (4), 438–446.

Happell, B., Manias, E. and Pinikahana, J. (2002) The role of the inpatient mental health nurse in facilitating patient adherence to medication regimes. *International Journal of Mental Health Nursing*, 11 (4), 251–259.

Newell, K. (2006) Concordance with asthma medication: the nurse's role. *Nursing Standard*, **20** (26), 31–33.

Snelgrove, S. (2006) Factors contributing to poor concordance in health care. *Nursing Times*, **102** (28), 28–29.

Walsh, M. and Walsh, A. (1999) Measuring patient satisfaction with nursing care: experience of using the Newcastle Satisfaction with Nursing Scale. *Journal of Advanced Nursing*, **29** (2), 307–315.

Weblinks

CE-Today	http://www.np.ce-today.com/ce-today/np/live/bb0403.htm	Audio that has been recorded live which looks at improving patient adherence in chronic heart failure. Also included are guidelines for nurses.
The Royal Pharmaceutical Society of Great Britain	http://www.rpsgb.org.uk/informationresources/museum/	Typing in the terms adherence, concordance and compliance will result in many research and policy documents looking at these issues.
Up To Date Patient Information	http://patients.uptodate.com/topic.asp?file=asthma/5578	Up-to-date patient information website that takes an in-depth look at adherence as well as enhancing adherence to asthma therapy.
Public Health Training Network	http://www.phppo.cdc.gov/PHTN/tbmodules/modules6-9/m9/9-27.htm	A module that looks at patient adherence to tuberculosis treatment with interactive exercises. Is also useful for general information concerning patient non-adherence, e.g. how it can be improved.
The Pharmaceutical Journal	http://www.pjonline.com/editorial/20031011/concordance/whatisconcordance.html	Patient concordance explored in detail.

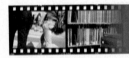

Media example

News reports from the BBC have highlighted antibiotic resistance: http://news.bbc.co.uk/2/hi/health/6283530.stm

Chapter 17
Communication and counselling skills

Learning outcomes

When you have read through this chapter you should understand:

- How communication skills and models can be applied to the nurse–patient relationship.
- How non-verbal communication can influence the communication process between nurse and patient.
- The verbal communication skills required to fully understand the patient.
- How counselling framework models can be applied to the nurse–patient relationship.
- What different types of communication strategies can be used to meet the differing needs of patients.
- How to use goal setting effectively.
- How to effectively communicate with patients who may be enduring stress, anxiety, confusion or different types of emotion.
- How to tailor communication according to age and health state.

Case study

Amarjit Singh (age 34) has been referred by his GP to the prostate cancer ward for a biopsy, after he noticed blood in his semen. The prostate cancer specialist nurse asked Amarjit some general questions about his health, before they commenced with the biopsy.

It soon became apparent to the nurse that the patient would not look at her when talking. He would answer questions while fidgeting constantly. He also sounded distraught. The nurse decided to stop asking questions and talk to the patient so that she could address his anxiety.

The nurse began by asking Amarjit if he enjoyed his job. It was clear that Amarjit's profession as a salesman was very much male dominated. Amarjit still did not relax, even when having a conversation about non-medical topics. The nurse decided to confront Amarjit's anxiety by embracing the subject of prostate cancer. Amarjit became even more distraught and began crying. It was clear to the nurse that the patient was distressed. As a result, she moved away from her desk and sat at the side of the patient, where she sat in silence and touched his hand while he cried. The nurse did not say anything until he started to confide in her.

Amarjit told the nurse that he had mentioned the symptoms to his friend who laughed at him and questioned his fertility. The nurse informed Amarjit that there is a lack of awareness of prostate cancer among younger men, which may have resulted in his friend laughing. The nurse reassured Amarjit that he did very well to seek help promptly. Amarjit looked even more distraught. The nurse confronted the patient by asking, 'Why do you feel so emotional?' After a long pause, the patient told the nurse that apart from the friend who laughed at him and his GP, no one else knew about his symptoms. The nurse reassured Amarjit that it was very common to have patients who did not confide in many people if they had discovered something unpleasant, especially men. Amarjit then told the nurse that he had lied to his GP, and the blood had been present in his semen for several months. It was only when his general health began deteriorating that he decided to seek help. The nurse praised Amarjit for seeing his GP, and told him about the importance of putting this down on his medical record.

Amarjit now began to appear calmer. The nurse was confident that she had equipped Amarjit with the appropriate information, which had eased his anxiety. The nurse also asked if he needed to know anything else before they carried out the biopsy, which was important as it would determine whether the prostate cells were cancerous.

Three months later, Amarjit sent a thank you letter to the nurse who had taken time to talk to him. The cells were cancerous and he had a prostatectomy. Amarjit opened up to people around him about his prostate cancer. He will always be thankful to the nurse who made sure that he had his biopsy, rather than turning away from the waiting room, which he was so close to doing.

Why is this relevant to nursing practice?

The case study of patient Amarjit Singh highlights many issues in relation to how a nurse communicates effectively with a patient who is upset. What would have happened if the nurse had carried on with the standard health questions? Would the patient's anxiety have remained the same, increased or, worse still, would the patient have walked out before the scheduled biopsy?

This case study exemplifies how the nursing role reaches far beyond the standard care practice or procedures that need to be followed. In addition to basic care, nurses will be in situations that require them to communicate with patients who have high anxiety levels, feel emotional or just need to talk. All of these scenarios bring into focus the importance of how a nurse effectively communicates within the nurse–patient relationship. Without effective communication, a patient will not be helped to move away from their current thought patterns.

It could be argued that the fact that an interaction between the nurse and the patient occurs means that communication has taken place. However, to be an effective communicator, a nurse needs to acknowledge the different counselling and communication framework models, as these can distinguish between nurses who just communicate and nurses who *effectively* communicate. In the case study above, the nurse is a clear example of an effective communicator. It is evident that the nurse was aware of the patient's verbal and non-verbal communication, which resulted in her changing her interaction with him. Had she not been aware of the patient's non-verbal communication, she may have not addressed all of the issues that were brought to light.

There may be many questions a nurse will think about when in a similar situation. Do I confront Amarjit's behaviour? What appropriate **strategies** can I use, so that the patient will 'open up' to me? How can I make sure that I 'don't put my foot in it'? How do I prevent the patient becoming dependent on me for answers? How can I decrease the confusion that the patient has? Or simply, where do I start and how can I move the patient out of their current negative thinking pattern?

These are some of the questions that may have crossed your mind when reading the case study and thinking about how you would effectively communicate with a patient in a similar situation. Being aware of the counselling and communication models and skills that are available and then applying them to the nurse–patient context, as well as being able to choose the most effective and appropriate strategies, will result in a nurse communicating more confidently within situations such as the one above. This chapter will examine particular strategies and skills highlighted in communication and counselling models. These will be considered in relation to the nurse–patient relationship.

Communication awareness among nurses

Communication skills training has become increasingly important within medical education worldwide (Simpson *et al.*, 1991); this has been associated with an improvement in reported satisfaction among patients. For example, nearly 74 per cent of patients in 2004 felt that they had been listened to by doctors and nurses within accident and emergency wards and 67 per cent of patients felt that they had adequate explanation about their condition or treatment (Healthcare Commission, 2005b). Nonetheless there is still room for improvement; 11 per cent of patients surveyed in 2004 felt that they had been talked to 'in front of' and 39 per cent of patients felt that the staff did not even introduce themselves (Healthcare Commission, 2005b).

The need to further raise communication awareness among nurses has been reflected by the Healthcare Commissioning Body; the top complaint is 'poor communication with patients and relatives' (Meeting of Healthcare Commission, 2005, p. 3). Despite emphasis on communication within training and increased patient satisfaction in relation to communication

(Healthcare Commission, 2005b), major problems still continue to exist (Castledine, 2002). The UK Audit Commission's (1993) report highlighted the inadequacies in communication between health professionals and patients, as the root cause of patient dissatisfaction (see Chapter 16). In turn, practitioners who use 'effective' communication skills will identify patients' problems more accurately, and patients will be more satisfied with the care they receive (Maguire and Pitceathly, 2002). The proposed plan entitled 'Creating a Patient-led NHS' (Department of Health, 2005a), which has set working targets to be achieved by 2008, emphasises that communication training among nurses will have to be given top priority to ensure a truly 'patient-led NHS'.

What is communication?

One-way versus two-way communication

The basic unit of communication involves the sender, message and the receiver. This is referred to as **one-way communication**:

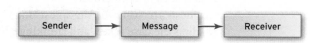

During one-way communication, the emphasis is on the sender (nurse) providing a message (e.g. instruction) that the receiver (e.g. patient) will listen to and not respond to (e.g. no questions). This process solely lies with the sender, who conveys a message that does not require any extensive feedback. For example, in the above case study, the nurse asked the patient standard general health questions, which warranted yes or no answers, during the beginning of the consultation. One-way communication is required when communicating in certain situations, especially those that require information immediately. For example emergency situations, the standard discharge procedure, standard drug administration or instructing a patient to follow instructions.

When we need to know more about the patient, require disclosure of information or need to ensure that the patient has understood the information, the nurse has to use **two-way communication**, e.g. when the nurse was talking to Amarjit about his anxiety.

One-way communication results in the receiver being prompted to give a simple yes or no answer. Hence, the sender conveys a statement with the emphasis on **closed questions** that warrant a yes or no response without any further clarification. The emphasis on being more 'patient-centred' has resulted in communication awareness training emphasising the need for nurse–patient communication to ideally be two-way communication:

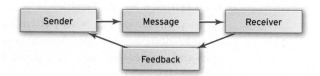

The difference between one- and two-way communication is that within two-way communication, there is the opportunity for the receiver to clarify, pose a question or elaborate on what the sender has said. This is evident in the feed-back loop in the figure above. By making a statement or posing a question that is open the sender facilitates two-way communications. **Open questioning** warrants the receiver to elaborate, clarify and further pose questions to the initial sender.

Think about this

Have a look at each of the scenarios below and decide if they are one- or two-way communication.

- You will be 'nil by mouth' for the next 48 hours.
- How has the management of your diabetes at home been since your last visit?
- Are you allergic to any medication?
- Is it right to say from what we have found in your unconscious wife's handbag that she is a Jehovah's Witness and will not have any blood administered to her?

In reality, those who assent to two-way communication may not practise it all the time. Bradley and Edinberg (1990) state that there are three main reasons why this occurs:

- In one-way communication the communicator is in control. Listening to a response makes demands on the nurse's capacity to adapt to the unexpected and they may feel more vulnerable or intimate with the patient as a result.
- One-way communication can take place more easily while doing something else, e.g. while making a bed. Full attention on the receiver is not always necessary.
- Nurses feel under pressure to do lots of tasks. Two-way communication may take time away from other important aspects of patient care.

Most definitions of **communication** refer to two-way communication (Coutts and Hardy, 1985). Le May (2004) defined communication as 'a complex two-way process that involves passing a message intentionally or unintentionally, between two or more people using either (or both) verbal or non-verbal communication strategies' (p. 488). Or Stanton (1990) simply defines communication as being an act of imparting a message, an idea or information between two or more people.

Models of communication

Researchers who explore communication refer to the process as cyclical and dynamic. This can be seen in the two-way communication process, where the sender assesses whether the recipient has understood the message (for example, can you repeat back how many times a day I told you to take the medication?). This dynamic process is referred to in much of the literature (e.g. Ellis *et al.*, 2001). Researchers have highlighted the importance of attending and listening within communication models to ensure effective communication between the speaker and the listener.

Non-verbal communication

Non-verbal communication can be defined as 'all behaviours that help us to understand a message, without the use of a verbal language, which is experienced consciously and unconsciously every time people interact' (Le May, 2004, p. 489). There are many types of non-verbal communication which will be considered below, beginning with attending and listening.

Attending and listening

Part of listening to a patient involves attending to them. **Attending** refers to the way in which the nurse listens and is present with the patient, both physically and psychologically (Egan, 1994, 2002). There are situations whereby just being present, e.g. during the final stages of an illness or bereavement, can provide comfort. Within such a situation, the patient will require a certain intensity of presence, so they feel cared for, and attended and listened to. The way nurses orientate and position themselves, as well as paying attention, listening and responding appropriately contribute to making them active attenders and listeners.

Think about this

In the opening case study, how did the nurse actively listen and attend? How did this result in a positive outcome with Amarjit? If the nurse had not actively attended, would the outcome have been different?

There are various levels of attending. If these are achieved, the patient is more likely to open up with any anxiety, issues or problems they may be facing. Had the nurse in the case study not actively attended to Amarjit, he may not have confided in her.

According to Egan (1994, 2002), attending can be divided into three levels: (1) the micro-skills level, (2) the body language level and (3) the human presence level.

The micro-skills of attending

Egan suggested that there are certain micro-skills that nurses can use when attending to their patients, which are summarised in the acronym **SOLER**.

- S: Face the patient *squarely*; adopt a posture that indicates involvement. This portrays to the patient that you are fully involved. The aim here is for the person not to feel threatened, which can happen when sitting directly opposite a person. An angled position can be beneficial. This could be seen with the nurse in the opening case study, who moved away from her desk to an angled position next to Amarjit when he began to cry.

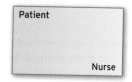

- **O**: Adopt an *open posture*. This means not crossing legs or arms (even though this may feel comfortable). An open posture is a sign that you are open to the patient and what they have to say. At the same time, the nurse should be aware of the patient's posture. In the case study the nurse was aware that Amarjit had a closed posture when stating, 'I'm fine', which suggested incongruence (see Chapter 3).
- **L**: At times *lean* forward to the patient. The upper part of the body is on a hinge, it can move towards a person and back again. However, the nurse has to be aware not to lean too far forward, as this could be interpreted by the patient as being intimidating, which could result in the patient not opening up. Leaning forward indicates to the patient that the nurse is concerned and interested, as well as willing to take time out to listen.
- **E**: Maintain good *eye contact*. Maintaining steady eye contact is a way of conveying to the person speaking that, 'I am with you, listening and wanting to know what you have to say'. A common belief is that when an individual is not maintaining steady eye contact, there is a possibility that he or she is not being truthful or is feeling anxious. This common belief needs to be considered in light of the diversity of patients (Sue, 1990). For example, certain cultural groups may look away from a nurse as a sign of respect. Gender may also influence the duration of eye contact (see Chapter 9). While maintaining eye contact is generally beneficial, a constant stare could result in the other person feeling uneasy and threatened. The general rule of thumb is to maintain eye contact which is not too prolonged with the help of natural 'glances away'.
- **R**: Attempt to *relax* and incorporate the above in the most natural and relaxed way. If the nurse is perceived as relaxed it will put the patient at ease when they are disclosing information. At the same time the nurse should be aware of the patient's posture. For example, the nurse in the opening case study was aware that Amarjit was constantly fidgeting, which resulted in the nurse easing Amarjit's anxiety by encouraging discussion about his possible concerns.

Non-verbal communication skills

Active listening is just one aspect of non-verbal communication. Argyle (1994) lists the main forms of non-verbal communication as: facial expression, gaze, gesture, body movement, posture, touch, spatial behaviour, clothing and appearance. Edwards and Brilhart (1981) also included the timing of communication within non-verbal communication.

It is very important that nurses are aware of non-verbal communication as it can provide a lot more valuable information than words alone. This is shown in an early study carried out by Mehrabian (1971), who wanted to know what cues people use to judge whether another person likes them or not. He and his associates discovered that the other person's actual words contributed to only 7 per cent of the impression of being liked or disliked;

voice cues contributed 38 per cent and facial cues, 55 per cent. They also discovered that when facial expressions were inconsistent with spoken words, facial expressions were believed more than the words.

Nurses should be aware that certain patients may find it difficult to express themselves because of certain states of health, illness or even age (e.g. elderly, having a disability affecting hearing, anxiety with regard to the management of illness). The key for nurses is to understand and read these messages without distorting or over-interpreting them and not using general rules of non-verbal communication for such patients.

Think about this

Was the nurse in the opening case study aware of Amarjit's non-verbal communication? How did any awareness of the patient's non-verbal communication help the nurse to understand Amarjit better?

Types of non-verbal communication in more detail

Facial expressions

Seven main facial expressions have been identified by Ekman *et al.* (1972): happiness, surprise, fear, sadness, anger, disgust and interest. These serve to reinforce what a person is saying. For example, 'I am feeling really happy today' is supported by non-verbal signals including a very big smile and raised eyebrows. The main function of facial expression is to communicate emotional states and attitudes, such as liking and hostility (Argyle, 1994; see picture). They can act as aids when attempting to understand what a patient is feeling and if this is the same as or differs from what they are expressing verbally. For example, the patient in the opening case study clearly displayed a expression facial of confusion and despair but verbally stated that he was fine. A classic way of disguising how we feel is to hide our real facial expressions behind another (Le May, 2004); for example 'I'm fine', would be consolidated by a quick and temporary smile. When applying to practice, it should be noted that certain illnesses or pain may result in the patient not being able to express themselves as freely as other patients. For example, damage to the face, facial nerves or muscles or a disease may alter our facial expressions: people with Parkinson's disease often have an expressionless, mask-like face (Le May, 2004).

Gaze

Gaze is useful when assessing how the patient reacts to what the nurse is saying. In essence, the eye and eye gaze are both good indicators of where the patient's attention lies. For example, in the opening case study, after the patient stated that he was fine he looked away and gazed towards the window with a despairing expression. It was clear to the nurse that the patient was preoccupied with his own thoughts, which resulted in heightened anxiety. The nurse then took this as a cue to change her interaction with Amarjit, as it was clear to her that the patient needed help.

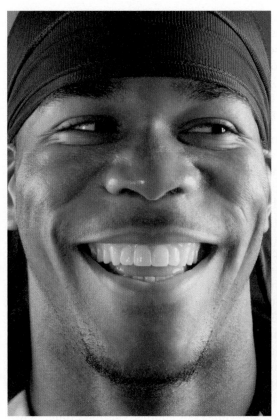

Facial expressions can state far more than words.

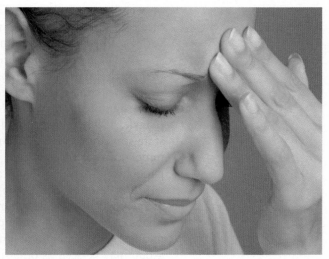

© Heide Benser/zefa/Corbis

Christopher Baines/Alamy

Gaze is also an important non-verbal communication tool when dealing with a loss situation or the delivery of bad news. A patient sustaining a prolonged gaze within the loss context is normal and is clearly indicative of contemplating and digesting the 'bad' news. Out of this context, a prolonged gaze, particularly when directly at someone, can cause embarrassment and feel unpleasant (Argyle, 1994), or even threatening. What should be remembered is that eye contact or eye gaze is rarely maintained for more than three seconds. We generally begin an utterance by looking away, and end it by looking back to the listener. While speaking, we alternate between gazing and gazing away (e.g. Kendon, 1967).

Cultural variations need to be taken into consideration. For example, in Japan, listeners are taught to focus on the speaker's neck in order to avoid eye contact, while in the United States listeners are encouraged to gaze into the speaker's eyes (Burgoon *et al.*, 1989).

The eye and eye contact

The eye reveals a great deal about the individual's emotions, convictions and moods (Givens, 2005). Eyes accurately reflect how we feel about and relate to the people. Eyes convey unpleasant feelings through closed eyelids and an averted gaze. Positive or provocative feelings show in opened eyelids, dilated pupils and direct gaze (Givens, 2005). A common inference made is that when an individual looks away, they are not disclosing everything or are not telling the truth. This interpretation should be used with caution, especially considering cultural variations. For example, for certain women not maintaining eye contact is a sign of modesty. This is especially heightened when talking to a nurse of the opposite sex. For other cultural groups, not maintaining eye contact is a sign of respect towards a person in authority, which can be the nurse.

Gestures and bodily movement

Gestures and bodily movement are important in making speech more expressive and interesting; they are closely coordinated with speech and form part of overall communication. They also express emotional states – for example, face touching may signify anxiety (Argyle, 1994). The extent of gesture use varies across different cultural groups.

Certain cultural groups are more expressive when using gesture to support their verbal communication. In practice, perceiving an individual as 'very expressive' can be misinterpreted as a sign of aggression, when in actual fact it is a sign of sincerity. *Head nods* reinforce of what has been stated verbally (Argyle, 1994). This is useful for the nurse to know; when he or she needs to state something that is of importance, head nodding will help reinforce the importance of the message. Head nods are also useful in encouraging the patient to talk, rather than stating that they should, or need to, talk.

Other gestures such as the use of certain hand signs are used independently of speech. For example, 'thumbs up' within Western society is taken to mean 'that's fine' or that 'I am happy with that'. However, this may not have any meaning for other cultural groups. A gesture used daily by many in one cultural group may be seen as offensive to members of another cultural group. When time is of the essence it is very easy to use such gestures, but they should be used with awareness, especially if there is a cultural diversity in the audience.

Waving a small white cloth: a sign of peace historically but for others a sign of anger and outrage!

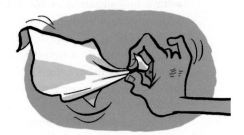

Posture

Literature suggests that posture is not indicative of a person's emotions. There are some exceptions, however, which are important when a nurse is attempting to understand how a patient may be feeling. For example, Bull (1987) found that boredom and interest were shown via the individual's posture. An individual who is tense tends to have shoulders and arms that are closed; those who are at ease tend to have their shoulders relaxed back and arms uncrossed. Depressed individuals have a particularly drooping posture. Leaning forward (as exemplified with SOLER) displays interest. Heightening shoulders, head and chest displays confidence in one's ability when verbally stating something. In the opening case study, the nurse perceived Amarjit's dropped shoulders and overall closed posture as indicating that the patient was uneasy.

Think about this

How did the nurse use her non-verbal communication to show Amarjit that she was there to listen and help him? What types of non-verbal communication did the nurse take into account when observing Amarjit? How did this help the nurse communicate more effectively with the patient? How did Amarjit display heightened anxiety via the non-verbal channel of communication?

Non-verbal communication in nursing

Non-verbal communication can also be used to punctuate verbal messages in the same way we use a question mark or exclamation mark when punctuating written language. Non-verbal behaviour can punctuate or modify interpersonal communication in the ways shown in Table 17.1 (Egan, 2002; Knapp, 1978).

Table 17.1
How non-verbal communication affects interpersonal communication

Type	Description	Example
Confirming or repeating	Non-verbal communication that confirms or repeats what is being stated verbally.	A pre-operative assessment nurse asks a patient how they are feeling about their forthcoming surgical procedure. The patient replies, 'I'm fine'. This verbal statement is confirmed by the patient's facial expressions, with a smile, lifting of eyebrows and dilation of eyes.
Denying or confusing	Non-verbal communication can deny or confuse what is being said verbally.	The same pre-operative nurse asks her patient how they are feeling about their forthcoming surgical procedure. This patient also replies, 'I'm fine'. However, this is voiced in a low tone pitch, voice which begins to falter and the patient looks away when this particular statement is made. In addition, the patient crosses their arms.
Strengthening or emphasising	Non-verbal behaviour can strengthen or emphasise what is being said.	The first patient strengthened the statement, 'I'm fine', with hand gestures and open posture, i.e. arms uncrossed (see picture).
Controlling or regulating	Non-verbal cues are often used in conversation to regulate or control what is happening.	The pre-operative nurse asks her third patient, 'how do you feel about surgery tomorrow?' The patient replies, 'I'm not feeling too good'. The patient then looks at the nurse who maintains eye contact and nods her head in anticipation that the patient will elaborate on their disclosure of not feeling 'fine' about surgery.

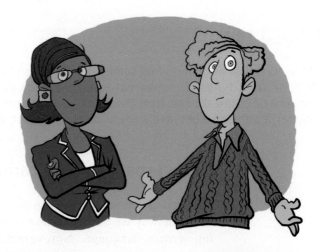

Who is telling the truth? Both of these individuals are stating verbally that they are fine but which person out of the two is actually 'fine'?

Think about this

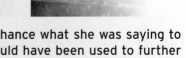

How did the nurse use non-verbal communication to further enhance what she was saying to the patient? Which other type of non-verbal communication could have been used to further enhance the help she was providing for Amarjit? How did she control and regulate the conversation via the non-verbal communication channel?

Verbal communication

Nurses will communicate with patients on a daily basis. The interactions will vary depending on the end goal. This can range from taking routine blood pressure and providing necessary information, to providing information that causes high anxiety or the patient needing to talk. The latter two interactions warrant enormous sensitivity in order for the nurse and patient to receive as much information as possible, as well as relieving any anxiety. Even though nurses are not counsellors, such interactions will involve the nurse providing enormous psychological support, which can be aided by knowledge and use of some basic counselling skills.

According to Burnard and Morrison (1991), nurses have difficulty in establishing and maintaining a facilitative relationship, where the patient is encouraged to talk and disclose information to the nurse in a trusting relationship. With an awareness of the basic verbal skills, the nurse will be able to facilitate and support patients more effectively.

Open and closed questions

Earlier in this chapter we briefly examined open and closed questions. Closed questions will usually be used in emergency situations or questions relating to a regular drug routine, e.g. is this your date of birth. Open questioning allows the patient to talk and elaborate, with the nurse listening and further **probing** the patient to carry on disclosing how they feel or the perspective they have. Probing can be achieved by the use of further open questions. Table 17.2 gives examples of opening questions, which tend to begin with: how, why, what, when and where.

Opening word	Example
How	How do you think this treatment/new outlook will help you?
Why	Why do you think you are feeling this way?
What	What do you think could be a possible cause/solution?
When	When do you think this all began?
Where	Where do you think you could find a support group to help you when you return home?

Table 17.2
Table of open questions

The use of leading questions such as 'don't you think?' is inappropriate, as this will lead the patient to answer in a particular way. In addition to this, negative 'whys' should be avoided, e.g. why don't you want to ...', as this suggests advice from the nurse, rather than the patient exploring their own solutions.

Think about this

How did the nurse change the way she communicated with Amarjit once she recognised that he was not at ease? How could other open questions have been used, if the conversation between the nurse and Amarjit had carried on?

Paraphrasing, clarifying and summarising

There will be instances where a patient may become confused or has not fully understood the information the nurse has provided. The skills of **paraphrasing**, **summarising** and **clarifying** combined with the use of open questions, will decrease the probability of any misunderstandings occurring.

Paraphrasing

Paraphrasing occurs when the listener (the nurse), reiterates back to the talker what they have said (the patient). The nurse rephrases but in fewer words, rather than repeating their words in parrot fashion. Take the example below:

A correct way of paraphrasing:

> Patient: I am feeling confused and down today.

> Nurse: I take it that you are not feeling very good today.

An incorrect way of paraphrasing:

> Patient: I am feeling confused and down today.

> Nurse: Am I right in saying that you are feeling confused, depressed and down today?

Paraphrasing is helpful as each part of the interaction is checked for understanding. It also ensures that the information shared is fully understood by the nurse and the patient as being the same; this results in a decreased probability of misunderstanding.

When paraphrasing, the nurse (listener) should pay attention to what the patient (speaker) expresses in terms of emotional words or feelings. These are then concentrated on by the nurse, who will paraphrase these back to the patient. For example, the nurse encouraged Amarjit to reflect on his confused feelings. By paraphrasing these back to Amarjit, the nurse enabled him to become more aware of his own feelings.

A nurse paraphrasing the feelings of the patient is very much like holding up a mirror. In states of anxiety, we often tend to be confused or are blind to what we are feeling. It is only when feelings are reflected upon (looking in the mirror) that these feelings become obvious. Think about the last time your feelings or behaviour were not obvious to you, until someone stated what you were feeling or commented on the way you were conducting yourself.

The reflection of feelings in paraphrasing can be referred to as a type of **mirroring.**

Summarising

When summarising the nurse will pull together everything that has been said; this usually comes towards the end of an interaction. There are many advantages in summarising, both for the nurse as well as for the patient. The patient will be able to understand what has been explored. The summary also acts as a conclusion to what has been said, which has the advantage of making the feelings and thoughts discussed clearer for both parties. The nurse in the case study used summarising by linking information back to the way Amarjit was feeling. This resulted in concluding what has been discussed and had the advantage of moving Amarjit 'away and out' of his current thinking pattern and then preparing for the biopsy with less anxiety.

Paralinguistics: the third component of communication

Another aspect of communication that is important to take into account is a **paralinguistic message,** or para-verbal message. This refers to what is verbally expressed, other than words. Tone of voice, the speed at which words are paced and pitched, and other verbal expressions that are not words, such as 'ums and ahs' are all examples of paralinguistic communication.

It has been suggested that up to 38 per cent of communication consists of paralinguistic messages. They will be most often used when you are very busy but have to listen to someone at the same time. Paralinguistics are important as they convey the impression of listening. Within an interaction where emotional information is being disclosed, head nods and ums are recommended. These act as a prompt for the patient to carry on talking without the need for a verbal probe. Table 17.3 demonstrates some general rules of thumb when it comes to paralinguistic communication and how this can aid a better understanding of a patient.

Type of rule	Example
Speech becoming rapid and highly pitched	This usually occurs when angry or excited: ' I am so excited that the results are negative!'
Speech becoming slow and lower pitched tone	Occurrence is indicative of depression: 'I ... don't feel so ... good ... but I'll have ... a go today'.
Speech becoming abrupt	Occurs when an individual is defensive: 'But I told you! I have taken such good care of myself! The test results have definitely been mixed up!'

Table 17.3
General rules for paralinguistics

Think about this

How did the nurse use paralinguistics when listening to Amarjit expressing his emotions?

Counselling framework models

Counselling framework models enable the nurse to see how the recognition and application of verbal and non-verbal communication and paralinguistics can be put together in practice.

The skilled helper model

Egan's **skilled helper model** (1990) covers the basic skills that are involved when helping a patient. The model is dynamic in its application and is useful for health professionals such as nurses, who are not qualified counsellors but need to use basic counselling skills to help patients. The model also allows the nurse to see where counselling and communication skills are placed during an interaction with a patient. The skilled helper model has the following steps:

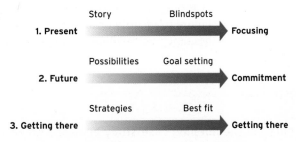

Source: From Egan. *The Skilled Helper*, 5E. © 1994 Wadsworth, a part of Cengage Learning, Inc. Reproduced by permission. www.cengage.com/permissions

Stage One: the present

Telling the story

This stage involves exploring the current situation/problem and clarifying what is happening from the patient's perspective. It also involves exploring possibilities and options or solutions. The main aim is to establish trust between the nurse and patient, and achieve clarity regarding the problem. This is achieved with the use of empathy (refer to Chapter 3), attending, listening and open questioning.

In the opening case study, the nurse clarified how Amarjit was feeling. By reflecting on his feelings, Amarjit could then see his situation in a clearer light.

Identifying and challenging blindspots

A patient who may be feeling down, depressed, anxious or confused will be unlikely to see any opportunities or engage with positive thinking. This will make it difficult for the patient to move forward. According to Egan, most clients need to move beyond their initial understanding of their current problem. An effective way a nurse can help a patient is to challenge or **confront** the patient's current negative thoughts, which are stopping him or her moving forward.

Confronting or challenging mental thoughts and processes has a different meaning from the everyday understanding of confronting or challenging. Confronting or challenging a patient within a therapeutic relationship means making them think about their current thought patterns or actions and making them reflect on them in order to change the way they behave or think. Egan refers to **blindspots**; the individual is not able to think about or see the positive aspects of their current life or the strengths within themselves. According to Egan, if challenges are successful blindspots are reduced and a new perspective is taken or unused opportunities come to light.

The following are common areas that tend to require the need for challenge and confrontation:

- failure to own problems;
- failure to define problems in solvable terms;
- faulty interpretations of critical experiences, behaviours and feelings;
- evasions, distortions and game playing;
- failure to identify or understand the consequences of behaviour;
- hesitancy or unwillingness to act on new perspectives (Egan, 2000, p. 161).

Think about this

How did the nurse in the opening case study confront Amarjit's thinking? Was the confronting obvious to the patient? Did this help Amarjit to move forward?

Focusing

Part of helping a patient to move forward is assisting the patient to become more focused. **Focusing** enables both the patient and nurse to identify and prioritise what needs to be explored. Breaking up a problem into smaller goals will result in greater confidence and motivation.

Think about this

How did the nurse in the opening case study use focusing so that Amarjit could understand what needs to be addressed first?

Stage Two: the future

Possibilities

Exploring possibilities is one way of encouraging the patient to change their current thinking. Challenging alone can result in a cycle of 'ifs' and 'buts'.

Goal setting

According to Locke and Latham (1984), helping clients set goals empowers them in four ways:

- Goals focus the client's attention and action.
- Goals mobilise the client's energy and effort.
- Goals stated in specific terms increase persistence.
- Setting goals motivates clients to search for strategies to accomplish them.

(Also see Chapter 3.)

The advantage of goal setting is that it inspires positive thinking and motivation in patients; this can result in the patient being increasingly proactive in their illness management. Nurses who are goal setting should set small achievable goals, which will increase the patient's self-esteem, before tackling the overall goal (see Chapters 5 and 6).

Choice and commitment

In this stage, initial and ongoing commitment to the goals set are explored. According to Egan, goals that have incentives associated with them are more likely to make a patient committed to achieving them.

Stage Three: strategies

Strategies

Patients may also need information regarding how to achieve set goals. Egan suggests several principles that can be taken into account when developing strategies to help the patient move forward. These range from brainstorming to highlighting skills that the patient will need to move forward. Nurses will need to provide different types of support in this stage, including informational, educational and behavioural support (see Chapter 16).

The six categories of counselling intervention

According to Heron's (1975) **six categories of counselling intervention model**, there are six possible interventions that a nurse can use when helping a patient:

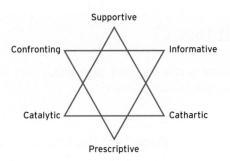

Source: Heron (1975)

The type of intervention chosen is dependent on the desired outcome of the consultation and the patient's needs. The six categories can be divided into two overall groups: **authoritative**, where the nurse is directing the focus of discussion, and facilitative, where the patient is involved in directing the conversation (see Chapter 16).

Authoritative and facilitative interventions

Table 17.4 defines and compares the authoritative and facilitative interventions that a nurse can use.

	Authoritative	Facilitative
Table 17.4 Authoritative and facilitative interventions	**Prescriptive**: a prescriptive intervention seeks to direct the behaviour of the patient, usually behaviour that is outside the practitioner–client relationship	**Cathartic**: a cathartic intervention seeks to enable the client to discharge, or release painful emotion, primarily grief, fear and anger
	Informative: an informative intervention seeks to impart knowledge, information, and meaning to the client	**Catalytic**: a catalytic intervention seeks to elicit self-discovery, self-directed living and problem-solving in the patient
	Confronting: seeks to raise client's consciousness about some limiting attitude or behaviour, which they are unaware of	**Supportive**: a supportive intervention seeks to affirm the worth and value of the client, their qualities, attitudes or actions

Communication across the lifespan

Different age groups require the use of different communication skills. Different knowledge, needs and issues are dominant at each particular stage of life. Below is a discussion of the particular communication strategies that are important for each age group.

Infancy and childhood

Newborns and infants communicate their needs in many different ways. For example, a newborn will communicate their need of hunger, or their experience of distress, through crying. The nurse or the child's parent can reduce distress by holding the child, touch and feeding. All of these should be carried out in a relaxed manner. The nurse should make the parent aware that panicking or being anxious will increase the distress of the child.

Building upon the earlier work of Erikson (1959) (see Chapter 7), Antai-Obong (2007) lists factors that need to be taken into consideration when communicating with children and parents who face fear and anxiety in relation to their state of health and have immature and vague communication skills. Antai-Obong lists nine factors that can strengthen interaction with children and their families:

- maintain eye contact;
- approach the child in a gentle and calm manner;
- use play therapy, story telling, painting and other strategies to understand the child's experience;
- encourage expression of feelings and fears;
- listen attentively;
- use words understandable by the child and parents;
- use age appropriate dialogue;
- avoid defensiveness with parents;
- validate assumptions about non-verbal communication.

A child's stay in hospital can be a highly distressing and anxious time for the parents and the child's family. Many factors, such as not being in control of their child's health, feeling helpless, or even guilt, can result in the child's family expressing their anxiety as anger towards the medical staff. It is important for the nurse to use empathy, listening, reassurance and reflection, as well as keeping calm both verbally and non-verbally, when communicating with the child's family. Working with children within the health care setting is discussed in detail in Chapter 7.

Think about this

How would a nurse calm a parent who is highly distraught and angry with medical staff as a result of feeling their son is receiving inadequate care? (The parents are anxious about test results that will be arriving to confirm if their child has leukaemia. As a result of their anxiety, the parents have reacted by being angry about the care that their child has been receiving, which they perceive to be inadequate).

Adolescence

During adolescence, many possible issues can influence the communication process. Peer pressure and family issues are at the forefront. Self-esteem and self-identity are critical during this stage. An illness that results in having to take 'time away from school' or 'taking medication' will impact on an adolescent's self-esteem and identity; adolescents do not want to look different from their peers. In addition to this, there will be many topics that the adolescent may not want their parents to know about, e.g. relationships. Hence, confidentiality and establishing trust are crucial when communicating with an adolescent. Skills such as empathy, reassurance and reflection all contribute to the adolescent feeling 'safe' and 'understood' in the relationship with the nurse. For more detail on working with adolescents, see Chapter 7.

Middle age

Middle-aged adults are usually in control of their lives but are meeting many challenges such as coping with growing children, careers, family needs, caring for parents and grandparents. A middle-aged adult may find the hospital a stressful environment, or struggle with the lack of control they have in hospital. This is a time that reflects age-related changes, which for some can be difficult to come to terms with. It is an even more concerning time for those who are diagnosed with a chronic or terminal illness, where life changes have to be made.

The nurse communicating with a middle-aged adult will have to be aware of changes that the adult is, or will be, facing. This may require the nurse to listen to the patient who is facing particular dilemmas as a result of changes that need to take place. Again, active listening and creating a trusting therapeutic relationship with the use of empathy and reflection will be paramount. In some cases, the middle-aged patient may confide in the nurse before any family member; this may result in emotional discharge, which the nurse will have to be prepared for. This is similar of the cathartic intervention that Heron proposes.

Think about this

How would you communicate with a middle-aged adult who has been diagnosed as being HIV-positive, has just 'broken down', and does not know how to break the news to their family? (Ensure that counselling and communication skills are incorporated.)

Older adulthood

With the advance of older age comes the inevitable gradual decline of sensory processes such as a decrease in hearing, vision and physical functioning. The negative effects of age-related changes can be minimised by speaking slowly, being more patient, allowing time to respond and directly facing the patient to ensure eye contact and understanding (Antai-Obong, 2007). A nurse acknowledging the possibility of sensory deficits can result in a better understanding of the patient and subsequent changes when communicating with them. At the same time, it is important for the nurse to be aware that old age does not necessarily mean sensory decline for the elderly patient. This can be interpreted by the elderly patient as patronising or being 'talked down to', or, as Ryan *et al.* (2000) state, spoken to inappropriately.

Cognitive decline or other sensory deficits may result in the elderly patient being confused or taking a long time to explain their state of health or pain. The elderly patient should not feel rushed, as this will only add to their confused state. **Silence** and attentive listening are the two most important communication skills that the nurse can use to ensure that the communication process is as smooth as possible for the elderly patient. Effective communication with the elderly patient will ensure the patient maintains their dignity and self-respect, which will result in their feeling secure within their relationship with the nurse (refer to Chapter 10).

Communicating with patients with differing health states

Working with patients with different states of ill-health will require different types of communication skills to meet the particular needs and impairments of that patient. The section below explores a few examples of states of health and the appropriate communication skills.

Stroke patients

According to Van der Smagt-Duijnstee *et al.* (2000), family members of stroke patients are often left out of the communication process, as nurses tend to be focused on the patient. They suggest that up to 95 per cent of relatives find the information provided by nurses 'very important'. It is therefore important for a nurse to provide information to relatives and address questions they have using the skills of empathy, open questioning, reflection and active listening. When providing information to relatives of a stroke patient, it is important that all questions are answered honestly while ensuring the confidentiality of the patient.

As for the stroke patient themselves, the nurse should be aware that the stroke may have affected their facial expressions as well as their voice. As a result, patience is required when talking to a stroke patient, as well as acknowledging that more emphasis will have to be placed on their verbal communication rather than their non-verbal communication. Head-nodding on the part of the nurse will encourage the patient to carry on talking irrespective of the time taken to express themselves.

Cancer patients

When communicating with a cancer patient, the patient may have episodes of being emotional and/or wanting to voice their concerns about their illness and future health. On the other hand, some cancer patients could be in a state of denial, especially during the initial stages of the diagnosis. Either of these scenarios will require the nurse to tailor communication so that the patient is emotionally supported and/or encouraged to come to terms with their diagnosis.

Research has provided evidence that despite communication being critical for cancer patients (e.g. Macleod Clark, 1982), nurses do not communicate well with them and few patients are satisfied with this area of care (Reynolds and Scott 2000).

The first step a nurse needs to take when attempting to effectively communicate with a cancer patient is to take 'time out' to listen to the patient. The second aspect of communication that a nurse needs to be aware of when listening to a cancer patient is that the issues discussed could be highly emotive. As a result, the nurse will need to make the best use of open questioning, empathy as well as sympathy, reflection and the cathartic intervention that Heron proposes. A nurse will also need to be attentive to when the patient wants to talk. Webster (1981) suggested that when cancer patients signalled signs of distress, nurses tend to use avoidance behaviours, which prevented the patients talking about their distress (refer to Chapter 4).

There are many reasons why blocking behaviours may be employed by a nurse. These could range from the nurse not having confidence in their ability to support the patient, to the nurse having their own particular beliefs or personal issues in relation to cancer (Wilkinson, 1991). Garcia *et al.* (2000), found that nurses who had communication training within their nurse education tended not to use blocking behaviour when patients wanted to talk about emotive subjects. Instead they used empathy and listening skills to best effect, which helped them to listen to and support cancer patients. The reverse was true for nurses who did not have any formal communication training. Self-awareness (see Chapter 6) allows nurses to assess their own beliefs, personal issues and agendas, which may be hindering the care they provide for a patient. Learning about self-awareness is even furthered in this application, as it may make the nurse aware of certain issues, of which they were previously unaware.

Think about this

In the opening case study, had the nurse had a negative attitude towards prostate cancer among young men, how would this have impacted on the support that she would have provided for Amarjit? Would the outcome have differed to the one in the opening case study?

Disability communication

For patients with a **disability communication**, family and carers are communicated with more than the patient themselves (Yeates, 1995). Lack of, or inappropriate, communication with a communication-disabled patient can increase the probability of the incorrect medication or dosage of medication being prescribed and, more worryingly, the wrong diagnosis (Howells, 1997).

Application of the above-mentioned communication skills are needed more than ever when working with this group. Studies have demonstrated a positive results when the nurse uses communication and counselling skills with patients with a communication disability, rather than relying heavily on the carers.

Research in focus

Murphy, J. (2006) Perceptions of communication between people with communication disability and general practice staff. *Health Expectations*, **9**, 49–59.

Objective

To explore consultation between people with communication disability and general practice (GP) staff from the perspectives of both patients and staff.

Background

Communication disability causes a particular problem in primary care. This issue has not yet been investigated from the perspective of both patients and GP staff.

Design

Eight focus groups were held – four with GP practice staff, two with people with an intellectual disability and two with people who had had a stroke. Picture symbols and talking Mats (a visual communication framework) were used to assist the participants with communication disability. Discussions were audiorecorded and analysed thematically.

Results

GP staff expressed frustration with not being understood and not understanding the patient; there was a lack of awareness of the reasons behind these difficulties. They recognised the significance of poor communication in terms of access to health services and agreed that the extent of the problem was greater than they had previously believed. People with communication disability described significant problems before, during and after the consultation. Although some acknow-ledged that they needed help from their carer, most objected to staff speaking to the carer and not to them.

Conclusions

The main priorities for GP staff were the need for relevant training and simple resources. The main priorities for people with communication difficulty were continuity of staff, trust, better GP staff communication skills and less reliance on carers.

Hearing-impaired patients

In March 2003, the UK Government recognised British Sign Language (BSL) as a language in its own right (British Deaf Association, 2005). As a result of this recognition, patients using BSL have the same rights as patients from an ethnic minority who do not speak English fluently and can request an interpreter. If a patient using BSL does not have an interpreter when one has been requested, this can be challenged in court (McAleer, 2006). There will be some point in a nurse's career where they will care for a patient who has a hearing impairment or is registered deaf. Figures suggest that 50 000–70 000 deaf people's first preference of language is BSL (RNID, 2004).

When communicating with a deaf patient who has requested BSL as a mode of communication, the nurse should take into account the following factors:

- Nurses who are not trained but have some knowledge of BSL should not act as interpreters (Elderkin-Thompson *et al.*, 2001).

- When planning patient-centred care, it is the responsibility of the nurse to organise an interpreter so that two-way communication takes place (Haskins, 2000). An interpreter has an important part to play when communicating a care plan to the patient.
- When you are carrying out a physical examination, be sensitive by ensuring that you ask the patient if they have any objections to the interpreter being present (Phelan and Parkman, 1995). If the interpreter is present, reassure the patient that confidentiality will be kept at all times. If the patient objects to an interpreter being present during the physical examination, ensure that extra effort is taken to explain information in the absence of the interpreter (Phelan and Parkman, 1995).
- Even if there is a shortage of interpreters, ensure that the family, who may be skilled in BSL, are not used as interpreters (Wood, 1999). One of the main reasons is patient confidentiality.

Learning disability patients

A patient who has a learning disability tends to have several differing health needs (Bristol and District People First, 2003). These can range from not being able to process and express information efficiently to having additional sensory and physical impairments (Godsell and Scarborough, 2006). Such needs have to be taken into consideration when communicating with the patient.

According to the two-way model of communication discussed earlier in this chapter, the sender of a message will want the recipient to hear what they are saying. It is not necassarily the case that a patient with a learning disability will want the nurse to understand their messages, or that they will understand messages that the nurse sends. A patient with a profound learning disability who is expressing themselves verbally or non-verbally, may not intend the message to be sent to a recipient; their expressions could be a response to their own body and feelings (Godsell and Scarborough, 2006). People with a learning disability also have a reduced ability to understand new or complex information (Department of Health, 2001). Simplicity of information and the use of non-verbal communication and pictures is important to consider. There are many factors which can act as a barrier to or confound the communication that takes place between the nurse and the learning disabled patient. Godsell and Scarborough (2006) list them as:

- limited understanding;
- limited vocabulary or difficulty in speaking;
- sensory impairments that limit ability to hear requests or instructions;
- poor understanding of health and healthy living;
- fear of people in uniforms;
- stress because of illness;
- dislike of new places;
- difficulty waiting and limited understanding of the concept of time or queuing;
- limited literacy and numeracy skills to read health advice and information, for example, instructions, letters, dosages;
- contact with nurses expected to be unpleasant because of previous experiences.

Nurses should be aware that all the above factors can influence communication. Setting extra time aside for a patient with a learning disability would be advantageous. In addition, simplifying conversation (while ensuring that it is not patronising) and using open-ended questioning, paraphrasing and repeating will improve patient understanding.

Conclusion

A nurse caring for a patient will be communicating with the patient at all times. In order to ensure that the communication process is effective, it is essential for nurses to be aware of the communication models and skills that exist. Not only will the nurse provide better care for their patient but they will understand the patient more fully. This will result in higher patient satisfaction and decrease the probability of misunderstandings occurring.

Counselling skills are fundamental to nursing practice as there will be patients who may need to disclose how they are feeling or the nurse may have to deal with a highly anxious patient. The use of counselling skills will ensure that the patient is helped to disclose information in the most appropriate manner and that the nurse remains objective at all times. Even though counselling skills are predominantly used by professional accredited counsellors, such skills need to be considered as part of nurse training, as the nurse may be in a situation that warrants the use of such skills. Further reading around this area will enhance the knowledge of nursing students. The student nurse's portfolio will also document communication skills practised on placements.

Summary

- Two-way communication is the ideal when striving towards being patient-centred. At the same time there will be particular situations where one-way communication will have to be used by a nurse.

- Facial expressions, eye gaze and body posture are all forms of non-verbal communication.

- Attending and active listening can be portrayed via the non-verbal channel. Egan (1994, 2000) highlighted this with his micro-skills, referred to as SOLER: Sitting squarely, Open posture, Leaning in, Eye contact and Relax.

- Non-verbal communication can help to punctuate verbal messages by making a statement a question, confirming a statement, denying a statement, strengthening what has been said or controlling a conversation.

- Open questioning can begin with the words how, when, what, where and why. As well as open ques-

tioning, summarising, clarifying and **reflecting** are all forms of verbal communication that can decrease misunderstanding and encourage the patient to disclose information and feelings.

- Verbal is the first mode of communication and non-verbal the second; paralinguistic is the third and final mode of communication, and makes up 38 per cent of communication.

- Egan's skilled helper model (1990) provides a three-step framework for counselling skills to be placed in. The first step is the present with focusing and blind spots. The second step is the future with commitment, goal setting and possibilities. The third step is getting there with strategies.

- John Heron's (1975) six categories of counselling intervention looks at what intervention is required, depending on the needs of the patient and the particular context. The six interventions can be

▶

divided into two categories. The first category is authoritative, comprising prescriptive, informative and confronting interventions. The second is facilitative, comprising cathartic, catalytic and supportive interventions.

● Knowing about lifespan developments and differing states of ill-health, disability and impairments can improve a nurse's communication skills, as barriers or hindrances to the communication process will be taken into consideration.

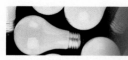

Check your understanding

1. What are the different forms of non-verbal communication that exist and what can they portray in terms of communication?

2. List the key verbal counselling and communication skills that can be used by a nurse when attempting to understand the patient.

3. Give two examples from states of ill-health, impairment or disability of factors that a nurse should take into consideration when communicating with the patient and their families.

4. Choose two phases of the lifespan and explain what issues/factors are important for a nurse to take into consideration when communicating with patients of this age.

5. List the three steps within Egan's (2000) skilled helper model. Explain each stage in relation to a nurse working with a patient who is attempting to lead a healthier lifestyle after a stroke.

6. With the help of Heron's (1975) six categories of counselling intervention model, design a care plan to help a patient out of continual negative thinking.

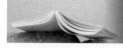

Further reading

Burnard, P. and Morrison, P. (1988) Nurses' perceptions of their interpersonal skills: a descriptive study using six category intervention analysis. *Nurse Education Today,* **8**, 266–272.

Dunne, K. (2005) Effective communication in palliative care. *Nursing Standard,* **20** (13), 57–64.

Garcia De Lucio, L., Garcia Lopez, F.J., Marin Lopez, M.T, Mas Hesse, B. and Caamano Vaz, M.D. (2000) Training programme in techniques of self-control and communication skills to improve nurses' relationships with relatives of seriously ill patients: a randomized controlled study. *Journal of Advanced Nursing,* **32** (2), 425–431.

McCabe, C. (2004) Nurse-patient communication: an exploration of patients' experiences. *Journal of Clinical Nursing,* **13** (1), 41–49.

Van der Smagt-Duijnstee, M.E., Hamers, J.P.H., Huijer, Abu-Saad H. and Zuidhof, A. (2001) Relatives of hospitalized stroke patients: their needs for information, counselling and accessibility. *Journal of Advanced Nursing,* **33** (3), 307–315.

Weblinks

British Association for Counselling and Psychotherapy	www.bacp.co.uk	Official website of the accrediting body for counsellors and psychotherapists in the UK. This site has links to many resources and information on counselling skills.
Royal College of Psychiatrists	www.rcpsych.ac.uk/mentalhealthinformation/olderpeople.aspx	This site provides information on appropriate communication across the lifespan when working with patients with differing mental health problems.
Cruse Bereavement Care	www.crusebereavementcare.org.uk/	A useful site for information about the counselling and communication skills that are vital within a bereavement situation.
Sign Station	www.signstation.org	A website that is dedicated to raising awareness of deafness and British Sign Language. This has an on-line BSL dictionary, supporting video clips and information about BSL interpreters.

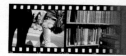

Media examples

British Telecom Advert The famous British Telecom advert begins and ends with the saying, 'it's good to talk', when promoting their phone-a-friend cut cost tariffs. This conveys the essence of communication and counselling; patients should disclose information rather than keeping thoughts and feelings bottled up.

Channel 4's *Big Brother* Series Contestants enter the Big Brother house where they are watched by viewers living their day-to-day life. Communication between the 'housemates' is a key determining factor in emotions, bonding and friendships. All of the *Big Brother* series to date have shown that when housemates openly discuss their problems to a listener who is attentive, it is less likely that arguments will occur and more likely that housemates will be happy during the remainder of their stay in the Big Brother house.

HSBC Advert During 2004 and 2005 the HSBC bank promoted their understanding of the nature of working with customers across many different ethnic minorities, as well as the ethnic majority living within the UK. This was portrayed very well, demonstrating how gestures that are used worldwide can have different meanings for different individuals.

Chapter 18

Being admitted to hospital

Learning outcomes

When you have read this chapter you should understand:

- How being admitted to hospital can have a negative psychological impact on the individual patient.
- How psychological support while in hospital can improve both mental and physical health.
- The anxiety-provoking nature of hospital admission and surgical interventions.
- The consequences of anxiety on post-operative recovery.
- The consequences of psychological interventions on improving post-operative recovery.
- The difference between 'monitors' and 'blunters' in their use of information.
- The importance of providing the correct amount of information for the individual patient.

Case study

Mrs Surinder Sharma is a 77-year-old grandmother with two grown-up children – Amir (aged 50 years) and Chunna (aged 55 years) who both now live away from home. Mrs Sharma was a university lecturer but retired from this job some 15 years ago. She currently lives at home with her husband and looks after both the house and Mr Sharma (a retired accountant), who was diagnosed with Parkinson's disease a number of years ago. He spends most of his day at home as he finds it difficult to get out. However, within the house he is relatively independent and can manage his own self-care activities, although there has been a recent deterioration and he requires some additional care.

Mrs Sharma has retained a high level of community involvement and is actively engaged in various clubs and societies around the locality. She is, for example, a volunteer with the local Women's Institute and helps out at the local community centre. She is a sociable woman and knows most of her neighbours, playing bridge with them on a regular basis.

Her children and grandchildren live locally and they visit regularly. They are all fit and have high-powered jobs within the neighbourhood. Mrs Sharma has a good quality **social support** from both her friends and her family. Despite her husband's illness, Mrs Sharma is content with life. She has some minor ailments, which she puts down to her age, but feels there is nothing serious she has to deal with.

One morning while Mrs Sharma was helping move some ladies and gentlemen at the luncheon club where she helped, she slipped and fell lightly. Mrs Sharma recalled that 'the fall was trivial but the pain was excruciating'. She could not stand and her friends at the Centre called for the local ambulance which took her to the local district hospital, 25 kilometres away. After an X-ray, the doctor on duty diagnosed a fracture to the neck of the femur and told him that she would need **surgery**.

Mrs Sharma was somewhat surprised that such a small fall could cause a fracture needing surgery she asked for some clarification from the staff at the hospital. Dr Sushil Gulam, an orthopaedic surgeon, explained that she had broken the head of her femur, commonly called a hip fracture, because of weak bones. When told that she required surgery, Mrs Sharma became extremely distressed – she had never been ill before and had only occasionally been to a hospital (for various tests but not an admission).

The surgeon operated and Mrs Sharma began a long and painful rehabilitation, during which her voluntary job was provisionally taken over by others. Mrs Sharma's hip fracture was a difficult injury to treat, especially since the bones involved were fragile and weak (probably a consequence of undiagnosed osteoporosis). In Mrs Sharma's case an orthopaedic surgeon performed the surgery, using metal devices such as plates and screws to stabilise the bone and hold it in place. Metal plates were used on the outer surface of the bone, and rods inserted through the marrow space in the centre of the femur. These methods of treatment were used to reposition fracture fragments precisely, enabling the bone to repair by 'knitting' together with new growth at the end surfaces of the injury. During the post-operative hospital stay, Mr Sharma was also rather concerned and asked for local home care support so that he could manage at home.

Mrs Sharma met with a physical therapist shortly after surgery to begin gently exercising her hip joint, first by simply getting up and later by walking with the help of crutches or a walker. Mrs Sharma was provided with an individually designed course of post-operative treatment that allowed her to gradually increase her realistic goals. However, her post-operative recovery did not go as smoothly as everyone hoped and she made slow progress. She was taught how to care for the injury as it healed, and arrangements were made for in-home or rehabilitative nursing care. Luckily, she was able to manage at home with support from the local services, combined with some family support.

Only after six months could she resume light exercise and meet friends, having followed the medical advice to the letter (as she reported). While on one of the evening walks recommended as part of her rehabilitation, Mrs Sharma made a quick movement to dodge a stray cat emerging from a hedge. She slipped, fell, and fractured her other hip. Again she saw the surgeon, and again she had a hip replacement surgery. But this time her rehabilitation was much more difficult.

Why is this relevant to nursing practice?

Obviously the case study of Mrs Sharma is not atypical for somebody with a fall and subsequent fracture of the hip. The nurse will probably be involved in each of the stages of the consequences of her accident, from her initial diagnosis on admission to the hospital, through to the surgical intervention and then to the care involved in her recovery from surgery. Much of the involvement with Mrs Sharma is in the hospital environment, including the major operation that she had to undergo. Although a nurse's role is far more than just being involved in hospital care, such care does represent a significant amount of work for a number of nursing professionals. However, more importantly, for the patient entering hospital there are a number of consequences: it can be an extremely stressful experience and can impact considerably on an individual's physical and mental health. How can entering hospital impact on the psychological health of the individual? How can the nurse assist the patient when they enter the hospital and how can they help minimise any psychological disruption encountered? It has also been shown that the psychological stress of surgery and hospitalisation can have a negative impact on physical health, so how can psychological factors be used to improve physical health and what psychological factors can the nurse use to improve the physical health of those entering hospital, having an operation or recovering from surgery?

There are numerous reasons why people enter hospital – not just for surgery. They may enter for assessment rather than treatment, for example. In the case of those entering with a mental health problem, there are a range of issues that can lead to admission (Bowers, 2005). These may include the following:

- *Dangerousness*: Patients may be admitted to hospital in order to prevent harm either to themselves or others and the underlying reasoning may be written into the legal criteria for compulsory admission in the United Kingdom (Houlihan, 2005). Hence, professionals may have a 'security' role (Bowers, 2005) along with preventing patients from harming themselves by acts of commission or omission using psychological support (Cutcliffe and Barker, 2002) which can be extremely complex and should not be underestimated (Johnson and Delaney, 2006).
- *Assessment:* An admission allows for an extended assessment period during which time extensive observations can be made. From this it will be possible to illuminate discrepancies between what the patient and significant others say and whether the problems exhibited are either situational or psychological. Abas *et al.* (2003) report that this was the major factor in some 43 per cent of psychiatric admissions.
- *Medical treatment*: Abas *et al.* (2003) suggests that almost a third of cases of admission are associated with non-compliance. Most of admissions for treatment are for physical treatment (e.g. medication or **electroconvulsive therapy**) but may also include the management of a physically ill person with a **concurrent mental illness** or the treatment of drug or alcohol withdrawal.
- *Severe mental disorder*: The provision of secure and containing environment is suggested as being important for those with severe symptoms of mental disorder (Sederer and Summergrad, 1993). This might include unpredictability, confusion, disorientation or delusional ideas, and the purpose of admission is to 'control, contain and manage these difficult behaviours' (Bowers, 2005).

- *Self-care deficits*: Sederer and Summergrad (1993) suggest that an 'inability to function' should be a criterion for admission to hospital and this means that mental health nurses may be involved in providing personal care, and provide rehabilitation, re-education and training.
- *Respite for carers*: Flannigan *et al.* (1994) in a large-scale study suggested that 29 per cent of all admissions in order to provide a major reason for admissions. In these cases admission becomes a form of stop-gap psychiatric supported accommodation in order to provide a temporary home for the patient until there is a resolution to the crisis.
- *Respite for the patient*: Sederer and Summergrad (1993) talk of the '**toxic support system**' and the need for the patient to be removed from such an environment that is worsening the mental illness, or is otherwise **psychologically noxious**.

In this case it is important that the nursing environment is tolerant, sympathetic and non-stressful.

Inpatient treatment beds for those with a mental illness are reducing (Delaney, 2006) and some have suggested that this may be due to the perception that inpatient care lacks relevance in the twenty-first century (Walsh, 2006). However, as we can see from the criteria provided by Bowers (2005) there still remains a need to provide such a service to those that are a danger to themselves or others, or whose symptoms impair their self-care skills and the support they or their relatives require.

Finally, it should be noted that some patients can be compulsory detained under the **Mental Health Act (1983)**. Currently this applies only to those who are suffering from a diagnosed mental disorder and aims to safeguard those who are not mentally disordered from wrongful detention (Fennell, 1996). There are three basic civil admission procedures that allow for a person to be compulsory detained:

- admission for assessment with or without treatment for up to 28 days which is not renewable (section 2);
- emergency admission for assessment for up to 72 hours (section 4);
- admission for treatment for up to 6 months, and thereafter renewable for periods of up to 12 months at a time (section 3).

There are powers and duties associated with the Mental Health Act which are too extensive to be discussed here, although Houlihan (2005) has produced a good review of its implications for psychiatric nurses. However, the Government has released plans to update the legislation published in 2006, which have been the subject of review and critique (Brown, 2006) and are currently under discussion, consultation and argument!

Entering hospital

Obviously being sick and unwell is not a pleasant experience and being seriously ill is even worse. However, entering hospital adds many other negative aspects: it is disruptive psychologically, socially and physically and can present many novel experiences that can be extremely distressing (Carr *et al.*, 2005; Caumo *et al.*, 2001). Hospital staff can have considerable influence on the individual patient's experience and they should take responsibility for improving the experience of the patient (Morris and Ward, 2003; Stirling 2006). At its most basic a hospital is an alien environment for most people whereas for the nurse it is a place of work and may simply be viewed as a normal experience. The patient is a stranger in the nurses' workplace and is likely to be unfamiliar and lost in the environment with its structure, procedures and language. Hence, the worry of the illness can be compounded by the hospital environment. The nurse can help alleviate some of these stressors.

Think about this

How can the nurse improve the admission to the hospital for the individual patient? What **psychosocial** factors come into play when a person enters hospital? What psychological, social and physical problems may become apparent? Think about how Mrs Sharma must feel when entering the 'alien' environment of the hospital. Think about the language, structure and procedures that you are used to but may be alien and stressful to patients being admitted.

Anxiety is probably the most common and all-embracing emotion of hospitalised people and this will probably be common to most patients irrespective of why they have been admitted (Marchevsky et al., 2000; Stoddard et al., 2005). If an individual's health problems have not yet been identified then they will worry about the problems, what they are and how the illness will influence their lives. If the diagnoses have been made, they may worry about many other matters such as what the treatment will be like and the degree to which it will be successful. Even those who are keen for their health problems to be resolved may still be anxious about the intervention and the outcome. Similarly, there may be a difference between elective and emergency surgery and between diagnostic and intervention surgery, but there will still probably be anxiety.

Many of the worries of patients stem from uncertainties that result from a lack of information or even basic understanding (Gillies and Baldwin, 2001). Although the lack of information may occur because tests have not yet been completed, sometimes it occurs because no health care professional has taken the time to inform the person. Hospitals are busy places, and the limited time of medical, nursing and associated personnel may account for their lack of the information provision to patients. But not providing information may lead to misunderstandings that may impair the person's adherence with the advice of the staff or cause unnecessary emotional suffering (Gillies and Baldwin, 2001). Hence it can have both psychological and physical complaints and unintended negative consequences.

Depersonalisation

The first potential pitfall that Mrs Sharma may face when entering hospital is being viewed not as a person but as a condition. A common characteristic of the way health care practitioners may interact with patients is called **depersonalisation**, or treating the person as if they were either not present or not a person. Goffman (1961), a sociologist, first described this characteristic as 'non-person treatment' – the patient is treated like a 'a possession someone has left behind' (pp. 341–342). This has been reported more recently, with Hornesten *et al.* (2005) suggesting that patients stressing their need to be viewed and treated as a person, not merely as a patient with a disease or 'as a case'. This had been previously reported by Kralik *et al.* (1997) who reported on 'detached nursing' with patients being treated as numbers (i.e. depersonalised), which led to patients feeling vulnerable and insecure.

Nurses may fall into the trap of treating patients as non-persons (akin to the reports of Kralik *et al.*, 1997) to distance themselves from the fact that the person they are dealing with belongs to a thinking, anxious and worried person who can observe what is going on, ask questions and behave in ways that can interfere with their work (Goffman, 1961). Nurses may attempt to save themselves and the patient trouble, awkwardness and anxiety by acting as if the person and the defective body were distinct: somebody had left the defective body at the hospital for repair and would pick it up when it was ready!

There are also many factors that lead nurses to treat patients in a depersonalised manner. Their role may entail heavy responsibilities and can be hectic, particularly during periods of emergencies. This can create high levels of stress and, in order to prevent this, the nurse may want to provide less personalised care since this helps protect them from the dysfunctional body and the potential consequences. Nurses (and other health care professionals) need ways to protect themselves emotionally when a patient takes a turn for the worse or dies, which can be a distressing experience. Depersonalisation probably helps practitioners feel less attached and emotionally affected when these events occur.

A classic study is that reported by Jeffrey (1979) who explored the reactions of accident and emergency staff to the admission of patients. He reported that patients were classified into either 'good patients' or 'rubbish'. Good patients were described almost entirely in terms of their medical characteristics, either in terms of their symptoms or the cause of their injury. Good cases were head injuries, heart attacks or road traffic accidents. In broad terms the good patients were related to medical considerations:

- If they allowed the health care professional to pass professional examinations: A person is guaranteed excellent treatment if they turn up with an unusual condition during a slack period. If it is a routine accident, or condition and one that is rarely seen then the interest is low.
- If they allow staff to practise their skills: The specific characteristics of a good patient were those that allowed practitioners to practise their skills or to use their skills in an advanced manner. Nurses, in particular, found it rewarding to fulfil the role of surgeon in particular patients.
- If they tested the general competence and maturity of the staff: The patients who were most 'prized' were those who stretched the resources of the department in doing the task.

In contrast, there appeared to be a range of patients who could be classified as 'normal rubbish'. The categories, as provided by Jeffrey (1979), were:

- Trivia: Normal trivia were those who had minor injuries – had banged their limbs or their heads, or 'didn't want to bother their GP with'.
- Drunks: Normal drunks were those who were abusive and threatening and came into the department shouting and singing after a fight or were sick all over themselves and the department.

- Overdoses: The normal overdose is female, and is seen as a case of self-injury rather than of attempted suicide.
- Tramps: Tramps can be recognised by the layers of rotten clothing and the smell. Normally they enter the department during the winter in order to get to a place of warmth and in order to do so will try to sham their symptoms.

Being classified as 'rubbish' resulted in punishment – the most common way to increase the amount of time that rubbish had to spend waiting for treatment in the accident and emergency department. Although this study was reported in the 1970s, it still stands the test of time and subsequent studies have indicated that nurses still maintain, categorise and regulate patient behaviour. As Hyde *et al.* (2006) report from their study: 'Findings from this documentation study suggest that nurses invigilated, monitored and regulated patients' capacity at performing ADLs [Activities of Daily Living], and created moral categories relating to such a capacity.' In such a way, nurses categorised their patients according to their behaviours: if they had an all-over wash they were perceived as cooperative, but if not they were seen as non-compliant and tarnished normal boundaries.

Think about this

Have you referred to, or have you heard a patient being referred to by their illness (e.g. 'the broken leg in bed 3', or 'An epileptic' or 'A depressive')? How can depersonalisation be avoided? What would be the psychological consequences of depersonalisation be on the patient? How can the nurse behave that would improve the experience of the patient?

Sick role behaviour in the hospital

Relations between patients and practitioners in the hospital are affected not only by the behaviour of the medical and nursing staff, but by the patient behaviour too. A hospital presents an unfamiliar and strange environment that requires psychological and social adjustments that many patients have difficulty making. They have to get used to a lack of privacy, rules and time schedules, having their own activities restricted, having little control over events around them, and being dependent on others. These things complicate their psychosocial transition to the **sick role**. How are patients supposed to behave in hospital or when they are sick?

We all have **social roles** – a role represents the way that someone is expected to behave in a particular social situation. Some of us have a role as a lecturer, or a nurse or a student and we usually know how each of these should react and behave in certain situations (and this may differ in different social situations). When people become ill, are defined as sick or enter the hospital, they have ideas about how they should behave: this is the so-called 'sick role'. Parsons (1951a), a sociologist, described the sick role as not simply a 'state of fact' or 'condition', it is a specifically social role. In Western societies the sick role implies major expectations which comprise both rights and duties/obligations (Parsons, 1951a, pp. 436–437):

- *Rights*
  - Sick person temporarily exempt from 'normal' social roles. The more severe the sickness, the greater the exemption.
  - Sick person generally not held responsible for their condition (absence of blame). Illness considered beyond individual's control therefore not simply curable by willpower.
  - Sick person has a right to be taken care of.

- *Duties/obligations*
  - Sick person expected to see being sick as undesirable, thus they have an obligation to try to 'get well'. In this context exemption from normal responsibilities is temporary and conditional upon wanting and trying to get better.
  - The sick person has an obligation to seek technically competent help from a suitably qualified professional and to cooperate in the process of trying to recover.

There are two underlying themes to the sick role: vulnerability and **deviance**. A person entering the sick role is seen as vulnerable because they have threatening symptoms, they are passive, trusting and prepared to wait for medical help and therefore they are open to exploitation by others. For example, patients must submit to bodily inspection which has a high potential for intimacy and consequently may breach social taboos. As a consequence there is an unequal relationship between the health care professional and the patient, with the practitioner having immense power. This requires a high level of trust on behalf of the patient and, of course, some form of social and political regulation of their activities.

But what about deviance? Why is this an underlying theme for the sick role? Becoming ill can be viewed as a threat to society and to social way of life: people who are sick are relieved of their social obligations and are able to avoid their responsibility. Furthermore, society may be exploited and hence there must be some form of protection for society – the medical profession acts in this way as providing a form of '**gate-keepers**' against this form of deviance.

Lorber (1975), in an old, albeit classic, study, reported on the sick-role behaviour of over 100 patients, mostly over 40 years of age, who entered a hospital for elective surgeries. These surgical interventions ranged from the routine to the extremely serious. At both the start of their stay, and at the end of their admission, patients were interviewed. The interviews assessed the role patients felt they should play: should they be active, passive or conforming? A finding from this study, not surprisingly, was that those people with passive beliefs on entering hospital were less likely to complain and ask for reassurance about minor discomforts.

Not only did this study explore the patient's view of sick role, but it also looked at the reactions of the medical staff to the patient's sick-role behaviour. At the end of each day, respondents were asked to rate the individual patient as a 'good patient', 'average patient' or 'problem patient'. The staff were also requested to provide a description of the patient's behaviour and their individual reactions to it when the behaviour occurred.

When the researchers explored the characteristics of good patients they found that individuals described behaviour such as 'passive, cooperative, uncomplaining and stoical'. Those rated as problem patients were seen as 'uncooperative, constantly complaining, dependent and over-emotional'. An example was provided in the paper – an overly passive 'good patient' who 'didn't want to bother the nurses'. However, the nurses' routines were constantly disrupted because they had to make sure that she was all right and well. On the other hand, an example of a 'problem patient' was a man who had both medical and psychological complications after his gall bladder was removed.

The influence of medical conditions on patients' behaviour was also investigated. Lorber reported on two types of problem patients: one type were seriously ill and have severe complications or poor prognosis. Because of their poor medical condition the staff often forgave their behaviour (e.g. requiring considerable attention). On the other hand, the other type were those who were not seriously ill but took up more staff time than was considered necessary, and they were either uncooperative or complaining. This behaviour may not necessarily be related to the seriousness of their condition but may simply be a reaction to their loss of freedom and control. For example, a patient with a leg injury may not be able to walk or a person with a hearing difficulty may want to have their radio/television turned up, but this will disturb other patients and the work of the medical/nursing staff. Being upset or angry at being controlled or with a lack of freedom is called reactance. Although the medical and nursing staff were usually pleasant and patient, sometimes they responded by administering sedatives and even arranging a premature discharge (Lorber, 1975).

The majority of patients were not problem patients (and, indeed, are not!) and most hospitalised patients recognised the hard and difficult work being undertaken by the medical and nursing staff. As a consequence they behave as 'good patients' rather than being perceived as 'troublemakers' and being disliked by staff. They think that they will anger staff who would consequently 'refuse to answer your call' or 'refuse to make your bed'. As a result these patients may have increased anxiety about not disturbing the staff (Lorber, 1975).

Emotional adjustment in the hospital

As we have seen, most hospitalised patients must cope with a number of significant issues both physically and emotionally with the over-riding emotion usually being anxiety. This may change over the course of the admissions but adjustment may be gradual. For example, most surgical patients experience anxiety levels that are especially high when they are admitted, remain quite high prior to their intervention and then decline steadily during the rest of their stay. But sometimes the anxiety levels of patients increase with time – as the condition worsens, or as test results become clear (and negative), or as the full realisation of the importance of the conditions becomes clear. Others with mental health issues may start with high anxiety, but with the structure and support of hospitals this may reduce during admission and increase just before discharge. How a patient adjusts to his or her health problem and treatment in the hospital depends on many factors, such as the person's age, gender and perceived characteristics of the illness or injury (Kincey, 1995; Moos and Billings, 1982). For instance, young adults often have more difficulty coping with serious illnesses than older individuals do. Also, men tend to be more distressed than women by illnesses that reduce their vigour and physical abilities, but women often have an especially difficult time adjusting to disfigurement such as facial injuries, losing a breast or undergoing gynaecological surgery (Walsgrove, 1999).

Think about this

What sort of issues does Mrs Sharma have to deal with? How do these relate to her physical, psychological and social condition?

Coping in hospital

Two broad ways of coping with stress have been discussed previously (see Chapter 13) and these may be applied to the stress of entering hospital. Firstly, the cause of the stress can be altered and the emotional response to the situation can be regulated. Some situations that produce stress in the hospital can be altered by the patient's taking action, such as by asking for medication to reduce pain or by reading information about their condition. Because these actions can reduce the demands of the **stressor** or expand the person's resources for dealing with it, they are examples of **problem-focused coping**.

Patients in hospital may experience many stressors they believe they cannot change (Kindler *et al.*, 2000). In some cases these beliefs are correct, as when a person whose spinal cord was severed in an accident must cope with not being able to walk. But in other cases they are incorrect, as when a patient does not realise that it may be possible to use another medication if the current one produces discomfort or other side effects. People who believe they can do nothing to change a stressor usually try to cope with their emotions and the situations by using methods classified as **emotion-focused coping**. Secondly, patients may try to regulate their emotions by denying unpleasant facts, performing distracting activities, or seeking social support, for example. Finally, there is social support which has previously been highlighted as important in buffering the effects of stress. Social support refers to the various types of support that people receive from others and is generally classified into two (sometimes three) major categories: emotional and instrumental (and sometimes informational) support (see Chapter 13) and this form of support can assist with recovery from hospital admission (see Stirling, 2006, for an overview).

Preparing patients for stressful medical procedures

Mrs Sharma is rushed from the accident and emergency department to orthopaedics to undergo emergency surgery to repair the fractured neck of her femur. This is an emergency operation that is required in order to prevent any long-term damage, and, importantly, to reduce the pain that Mrs Sharma is currently suffering. Obviously the preparation that Mrs Sharma undergoes will be different from that of somebody having elective surgery (furthermore, there may be differences among those undergoing different types of elective surgery). However, psychology can help all these different types of patients be prepared for their surgery – but how? What has psychology research demonstrated about the effects of surgical intervention and how can patients be best prepared? How can the nurse use this psychological research to improve the lot of the patient?

Preparing people psychologically for surgery has important implications for their recovery: generally the greater the pre-operative anxiety they feel before surgery, the more difficult their adjustment and recovery are likely to be after surgery. People with high pre-operative anxiety tend to report more pain, use more medication for pain, stay in the hospital longer, and report more anxiety and depression during their recovery than patients with less pre-operative fear. What can nurses do to reduce the stress people experience in conjunction with medical procedures? This will be the focus of the next section.

What makes the surgical situation stressful?

There are many obvious potential threats for the surgical patient: anaesthesia, pain, physical restriction, life-threatening procedures, being away from home, disruption of routines and sleep deprivation, post-operative pain, incapacitation, financial strain, and fear of death and the actual surgery (Egan *et al.*, 1992; Kindler *et al.*, 2000; Stirling, 2006). To some extent each of these contributes a similar amount but Volicer (1977), in an early study of the anxiety levels in surgical patients, found them to be more distressed by the unfamiliarity of their surroundings, loss of independence, the threat of severe illness and, as a consequence, an inability to cope (Michell, 2000). More recent evidence suggests that the lack of predictability and control are significant contributors to the stressful experience of surgical patients (Michell, 2000; Slangen *et al.*, 1993). There is a high proportion of people who experience anxiety prior to surgery and the prevalence has been reported to range from 11 per cent to 80 per cent among adult patient populations (Hollaus *et al.*, 2003; Maranets and Kain, 1999). It is usually the case that we need to be able to predict an event in order to be able to control it: how much is this the case with surgery? What about elective surgery? How does this relate to Mrs Sharma and her experience? Control does not always imply predictability. Such is the case for elective surgery, which accounts for the vast majority of surgical interventions.

This evidence confirms that there are common characteristics of the surgical situation which are identified by most patients as stressful. Kindler *et al.* (2000) have outlined three areas of pre-operative anxiety: fear of the unknown; fear of feeling ill; and fear for one's life. For example, there will be a perceived loss of the sense of security and control over life (Fyfe, 1999) or being removed from the family unit (Kanto, 1996; Kiecolt-Glaser *et al.*, 1998), or being uncertain about the future (O'Rourke, 1993) which could lead to inability to cope with the experience (Michell, 2000). Other sources of anxiety include the fear of drugs (Zvara *et al.*, 1994), fear of dying (Kiecolt-Glaser *et al.*, 1998) and fear of pain (Brunner and Suddarth, 1993; Dodds, 1993) and body image (Cheung *et al.*, 2003).

It seems likely, however, that different types of surgical procedures produce different types of stress. Weinman and Johnston (1988) suggest that a useful way of distinguishing among the various procedures would be by considering the function of the procedure (diagnostic, treatment or both) and the timeline and nature of stress associated with the procedural stress (i.e. the stress associated with the negative aspects of the actual procedure itself) and outcome stress (i.e. longer-term fears and concerns related to the results of the treatment or procedure). To illustrate the latter point, some operations, for example, may have positive characteristics in terms of their expected outcome than others, such as restoration (e.g. hip replacement) versus removal of physical function (leg amputation). Other forms of surgery may have different potential consequences. For example, gynaecological or breast surgery may have threats to a female patient's self-concept, role functioning, fear of alteration to body image (Cheung *et al.*, 2003).

Think about this

What aspects of Mrs Sharma's current predicament can she control? What elements of her current hospital experience can she not control? How can the nurse increase the amount of control patients have during their stay in hospital?

The negative impact of pre-operative anxiety on outcome

Considerable research has investigated the consequences of pre-operative anxiety on the outcomes from surgery and many of these studies have, over a number of decades, indicated that pre-operative anxiety can have a detrimental affect on both psychological and physical outcomes. For example, studies have indicated that anxiety can impact on quality of life, use of medical resources and general comfort. As a result of such studies, there has been considerable research into both the effects of pre-operative anxiety and potential anxiety reducing interventions (Stirling, 2006; Stoddard *et al.*, 2005). In particular, the role of the nurse in reducing anxiety and thereby improving post-operative outcome cannot be underestimated.

There are several reasons why nurses (and other health care professionals) should be interested in the psychological investigation and intervention for pre-operative surgical patients (Stoddard *et al.*, 2005). Firstly, the majority of operations undertaken are planned (or elective), and nurses can therefore have a considerable impact on the health of patients in a planned and considered manner. Secondly, patients at a high risk for anxiety can be identified and appropriate interventions put in place. As a consequence, improvements to surgical outcomes can be made. Finally, from a research perspective, surgical interventions offer a useful model of stress so that appropriate, controlled studies can be undertaken into useful methods of stress reduction. This can have considerable benefits in other areas of stress research and health care.

The consequences of pre-operative anxiety are significant and wide-ranging. The impact covers both physical and psychological consequences as well as having an impact on the recovery from the surgery and medical variables as well. Raised anxiety has important clinical implications as it can have a negative impact upon anaesthetic requirements and post-operative nausea and vomiting (Osborn and Sandler, 2004; Van den Bosch *et al.*, 2005). For example, Carr *et al.* (2006) report that women undergoing (gynaecological) surgery expressed more worry before their surgery and displayed greater heart rate and blood pressure changes before and during surgery and were more difficult to anaesthetise and were more likely to suffer headache, vomiting and pain afterwards. Some of the other negative consequences associated with high levels of pre-operative anxiety are outlined in Table 18.1. In addition to those short-term consequences listed in the table, studies have also indicated that there can be longer cognitive and behavioural sequelae which can have an impact on recovery in the long term (Kiecolt-Glaser *et al.*, 1998; Wilson-Barnett and Batehup, 1988).

Most of the studies have indicated that psychological factors are most important when considering outcomes from surgery. There are, of course, physical variables that can be considered – for example extent of tissue damage caused by the surgery – but there is substantial variability among patients who have had the same operation in terms of the physical and psychological outcomes irrespective of physiological or anatomical variables. Since there is this variability across patients who have undergone the same operation with the same tissue damage, with the same physiological outcome, then it is assumed that the variability must be down to some other factor. Research has indicated that it is these psychosocial factors that are fundamental. Hence the suggestion that psychological variables such as anxiety and depression may have a significant part in determining the duration and characteristic of post-operative recovery. Other variables that may impact on anxiety, depression and physical health outcomes include coping style, **neuroticism**, social support, gender, age, socio-economic status or age.

One of the first studies to investigate the potential role of psychosocial factors on post-operative recovery was completed by Janis (1958) who assessed recovery status post-operatively after measuring anxiety and fear before the

Table 18.1
Consequences of
pre-operative anxiety

Psychological factors

Anxiety (Auerbach, 1973)

Depression (Timberlake *et al.*, 1997)

Medical and surgical factors

Greater intra-operative anaesthetics (Maranets and Kain, 1999)

Post-operative pain (Kain *et al.*, 2000)

Greater demands for post-operative analgesics (Bachiocco *et al.*, 1996; Thomas *et al.*, 1995)

Less ability to make appropriate treatment decisions (Caumo *et al.*, 2001)

Less ability to comply with medical instructions (Caumo *et al.*, 2001)

Impaired wound healing (Kiecolt-Glaser *et al.*, 1998)

Impaired immune function (Kiecolt-Glaser *et al.*, 1998)

Slower post-operative recovery (Salmon and Hall, 1997)

Inactivity (Salmon and Hall, 1997)

Morbidity (Salmon and Hall, 1997)

Increased medical use (Home, 1994)

surgical intervention. He suggested, on the basis of his results, a type of **inverted-U relationship** between anxiety and optimal post-operative recovery (Figure 18.1). Hence, moderate levels of anxiety or 'distress' prior to surgery resulted in optimal post-operative recovery. In contrast, excessively low or very high levels of distress are associated with lesser levels of recovery. Janis termed this the 'work of worry' and suggested that a certain amount of anxiety was required in order for optimal recovery. This study, not surprisingly, led to considerable further research investigating the effects of psychosocial variables on post-operative recovery and how best to prepare patients for their surgery.

Very few (if any) studies, however, managed to replicate this inverted-U relationship and most have found a **linear association** between pre-operative anxiety and recovery success, such that the greater the level of anxiety, the poorer the outcome (and obviously the converse – the lesser the anxiety level, the better the outcome). Furthermore, De Bruin *et al.* (2001) report that pre-operative anxiety is related to intra-operative adjustment, although this is a one-off study and the results are far from conclusive.

Personality and outcome from surgery

In terms of personality variables, it has been demonstrated that neuroticism has been associated with poorer surgical outcome, with higher levels of neuroticism being associated with increased post-operative pain and medical complications. Other personality variables such as optimism have also been associated with post-operative recovery – in particular recovery from coronary artery bypass surgery. Scheier *et al.* (1989) reported that those men high in optimism reported better post-operative outcome than pessimistic men. As would be predicted they also had better outcomes in terms of exercise following surgery, returned to work faster and were rated by their therapists as showing a more favourable physical outcome.

There are, of course, interactions between the psychological factors and other variables. For example, Linn *et al.* (1983) suggested that there was a relationship between age and anxiety such that the younger patients had a

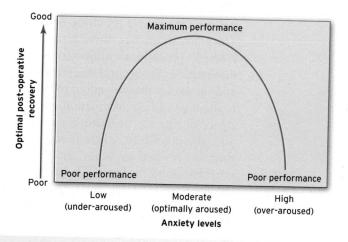

Figure 18.1 Inverted-U relationship between anxiety and recovery.
Source: after Janis (1958)

significantly better outcome than older adults. There are, consequently, a number of psychosocial factors that are associated with higher levels of pre-operative anxiety. Some of these may not be subject to change and most patients attempt to prepare themselves for surgery and potentially painful medical procedures in the best way they can. However, as we have seen, in a large proportion of these patients there is a high level of anxiety that can impede successful recovery.

Interventions to reduce pre-operative anxiety

In light of the range of serious negative consequences associated with high levels of pre-operative anxiety a number of methods have been developed in order to help patients reduce their anxiety levels. Janis (1958) was one of the first to investigate how patients could be helped to cope with their pre-operative anxiety. His early investigations found that those patients that had received additional information on the procedures they were undergoing made fewer requests for pain medication, made fewer demands on staff and were discharged earlier than those receiving the usual information. Another early study found that the medical anaesthetists visiting the patient the night before the surgery and told the patient about typical post-operative physical consequences had fewer reports of pain and were discharged nearly three days (2.7 days to be exact) earlier than those receiving routine care. Furthermore, these patients had less pain medication and, all in all, a better outcome than those with 'normal' care (Egbert et al., 1964). As a consequence, in the following 40 or 50 years a considerable number of studies have investigated a range of intervention techniques on a range of outcome measures.

The research since the time of Janis has generally supported the effectiveness of pre-surgical interventions (e.g. Alberts et al., 1989; Cooke et al., 2005a; Horne et al., 1994; O'Halloran and Altmaier, 1995; Stoddard et al., 2005; Stirling, 2006), although a few studies have failed to demonstrate an effect or even the converse – have increased the levels of anxiety (e.g. Johnston, 1988; Johnston and Vögele, 1993; Mathews and Ridgeway, 1984).

There are several forms of pre-surgical intervention that have been investigated in terms of reducing anxiety. The most common form of intervention has been the simple provision of information about the forthcoming surgery. There are, in essence, three forms of information provision that can be considered: procedural information, **sensory information** and behavioural information. Procedural interventions are those that describe the procedure and the events that are going to occur in detail, whereas sensory information is about providing information on the sensations the patient is likely to experience during the procedure, such as the type of pain they will experience after the procedure, where it will occur and how long it will last. A further form is provided by behavioural interventions which provide patients with instructions on the type of behaviours they should perform in order to speed recovery; for example, walking, eating or breathing in a particular manner. Although these three forms of intervention appear distinct, interventions designed and implemented are primarily a combination of all three (it should be noted that most intervention, despite the combinations, are relatively short and last approximately half an hour or less). Indeed, the evidence has suggested that the combination of interventions is considerable and more than a sum of its parts (Suls and Wan, 1989). Suls and Wan (1989) conducted a **meta-analysis** of the results and they found that there were significant benefits from sensory information but not from procedural information. However, combined sensory and procedural information appeared to provide the most benefit in terms of reducing negative affect, pain reports and other measures of distress.

There are other forms of psychological intervention, including cognitive techniques to help patients reappraise the surgical intervention in a more positive way, **progressive muscle relaxation**, breathing techniques, **hypnosis** and emotionally focused interventions (e.g. see Chapter 13 for details of how these methods have been used for stress reduction) in order to increase relaxation and to decrease stress associated with the medical procedures. Research has shown support for each of the interventions mentioned. For example, Lobb *et al.* (1984) reported that **biofeedback** and relaxation training techniques reduced pre-surgical anxiety and, more importantly, improved recovery from hysterectomy. With a similar form of intervention, Holden-Lund (1988) reported that relaxation techniques using **guided imagery** reduced stress reactions (as measured psychophysiologically) and improved wound healing in surgical patients. Patients that have been trained in cognitive-behavioural stress-inoculation techniques have also been found to score significantly better on measures of pre- and post-surgical anxiety along with measures of post-surgical pain (Wells *et al.*, 1986). Other studies have reported the benefits of massage (Richards *et al.*, 2000), humour (Gaberson, 1995), aromatherapy (Jellinek, 1999), reflexology (Ernst and Köder, 1997), and guided imagery (Turk, 1997), all of which promote relaxation.

Think about this

How could you use sensory, procedural and behavioural information with Mrs Sharma? What psychological and physical methods would you measure and what would you consider a successful outcome?

On the other hand, some studies have suggested that providing information may not always be helpful. Indeed, it has been reported that providing information may actually be detrimental to some patients since it sensitises some patients to their pain and discomfort, allowing them to focus on their pain, thereby increasing arousal and anxiety and preventing recovery. For example, Miller and Mangan (1983) compared anxiety, depression and general discomfort levels of patients given 'large amounts' versus 'minimal amounts' of preparatory information. Patients in the high-information condition demonstrated significantly greater levels of anxiety, depression and discomfort than subjects in the minimal information condition. Similarly, Kerrigan *et al.* (1993) found that providing patients with information about risks and complications associated with medical procedures significantly increased self-reported pre-operative anxiety. Not only are a variety of interventions used but there are also a range of formats in which they have been and, can be, delivered. For example, some interventions have been delivered on a one-to-one basis, whereas others have been used in a more cost-effective manner in a group format, or booklets, manuals, audio-tapes or video-tapes (e.g. Doering *et al.*, 2000).

There have been several meta-analyses of the 200+ studies of psychological pre-operative interventions and most have testified to the success of the various forms and formats of the preparation techniques. Depending on the meta-analysis, 60–75 per cent of patients who received an intervention had a better outcome than untreated controls and the size of improvement ranged between 2 and 28 per cent. Consequently, it can be concluded that psychological interventions are successful and should be implemented in order to improve the outcome of the patient, both psychologically and physically.

Explanations for the effect of psychological preparation

Researchers have attempted to explain how psychological preparation for surgery actually promotes physical recovery and some interesting suggestions have been made. In short, two forms of explanation have been outlined. In the first, it is assumed that the physiological changes associated with stress reduction improve the immunological responses of the individual (Kiecolt-Glaser *et al.*, 1998) and the endocrine function, which consequently improves physical recovery. The alternative explanation is that the psychological preparation either improves the behaviour and/or reduces the maladaptive behaviour of the individual patient. Obviously, these two explanations are not mutually exclusive – both could operate (Kiecolt-Glaser *et al.*, 1998).

Numerous studies have reported beneficial outcomes with a number of different conditions and a number of different procedures. These interventions are consistent with three major psychological theories that explain preferences for information. For example, the **safety-signal theory** (Seligman, 1971), **preparatory-response theory** (Perkins, 1968) and **information-seeking theory** (Berlyne, 1960) all suggest that lowered arousal will result when **aversive events** are predictable. Hence, according to all these theories, providing pre-operative information should reduce anxiety (or lower arousal) when aversive events are predictable. According to these theories, pre-operative information should reduce anxiety because it allows patients to discriminate safe situations from unsafe ones, make a well-timed preparatory response, or reduce uncertainty and conflict. Intervention studies have provided evidential support for these theories. For example, Roach *et al.* (1995) trained nursing staff to provide patients with information about joint replacements and found that patients' length of hospital stay was shortened and health care costs were reduced as a result.

Think about this

When designing information giving procedures for Mrs Sharma, what types of information should be the focus? How should more, potentially negative, information be provided? How should the information be framed and in what order should it be presented?

In light of the heterogeneity of intervention, however, intervention formats, surgical procedures and the potential of individual differences to interact with treatment outcomes, the results achieved by psychological preparation for surgery are generally positive and can be considered a robust effect. A number of reviews and meta-analyses have reported on this and have delineated some of the individual elements which are the most successful. For example, Johnston and Vögele (1993) found that procedural information and behavioural instructions demonstrated the clearest of effects with both forms of intervention having a positive impact on all forms of reported outcomes: for example, negative affect, pain, pain medication, length of stay, behavioural and clinical indices, and satisfaction. Relaxation training (of various forms) is also highly effective and showed positive benefits on nearly all measures of outcomes. Finally, they found sensory information, hypnotic and emotion-focused approaches to be rather less effective in improving outcome. However, these interventions have been explored in fewer studies and the procedures may be less well developed. In a more recent study comparing the effects of structured attention, self-hypnotic relaxation and standard care in a group of patients undergoing percutaneous vascular and renal procedures (angiographies), hypnosis had more pronounced effects on pain and anxiety reduction (Lang *et al.*, 2000).

Other simple interventions may also be effective in improving clinical outcome. For example, Ulrich (1984) reported that even small changes, such as having a room with a view, can result in improved outcome (shorter stay in hospital, less pain medication requested). In another interesting study, Kulik *et al.* (1993) compared the outcomes from cardiac surgery between those in a room with somebody who had either undergone cardiac surgery or who was waiting for surgery. Patients with a post-operative room-mate were less anxious before their operation and had a smoother recovery (ambulation, length of stay) than their counterparts. In addition, it made no difference whether the room-mate had a similar surgical procedure. In a follow-up to this study (Kulik *et al.*, 1996), the authors could show that patients without a room-mate had the slowest recovery of all. Parent and Fotin (2000) reported that patients who received support from former patients recorded less anxiety pre-operatively and increased physical activity post-surgery. Similarly, Carr *et al.* (2006) reported that fellow patients were used as a source of information, as a distraction from current worries and, most importantly, as a 'forum for discussion and validation of emotions and physical symptoms' (p. 349). Hence, this suggests one method for reducing the anxiety before surgery and improving post-operative recovery.

Obviously, this relates to the positive benefits of social support that have been reported in Chapter 13. There is ample evidence that social support has a stress buffering effect (see Chapter 13), and it may be that the benefits associated with psychological preparation for surgery can at least partly be explained by the effects of face-to-face contact provided in studies using a personal approach (as opposed to using a booklet or audio-tape). Whether pre-surgical interventions have any effect over and above the interpersonal support provided by the health care worker administering the intervention would have to be investigated in studies including an attention-placebo group.

Coping and information-seeking: monitoring versus blunting

As we have seen in Chapter 13, coping refers to those cognitive or behavioural efforts to master, reduce or tolerate the emotional and/or situational demands arising from a stressful event. Obviously we could define undergoing a surgical intervention as a stressful procedure and, consequently, we can assume that people will use their coping strategies to deal with the consequences of this stress. The strategies that people use will differ from individual to individual. A particular area of importance for those about to undergo surgical intervention is those that use information and those that try to avoid all the information: information seeking versus information avoidance.

Research has highlighted that when faced with an impending threat (the 'operation') an individual's information-seeking behaviour varies along two dimensions. The first is the amount of information sought by the individual and the extent to which they attend to the threat-relevant information. This is termed 'monitoring'. The second dimension is the extent to which an individual avoids and/or ignores the threat-relevant information. This is termed 'blunting' (Miller, 1980, 1987).

The way that people deal with information differs depending on whether they are monitors or blunters. Monitors will seek out information and if it is not available then they tend to become highly anxious. On the other hand, 'blunters' are those who avoid or ignore information and become anxious when provided with it (e.g. Ludwick-Rosenthal and Neufeld, 1993). In one particular study, for example, Miller and Mangan (1983) studied gynaecological patients at risk of cervical cancer just before they underwent a diagnostic evaluation. In the study, they found that blunters demonstrated lower psychophysiological arousal (i.e. a physiological measure of stress) when provided with low information, and monitors demonstrated lower psychophysiological arousal when provided with high information. Hence, the requirement is to provide the correct amount of information for the type of person undergoing the intervention. So, for example, Ludwick-Rosenthal and Neufeld (1993) reported on a study that matched the amount of information with the desire for information in a group of patients. The study found that there was less anxiety and more problem-focused coping (coping directed at moderating the situation), and less emotion-focused coping (coping directed at regulating emotions and distress) in those who had their information matched with their coping strategies. Thus, medical patients appear to fare best when their coping styles are matched with the amount of information provided to them.

There are a couple of methods that have been developed to measure monitor-blunters. The first was devised by Miller (1987) and has been used in many studies. However, a more recent and up-to-date questionnaire is that reported by Van Zuuren *et al.* (1996) – the threatening medical situations inventory (TMSI). The TMSI was developed mainly to be used in research with medical patients in order to establish possibly modulating effects of coping style on variables such as symptom perception, patient delay and disease outcome and on the outcome of the provision of different types of information and other types of psychological interventions. Examples of the types of questions in the TMSI are presented in the box.

The threatening medical situations inventory

Imagine you have been suffering from headaches and dizziness for some period of time. You visit your doctor. He or she tells you things don't look too well and refers you to a specialist for a rather trying medical examination.

Please indicate for each statement below to what degree it is applicable to you (on a scale from 1 - not applicable to 5 - strongly applicable), by circling your answer:

	Not applicable		Applicable		Strongly applicable
1. I plan to ask the specialist as many questions as possible	1	2	3	4	5
2. I think things will turn out to be all right	1	2	3	4	5
3. I determine to inform myself at other instances and doctors first	1	2	3	4	5
4. I plan to start reading about headaches and dizziness	1	2	3	4	5
5. For the time being I try not to think of unpleasant outcomes	1	2	3	4	5
6. I am not going to worry: such an examination is not as bad as suffering from headaches all the time	1	2	3	4	5

Source: Van Zuuren *et al.* (1996)

Think about this

How would you measure Mrs Sharma's style of information coping? Would you consider her a monitor or a blunter?

Conclusion

In summary, a considerable proportion of pre-operative patients report anxiety – in some studies up to 80 per cent. This pre-operative anxiety has been associated with poor medical and psychological outcomes, and increased costs associated with these poorer outcomes. A number of psychological methods for reducing anxiety have been devised and implemented (e.g.

information provision, relaxation training, cognitive techniques). These psychological methods have been associated with decreased anxiety and improved medical outcome. In particular, studies have demonstrated that such interventions result in shortened lengths of hospital stays, decreased anaesthesia/analgesic use, improved medical outcome, quicker healing and decreased medical expenditures.

Finally, monitor-blunter coping style may moderate the impact of information on anxiety, and the provision of information and determination of coping style can be accomplished with minimal time, effort and expense. Thus, it may be that the most beneficial health outcomes (to patient and establishment, alike) result from matching coping style with intervention type, which may have important implications for the medical field.

Research in focus

Cooke, M., Chaboyer, W., Schluter, P. and Hiratos, M. (2005) The effect of music on pre-operative anxiety in day surgery. *Journal of Advanced Nursing*, **52** (1), 47-55.

Background
As has been demonstrated in many other studies, people awaiting surgery experience anxiety and this may be more pronounced in those undergoing day surgery. Anxiety may impact both emotional upset and physical discomfort and adversely affect such patient recovery/recuperation. It is suggested that waiting time prior to surgery may allow for brooding, thinking, worrying and fearing the forthcoming surgery, and this consequently increases the anxiety. Thus if the nurse could create a supportive and interactive environment during this time then this may be important in ameliorating distress and improving psychological and physical outcomes. In this study the impact of music as a physiological relaxation technique was explored.

Method
Participants: 180 individual day case surgical patients undergoing a range of procedures (e.g. orthopaedics, cystoscopy, biopsy) were involved in the study.

Intervention: Participants were randomly assigned to one of three groups: control (no intervention), placebo (wore headphones but listened to no music), intervention (listened to their choice of music through portable CD player). Those in the intervention group chose their preferred music (classical, jazz, country and western, new age, easy-listening and other). Participants in the intervention group listened to their choice of music for 30 minutes, whereas the placebo group wore the headphones but received routine care only.

Results
The mean difference in anxiety scores (as measured on the Speilberger's state anxiety form; Speilberger *et al.*, 1977) between intervention and control/placebo patients was statistically significant but no such difference emerged between the means of control and placebo patients. Thus listening to music statistically significantly reduced mean anxiety scores compared with not listening to music. Music type was not statistically significantly associated with the anxiety scores.

Implications
Nursing management of pre-operative anxiety and stress is important and providing evidence-based interventions that meet psychosocial needs is a crucial aspect of nursing care. This study

demonstrated that patients having day surgery who listen to their choice of music while waiting for their procedure have reduced anxiety level, thereby enhancing their comfort and overall well-being. This finding is important because it provided clear evidence for the use of music in the day surgery area. Music is one of the few strategies for enriching the environment that is adult-orientated and provides a positive relaxing experience. It is also a relaxation intervention that nurses can initiate independently. It is important to note that individual preference is important as there is a potential risk that music could be seen and treated as a routine rather than used as a patient-centred nursing intervention.

Summary

- People are admitted to hospital for a number of reasons: assessment, treatment, both surgical and medical, and psychological.

- A range of mental health issues may lead to hospital admission and some patients can be compulsory detained under the Mental Health Act (1983).

- Anxiety is a common reaction to entering hospital and the nurse has a key role in smoothing entry into hospital and reducing anxiety.

- Interactions with patients should avoid depersonalisation, that is, to ensure the patient is treated as a person rather than a number.

- Nurses may categorise patients according to their own values and moral compass and it is important that this does not interfere with the care and treatment provided.

- People can enter the 'sick role' when they become ill and 'a patient' and this comes with rights and responsibilities.

- Pre-operative anxiety (which can occur in up to 80 per cent of patients) can have significant impact on the psychological and physical recovery of the individual patient.

- Pre-operative anxiety can have long-term physical consequences in terms of impaired recovery time.

- A range of interventions have been implemented to reduce pre-operative anxiety including relaxation, information provision or physical activity.

- Meta-analyses have indicated that psychological pre-operative interventions are broadly successful.

- Coping with surgery can be classified as either monitoring or blunting and these different forms of coping have different forms of preparation needs.

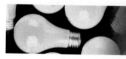

Check your understanding

1. What is stressful about being admitted to hospital and undergoing surgery?

2. How does pre-operative anxiety affect post-operative recovery?

3. Discuss the different forms of psychological preparation for surgery.

4. What benefits can be achieved by psychological preparation for surgery?

5. What individual characteristics should you take into account when preparing somebody for surgery and how can they impact on post-operative recovery?

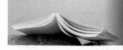

Further reading

Carr, E., Brockbank, K., Allen, S. and Strike, P. (2006) Patterns and frequency of anxiety in women undergoing gynaecological surgery. *Journal of Clinical Nursing*, **15**, 341-352.

Jeffrey, R. (1979) Normal rubbish: deviant patients in casualty departments. *Sociology of Health and Illness*, **1** (1), 90-107.

Johnston, M. and Vögele, C. (1993) Benefits of psychological preparation for surgery: a meta-analysis. *Annals of Behavioural Medicine*, **15**, 245-256.

Kain, Z.N., Mayes, L.C., Caldwell-Andrews, A.A., Karas, D.E. and McClain, B.C. (2006) Preoperative anxiety, postoperative pain, and behavioural recovery in young children undergoing surgery, *Pediatrics*, **118** (2), 651-658.

Stern, C. and Lockwood, C. (2006) Knowledge retention from preoperative patient information. *Evidence Based Medicine*, **3** (3), 45-50.

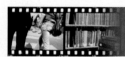

Weblinks

| UK Society for Behavioural Medicine | http://www.uksbm.org.uk/ | The UK Society for Behavioural Medicine (UKSBM) works towards integrating knowledge of biology, behaviour and the environment to prevent and treat disease. |
| Encyclopaedia of Surgery | http://www.surgeryencyclopedia.com/index.html | The Encyclopaedia of Surgery has been written by various experts in the field of surgery and has been written specifically for health care students and patients. |

Media examples

Carry on Doctor/Doctor in the House A range of films (from the 1960s) that demonstrate (historically) the problems associated with being in hospital. However, at least they will cure the stresses with humour!

Paper Mask (1990) A hospital porter impersonates a recently deceased doctor and goes to work in the busy accident and emergency department of a small hospital where he meets and befriends a nurse who slowly figures out his secret and helps him maintain his charade. A film to increase the anxiety...!

One Flew Over the Cuckoo's Nest (1975) An excellent film, although a rather negative view on the psychiatric hospital.

Part 4
Practical applications

Chapter 19

Applying psychology to specific conditions: Part I

Learning outcomes

When you have read this chapter you should understand:

- How psychology plays a role in the development, maintenance and adaptation to serious chronic illnesses.
- The influence of psychological factors on the aetiology of cancer and coronary heart disease.
- How psychological factors impact on the development of cancer and coronary heart disease.
- How psychology can be used throughout the course of cancer to assist patients in coping with their condition.
- How altering the perception of symptoms can reduce the physical consequences of CHD and myocardial infarction.

Case study

The difficulties faced by Mr Thomas Lynch and his three children, Cameron, Jerome and Natalie, are considerable. Mr Lynch's wife recently died from breast cancer and since then he has been coping as a single parent as well as attempting to hold down a full-time job. Cameron, the eldest son, was born with severe learning difficulties and was cared for by Mrs Lynch before her death. Now, Mr Lynch is considering applying for longer residential care for Cameron as he has to cope with a full-time job (he is a community psychiatric nurse) and the two other children. The family has suffered from a catastrophic life stress: there was an elder brother – Alexis – who was killed in a mobile phone mugging some three years ago. Two years after Alexis's death, Mrs Lynch developed some non-specific symptoms and later (after a delay in reporting these symptoms) died from breast cancer. Following the death of his eldest son and his wife, Thomas has suffered considerably and is finding it hard to continue, but does so because of the needs of his other children. He has rather a lonely time – he has few friends and limited contact with his family. He has trouble making friends either outside or within work and this is mainly due to his personality which some have described as rather 'aggressive' and, in particular, seems to always be in a rush.

By the time Mrs Lynch was seen by the GP and hospital consultant, she had secondary tumours (from the primary site of her breast). Ultimately, despite considerable chemotherapeutic and radiotherapy treatment she succumbed to the illness and died.

While at work one day, Thomas suffers from severe chest pain and is rushed to hospital with a suspected heart attack. He is treated immediately in the accident and emergency department before being sent to cardiology where he, eventually, undergoes a triple bypass operation. After the successful surgery he enrols on a rehabilitation programme while at the same time returning to work.

Why is this relevant to nursing practice?

The case of Thomas is a relatively simple one (although no less distressing for that): he has a heart attack, has surgery and then undergoes rehabilitation before, hopefully, experiencing a long and successful remainder of his life. However, this omits the experiences of Thomas: why did he have a heart attack? How did he come to enter hospital? How did he feel when he got there? How did he cope with the experience of entering hospital? What about dealing with the rehabilitation process? How is psychology implemented in each of these steps? How can the nurse use their knowledge of psychology to smooth the transition of Thomas through his health care crisis? This will be the focus of this, and the following, chapter.

What about his wife: why did Mrs Lynch develop breast cancer? What psychological factors are involved in the development of cancer (indeed, are there any)? Why did she delay seeking treatment? What happened when she entered hospital? What was her experience? How could psychology help her cope with the condition when she was being treated? What about during her final days? This, again, will be the focus of this and the subsequent chapter.

The case study is relevant to nursing practice as, although uncommon and relatively catastrophic, the case example has been chosen to illustrate how psychology may be implicated in health and illness throughout the whole of the health care system and 'career' of the individual patient/client. The role of the nurse in each of these stages will be explored and how the psychological knowledge that has been explored and explained earlier in this text can be used in day-to-day practice highlighted.

Alan Ball who died from a heart attack, reportedly never recovered from the death of his wife from cancer three years previously

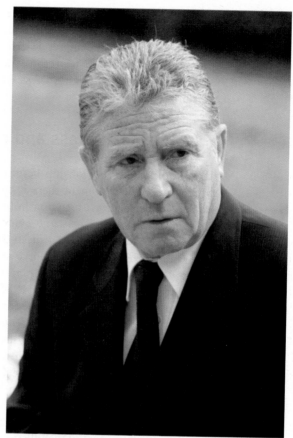

Chris Ison/PA

The two major killers present in the Western world are cancer and heart disease. These two chronic illnesses are also a major cause for concern for the individual patient and the health care system – they cause considerable pain, discomfort and impact negatively on quality of life. The focus of this chapter will be on psychology's role in both cancer and heart disease and applying psychology to professional nursing practice.

Think about this

What psychosocial variables do you think impact on the development of heart disease and cancer? List those variables you consider important and those you think the nurse could influence. Explore those variables that have a bearing on the Lynch family.

Psychology and cancer

Let's start with Mrs Lynch: what psychological variables are implicated in the development of her breast cancer? If we examine the case study we can see that it has been a stressful time – could these stresses be implicated in the development of the breast cancer? Is there any evidence linking **life events**, or stress, with the development of cancer? Before exploring this further, the first point to note is the difficulty in defining and measuring stress – this concept has been discussed in Chapter 13. However, with this caveat in mind, what is the relationship between breast cancer and some of these stressful events? What evidence exists linking stress with the development of cancer, in particular breast cancer?

Psychosocial stress and cancer

If we look at the relationship between the life events of Mrs Lynch and her breast cancer development there is compelling anecdotal evidence to link her adverse experience with the pathological development of the cancer, but is there any substantial *research* evidence? As we have noted in Chapter 13 there are a number of life event studies (as usually measured by the Holmes and Rahe, 1967, scale) that have shown a relationship between these life events and several health complaints, such as infectious diseases (e.g. the common cold, Cohen and Wills, 1985). Hence, the argument goes if there is a relationship between mild illnesses and life events surely there must also be a relationship between severe life events and severe illnesses?

One piece of evidence that may be relevant to Mrs Lynch is that provided by Garssen (2004) in a thorough review of the relationship between psychosocial factors and breast cancer. Garssen (2004) reports on several studies that have explored the relationship between total number of life events and survival, period of being free from disease, or relapse in cancer. Some studies have found a relationship (Forsen, 1991) and others found no relationship (e.g. Maunsell *et al.*, 2002). Lillberg *et al.* (2003) highlighted the relationship between stressful life events and risk of breast cancer in a large-scale study of over 10 000 women. The authors reported a relationship between the accumulation of life events during the 5 years before baseline and an increased risk of cancer development at 15 years follow-up. This **prospective** study reported that divorce/separation, death of a husband and death of a close relative/friend were each associated with increased risk of subsequently developing breast cancer.

However, this is a rather simplistic study: counting the number of life events and then merely correlating this with the occurrence (or otherwise) of an illness. However, the problem with any study merely totalling the life events is the issue discussed in a previous chapter: do a series of life events have a significant impact? Does the relative impact of a series of minor events have the same impact as the most serious of events? Do individual differences play a part? How can an individual's personality or coping strategies play a part in mediating the effects of life events? A more sophisticated approach would be to explore the relationship between life stressors and cancer progression/aetiology with other psychological factors (e.g. coping style, personality) taken into account. With such studies a prospective study design is preferred, for it allows for the impact of various factors to be singled out and any potential bias to be minimised. What about the serious life event that has been suffered by Mrs Lynch? Could that have been influential in the development of her breast cancer?

Mrs Lynch suffered an acute severe life event – the death of her son in a violent episode – and was caring for another son with severe learning difficulties, which can be considered a chronic stressor. Could either of these (or both) lead to the development of her illness? (Indeed, could they have contributed to the development of Mr Lynch's heart attack?) It might be assumed that the severest of life events would place a heavy burden on the coping resources of Mrs Lynch, perhaps leading to a state of depression or hopelessness which might promote cancer development or progression. This has been studied in a number of large scale studies (e.g. Jones and Goldblatt, 1986; Martikainen and Valkonen, 1996). The results from these studies have been equivocal: some have found no effect, some minor, and others a significant influence of bereavement.

Duijts *et al.* (2003) in a summary and evaluation of the literature suggested that there was an association between stressful life events and breast cancer risk, with the risk being increased in light of a more severe life event. For example, the death of a family member or close friend such as that suffered by Mrs Lynch has a greater impact than other stressors (e.g. change in marital status or financial state). Direct evidence also comes from Jiong *et al.* (2003) who reported that the death of a child was associated with an increased risk of cancer in their mothers. In this particular study, however, there was no relationship between stressful life events and breast cancer. However, there was a relationship between the death of a child and an increase in lung carcinoma. Hence, it could have been a consequence of an increase in smoking behaviour as a result of trying to cope with the stresses of bereavement rather than other factors. For example, there was no increase in alcohol-related malignancies, or hormone-related malignancies. What was also interesting in this study was that there was no relationship for fathers, only for mothers, with the authors suggesting that this was a consequence of mothers experiencing more stress than fathers after the loss of a child. This study was useful since the death of a child is a severe stressor, regardless of personality, coping style, social support or social network (or other variables associated with mediating stress). It consequently suggests that there is an increased risk of developing a malignant disease in bereaved mothers, probably due to lifestyle behaviours after parental bereavement. Taken overall, the evidence does seem to suggest a link between stress and the development of breast cancer.

How could this happen? How could a stressor be linked to the development of cancer? One explanation that has already been touched upon is the link between cancer and behaviour, with the suggestion that a stressor compromises behaviour; hence in the Jiong *et al.* study (2003) there was an increased level of smoking following the death of a child and this resulted in a subsequent increased levels of lung cancer. However, Lillberg *et al.* (2003) report that life events increase breast cancer risk independently of body mass index (BMI), weight change, alcohol use, smoking and physical activity.

Another explanation is that stress disturbs aspects of the immune system and that an impaired immune system predisposes individuals to malignant tumour growth (Tosevski and Milovancevic, 2006). It has been suggested that various immunological changes among those with stressful life events could promote the development of breast cancer (Cohen and Herbert, 1996). The relationship between life events and breast cancer risk could also have a hormonal basis (Hilakivi-Clarke, 1997), but the exact mechanism is still unclear.

What about other variables that may be important in the development and progression of cancer? What variables might mediate the relationship between stressors and disease aetiology or progression? One such important variable is that of social relations, or social support. A number of studies have explored the relationship between social support measures and disease progression. Social support, as we have seen in Chapter 13 can include having social networks of friends and family, having confidants and being involved in networks (e.g. churches, social groups). A number of studies reported by Garssen (2004) show that those having better social relationships have longer, disease-free intervals and longer survival (e.g. Reynolds *et al.*, 1994, 2000). For example Maunsell *et al.* (1995) interviewed 224 women with newly diagnosed breast cancer and recorded whether they had a confidant (e.g. spouse, children, friends, colleagues or 'professional' confidants such as nurses) with whom they had discussed personal problems in the three months since surgery. Survival rate in women without a confidant was 56 per cent, but was 72 per cent for women who had at least one type of confidant. There was also a kind of dose–response relationship: survival rates at seven years increased stepwise in women reporting no, one or at least two types of confidants, respectively. Similarly, Osborne *et al.* (2005) found that marital status at diagnosis was related to long-term survival. That is, those who were married had a longer survival period than those who were not. The message is clear: those with better social networks survive longer. Interestingly, Lutgendorf *et al.* (2005) reported that better social support offered a biological protection against tumour development suggesting that stress, and putative stress protectors, influence the micro-environment of tumour development.

Think about this

What are the implications of social networks and social ties for improving the outcomes for women once diagnosed with the condition? What can the nurse do to promote social ties and social networks? How can the nurse behave to decrease social isolation?

Another variable warranting investigation is the relationship between negative emotions and cancer progression. Many studies have investigated this exploratory relationship with, not surprisingly, divergent findings. Some studies have found the expected and commonly reported relationship: more distress and psychological problems being associated with unfavourable disease outcomes. In contrast Garssen (2004) reported that six studies found the opposite – high levels of psychological distress being associated with better disease outcomes! A sizeable proportion of studies (some 50 per cent) have failed to find this relationship so there is no real research evidence to support this contention.

What about personality – does that have a part to play in the development of breast cancer? In terms of traditional measures of personality, a number of studies have explored the relationship between extroversion and neuroticism and disease-free intervals and survival. The results, not surprisingly, have been equivocal with most studies reporting no such relationship (e.g. Dean and Surtees, 1989; Schapiro *et al.*, 2001). However, one study showed that having a reserved personality was a risk factor for death from lung cancer. This study also found an association for the two extremes of one personality scale: being very sober or very enthusiastic versus being average increased the chance of dying from lung cancer (Stavraky *et al.*, 1988).

Another measure which has been investigated is the health locus of control (HLC) or locus of control (LoC). As outlined in Chapter 1, LoC is a measure of how much control people believe they have over their situation – those with an internal LoC believe that they are responsible for controlling their condition (compared with those with either an 'external' or 'powerful others' LoC). It might be predicted that the negative consequences of cancer are dampened in people with an internal LoC (persons with an internal LoC believe that they have control over their destinies). Some studies failed to find a relationship between LoC and disease outcome but in one study an internal LoC was associated with a longer disease-free interval (Hislop *et al.*, 1987) and more recently the relationship between locus of control and attending screening has been stressed (e.g. Rowe *et al.*, 2005).

Think about this

How can health locus of control (see Chapter 1) help explain why people delay reporting symptoms? How would you promote breast cancer identification in those with high and those with low, health locus of control?

Delays in seeking treatment

One of the major issues concerning Mrs Lynch and her cancer is the fact that she delayed seeking treatment even after symptoms appeared (see box for symptoms of breast cancer).

Symptoms of breast cancer

- A lump or thickening.
- A change in the size or shape of a breast.
- Dimpling of the skin.
- A change in the shape of your nipple, particularly if it turns in, sinks into the breast or becomes irregular in shape.
- A blood-stained discharge from the nipple.
- A rash on a nipple or surrounding area.
- A swelling or lump in the armpit.

Breast cancer is a serious illness and affects thousands of women every year – it is predicted that approximately 35 000 new cases of breast cancer are diagnosed each year in the United Kingdom. In younger women aged 35–54 years, breast cancer accounts for 17 per cent of all deaths, the most common cause of death in this age group. Furthermore, the mortality rate from breast cancer is high particularly in the UK and this may relate to any delay in diagnosis.

Figure 19.1 shows that the later the diagnosis (i.e. the later the stage) the poorer the survival rate. Consequently, there have been considerable attempts

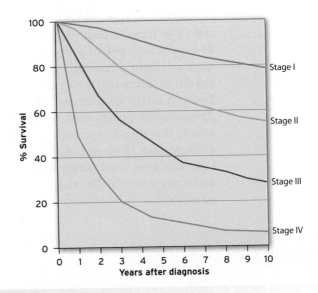

Figure 19.1 Relationship between survival and stage of diagnosis.

Source: Cancer Research UK, http://info.cancerresearchuk.org/cancerstats/types/breast/survival/, (accessed November 2007)

at highlighting the importance of having regular screening and breast self-examination: both can decrease the time before diagnosis. However, despite the success of some of these processes and education attempts there is concern that there is often a delay between the discovery of symptoms and their reporting (Mohamed *et al.*, 2005). Facione *et al.* (2002) suggest that approximately one-third of women delay for three months or more prior to reporting their symptoms. Since the majority – some three-quarters – present to the health care after spotting the symptoms themselves rather than through an NHS screening service (Richards *et al.*, 1999) it is important to get women to self-examine and to report their symptoms once they have been spotted. How can we explain why Mrs Lynch delayed reporting her symptoms? Why did she not report them when she first spotted them? There are a number of psychological models that we could apply to this observation and some of these were outlined in Chapter 15. However, it could also be useful to understand both the cognitive representation of the disease and the associated symptoms, along with the beliefs regarding the treatment for breast cancer and how this has implications for the individual in seeking health care. One such model that attempts to explore these variables in further detail is the self-regulation model proposed by Leventhal *et al.* (1984). This model proposes that people construct cognitive representations of an illness or disease in order to understand and cope with it.

Self-regulation model

The model of Leventhal *et al.* (1984) is based on the assumption that people deal with the problems of illness in the same way they would deal with any other problem. The model suggests that faced with a problem, or some potential disturbance of status quo, the individual will be motivated to solve the problem and re-establish their normal state.

The model consists of a number of stages – interpretation, coping and appraisal (Figure 19.2) – and these three components interrelate in order to maintain the status quo. So, for example, interpretation and symptom perception may result in an emotional shift, or the coping strategy will result in a change in symptom perception.

Interpretation

At the onset of a symptom an individual will realise that they have a potential illness through two potential routes: symptom perception ('I have a lump in my breast') or a social message (the doctor tells you, 'I can feel a lump' on examination). This is the first stage. Once the individual has received either (or sometimes both) of these messages, the individual can be classified as having 'a problem' and will want to resolve (according to this problem-solving theory) this and return to a 'problem-free' state. In order for this to happen, the meaning of the problem must be understood by the individual and this obviously involves cognitions. Therefore, the symptom perception and external messages will contribute towards the development of the cognitions (or thoughts) about the illness. There is evidence that illness representations consist of five distinct but interrelated components:

- *Identity*: Label that the individual uses to describe the condition and associated symptoms (e.g. 'cancer' and breast lump).
- *Cause*: Individual's beliefs about the cause of the condition (e.g. 'I think the lump is a cyst like my friend had').
- *Timeline*: Expectations about the conditions length (e.g. 'This has been going on for some time').
- *Consequences*: Physical, social and psychological (e.g. 'I am scared of any potential diagnosis').
- *Control/cure*: Beliefs about the possibility of cure or control of the condition (e.g. 'This condition will go away by itself').

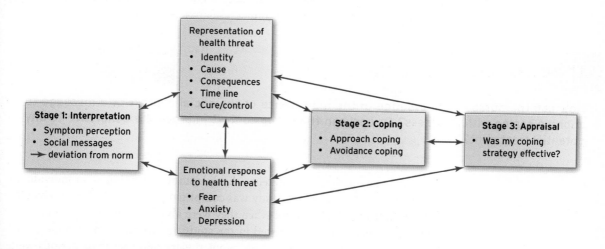

Figure 19.2 Leventhal's self-regulation model.

Source: Ogden, J. (2004) *Health Psychology: A Textbook*, 3rd Edition, Open University Press. Reproduced with the kind permission of the Open University Press Publishing Company

These cognitive representations of the 'problem' will give the problem meaning and will enable the individual to develop and consider suitable coping strategies. Symptom perception is not as straightforward as people initially imagine (as we saw in the case study in Chapter 1). We all have non-specific symptoms from time to time, for example a slightly raised temperature, a runny nose, a slight pain or the like. However, how each of us interprets this may differ according to a number of factors. What to one person is a runny nose, to another is a mild cold and to another the forbearer of flu! There are a number of individual differences that may contribute to these perceptions. For example, some people may be more internally focused and therefore more sensitive to symptoms whereas others may be more externally focused and less sensitive to internal changes.

Think about this

What social factors may influence the perceptions of symptoms? For example, are men or women more likely to have an internal focus? What about other social factors? Why should this be? You may like to re-consider the material presented in Chapter 6.

Symptom perception is not only a consequence of some of these individual differences, it may also be a consequence of factors such as mood, cognition and the social environment. In terms of mood, the clearest example is the consequence of anxiety. Anxiety can influence the perception of pain (as we have seen in Chapter 14) but can also influence the perception of symptoms with those higher in anxiety more likely to perceive a symptom.

Other studies (e.g. Stegen *et al.*, 2000) have indicated that what individuals are told about the symptoms and the context in which they are given will influence their perception of that symptom. For example (and perhaps not surprisingly) if people are told that the symptom is meaningless or mild then they are less likely to worry about it and consider it a symptom. Similarly, if people are directed towards a symptom then they are more likely to perceive it as important, which is likely to increase anxiety.

Think about this

How can the nurse use knowledge of the importance of the social context of a message to improve coping with an illness? Or how can the social context improve the adherence to any potential treatment?

Another factor that can influence the symptom perception is an individual's cognitive state. An interesting study was completed by Ruble (1977) who manipulated women's expectations of when they were about to start menstruating. She gave the women who participated in the study an 'accurate physiological test' (which was, in reality fictitious) and women were told that their periods were either very close or a week away (which was randomly assigned). The results showed that women who believed they were about to start menstruating (although they were not) reported more premenstrual symptoms.

Finally, environment (or social context) may also influence symptom perception. The most well-known example of this is the so-called 'medical student's disease' (Mechanic, 1962). Since medical students spend most of their time learning about different illnesses and symptoms it has been reported that two-thirds of medical students have incorrectly reported that they have symptoms they are being taught about.

Think about this

What about the nurse? Do you think they could suffer from 'medical students' disease'? What sort of factors could influence the symptom perception of nursing and medical students? How can mood, cognition and social factors influence such a condition?

The other factor that can influence symptom perception is the social message. The information that people receive about their illness may come from somebody else – a health care professional, for example. So an individual may get a diagnosis following screening or a health check even though they may be asymptomatic. In this case the information a person receives comes from the health care professional and then subsequently perhaps from friends and family (e.g. 'a friend of mine had this and it was good/bad ...'), or from some other information resource such as the medical literature or, increasingly, the Internet. The illness cognitions are not the only consequence of receiving a social message, there is also an emotional result. For example, Mrs Lynch may have felt the lump in her breast, been told that it may be cancer and this will result in both a cognitive representation of the problem and an emotional consequence – for example anxiety. Thus, Mrs Lynch (or any individual according to the model) will have to develop coping strategies for both the illness cognitions and their own emotional state.

Implications of illness representation

Differences in illness representation have been reported between those who intend to seek help for potential breast cancer symptoms and those who were potential delayed help-seekers (Hunter *et al.*, 2003). These authors suggest that the identification of symptoms as potential signs of breast cancer (identity) was the variable that most strongly predicted intention to seek help for breast cancer symptoms. This supports the view that cognitive representations are the key factors in the initiation of the self-regulatory process.

One of the issues, of course, is the knowledge that women have of breast cancer symptoms and this is a well-established predictor of delayed behaviour. In particular, a patient with a non-lump breast symptom is over four times more likely to delay seeking medical help than an individual with a breast lump (Burgess *et al.*, 1998; Ramirez *et al.*, 1999). It is possible that those who delay reporting their symptoms have misattributed their symptoms to a rather benign process. Obviously this suggests that health education campaigns (either at an individual or community level) should highlight the range of different symptoms so it provides the 'cancer knowledge' of the patient. It is important to encourage women to be aware of non-lump symptoms as this will have implications for the early reporting of symptoms and consequently survival.

Coping

The next stage, according to this model, is the development of appropriate coping strategies. If we assume that the illness can be perceived as a stressor then the models of stress that we have previously discussed (see Chapter 13) can be applied and this approach has been most developed by Moos and Schaefer (1986). One of the key issues in this model is coping and there are a considerable number of forms of coping that individuals can engage in (again, see Chapter 13). The ultimate aim of all these different coping strategies is to return the individual to a state of healthy normality or positive affect.

These coping strategies are similar to those with any stressor and can be categorised into one of three forms:

- *Appraisal-focused*:
  - logical analysis and mental preparation: turning the event into a series of manageable events;
  - cognitive redefinition: accepting the situation by redefining it in a positive manner;
  - cognitive avoidance or denial: minimising the seriousness of the illness.
- *Problem-seeking*:
  - seeking information and support: accessing information and support;
  - taking problem-solving action: learning specific skills associated with the condition;
  - identifying rewards: attempt to find events that will offer positive rewards.
- *Emotion-focused*:
  - affective regulation: attempting to maintain hope in light of the stressful situation;
  - emotional discharge: venting feelings of anger, despair or depression;
  - resigned acceptance: coming to terms with the outcomes of an illness.

Think about this

Do you think any of the above coping strategies are particularly positive or negative? Is it possible to identify a more efficacious strategy for coping with breast cancer? If so, how do you think you could promote it?

Is there any evidence linking coping strategy to outcome? A number of studies have investigated this relationship. For example Greer *et al.* (1990) explored the relationship between coping and survival from breast cancer in a 15 year follow-up study. They reported that women who had a coping style of fighting spirit (i.e. affective regulation) or denial survived longer after surgery than those who reacted with either stoic acceptance or helpless attitude (i.e. resigned acceptance). Similarly, Watson *et al.* (2005) reported that those patients who showed a helpless/hopeless response had greater mortality rates at 5 and 10 years follow-up compared with those with other forms of coping strategy.

These reports gathered considerable media attention and were reported in a rather simplistic fashion: having a fighting spirit promotes survival in those with cancer. Unfortunately, the evidence of other studies has not always been supportive of this position although there is some general support (Tschuschke *et al.*, 2001). The converse has also been found: people with a hopelessness or pessimistic view are reported to have a poorer outcome (e.g. Watson *et al.*, 2005).

When other forms of coping have been explored, a rather unexpected finding has been reported: many studies have found that those that deny or minimise the impact of the cancer have a better prognosis. This may be related to either severe denial (e.g. attempting to describe the cancer or a mastectomy as a minor inconvenience) or a less extreme form of denial by attempting to adopt a position of minimising the impact of the cancer. This is a milder and probably a more realistic form of denial (Butow *et al.*, 2000) which has been associated with longer survival (Butow *et al.*, 2000).

Other studies have explored the effectiveness of active coping strategies. The results of these studies have been rather mixed: some studies (e.g. Faller *et al.*, 1997) have reported a positive relationship between use of these coping strategies and survival at three to five years, although this had disappeared at a longer follow-up of seven to eight years (Faller *et al.*, 1999).

Hence, these coping studies suggest that, although the evidence is mixed, the form of coping strategies a person employs can have an impact on their physical health.

Think about this

Consider the evidence about the coping strategies provided above. What, as a nurse, could you do to help a women better cope with breast cancer?

Appraisal

The third stage is the appraisal, which involves the individual evaluating the effectiveness of the coping strategy and determining whether to continue with the strategy or not.

We have shown that, although there is conflicting research evidence on the extent, psychological variables play an important role in the development and coping with cancer. In particular how symptoms are represented by the individual patient can impact on the development and understanding of the condition. How other psychological factors can impact on the other major killer – heart disease – will be explored in the next section of this chapter.

Psychology and heart disease

When we look at the experiences of Mr Lynch and his heart attack, what psychosocial factors could be linked to the development of his heart disease and subsequent **myocardial infarction** (MI)? Coronary heart disease (CHD) refers to the dysfunction associated with the coronary arteries which may result in three different conditions/diseases: angina (pain in the left-hand side of the chest sometimes radiating down the left arm, caused by a lack of oxygen as a result of blood flow being restricted), acute MI (which occurs when blood flow is restricted to such an extent that heart tissue death occurs) and sudden death (usually occurs in patients that have a history of angina and/or MI). All of these are a consequence of the thickening of the arteries – atherosclerosis.

CHD is the major cause of illness and death in the United Kingdom and the developed world, being responsible for approximately one-third of all deaths. It has been estimated to cost the NHS some £400 million a year. In 1999, an estimated 17 million persons worldwide succumbed to heart disease (Bonow *et al.*, 2002) with 2.6 million people in the United Kingdom living with heart disease. But more than this, it has an impact on the individual and their friends and family. Hence, it is worth exploring how psychology can play a part in the aetiology and progression of CHD and then how psychology can be used to improve health and return the individual to full fitness and functionality.

Traditional risk factors associated with CHD include smoking, high blood pressure, high cholesterol and diabetes (all of which may have some form of lifestyle component as discussed in Chapter 12). There are, however, several other risk factors that may be important from a psychological perspective. When looking at potential risk factors for CHD, studies have concentrated on stress, social support, low sense of coherence and hardiness (see Chapter 13) along with the lifestyle factors previously discussed. Indeed, clinical anecdotes and historical observations have ascribed the importance of emotional and personality factors in the development of CHD (Everson-Rose and Lewis, 2005). When we look at Mr Lynch we notice that there are some classic signs that we would want to explore further:

- type A personality;
- chronic psychosocial stressors;
- social factors – social support and social networks.

These three factors will be explored in this section, not only examining how these psychosocial factors play an important role in the aetiology of the CHD but how they can be used in the rehabilitation context.

Type A personality (deconstructed)

The concept of Type A has been briefly outlined in Chapter 13 but it is worth spending some time here exploring the link between this behaviour pattern and CHD, along with the more interesting concept of hostility.

The term 'Type A personality' or 'Type A behaviour pattern' has almost become a household term and is common in everyday speech on the radio, television and other forms of media. The perceived relationship between Type A personality and heart disease has become an accepted part of everyday knowledge – a simple relationship, with the greater the Type A behaviours, the greater the risk. However, does the research support this perception?

In spite of its wide publicity and media attention, criteria of Type A behaviour or personality still remain vague and the relationship has not stood up to strict scientific scrutiny. There are three elements of Type A that we must remember:

- time urgency or time-impatience;
- pervasive hostility;
- competitive ambition.

When asked to describe Thomas Lynch, from the opening case study, one of his colleagues suggested that the following description was an accurate one:

> Thomas Lynch speaks at great pace and some have estimated it to be at the rate of between 130 and 150 words per minute. His colleagues have described his voice as grating, harsh, irritating, excessively loud, and just generally unpleasant – hence one of his difficulty in making friends at work. You can hear his breath as he continuously sucks in air to speak rapidly. He sighs as he exhales, which is not a sigh of relief but a sigh of frustration and emotional exhaustion. In addition his posture is described as tense and he has a number of idiosyncrasies (for example he raises his eyebrows, pulls back one or both shoulders and blinks in a tic-like fashion). He frequently exhibits beads of perspiration on his forehead and upper lip even at normal room temperature.
>
> His facial expression with glaring eyes and lowered eyebrows make him look hostile. His lower eyelid is raised permanently which makes him look like he's staring at you. He looks aggressive and determined because the muscles surrounding his mouth are always tight. His thin lips are slightly pulled on both sides, and a visible bulge is created by tense jaws which make him look angry with an artificial smile.

Thomas Lynch exhibits all of the noted physical signs of Type A behaviour pattern (TABP). In fact, consider Thomas as the personification of TABP.

But how can we assess whether the person we are dealing with has TABP? Initially Friedman and Rosenman (1959) used a semi-structured interview and identified three personality types: A1 (as described above), A2 (less extreme than A1) and B (relaxed, showing no interruptions and quieter). Later on, a survey instrument – the Jenkins Activity Survey (JAS) – was developed (Jenkins *et al.*, 1971). Both the semi-structured interview and the JAS are psychometric instruments that have been developed to ensure both reliability and validity. However, a few questions are provided below that have been adapted from these assessment techniques to provide some indication of the sort of behaviours you would expect from anybody presenting with TABP (adapted from Friedman and Rosenman, 1959 by Sharma, 1996):

- *Time-impatience*
    1. Do you eat fast and leave the dinner table immediately?
    2. Does your partner or any close friend tell you to slow down, become less tense, or take it easy?
    3. Does it bother you a lot to wait in line at a cashier's counter or to be seated in a restaurant?
    4. Do you usually look at television or read the paper while eating?
    5. Do you examine your mail or do other things while listening to someone on the telephone?
    6. Do you often think of other matters while listening to your partners or others?
    7. Do you believe that usually you are in a hurry to get things done?
- *Hostility*
    1. Do you often find it difficult to fall asleep or difficult to stay asleep because you are upset about something a person has done?
    2. Do you believe that most people are not honest or are not willing to help others?

3. Do you become irritated when driving or swear at other drivers?
4. Does your partner, when riding with you, ever tell you to cool or calm down?
5. Do you often have a feeling that your partner is competing against you or is too critical of your inadequacies?
6. Do you grind your teeth or has your dentist ever told you that you have done so?

The classic initial studies exploring personality variables and CHD are the Western Collaborative Group study (Friedman and Rosenman, 1974) and the Framingham heart study (Dawber *et al.*, 1957). These studies seemed to link TABP as a risk factor for cardiovascular disease. However, subsequent studies (e.g. the Multiple Risk Factor Intervention Trial – MRFIT: Kjelsberg *et al.*, 1997) found no association and the Western Collaborative Group study found that the association was rather more complex than initially suggested. Hence, it is rather a complicated picture despite being systematically explored over the past 50 years or so. But let's explore some of these individual elements in more detail and see how they relate to the experience of Mr Lynch.

Rosenman *et al.* (1975) suggested that men with Type A (time urgency, hostility, achievement striving) were twice as likely as their Type B counterparts to develop CHD over an eight year period. However, subsequent research demonstrated that there was no consistent relationship between Type A behaviour and CHD which is probably a consequence of the multi-dimensionality of the construct. Hence, researchers have tried to disentangle the concept and come up with the main factor. Of the three interrelated components hostility has been the most extensively studied and a meta-analytical study reported that hostility was an independent risk factor for CHD and mortality (Miller *et al.*, 1996) hence the more hostility reported, the greater the risk of hypertension, MI and mortality.

Hostility

Hostility is characterised by a suspicious, mistrustful attitude or disposition towards interpersonal relationships and the wider environment; it is considered to be enduring. Hostility is usually measured using the Cook Medley Hostility Scale (Cook and Medley, 1954) using statements such as the following:

- I have often met people who were supposed to be experts who were no better than me.
- It is safer to trust nobody.
- My way of doing things is apt to be misunderstood by others.

Agreement with such statements is an indication of high hostility. Hostility is usually higher in men than in women and in those of lower socio-economic class. It is suggested that hostility is a social manifestation of this heightened reactivity. For example, Frederickson *et al.* (2000) demonstrated that hostile people showed larger and longer-lasting changes in blood pressure when made to feel angry. Therefore hostility and stress reactivity seem to be closely linked.

The other component demonstrating a strong link with CHD is time urgency which has consistently been shown to be related to CHD and MI (e.g. Hart, 1997). Time urgency has a number of components and includes such elements as:

- eating too quickly;
- hard driving and competitive;
- going 'all out';
- setting deadlines;
- bossy or dominating;
- putting words in another's mouth;
- speak louder than others;
- talk rapidly;
- trying to persuade others;
- working fast;
- often feel very pressed for time;
- often in a hurry.

Interventions to reduce Type A behaviour

A large-scale study – The Recurrent Coronary Prevention Project – investigated whether a Type A training programme could reduce mortality and morbidity from cardiac events. A total of 862 patients who had recently suffered an MI were either provided with Type A counselling plus cardiac counselling or simply cardiac counselling alone (Friedman *et al.*, 1986). The results, after a three year period, showed that the Type A counselling group had a greater decrease in Type A behaviour than the cardiac counselling group. Importantly, however, further follow-up (four years after the treatment ended) demonstrated that those in the Type A counselling group had reduced cardiac events (Mendes de Leon *et al.*, 1991). It has been reported that those who had Type A counselling also had improved hostility, anger, depression, self-efficacy and well-being, and consequent improved morbidity and mortality (Scott *et al.*, 2005). While this is a positive outcome, it also means that we cannot be certain which aspect of the programme was responsible for the improvement in heart disease.

In another study (Gidron *et al.*, 1999) post-MI patients were allocated to either hostility reduction training or usual care. Patients in the hostility reduction group showed larger decreases in both self-reported and behaviourally assessed hostility than patients randomised to usual care. Again, this is a finding that is not unexpected – this is what the programme set out to do. What was interesting was that blood pressure readings reduced as a result of the hostility control training – the diastolic blood pressure decreased by an average of 8 mm Hg at two months following the intervention, compared with an increase of 6 mm Hg in the usual care group. Finally, there was also a dose–response effect, with larger decreases in self-reported hostility from pre- to post-training associated with larger decreases in blood pressure at two months follow-up.

Think about this

Although there has been a statistical drop in blood pressure is this clinically relevant?

Chronic psychosocial stressors

Research exploring the link between psychosocial stressors and CHD has a long history with researchers highlighting the link between heart disease and psychosocial stressors such as poverty, poor housing and work conditions. When we explore the case of Mr Lynch we notice that there are two major stressors in his life that may be impacting on his health: his occupation and the recent bereavements. Let us explore the research on work-related stressors first.

Two potential models of work-related stress have been suggested. The first is the job strain model, which suggests that high demand coupled with low job control have a deleterious effect on cardiovascular health. Another similar model suggests that it is the effort–reward imbalance that is influential. Hence, those jobs that have high efforts (high demands and/or high involvement) in the presence of low rewards (low pay, low esteem, few career opportunities and/or job insecurity) may have a hazardous influence on health. Although Mr Lynch was well educated and had a good, respected job, he often felt a lack of control. His line manager had relatively little time for discussion and usually barked out orders in the morning for his staff to follow throughout the day and, despite being responsible for a number of patients, felt unable to discuss any issues with senior colleagues from either nursing or medicine.

A number of large-scale prospective **epidemiological studies** (e.g. Kuper and Marmot, 2003) have indicated a positive link between job strain and morbidity and mortality from CHD. In particular the impact of low control aspects of the job strain model have demonstrated to have a consistently poor impact on CHD health. For example, in Figure 19.3 the relationship between control (either rated by the individual themselves or by an external assessor) and mortality from coronary heart disease indicates that those with low job control had a greater level of mortality.

Think about this

What aspects of nursing can cause stress? Do you notice that in certain situations, where you have high demands, but low levels of control, you feel more stress? What situations are these characteristics most apparent?

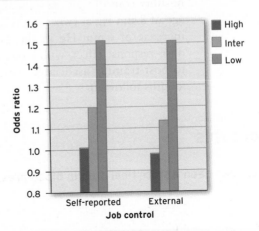

Figure 19.3 Relationship between control and mortality.

Bosma *et al.* (1998) in a sample of nearly 7000 men and 3400 women from the Whitehall II cohort (see box) found that low job control independently predicted cardiovascular outcomes with a 1.56–2.38-fold greater risk of new coronary heart disease over five years follow-up.

What is the Whitehall II study?

The Whitehall II study was set up to explore the factors underlying the social gradient in death and disease. In 1985, all non-industrial civil servants aged between 35 and 55, in Central London were invited to a cardiovascular screening of which almost three-quarters took part (10 308) in the baseline survey. Not only did the civil servants have a medical screening but they also completed several questionnaires covering a range of topics. The factors recorded at baseline have been related to the health status of the civil servants in many subsequent studies.

Other types of psychosocial stressors also predict death from CHD and this is certainly clear from both anecdotal and research evidence. For example, bereavement has been associated with an increased mortality from ischaemic heart disease and CHD in a sample of more than 95 000 men and women (Kaprio *et al.*, 1987).

In terms of chronic stressors there are relatively few studies that have explored this. However, two reports from the Nurses Health Study have shown a strong association between the chronic stressor – caregiving – and incident CHD, including mortality in women. Women caring for an ill spouse for nine or more hours a week had nearly twice the risk of incident of CHD over four years (Lee *et al.*, 2003a). Women who reported high levels of caregiving for non-ill children (more than 21 hours a week) or grandchildren (more than 9 hours a week) also experienced increased CHD risk (Lee *et al.*, 2003b) compared with women with no child caring responsibilities.

Social factors: social support and social networks

Many studies have found an association between social ties and the development of CHD. For example, people who are socially isolated (for example living alone, being unmarried or having little family contact) have higher rates of mortality and morbidity associated with CHD (Brummett *et al.*, 2001; Eng *et al.*, 2002; Kaplan *et al.*, 1988; Orth-Gomer *et al.*, 1998). In one particular study, for example, the risk was twofold greater in socially isolated men (Eng *et al.*, 2002; Kawachi *et al.*, 1999). In a similar study coronary patients who had small social networks (three or fewer individuals) had over a twofold higher rate of mortality compared to those with larger social networks over a five year period. These studies have merely reported on objective measures of social networks – for example, counting up the social contacts or simply recording whether the individual is married or not. However, an interesting study (Herlitz *et al.*, 1998) asked coronary bypass patients to simply report whether they were lonely or not. Those that reported that they were lonely were nearly twice as likely to have died from coronary-related conditions after five years.

As we saw in Chapter 13 there is a difference between social ties (the mere quantitative measure) and social support (the qualitative aspects of the social ties). Research exploring social support has generally linked into emotional support. Emotional support (characterised by high degrees of caring, understanding and esteem support) has been shown to be protective of further CHD difficulties. On the other hand, low levels of social support have been found to be associated with a high number of poor CHD outcomes. For example, in one study, there was a three-fold increase in MI in those with low levels of emotional support from close friends (Berkman *et al.*, 1992; Krumholz *et al.*, 1998).

Not only are there positive consequences of social networks and social support, there is also awareness that such relationships may have negative consequences. For example, marital conflict may be associated with CHD ill-health and subsequent mortality. In a study of nearly 300 women patients recovering from coronary events those with marital distress had a three times greater likelihood of recurrent coronary event over a four year follow-up (Orth-Gomer *et al.*, 2000) compared with women with no marital conflict. Matthews and Gump (2002) found that divorce in men was associated with an increase in mortality over a nine year period.

Overall, therefore, the literature suggests that social factors will have a strong impact on coronary health and in particular those that have previously suffered from some form of coronary morbidity.

Think about this

What psychosocial stressors can be implicated in the development of Mr Lynch's heart attack?

Psychosocial interventions to reduce CHD morbidity and mortality

Programmes that aim to reduce risk factors have been demonstrated to be successful in reducing the atherosclerotic process and several non-drug interventions have demonstrated their effectiveness at reducing or controlling blood pressure (Esselstyn, 1999; Kaati *et al.*, 2006; Scott *et al.*, 2005).

Kaati *et al.* (2006) reported on a prospective study of almost 2500 patients with the main components of the programme as listed in Table 19.1. The programme took place in a residential setting and then followed up at a later date. At both outset and follow-up blood pressure, pulse, weight and BMI were recorded. The outcomes reported that there was an improvement in most of these measurements after the intervention. For example, there was a 10 per cent reduction in both systolic and diastolic blood pressure and a 5 per cent reduction in weight (with consequent reduction in BMI). Importantly, the blood pressure measurements were achieved in both males and females and demonstrated that a simple psychosocial educational programme could have a positive impact on coronary health.

There are other programmes, of course, and one that uses illness perceptions is presented in the research in focus box. This uses Leventhal's self-regulatory model of illness perceptions previously described in relation to

Table 19.1
Elements of programme

Element of programme	Underlying component
Ability to plan own health	To maintain programme after residential period
Ability to manage stress	Knowledge about stress and relaxation
Ability to manage own body	Breathing, body language exercises
Improved self knowledge	Group sessions
Improved physical status	Physical exercise
Development of health skills	Diet, relaxation
Improved knowledge about diseases	Lectures on CHD

breast cancer. From the example it shows how psychological models can be applied to a variety of conditions with consequent benefits in terms of both psychological and physical health.

Research in focus

Petrie, K.J., Cameron, L.D., Ellis, C.J., Buick, D. and Weinman, J. (2002) Changing illness perceptions after myocardial infarction: an early intervention randomised controlled trial. *Psychosomatic Medicine*, **64**, 580–586.

Background
A large number of patients recovering from MI fail to return to work and normal functioning despite being physically well and it may be that patients' perceptions of their illness are important in recovery. In this study, Petrie *et al.* (2002) tested whether a brief psychological hospital-based intervention designed to change inaccurate and negative illness perceptions of MI would result in an earlier return to work, less long-term disability and improved cardiac rehabilitation attendance.

Method
Participants: 65 first time MI patients aged over 65 years of age over a 12 month period were entered into the study and were randomly assigned to receive either standard care, which involved cardiac rehabilitation nurse care, or three 30–40 minute intervention sessions conducted by a psychologist along with a nurse.

Intervention: The intervention consisted of three distinct psycho-educational sessions. The first session consisted of the pathophysiology of MI, which included a distinction between cardiac and non-cardiac symptoms. This session also contained an exploration of the patient's beliefs about the cause of the MI, to try and improve the participant's personal control and management of their condition.

The second session built on the causes identified by the patient and then developed an action plan and how they could reduce future risk by changing the patient's risk factors and increasing beliefs about control of their condition. In particular, highly negative beliefs about the consequences of the MI, specifically the view that the patient will need to significantly reduce activities over the long term, were challenged and a recovery action plan developed.

▶

In the final session, this action plan was reviewed and symptoms of recovery were discussed. The difference between normal healing and recovery symptoms were distinguished from symptoms that may be a warning sign of a further MI.

Results
The intervention significantly altered patients' beliefs about their illness. Furthermore, intervention subjects were significantly less likely than control subjects to report angina pain at three months. Furthermore, the intervention group had a quicker return to work (some nearly 1.5 times quicker), increased patients' intentions to go to a rehabilitation programme, and a higher attendance at rehabilitation.

Implications
This study demonstrated that a brief inpatient intervention was successful in changing patients' perceptions of their illness. Before leaving hospital, the intervention group patients had significantly changed their views about how long their illness would last and the personal consequences of the MI on their life. Importantly:

- the programme was theoretically based;
- illness perceptions provided both an initial target for change;
- it was conducted within the patient's normal hospital stay;
- patients are most amenable to interventions immediately after a major illness or health threat such as an MI and are thus more receptive to change.

Conclusion

This chapter has demonstrated that psychological factors can have a major impact on the development of serious, life-threatening illnesses, whether these be 'internal' cognitive factors, personality traits, or social factors such as friendships and social ties. Knowledge of these factors can help the nurse in the development of their role – from understanding and appreciating how a patient's career has developed to using these factors to improve the physical and psychological health of their patients.

Summary

- Personality variables have been implicated in the development of both cancer and coronary heart disease.

- Similarly, stressful life events have been implicated in the development of CHD and breast cancer. Generally, the evidence has indicated that the more severe the life event the greater the risk.

- Stress can disrupt both healthy behaviours, the immune system, and neuroendocrine processes which have all been implicated in the development of cancer or heart disease.

- Delays in seeking treatment can be explained, in part, by the interpretation of symptoms.

- Having a strong, fighting spirit can impede the development of breast cancer. In contrast, having a hopelessness or pessimistic view has a poorer outcome.

- Type A personality, in particular hostility, can contribute to the development of coronary heart disease.

- Psychological interventions have been developed which can help reduce Type A behaviour patterns and has a consequent positive impact on blood pressure.

- Having low control but high responsibility in your workplace can lead to work-based strain - a potential contributor to heart disease.

- Lack of social ties and networks can lead to increased mortality from heart disease.
- Interventions have been developed that can improve psychosocial factors and have a consequent impact on physical health.

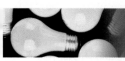

Check your understanding

1. Discuss the role of psychology in the aetiology of breast cancer.

2. Why do people not report their illness at the first onset of symptoms?

3. What psychological variables can contribute to the development of breast cancer?

4. How prominent is the role of psychosocial variables in the aetiology and development of coronary heart disease?

5. What psychosocial variables are influential in the development of both breast cancer and heart disease?

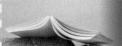

Further reading

Everson, S.A. and Lewis, T.T. (2005) Psychosocial factors and cardiovascular diseases. *Annual Review of Public Health*, **26**, 469–500.

Garsson, B. (2004) Psychological factors and cancer development: evidence of thirty years of research. *Clinical Psychology Review*, **24**, 315–338.

O'Rouke, W. (2006) *On Having a Heart Attack: A Medical Memoir*. Notre Dame, IN: University of Notre Dame Press.

Weblinks

Breast Cancer Care	http://www.breastcancercare.org.uk/	Breast Cancer Care is the UK's leading provider of information, practical assistance and emotional support for anyone affected by breast cancer.
British Heart Foundation	http://www.bhf.org.uk/	The aim of the British Heart Foundation is to play a leading role in the fight against disease of the heart and circulation so that it is no longer a major cause of disability and premature death.
Whitehall II Study	http://www.statistics.gov.uk/STATBASE/Source.asp?vlnk=1327	Details of the methodology and the results obtained so far.

▶

Whitehall II Study	http://www.ucl.ac.uk/whitehallII/	Home page of the Whitehall II study
Royal College of Physicians (RCP)	http://www.rcplondon.ac.uk/pubs/books/minap04/	How the NHS manages heart attacks as prepared by the RCP.
Cancer Research UK	http://www.cancerhelp.org.uk/default.asp	CancerHelp provides a free information service about cancer and cancer care for people with cancer and their families.
Framingham Heart Study	http://www.nhlbi.nih.gov/about/framingham/	In 1948, the Framingham Heart Study started to explore the general causes of heart disease and stroke. This website presents an overview of the study with all the publications since 1954 being listed.

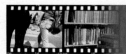 ## Media example

The Inner Circle A film about a woman who survives breast cancer and has gone through a mastectomy. The film is about the interplay between sexuality in the larger cultural experience and how the disease affects the woman and her inner circle, her husband and friends – both psychologically, emotionally and socially.

Chapter 20

Applying psychology to specific conditions: Part II

Learning outcomes

When you have read this chapter you should understand:

- The consequences of treatment for physical conditions on psychological functioning.
- The impact of psychological interventions on physical functioning.
- The psychological impact that medical treatment for breast cancer can have on both the individual patient and their immediate family.
- The role of the nurse in improving psychological and physical outcomes after treatment.
- How the reactions of the patient's family can impact on adjustment to both illness and treatment.
- How psychology can be used by the nurse to help prepare the person with breast cancer for surgery.
- How the psychological concepts introduced in previous chapters can be applied to real life situations.

Case study

We met the Lynch family in the previous chapter and we can recall that Mrs Lynch was diagnosed with breast cancer (after some delay) and subsequently underwent treatment for her condition. In the previous chapter we explored how psychological factors contributed to the onset and development of her cancer. In this chapter we will shift our focus onto the treatment that Mrs Lynch underwent and her experience of living with cancer. The treatment consisted of surgery: initially conservative, but ultimately a radical mastectomy had to be undertaken. In addition to this surgical intervention, she also underwent both **chemotherapy** and **radiotherapy.** Prior to her surgery Mrs Lynch had some chemotherapy in order to shrink the tumour. During her chemotherapy treatment the nausea and vomiting was severe.

Mrs Lynch also had radiotherapy after her surgery as she was concerned that the cancer may have returned and radiotherapy lowers the risk of the cancer coming back. Mrs Lynch was considered for conservative surgery but in light of the extent of the cancer when she was diagnosed she both requested, and was recommended, a (modified) radical mastectomy. The modified radical mastectomy removed the breast and lymph nodes under the arm but left the major chest wall muscles intact.

This additional removal was to check whether the cancer cells had spread from the breast – results from this investigation revealed that it had. On this basis the doctor decided that she needed further treatment after surgery and as a consequence Mrs Lynch was also sent for radiotherapy. The radiotherapy was used as a back-up to her breast surgery. A Cochrane review of trials conducted over the past 40 years has shown that this treatment lowers the risk of the cancer coming back either in the remaining breast or in any lymph nodes that are treated – consequently both Mrs Lynch and her oncologist decided that she had to undergo further treatment as a 'belt and braces' approach. Her radiotherapy was organised by a radiologist and radiotherapist, and was supported by various other health care professionals. In terms of her treatment, Mrs Lynch spent some time travelling to hospital for her radiotherapy treatment as an outpatient. She had her treatment once a day, from Monday to Friday, with a rest at the weekend and this treatment continued for six weeks.

Her daily treatment took only a few minutes with the radiographer making Mrs Lynch comfortable under the simulator and the sessions being as pleasant as they could be under the circumstances. As a result of the support provided by, among others, the nurses on the radiotherapy unit she had few problems undergoing the treatment. However, there were some physical side-effects of the radiotherapy itself including reddening and soreness of the skin and some other problems.

Unfortunately, as mentioned, Mrs Lynch suffered from some physical side-effects of the radiotherapy. Although radiotherapy destroys malignant tissue, it also affects normal tissue. She suffered from fatigue, skin irritation at the site of the tumour, nausea, diarrhoea and gastrointestinal symptoms, and these continued for a number of months after her treatment finished. Mrs Lynch's treatment with radiotherapy was delivered in a series of treatments over a period of six weeks on a daily basis, which meant that her work was disrupted, although her family life was not (by the treatment at least – it was, not surprisingly, influenced by her disease and the physical side-effects).

Despite the significant medical and surgical interventions there was no improvement. The cancer spread and Mrs Lynch ultimately died from her cancer. This led to Mr Lynch becoming ill and having a heart attack. Mr Lynch has suffered considerably during the preceding couple of years – he had experienced several severe life events, not least the most recent death of his wife. When he recovered from the acute phase and a period of recovery he was sent for more long-standing treatment and this consisted of both behavioural and surgical interventions.

Why is this relevant to nursing practice?

The cases of Mr and Mrs Lynch are distressing and highlight a number of physical and psychological issues and how these two may be related. In this chapter we will explore how psychology can be used with patients/clients such as Mrs Lynch, in particular, the role of the nurse and psychology in improving both the physical and psychological experience those individuals undergoing treatment.

In this particular example there are several forms of treatment that we should explore: surgical interventions for breast cancer; chemotherapeutic and radiotherapeutic interventions for Mrs Lynch's cancer. We will explore each of these in turn and examine how these medical and surgical treatments can influence psychological well-being and how the nurse can use their psychological knowledge and skills to improve both the psychological and physical outcomes from such medical interventions.

This case study is relevant to nursing practice as, although the role of the nurse is greater than simply dealing with surgical interventions in a hospital-based setting (indeed this is a minor role), the principles and techniques mentioned will be useful to most forms of nursing interventions, and the psychological principles relevant to the majority of nursing. It will also be important for you to appreciate how the psychological principles outlined throughout this text can be incorporated in practical, day-to-day examples. It should be emphasised that the individual case study has been developed to present a catastrophic case study – it would be most unfortunate for any one family to suffer to the extent of the Lynch family.

However, cancer causes significant concern for the individual, as does their treatment and they can cause considerable pain, discomfort and impact negatively on **quality of life**. Breast cancer accounts for some 16 per cent of all cancers, with each year almost 44 100 women being diagnosed in the United Kingdom (and around 335 males). Overall, breast cancer causes more than 12 400 deaths each year in the United Kingdom (Office for National Statistics, 2004). Thus, the focus of this chapter will be on psychology's role in the treatment of cancer and applying psychology to professional nursing practice in breast cancer. However, it is hoped that some of the concepts, models and applications discussed will be of value to a range of health care areas.

Think about this

What psychological factors do you think that Mr and Mrs Lynch will have to deal with when they receive the diagnosis and start to undergo treatment?

Consequences of the diagnosis of cancer

We explored in the previous chapter the experience of Mrs Lynch when she initially noticed her primary symptoms and the path from this through to her receiving her diagnosis of cancer. For Mrs Lynch, and for most (if not all) people diagnosed with a chronic condition – cancer particularly – there may be significant distress. At the time of diagnosis there may be considerable stress and some disruptions to major life areas. Indeed, many women report 'feelings of intense fear, helplessness, or a sense of horror' with the diagnosis which may equate with a diagnosis of **post-traumatic stress disorder** (Amir and Ramati, 2002). Studies have indicated higher rates of anxiety and depression in women with breast cancer in the early period after diagnosis (e.g. Burgess *et al.*, 2005).

But what about during the treatment or when the intervention has been completed (hopefully) successfully? Considerable research has investigated this and the studies have reported that even after the lengthy and disruptive medical treatment has finished, individuals with a diagnosis of 'cancer' or 'remission' still report disruptions in major life areas and chronic stress (e.g. Stanton, 2006). This chronic stress can lead to emotional distress and lower quality of life even though the immediate physical difficulty may have been either removed or alleviated.

Cancer diagnosis is the beginning of a process that is not simply another chronic disease journey. The individual may suffer a series of experiences that can profoundly affect themselves, alter the view on their life and the views and perspectives of their family and friends. As many as 50 per cent of patients with cancer have psychological distress at some stage of their disease (Burgess *et al.*, 2005) and this may be related to a number of variables. The exact nature of this psychological distress will, however, alter over the course of the disease and its treatment and is related to both physical and psychological factors (Bardwell *et al.*, 2006).

A model has been proposed that attempts to highlight the relationship of a range of variables impacting on a physical ailment – in this case breast cancer (see Figure 20.1). Applying this to the case of Mrs Lynch, we can note the consequences of her treatment on intimate relationships, social support, emotional distress, financial difficulties and lessened employment prospects. This can then, ultimately, impact on the disease progression along with influencing psychosocial factors. In summary, therefore, a history of cancer can result in chronic, stressful and lowered quality of life (Green *et al.*, 2000). It is worth exploring some of the variables highlighted in the model to see how the factors interrelate and how they can influence the disease progression faced by Mrs Lynch.

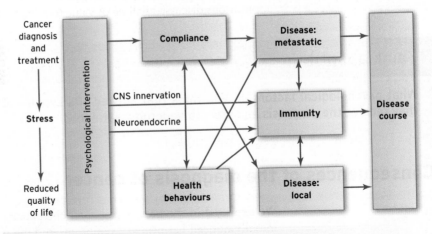

Figure 20.1 Relationship between psychological, behavioural and biological factors and cancer stressors.

Source: Andersen *et al.* (1994)

Concordance with medical advice

As we have seen in Chapter 16 there is considerable evidence of poor patient adherence (the difficulties of definition and the differing terminology used – concordance, adherence or compliance are explained in greater detail in Chapter 16 to most forms of medical and psychological treatment. Studies have indicated that concordance with treatment in people with cancer is usually higher than other chronic conditions (DiMatteo, 2004) but is still relatively low given its potentially serious consequences. Despite the potentially fatal condition, between 20 and 30 per cent of people are not adhering to the recommended medical treatment (DiMatteo, 2003), although Atkins and Fallowfield (2006) reported that 55 per cent of their sample were not adhering to the recommended treatment regimen. The model suggests that there is a relationship between following medical/nursing advice and disease outcome – which is not a surprise and does suggest a potential intervention to improve adherence may result in improved physical outcome.

The actual form and nature of the treatment may, of course, influence the level of concordance with medical advice. The unpleasantness of the treatment may influence the level of adherence to it: the more severe the side effects, the lower the level of adherence (although, this relationship is not a simple linear one). In cancer this may be particularly important since both chemotherapy and radiotherapy may come with unwanted and severe side effects which can reduce concordance with this treatment (DiMatteo, 2004). However, there are a number of psychosocial interventions that may be of benefit, for example, better patient education or improvements in psychological state (e.g. anxiety or depression) may improve adherence (see Chapter 16), as will psychological interventions that can reduce the occurrence or severity of treatment side effects (e.g. nausea or vomiting) so that patients are more tolerant of the treatment regimes (Atkins and Fallowfield, 2006). It is obvious that if treatment is refused then this can hasten the progression of the disease and, as consequence, potentially death.

Think about this

Why wouldn't somebody with cancer follow their treatment advice? What could prevent them from following appropriate medical advice? What psychological interventions can the nurse use to improve adherence to treatment in the case of Mrs Lynch? You may have to refer back to Chapter 16.

Health and lifestyle behaviours

The model reproduced in Figure 20.1 highlights the value of health behaviours in the link with cancer and the subsequent treatment. As we have seen in Chapter 12 there is a strong relationship between most of these lifestyle behaviours and morbidity and mortality from a host of different conditions. Individuals who are undergoing treatment for cancer may have a range of negative health behaviours which can impact upon both their health and, as a by-product, the treatment for their condition.

So, for example, studies have indicated that diet and exercise can slow the progression of the cancer and improve outcomes (e.g. Campbell and McTiernan, 2007; Sprague *et al.*, 2007). Galban *et al.* (2000) report that improvements in nutrition can enhance immune responses, reduce rates of infection and improve mortality rates in those with cancer. Similarly, physical exercise can have a positive impact on the immune and endocrine systems which also improves infection resistance and consequent mortality rates. Campbell and McTiernan (2007) suggest that 'adoption of lifestyle changes by individuals and populations may have a large impact on the future incidence of cancer' (p. 161), a conclusion supported by other studies (e.g. Mutrie *et al.*, 2007).

For instance, it has been highlighted that those who are distressed or undergoing some form of treatment for their cancer may have a disturbance in diet or appetite (Rock and Demark-Wahnefried, 2002). Eating habits may change because of treatment (e.g. because of the consequences of nausea or taste aversion from chemotherapy) or because of the alterations in appetite as a consequence of stress (see Chapter 13). The change in appetite may be in one of two directions: either over-eating or under-eating. However, both result in weight change – either gaining or losing weight, neither of which may be ideal. Because of this change in appetite, vulnerability to further ill-health may be heightened. This indicates the interplay between the disease, the treatment, psychological factors and health behaviours, all of which have to be considered when treating a woman undergoing treatment for her cancer.

Another case is smoking. Obviously any woman who is diagnosed with breast cancer and smokes is strongly counselled to quit (as indeed should any smoker). However, there are two competing effects here – on the one hand the women may want to quit because of the cancer and the advice being provided by the health care professionals. Conversely, for some women smoking may increase because of its use as a (perceived) stress reducer and a coping mechanism to deal with the stresses of the cancer and its diagnosis and treatment. Indeed, recent evidence (Siahpush and Carlin, 2006) has suggested that 'smokers with more financial stress were less likely to quit' (p. 121). Again, the complex interplay between health behaviour, the physical condition/treatment and psychosocial factors is apparent.

In addition to the increase in negative health behaviours there also may be a decrease in some positive health behaviours. So, for example, positive health behaviours such as physical exercise may decrease because the patient feels they have neither the time nor the energy to exercise as they undergo or recover from their treatment. However, physical exercise can have a positive impact on the psychological adjustment to cancer and its physical consequences and hence should be encouraged.

Numerous studies have explored the impact of interventions aimed at improving health behaviours. One such example is that of Mock *et al.* (1997) who conducted a trial of a walking programme offered to women with breast cancer undergoing chemotherapy. Women in the intervention group were instructed to walk 20–35 minutes per day and record their experiences. The findings of the study for the intervention group, compared with the control group, suggested that there were positive outcomes: decreases in anxiety, sleep disturbance and fatigue, and improvements in physical health. Similarly, Segal *et al.* (2001) completed a randomised trial with breast cancer patients (those with either stage I or II) undergoing treatment comparing two exercise groups (self-directed and supervised) and a control group. The supervised group attended three exercise sessions per week whereas the other exercise group were provided with written exercise instructions. Overall, there was an improvement in the physical status in the exercise groups. These studies indicate that physical exercise can have positive psychological and physical benefits – a finding confirmed in more recent studies (e.g. Midtgaard *et al.*, 2006).

Finally, exercise can have a positive impact on the experience of chemotherapy. Andersen *et al.* (2006) report that a six week multi-dimensional exercise intervention undertaken by cancer patients with or without residual disease while undergoing chemotherapy led to a reduction in treatment-related symptoms.

Taken altogether the results of the various studies indicate that health behaviours can impact on morbidity and mortality and that focused interventions can make a positive contribution to improving the physical consequences of both physical conditions and their treatment.

Think about this

What psychological techniques could you use to improve the health behaviours of Mrs Lynch during her various forms of treatment? What behaviours would you want to promote and what would you want to reduce? You may want to refer to Chapter 12.

Pain from cancer

Between 50 and 90 per cent of patients with cancer get some form of pain from either the disease or the treatment and the evidence suggests that despite considerable advances in this area there are still areas of inadequate pain control (estimated to be between 16 and 91 per cent of all patients, depending on study). The pain that the individual patient suffers can influence quality of life and can be an important predictor of survival (Gordon *et al.*, 2005).

When developing intervention programmes for a woman experiencing pain and trauma from her cancer and its treatment, a comprehensive evaluation of all factors associated with the pain is required. As we have seen from Chapter 14 the identification of all the relevant psychosocial factors in the experience of pain is important since it is not merely physical factors that contribute to pain. Once the complete range of psychosocial factors has been identified, they can be addressed in an individualised treatment plan. This plan has to take into account the biopsychosocial aspects identified in the gate control theory of pain. This model, as we have seen in Chapter 14, indicates that pain is a complex interaction between physiological, psychological, cognitive, social and other factors.

It is now recognised that tactics to reduce pain for women undergoing treatment for breast cancer should include psychological factors as well as drug therapy. The biomedical model still predominates in both the assessment and management of cancer pain. Indeed, psychosocial interventions are not extensively used or recommended – although the situation is improving with the realisation of its value and importance (Gordon *et al.*, 2005). Much of this can be a consequence of the limited focus on psychosocial assessments associated with cancer pain. The relationship between psychosocial factors and chronic cancer pain has not been extensively examined. However, in those studies that have been reported (Zaza and Baine, 2002) a comprehensive chronic pain assessment has been enhanced by screening for psychological distress. Psychosocial interventions (as outlined in Chapter 14) have been shown to be effective and to reduce health care costs to both patients and those delivering the service. Furthermore, the social support available to patients can be of considerable benefit and this is outlined in Chapter 14 and subsequently in this chapter.

Think about this

Reviewing the material presented in Chapter 14, how can the nurse assist with the pain experienced by Mrs Lynch from her treatment? What psychological factors are important in this area?

The impact of chemotherapy

Mrs Lynch, along with the majority of women with breast cancer, underwent chemotherapy. It is not just the cancer and its diagnosis that can distress the individual but the various treatment methods employed to treat the conditions (Michael and Tannock, 1998; Moynihan *et al.*, 1998) can also lead to worry and distress. Obviously given the toxic regimens of chemotherapy that are often used, the impact of such treatment has to be considered fully when caring for the women with breast cancer. The side effects of chemotherapy may include such physical side effects as nausea, **alopecia**, **anorexia**, constipation, diarrhoea, fatigue and **mucositis** – as we have noted Mrs Lynch suffered from many of these.

In addition, several authors (Del Mastro *et al.*, 2002; Jacobsen *et al.*, 2002) have found that chemotherapy is related to social and psychological problems. For example a study involving 12 patients who received chemotherapy for the first time reported on the feelings of the individual patients. They noted that respondents attributed feeling aggressive, depressed, angry and suffering mood swings to the chemotherapy (Dikken and Sitzia, 1998).

It is obvious that the psychological care that individuals with cancer receive should be a priority and this is one role (of a number!) that the nurse can play. Nurses, as other health professionals, need to consider the whole person and assess side effects from biopsychosocial perspective (Priest, 1999). Despite this being actively acknowledged, Tanghe *et al.* (1996) found that nurses did not document anything related to the distress patients may have felt in relation to chemotherapy, their psychological needs or the information they received. This is in line with Voogt *et al.* (2005) who comment that the psychosocial aspects of cancer are not routinely treated and that patients are less satisfied with information about psychological needs than information about diagnosis and treatment (Cox *et al.*, 2006).

Furthermore, Iconomou *et al.* (2002) report that only 37 per cent of their sample of patients with cancer did not know that they had cancer. This is a surprisingly low figure but one that has been recorded in other studies (Caruso *et al.*, 2000; Pronzato *et al.*, 1994). On this basis, therefore, how can the psychological needs of patients be assessed if a substantial minority of them don't know their own condition? A further step consequence is that the nurse cannot deal with the psychological consequences as they are unknown, or at least the psychological consequences of the diagnosis are unknown and unassessed.

What do nurses think the needs are and how do they meet these needs? One study (Arantzamendi and Kearney, 2004) indicated that in addition to the needs of cancer, patients have additional needs that are a consequence of the treatment. Patients undergoing cancer treatment are generally anxious, distressed, scared and feeling isolated and therefore need social and financial support with clear information about the disease and the treatment in order to support both themselves and their families. This is probably because the anxiety is based on a lack of information. Hence, in order to cope with the uncertainty of cancer and treatment they need informational support (see Chapter 18).

Furthermore, the needs associated with chemotherapy also need to be explained as they can increase distress and affect a patient's quality of life. The nurses in the Arantzamendi and Kearney (2004) study also reported that patients receiving chemotherapy have psychological needs, which need to be borne in mind by all involved in the care of such women. This is especially the case when caring for patients with cancer receiving chemotherapy; especially at the two stages identified by the nurses as the most psychologically demanding for the patients: the beginning and the end of the chemotherapy. Of course, there are many demands on an individual nurse's time and work commitments and these may influence the psychological support that patients receive but it is important to provide information and support to women undergoing treatment throughout the progression of their disease.

Think about this

What sort of information do you think Mrs Lynch requires about her treatment? How does this change over the course of her disease, from diagnosis, through to treatment to palliative care? You may want to consider the information presented in Chapter 18.

Chemotherapeutic treatment of cancer

During her chemotherapy Mrs Lynch suffered some typical side effects – she experienced nausea and vomiting, and other common consequences of her form of treatment. Although she was treated with **anti-emetic** therapies she was also considered for non-pharmacological interventions. So, what are these forms of treatment and how successful are they? How can psychology help in such cases? Some patients are sceptical about the effectiveness of such non-pharmacological interventions and the nurse should always consider the views of the individual patient when designing such interventions (Roffe *et al.*, 2005). However, four reasons have been proposed to explain why non-pharmacological interventions are likely to be useful:

- They can decrease affective and psychological arousal and reduce general feelings of distress.

- They can serve as cognitive distracters, redirecting patients' attention from conditioned stimulus and refocusing it on neutral or relaxing images.
- They can promote feelings of control and reduce feelings of helplessness by demonstrating to patients that they can successfully help themselves reduce treatment side effects.
- They can easily be administered and learned within the chemotherapy environment and have few, if any, side-effects.

There are a number of psychological interventions that can be employed and these have a number of potential benefits: they are relatively inexpensive, easy to learn, free from side effects, and, probably most importantly, allow the individual patient to be in control of their own treatment (Roffe *et al.*, 2005; Wilson *et al.*, 2006). Despite these benefits the majority of patients have not had them incorporated into their usual care by health care professionals (Dibble *et al.*, 2000).

These interventions include **progressive muscle relaxation** (PMR) training, **guided imagery, biofeedback** and cognitive distraction. All of these have been highlighted as stress management techniques (see Chapter 13) and their use with those being treated for cancer can be seen as allowing for the reduction of the stresses and strains associated with both the diagnosis and the treatment.

Progressive muscle relaxation training

As we have seen, PMR is the conscious relaxation of various skeletal muscles (see Chapter 13). The individual is taught to recognise tension in various muscle groups and then subsequently to relax the muscles, to learn to differentiate between tension and relaxation. Consequently, the individual patient should be able to learn and ultimately achieve the deepest degree of relaxation possible (King, 1997; McCallie *et al.*, 2006). With training the patient will be able to apply the learned relaxation when required and be able to enter a state of deep relaxation when required (Redd *et al.*, 2001). Obviously, this strategy can be used during the negative experiences associated with cancer and its treatment, whether this be the cognitive worries associated with the diagnosis or the physical impact of the disease and/or its treatment or indeed whenever the patient is feeling tense or anxious (Post-White, 2002; Redd *et al.*, 2001). There are a number of benefits associated with PMR including its low cost and ease of learning. It has been suggested by King (1997) that if PMR is taught and used before the initial chemotherapy then it may either prevent or delay the onset of symptoms – a conclusion supported by empirical evidence (e.g. Molassiotis *et al.*, 2006). Wilson *et al.* (2006) reported that a self-administered stress management programme had positive benefits for people with cancer during their treatment with improvements in pain and mental health following the intervention. Furthermore, Arakawa (1997) reported on a study of 60 patients receiving chemotherapy who received either PMR or control treatment. The study indicated that PMR was effective in reducing the nausea and vomiting associated with chemotherapy.

Guided imagery

Another form of stress reduction through relaxation is guided imagery. In this psychological intervention the individual patient is asked to focus on pleasing, relaxing images (Roffe *et al.*, 2005). It is suggested that the patient's attention to aversive stimuli is blocked by their attention to these pleasing and relaxing images (Post-White, 2002; Roffe *et al.*, 2005). Results from studies have indicated that the positive effects of distraction usually last only as long as the patient is actively engaged in the distraction task (Redd *et al.*, 2001).

Furthermore, studies have suggested that those patients receiving chemotherapy had reduced occurrence and distress associated with nausea, vomiting and retching. In addition, results from some studies (Troesch *et al.*, 1993) show that those patients having guided imagery felt significantly more in control, more powerful, more relaxed and more prepared than the control group. However, in a more recent review, Roffe *et al.* (2005) suggested that although there was an increase in psychological status following the intervention there was no strong evidence for positive effects on physical symptoms.

Biofeedback

Biofeedback involves patients learning to control a specific physiological response by receiving information about moment-to-moment changes in that response. The two most frequently used forms of biofeedback are electromyographic (EMG) biofeedback – which induces a deep state of muscle relaxation – and skin temperature (ST) feedback, which records skin temperature changes such as those that precede nausea and vomiting (King, 1997). Some studies have indicated that PMR training resulted in patients having less nausea and vomiting than those patients who had no such training. However, those that had biofeedback did not improve as much as those with PMR.

Cognitive distraction

A further form of psychological intervention is cognitive distraction (also known as attentional diversion). In this form of intervention the patient is simply told or encouraged to engage in another form of activity – for example, playing games or using computer games. It is thought that this is of use since it focuses the patient's attention away from nausea and vomiting (King, 1997). The results from studies have indicated some benefit and that lower levels of nausea and vomiting result.

Although there are a number of potential methods for reducing the stresses and strains of both cancer diagnosis and its treatment the most effective method for dealing with the adverse consequences of chemotherapy is suggested to be PMR. Consequently, any form of psychosocial intervention for individuals undergoing cancer treatment should involve this form of psychological intervention.

Think about this

What form of intervention would you recommend for Mrs Lynch? Looking back at previous information (see Chapters 13 and 18), what different elements would you include? How could you actively engage Mr Lynch in the process?

Coping with breast cancer treatment

In the previous chapter we noted the benefits of a range of coping strategies for women with breast cancer. Studies have also explored the coping strategies employed by those dealing with chemotherapy and related these to a range of demographic and disease variables (e.g. Costanzo *et al.*, 2006). For example, Manne *et al.* (1994), in a study of 43 women in chemotherapy, found different coping strategies to be associated with positive or negative mood. Patients with low mood used more escape-avoidance coping, while those with better adjustment used more distancing, self-controlling coping and positive reappraisal. Lerman *et al.* (1990) found that those who used an information-seeking or monitoring style of coping had higher anxiety and more nausea before and during treatment (i.e. the more they tried to find out about the treatment before undergoing the treatment the worse they felt!), although Ransom *et al.* (2005) found the converse. Heim *et al.* (1997) found a stage-dependent relation between coping and psychosocial adaptation in three stages of adjustment – hospitalisation, chemotherapy and rehabilitation. Thus, research on coping styles has had some equivocal results but suggests that certain coping strategies lessen the psychological repercussions of diagnosis, surgery and treatment for breast cancer, depending upon the stage of disease and treatment process (Costanzo *et al.*, 2006). Most patients use several coping strategies and these vary over time and it is important that nurses recognise this.

Think about this

How do you think Mrs Lynch's coping strategies will vary from diagnosis, to her different forms of treatment (radiotherapy, chemotherapy and surgery)?

Surgical treatment of breast cancer

Mrs Lynch underwent a mastectomy as one of the options for her treatment. After breast cancer surgery, rates of depression have been found between 10 and 55 per cent of women (Burgess *et al.*, 2002, 2005). Psychological morbidity in women with breast cancer peaks between one and three months following surgery and persists for a further 16 months. However, this may not be the end of the psychological difficulties: anxiety, depression, social disruption and reduced attractiveness affect women for at least another five years (Burgess *et al.*, 2005). For example, Burgess *et al.* (2005) report that 50 per cent of women in the first year following diagnosis experience depression, anxiety or both and this continues in a substantial proportion (15 per cent) in the fifth year. As we have seen, distress about symptoms and impaired function due to adjuvant chemotherapy and radiotherapy also contribute to psychological morbidity (Pasacreta, 1997). There are a number of psychological factors that may also contribute to psychological state following surgery – coping, optimism, self-efficacy are some examples (Carver *et al.*, 1993;

Costanzo *et al.*, 2005). Other factors may include the consultation process, the decision-making involved, lack of information and uncertainty, and patient values and expectations.

We saw in Chapter 18 that psychological preparation for surgery was essential in reducing post-operative anxiety and enhancing the physical and psychological outcomes following the hospital stay. The evidence presented in the chapter, based on the research evidence, was that there are common characteristics of hospitals and surgical interventions that patients view as stressful. Some of these characteristics (the environment, the language and so on) may be common to all hospital interventions, whereas others may be specific to the form of surgery. As we have noted previously those undergoing breast surgery have specific stressors in terms of body image alteration, role functioning and self-concept damage.

In terms of pre-surgical intervention for Mrs Lynch's mastectomy a variety of forms of intervention have been reported on. As we have noted, the most common, and probably the most useful, form of intervention is simple information on the surgery. There are, in essence, three forms of information provision that can be considered: procedural information (information on the process of the surgery), sensory information (information on the sensations likely to be experienced) and behavioural information (information on behaviours likely to improve recovery). Together, all these forms of information can provide impact and improvement in outcome.

Think about this

How might the nurse be able to positively influence the views of the patient towards surgery for breast cancer? Exploring Chapter 19, how could the health care team best prepare Mrs Lynch, psychologically, for her mastectomy? What type of information would help Mrs Lynch cope with her surgery?

Body image

Given that Mrs Lynch had a mastectomy and this typical procedure for breast cancer involves the alteration of part of her body and her physical appearance – of great value in Western society – it is not surprising that women with breast cancer, Mrs Lynch included, often present concerns regarding body image. Hence Ganz *et al.* (1998) and Avis *et al.* (2005) reported that some two-thirds of women reported being unhappy with their body appearance following breast surgery. Ganz *et al.* (1998) did, however, note that there was a difference in women with different forms of surgery, such that those with mastectomy were the most distressed, followed by those with mastectomy and reconstruction, followed by those women with a lumpectomy. Obviously, the psychological distress appears to be related to the extent and consequence of the surgery.

There are some putative explanations for these findings relating surgical interventions to psychological distress. It may be, for example, that as physical beauty is greatly valued in our society, women are likely to become distressed when they lose their breast or their appearance changes. Some studies have found that those women who prior to surgery reported a higher level of investment in physical appearance demonstrated more emotional distress following their breast surgery (Carver *et al.*, 1998). Similarly, Wai Ming (2002) reported that the husband's evaluation of his wife's physical appearance was a good predictor of her marital satisfaction than was her own perception of her body image. In summary, it does appear as if the psychological consequences of surgery can be negative for both the woman and her partner. However, the partner's reaction (usually the male partner) can be influential in the woman's reactions. This brings us on to another important area for consideration – the support from the woman's partner during treatment and the impact this may have on her psychological adjustment to the condition.

Sexual functioning

When Mrs Lynch underwent her breast cancer treatment she suffered from a number of physiological changes that interfered with her adaptive sexual functioning. For example her breasts were sore and tender and her skin became red, tender and irritated. Although this subsided over time Mr Lynch was unaware of what was painful to his wife and how long it would last. It appeared as if they started to avoid sexual activity on a short-term basis and this continued on an ongoing basis. As they approached the possibility of sexual interaction, a common pattern was that either Mr or Mrs Lynch experienced anxiety and tended to withdraw from sexual interaction. This avoidance decreased anxiety and thus avoidance was reinforced over time.

Think about this

Consider the behavioural approach to understanding human interactions (see Chapter 2): how can this be used to explain the decrease in sexual functioning of Mr and Mrs Lynch?

Physical treatments can also induce physical problems which may impact on the sexual functioning of the woman. For example, chemotherapy can induce premature menopause with the attendant symptoms of hot flashes, reduced libido, vaginal and vulval dryness and atrophy. Not only do these changes directly contribute to a loss of sexual desire and discomfort during intercourse, but the fatigue that accompanies treatment also can contribute to less interest in these sexual activities. The findings from a number of investigations confirm that sexual difficulties occur at a substantially higher rate for women with breast cancer (e.g. Avis *et al.*, 2005) and those undergoing chemotherapy. This may be a particular form of information that the couple may wish to be provided with as it could allow for the realisation that any difficulties experienced are understandable and predictable given the course of treatment the woman is undergoing.

Following treatment, a number of difficulties may be experienced by women with cancer and some of these may be related to the treatment as well as the condition itself and these may be experienced by the individual patient, and their partner (e.g. Henson, 2002; Tan *et al.*, 2002). In addition, overall, it appears that approximately one-third of both women with breast cancer and partners of women with breast cancer experience sexual difficulties and these difficulties can be long term (Bukovic *et al.*, 2005). For example, even some 5–10 years following diagnosis, disease-free survivors experienced sexual difficulties (Bloom *et al.*, 1998). Given that there may be an alteration in physical appearance and resultant body image following breast cancer treatment, it is not surprising that there may be an impact on the sexual functioning of the woman and her partner. Given that women's sexual functioning is influenced by her individual relationship, and physiological well-being, it is difficult to disentangle these factors in understanding sexual functioning after breast cancer treatment. Many women with breast cancer and their partners may experience depression and anxiety, particularly during the first year subsequent to breast cancer diagnosis. Loss of interest in sexuality is a common symptom of depression, and anxiety contributes to difficulties in sexual arousal. A partner's reaction to breast cancer can influence the relationship which can lead to sexual concerns.

Social support and couple functioning

As we have seen in Chapter 18 there is a relationship between social support and psychological adjustment in people with chronic illness. It is not surprising therefore to find that social support may be extremely useful in helping women come to terms with their breast cancer and the treatment.

Studies of social support and adjustment to breast cancer have examined support from several sources. For example in an early study, Bloom and Spiegel (1984) found that emotional support from the family and opportunities for social interaction were related to adjustment in a sample of women with advanced breast cancer. Bloom (1986) found that social support, including perceptions of family cohesiveness, social affiliation, and presence of a confidant, was related to adjustment to the diagnosis of breast cancer. Other studies have included medical and nursing professionals among the sources of support studied (e.g. Han *et al.*, 2005; Lepore and Coyne, 2006) and Hellbom *et al.* (2001) suggest that a course for nurses can be trained to provide this support more effectively.

Among married women who have breast cancer the support derived from their partners is viewed as the most crucial source of support. The presence of good social support may result in lower levels of depression and anxiety and better quality of life (Wimberly *et al.*, 2005). As outlined previously (see Chapter 13) partner support may include two forms: emotional support – listening and comforting ('a shoulder to cry on') – and practical support – performing tasks around the house, transporting the woman to hospital and outpatient appointments. Although both are extremely useful and beneficial, women with breast cancer tend to rate emotional support as the most useful in helping to address some of the major issues facing long-term survivors of breast cancer (Vivar and McQueen, 2005). Indeed, good emotional support has positive impact not just on psychological adjustment but also on long-term survival and, therefore, multi-disciplinary intervention programmes can be developed to improve quality of life for patients undergoing treatment (Rummans *et al.*, 2006).

Think about this

What form of emotional and practical support could the nurse provide Mrs Lynch with during her treatment?

How supportive, however, are the partners of women with breast cancer? Many married women report that their interactions with their husbands are dissatisfying (even if their relationship is satisfactory). For example, the partner may avoid discussions of fears and concerns in order to protect the other person and they may not be able to talk as freely as they would wish because of the 'protective buffering' that has occurred. Indeed, in some studies, it has been reported that the discussions held with other people are more useful than the discussions held with the husband (Pistrang and Barker, 1995).

Avis *et al.* (2005) reported that young women with breast cancer with high levels of marital problems reported lower levels of global, emotional and physical quality of life. Indeed, it was reported that these women fared worse than women with no partners. Therefore, the message from this particular study is for the woman to either have a good relationship or none! However, one study has indicated that the consequence of a diagnosis of breast cancer can result in separation or divorce. Walsh *et al.* (2005) found that in the two years following diagnosis, 12 per cent of young women were divorced or separated, with the majority of women reporting that their partners had initiated the great majority of these separations, primarily because they were unable to cope with the cancer diagnosis and treatment.

Manne *et al.* (2004a) observed the interactions between women with breast cancer and their male partners while discussing cancer-related topics. The results of the investigation highlighted that the critical factor in having a high-quality relationship was the extent of the disclosures that the male partners made to their wives. Thus, from this study, it is important not only for the women to express their feelings but also for their spouses to do so as well. If this is the case then women with breast cancer will have a greater likelihood of being accepted, understood and cared for by their partners. In contrast, the unhelpful interaction patterns included partner avoidance and criticism (Manne *et al.*, 1997). This indicates that it is not enough for couples to have, overall, a good relationship but they have a range of specific issues to deal with. These will include the male partner being faced with overwhelming demands, including tangible and emotional support to the patient as well as having to deal with their own emotional distress. Obviously if the relationship has children then there are additional demands in order to respond to the children's needs. Furthermore, investigations indicate that men have particular difficulty addressing interpersonal issues with their female partners and as a consequence they avoid or withdraw during the interactions. It should also be highlighted that spouses of cancer patients are often unaware of, or misinformed about, how best to assist their partner – or 'patient' as she has now become. They may try to minimise the situation or have forced cheerfulness but these are the actual behaviours that are most frequently reported as being unhelpful by patients with cancer (Peters-Golden, 1982).

Thus, the findings to date indicate that both women and their male partners are affected by the diagnosis of cancer and that each person's adaptation influences the other person. It also appears that having a good relationship 'overall' is not enough. Instead, learning specific ways to address the woman's cancer is important. Given that women particularly value social support from their partners, helping couples to learn to support each other during this stressful time is essential.

Manne *et al.* (2006) noted that there are certain communication difficulties in those couples where the woman has breast cancer. Sometimes there are communication difficulties. If these are identified, then a couple-focused intervention may prove useful. Such interventions may need to focus on reducing avoidance of discussion of issues and pressuring one another to 'talk' about cancer-related stressors, and working at enhancing constructive communication and problem-solving.

What about Mr Lynch's view?

As we have seen, there are many severe and extensive challenges that face women who are diagnosed with and are treated for breast cancer. Many women who are treated with early-stage breast cancer and have a good prognosis do not experience any severe long-term psychological problems. However, almost all experience some difficulties in adjustment, particularly in the early stages after the diagnosis (Nosarti *et al.*, 2002). The psychosocial consequences of breast cancer include emotional distress, sexual and relationship difficulties (Henson, 2002; Tan *et al.*, 2002), and concerns for the future stemming from both the possibility of relapse and the long-term impact of the cancer treatment (Moyer and Salovey, 1996; Spencer *et al.*, 1999).

It has to be remembered and emphasised, however, that the diagnosis of life-threatening illness such as breast cancer can interfere with the life of the patient and the lives of those closest to the patient. The cancer can be associated with a chronic and prolonged stress and the family must deal with a series of challenges related to the treatment process. These series of adverse events influence not only the patient but also the family members – especially those partners of the women affected, who often have to act as informal caregivers and the most frequent providers of informal support to their partners with breast cancer (Wagner *et al.*, 2006).

As we have seen, the role of partners in adjustment to breast cancer has consistently found that a better relationship is associated with better emotional adjustment (Coyne and Anderson, 1999). However, what impact does a diagnosis of breast cancer have on relationships? Not surprisingly, there is evidence to suggest that such a diagnosis can lead to stresses and strains on a relationship and hence lead (where the couple is married) to marital discord (Wai Ming, 2002). Northouse *et al.* (1998) report that when one partner has a chronic or serious illness then both partners in an intimate relationship can experience considerable distress, which can ultimately impact on the couple's communication and their sexual relationship (Ben-Zur *et al.*, 2001; Holmberg *et al.*, 2001; Lindholm *et al.*, 2002).

Think about this

What part can the nurse play in the adjustment of the *partner* of a patient with breast cancer? What informational and emotional support do they require? What sort of support would you provide to Mr Lynch?

Psychosocial treatments

But what about some forms of psychosocial interventions for those undergoing treatment for cancer? Zimmermann *et al.* (2007) in a meta-analysis, concluded that such interventions are generally useful for cancer patients, although not as useful for those with breast cancer as for other cancers. Interestingly, many of these interventions are offered to women *without* their partners being present. Hence, they were assuming that breast cancer be seen as an individual diagnosis and as a consequence the women had an individual treatment. However, on the basis of the material presented above it might be more helpful to consider the diagnosis a 'relationship diagnosis' highlighting that the diagnosis impacts on both the woman and her partner. Furthermore, there is a reciprocal relationship in that the partner's functioning influences the woman's adaptation: the two partners need to understand how to provide support to each other, both emotionally and practically. As we have noted previously, one important topic for discussion is sexuality: many couples may have sexual difficulties and find this is a problematic area for discussion. However, it is important that couples understand that there are both psychological and physiological reasons as a consequence of medical treatment that lead to decreased sexual desire, complications with sexual arousal, and pain during intercourse for women with breast cancer.

One study (Scott *et al.*, 2004) reported on a randomised control trial based on couple-based interventions to help couples address breast cancer. This intervention assessed the efficacy of a cognitive behavioural coping skills training for women with breast (or gynaecological) cancer. The intervention included: (a) communication skills training; (b) conversations about sexual concerns; (c) training in individual coping skills and stress management (e.g. relaxation training); (d) educational materials; and (e) challenging individuals' negative cognitions. The results indicated that couples began communicating more effectively as a team. In addition, women who received the intervention showed significantly better positive image and a reported subjective sense of greater intimacy with their partners. Similarly, Manne *et al.* (2005) have reported results comparing usual care with a couple-based group intervention for women with early-stage breast cancer. Their findings indicated that the couple-based intervention was generally more effective than usual care, and it appeared to be particularly effective for couples in which the wife viewed the partner as less supportive prior to intervention, hence, having a positive impact on communication within the couple and ultimately improving both psychological and physical outcomes.

Radiotherapeutic treatment of cancer

A major conclusion from the research literature on the psychological aspects of radiotherapy is that there is considerable variability in the results from the studies – nothing consistent but the inconsistency! However, some common findings can be gleaned from the disparate results. For example, before starting radiotherapy there is usually an increase in anxiety but this tends to decrease over the course of the treatment. After completion of radiotherapy there is a rather inconsistent set of results: some studies have indicated that there is a reduction in anxiety, some that there is no change and some that there may be an increase. However, the research has reliably indicated that there may be an increase in depression both during and after radiotherapy, although this seems to peak during the final weeks of treatment. There is also a trend for a positive relationship between physical problems including side effects and psychological distress. The more physical the side effect encountered by the patient, the greater the impact on psychological functioning (Stiegelis *et al.*, 2004).

Anxiety at the outset of radiotherapy may be related to a lack of understanding about the treatment and its consequences. At the start of treatment when there is more understanding of the treatment and its side effects the anxiety reduces, but may increase at the end due to uncertainties about the future. The anxiety may be related to these specific situations rather than a more general feeling. On the other hand, depressive symptoms are more general in nature rather than more difficult to ascribe to specifics of the situation. Thus, psychological treatment should be aimed at helping the patient cope with both the specific situational demands but also the general negative consequences of both the cancer and the treatment (Johnson, 1999). This process should continue following treatment to ensure that the psychosocial difficulties are not overlooked in the long term.

The nurse has a key role in the reduction of anxiety associated with radiotherapy. There are feelings of anxiety associated with a lack of information about the treatment, so the anxiety could be reduced by education provided by nurses. Furthermore, patients could be provided with information about radiotherapy and the misperceptions about radiotherapy – perhaps nurses could recruit other patients who are undergoing radiotherapy to act as role models and to guide patients through the treatment. This could obviously extend to the partner and family of the women with breast cancer.

Conclusion

This chapter has demonstrated that physical treatments for medical conditions and in particular cancer can have major psychological consequences. The psychological consequences of the treatment can be as significant as those experienced as a consequence of the underlying medical condition. Consequently, it is important that the impacts of both the condition and treatment are recognised, identified and taken into account by the nurse and other health care professionals.

Research in focus

Andersen, B.L., Farrar, W.B., Golden-Kreutz, D.M., Glaser, R., Emery, C.F., Crespin, T.R., Shapiro, C.L. and Carson, W.E. III (2004) Psychological, behavioural, and immune changes after a psychological intervention: a clinical trial. *Journal of Clinical Oncology*, **22**, 3570–3580.

Background

Previous research has indicated that psychosocial interventions for people with cancer can lead to significant improvements in emotional distress, with some studies indicating that this is also accompanied by improved survival rates. However, the process by which psychosocial interventions improve psychological distress and survival rates is unknown although it may be related to improved social support, improved health behaviours and/or improved **neuroendocrine** response. This randomised clinical trial attempted to unpick some of these factors by testing the hypothesis that psychological interventions could reduce emotional distress, improve health behaviours and also enhance immune responses in those with breast cancer following surgery.

Method

A total of 227 women who were surgically treated for breast cancer were included in the study. Before the intervention therapy, women completed interviews and questionnaires assessing emotional distress, social adjustment, and health behaviours. In addition, a blood sample was drawn for immune assays. Patients were randomly assigned to either the intervention group or assessment only group. The intervention was conducted in small patient groups, with one session per week for four months. The sessions included strategies to reduce stress, improve mood, alter health behaviours, and maintain adherence to cancer treatment and care. Reassessment occurred after completion of the intervention.

Participants: Women who were diagnosed with either stage II or III breast cancer who had been surgically treated.

Intervention: The intervention was designed to reduce stress, lower emotional distress and improve quality of life. The intervention was provided in small groups of between 8 and 12 patients. Each group met for 1.5 hours for 18 sessions over a four month period. Sessions included components on understanding stress and the stress response, relaxation training and positive coping, communication skills training, diet and exercise, social support and referrals, and disease and treatment information.

Results

As predicted, patients receiving the intervention showed significant lowering of anxiety, improvements in perceived social support, improved dietary habits, and reduction in smoking (all $P<0.05$). Immune responses for the intervention patients paralleled their psychological and behavioural improvements (all $P<0.01$).

Implications

These data show a convergence of significant psychological, health behaviour and biological effects after a psychological intervention for cancer patients. In short, a psychosocial intervention demonstrates improvements in psychological, social and biological variables in those women suffering from breast cancer.

Summary

- Psychology has a clear and significant impact on a woman's experience of breast cancer and its treatment.

- The diagnosis of cancer brings with it anxieties related to the uncertainties of both the condition and its treatment.

- The treatment for cancer brings with it chronic stress and disruption to social, employment and psychological relationships.

- Adherence to cancer treatment is not 100 per cent, and can be influenced by the psychological and physical consequences of the treatment. Psychosocial and educational interventions can lead to better concordance and ultimately, therefore, physical outcomes.

- Treatment for cancer can result in an increase in negative health behaviours (e.g. smoking and drinking) and decrease in positive health behaviours (e.g. exercise).

- Pain from cancer and the treatment can be considerable and biopsychosocial factors have to be taken into account when developing and implementing care plans.

- Chemotherapy brings with it a number of psychosocial consequences which should be considered and addressed by the nurse and health care professional.

- Psychological interventions can improve the experience of chemotherapeutic and radiotherapeutic treatments of breast cancer.

- Physical treatments for breast cancer – both medical and surgical – bring consequences for body image and, ultimately, close relationships.

- The partner of the individual with breast cancer has a role to play in improving the psychosocial outcomes of the woman. Furthermore, the impact of the woman's breast cancer on her partner can be considerable.

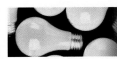 ## Check your understanding

1. Discuss the role of psychology in assisting the women undergoing chemotherapy for breast cancer.

2. How can a partner's reaction to breast cancer contribute to the sufferer's physical and psychological difficulties?

3. What role does the nurse have in promoting the psychological well-being of the husband of the woman with breast cancer?

4. What stresses are associated with the medical treatment of breast cancer? How can the nurse use their psychological knowledge to reduce the psychological impact of this treatment?

5. What information and emotional support can the nurse provide for the woman undergoing treatment for breast cancer?

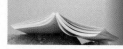

Further reading

Baucom, D.H., Porter, L.S., Kirby, J.S., Gremore, T.M. and Keefe, F.J. (2005/6) Psychosocial issues confronting young women with breast cancer. *Breast Disease*, **23**, 103–113.

European Journal of Oncology Nursing.

Metz, J.M. and Hampshire, M. (2006) *OncoLink Patient Guide to Breast Cancer*. Philadelphia, PA: Saunders.

Hewitt, M.E., Herdman, R. and Holland, J.C. (2004) *Meeting Psychosocial Needs of Women with Breast Cancer*. Washington: National Academies Press.

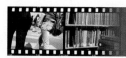

Weblinks

Cancer Backup	http://www.cancerbackup.org.uk/Cancertype/Breast	Backup cancer charity providing information and support on breast cancer.
Breast Cancer Husband	http://www.breastcancerhusband.com/	A website from an author of a book on being the husband of a woman with breast cancer. Although trying to sell the book, the website does include some relevant information and a message board.
Chemocare	http://www.chemocare.com/	Providing the latest information about chemotherapy to patients and their families, caregivers and friends.

Media examples

Before I Say Goodbye (1998) A book by Ruth Picardie on her journey through the diagnosis, treatment and, ultimately, death from cancer. The book is movingly written and provides an interesting and accurate description of how an average family deals with cancer and loss. Although the finality of death is threaded all the way through this book, it remains up-lifting with appropriate hope. It is a strong book but does provide some moving and meaningful sentiments (tissues should be at the ready!). The impact of the diagnosis and the treatments that Ruth has are felt by the reader and clearly written by Matt Seaton, who highlights from his perspective the impact on the family unit and the impact on the psychological and physical functioning of his wife.

Soap operas In recent years all of the major soap operas on TV have had a story line with a character suffering from either breast cancer or heart disease (for example, *Coronation Street* and *Eastenders*). It is worth watching these to see how people experience the condition, live with it and deal with its consequences. For most of the time the presentation is sympathetic and reasonably close to a real-life experience.

Glossary

ABC model: model put forward by Beck within cognitive restructuring – an acronym which stands for Antecedent (beginning), Behaviour (that is in question) and consequence (of the behaviour that is in question).

ABCDE'S delivery of bad news: put forward by Dyer, a framework for health practitioners who have to break bad news to the patient or family.

Abnormality: a subjectively defined characteristic, assigned to those with rare or dysfunctional conditions. Defining who is normal or abnormal is a contentious issue in psychology.

ACCESS model: Narayanasamy put together this model which acts as a framework for nurses to work within, so that they can effectively communicate with patients who may hold differing health beliefs.

Acute pain: pain that comes on quickly, can be severe, but lasts a relatively short time.

Adherence: patient commitment to the medical regimen. Negotiation and patient empowerment feature when the patient is adhering to medication as opposed to compliance.

Advocacy: working on behalf of the patient when pursuing their best interest.

Aesthetic needs: higher order needs on the hierarchy of needs.

Affective: relating to mood, emotion, feeling, sensibility or a mental state.

Affective care: provides one of the following aspects: emotional support, reassurance, concern and understanding.

Age stereotyping: fixed ideas based on an age group where all people within that group behave or should behave the same.

Ageism: treating people unfairly because of their age.

Ageist: behaviour in the form of a remark or treatment that is provided which results in the individual being treated unfairly because of their age.

Aggression: the intentional infliction of some form of harm on others.

Alameda Seven/Alameda Study: seven health habits, commonly referred to as the 'Alameda 7', were shown to be associated with physical health status and mortality in a pioneer longitudinal study initiated in 1965 in Alameda County, California. These habits are having never smoked, drinking less than five drinks at one sitting, sleeping 7–8 hours a night, exercising, maintaining desirable weight for height, avoiding snacks, and eating breakfast regularly.

Algorithms: mathematical procedures that are followed to solve a problem.

Alopecia: a form of hair loss from areas of the body, usually from the scalp.

Alzheimer's disease: a disease that results in the gradual loss of memory, speech, movement and the ability to think clearly. common especially among older people. Also known as dementia.

Anhedonia: an inability to experience pleasure from normally pleasurable life events such as eating, exercise and social/sexual interactions.

Anorexia: a psychiatric diagnosis that describes an eating disorder characterised by low body weight and body image distortion with an obsessive fear of gaining weight. Individuals with anorexia often control body weight by voluntary starvation, purging, vomiting, excessive exercise or other weight control measures, such as diet pills or diuretic drugs.

Anti-emetic: an agent that prevents or arrests vomiting.

Anxiety: a complex emotional state with apprehension and dread being the prominent features.

Appraising: combination of informing, advising and educating the patient.

Assertiveness: enables the individual to express themselves with confidence, without the inappropriate use of aggressive, passive or manipulative behaviours.

Atherosclerosis: a disease affecting arterial blood vessels. It is a chronic inflammatory response in the walls of arteries, commonly referred to as a 'hardening' or 'furring' of the arteries.

Attending: listening to a patient both physically and psychologically.

Attitude: a complex, hypothetical construct that represents an individual's beliefs, feelings, values and dispositions towards an item.

Attribution: (1) a concept in psychology whereby people attribute traits and causes to things they observe; (2) process of assigning a cause to one's own or others' behaviour.

Attribution theory: theory explaining how attributions are formed.

Authoritative: part of Heron's six category intervention model where the nurse is instructing the patient what to do or what they have to follow.

Autogenic muscle relaxation (AMR): learning to relax through associating a state of relaxation (learnt through progressive muscle relaxation) with a particular action or word.

Aversive events: negative stimuli that induce behaviour changes by causing avoidance of a situation, object or mode of response.

Ayuverdic: school of medicine based within naturalistic systems, which provides treatment according to the balance of the humors within the body.

Bad grief: where the individual experiences the different stages of grief with problems and could remain in one stage of grief work and have problems moving towards acceptance. Also referred to as abnormal grief work.

Behavioural activation: behavioural strategy intervention for depressed patients which raises awareness of current avoidance behaviours and then provides a platform from which non-avoidance behaviour is reinforced.

Behavioural coping: efforts that involve an action aimed at reducing the impact of a stressor.

Behavioural immunogens: health-protective behaviours, e.g. eating healthily, attending regular check-ups, exercising.

Behavioural methods: pertaining to changing behaviour patterns.

Belongingness and love needs: third level of Maslow's hierarchy of needs, which consists of family and friends as needs.

Bereavement: depriving someone of a beloved person through death.

Biofeedback: a form of alternative medicine that involves measuring a person's bodily processes such as blood pressure, heart rate, skin temperature, galvanic skin response (sweating) and muscle tension, and conveying such information to him or her in real-time in order to raise his or her awareness and conscious control of the related physiological activities. Based on the principles of operant and classical conditioning where an individual's behaviour is reinforced with immediate feedback.

Biomedical: origins of illness and health explained in the main from a physiological perspective.

Biopsychosocial: posits that biological, psychological and social factors all play a significant role in human functioning, including in mental processes.

Blindspots: encouraging a patient to think, discuss or reflect on issues that they have not acknowledged, ignored, denied or overseen. Part of challenging and/or confronting.

Blunting: the extent to which an individual avoids and/or ignores threat-relevant information.

Bottom-up process: analysis of the action of feature detectors in the sensory experience based just on what you see.

Brain stem: part of the brain, consisting of the medulla oblongata, pons varolii and midbrain; connects the spinal cord to the forebrain and cerebrum.

BSL: British Sign Language which is a recognised language for 50 000–70 000 deaf people living in the United Kingdom.

Buffering hypothesis: events, support of psychological characteristics act as a buffer against the negative consequences of stress.

Burnout: physical or emotional exhaustion, especially as a result of long-term stress.

Cartesian dualism: attributed to René Descartes, the first to clearly identify the mind, consisting of consciousness and self-awareness, and to distinguish this from the brain, which was the seat of intelligence. The central claim of Cartesian dualism is that the immaterial mind and the material body, while being ontologically distinct substances, causally interact.

Catalytic intervention: falls within the facilitative category of Heron's (1975) six categories of counselling intervention model. This intervention encourages the patient to problem-solve, elicit self-discovery and self-directed learning.

Catharsis: the process where an individual can disclose their feelings, thoughts and anxieties. Also referred to as being *cathartic*, which brings with it the therapeutic element that stems from such disclosure.

Cathartic intervention: falls within the facilitative category of Heron's six categories of counselling model. This intervention enables the patient to discharge pain, emotion, grief, anger and fear.

Cerebral artery: any of the arteries supplying blood to the brain.

Chemotherapy: the use of chemical substances to treat disease. In its modern-day use, it refers primarily to cytotoxic drugs used to treat cancer.

Chronic illnesses: long term, to be managed for the rest of the person's life.

Chronic pain: although there is no one clear definition, chronic pain is often defined as pain that lasts longer than 3 months (for some 6 months).

Chunking: Miller (1956) coined this term which refers to how one can exceed the capacity of short-term memory by grouping meaningless information into meaningful units.

Clarifying: counselling skill where the nurse seeks clarification as to what has been said by re-wording back to the patient what they initially said, which helps clarification both for the nurse and the patient (also part of Heron's six category intervention model).

Classical conditioning: the exploration of behaviour that occurs as a result of associations made with the environment (stimuli) and response.

Clinical iceberg: used to describe the phenomenon of many unreported levels of illness, as it is thought that only a small proportion of the population actually reach the health care services, i.e. the tip of the iceberg.

Closed questions: a question that warrants only a yes or no answer.

Cocktail-party phenomenon: an analogy that is used to describe how individuals attend to information when they are surrounded by distraction.

Cognition models: in cognitive psychology, a model is a simplified representation of reality. In cognitive science, a cognitive model is a model of cognitive processes. Briefly put, it is the use of computers to model cognitive behaviour.

Cognitions: The mental processes of knowing, thinking, learning and judging.

Cognitive appraisal: can be most readily understood as the process of defining an encounter or event, with respect to its significance for personal well-being.

Cognitive behavioural therapy (CBT): psychotherapy based on modifying everyday thoughts and behaviours, with the aim of positively influencing target emotions and behaviours.

Cognitive coping: cognitive coping involves the use of mental strategies to reframe the situation in a more favourable light.

Cognitive dissonance theory: put forward by Festinger (1957) which explains how individuals are in a state of tension when they have bits of information that is contradictory which is referred to as cognitive dissonance. The theory outlines how individuals strive to make information consistent so cognitive dissonance is not experienced.

Cognitive hypothesis model of compliance: put together by Phillip Ley (1981, 1989) which identifies patient understanding, recall (memory) and satisfaction as contributing factors to the adherence behaviour of a patient.

Cognitive impairments: impairments that have resulted from illnesses associated with ageing which result in a gradual loss of sensory channels such as hearing, sight. This results in a lower stress threshold and slower communication.

Cognitive needs: fifth level of needs in Maslow's hierarchy of needs which consist of the need for understanding and knowledge.

Cognitive psychology: (1) how people learn, structure, store and use knowledge; (2) perspective in psychology which explore mediators such as the mind, perception and thinking which influence behaviour.

Communication: a complex two-way process that involves passing a message intentionally or unintentionally between two or more people using either (or both) verbal or non-verbal communication strategies.

Compliance: extent to which the patient's behaviour coincides with the medical/health advice provided by the practitioner. Emphasis here is on the patient following advice and instruction without question.

Concordance: patient who is an equal with the practitioner who is offering advice and instructions, the outcome resulting from a shared decision-making.

Concurrent mental illness: a mental illness that occurs at the same time as another illness.

Conditioned response: a response to a conditioned stimulus which results in a new behaviour when the conditioned stimulus is present.

Conditioned stimulus: a neutral stimulus paired with a unconditional stimulus which, after several repeated pairings, becomes a conditional stimulus, since it evokes a conditioned response without the unconditional stimulus being present.

Conditioning: part of the process of learning where new associations are made which result in newly learned behaviour as a result of conditioning which features within the principles of classical conditioning.

Conformity: a deep-seated private and enduring change in behaviour and attitudes due to group pressure.

Confront: Encourage patients to think about their thought patterns or actions and encourage them to reflect on their current thinking in order for them to change the way they currently think or behave. Also known as challenging.

Confronting intervention: the third intervention within the authoritative category of Heron's six categories of counselling intervention model. This intervention requires the practitioner to raise the patient's consciousness about some limiting attitude, behaviour, which they are unaware of.

Congruence: being genuine in a relationship. Congruence is displayed when verbal and non-verbal behaviour are in agreement. A core value on a counselling/helping relationship.

Conscious: first level or part of the mind that contains thoughts and feelings which the individual is fully aware of.

Context-dependent learning: recalled information, associated with external cues that were there when learning took place.

Coping strategies: coping strategies refer to the specific efforts, both behavioural and psychological, that people employ to master, tolerate, reduce, or minimise stressful events.

Correspondence bias: when behaviour is attributed to internal rather than external causes which is also referred to as fundamental attribution error.

Covariation model: put forward by Kelley, which outlines attributions being based on information that is consistent, distinctive and consensual.

Cross-sectional studies: An approach to research where groups of subjects are studies at one point in time.

Cue reactivity: behaviour that occurs as a result of stimuli related to the behaviour, which can be internal or external, which results in the onset of the behaviour.

Culturally competent: being self-aware of cultural and diversity issues when working with patients.

Culture: rules, way of behaviour, which are learned from birth and throughout life. This is dynamic and is forever changing when adapting to situations.

Death: the irreversible cessation of life.

Debridement: the act of debriding (removing dead, contaminated or adherent tissue or foreign material).

Defence mechanisms: employed by the ego which represses thoughts and feelings into the unconscious part of the mind.

Deficiency needs: the four basic needs levels in Maslow's hierarchy of needs, which are physiological, safety and security, love and belonging and esteem levels of needs.

Denial: type of defence mechanism where there is a refusal to acknowledge the existence of a real situation or the feelings associated with it.

Dependence: dependence is compulsively using a substance, despite its negative and sometimes dangerous effects.

Depersonalisation: a feeling of unreality or of being 'outside' your body.

Desensitisation: process that takes place where there is a gradual exposure to an individual's fears; in turn, a de-conditioning process takes place.

Deviance: differing from a norm or from the accepted standards of a society.

Diastolic blood pressure: the lowest pressure in the arteries (at the resting phase of the cardiac cycle).

Dignity: the opinion that you have of the standard of your own importance and value.

Disability communication: the inability of an individual to express themselves fully either via the verbal or non-verbal channel.

Displacement: defence mechanism also known as 'kick the cat syndrome' where energy such as anger, frustration and hostility are displaced on to a non-threatening object or person.

Diversity: variation within and across groups.

Drug resistance: becoming immune to medication.

EdFED questionnaire: Watson's questionnaire which incorporates questions that can be addressed by nurses when assessing possible malnutrition or if the patient has been consuming food on a regular basis.

Ego: a component of personality which mediates between the needs of the id and superego. The ego is based on the reality principle which aims to get rid of any tension or anxiety that results from the conflict that occurs between the id and superego.

Ego defence mechanisms: employed by the ego to repress wishes, thoughts, needs, etc. into the unconscious mind when there is anxiety and tension between the id and superego.

Elaborative rehearsal: the linking of new information in short-term memory to familiar material stored in long-term memory.

Elder abuse: can range from not meeting needs of the elderly patient when in a position of trust as well as invasion of privacy, dignity and lack of respect to verbal and physical abuse.

Electroconvulsive therapy (ECT): a controversial psychiatric treatment in which seizures are induced with electricity. Also known as electroshock.

Electromyography (EMG): a medical technique for evaluating and recording physiological properties of muscles at rest and while contracting by means of an electrode inserted into the muscle or placed on the skin.

Emotion-focused coping: these skills reduce the symptoms of stress without addressing the source of the stress. Consuming alcohol, sleeping or discussing the stress with a friend are all emotion-based coping strategies. Aimed at regulating emotions.

Empathetic understanding: third core value of counselling which, through counselling skills, enables the practitioner (nurse) to attempt to understand where the client (patient) is coming from, or perceiving their treatment and illness from the patient's perspective.

Empathy: whereby the nurse lays aside their own feelings and responds to their patient's experiences and perception of themselves as if they had originated in themselves.

Empowerment: means by which individuals gain some control or mastery over their lives.

Encoding: information that is attended to and then processed.

Endogenous: illnesses developing, originating or arising from causes within the human body.

Epidemiological study: study on human populations, which attempt to link human health effects to a cause.

Equilibrium: condition in which all acting influences are cancelled out by others resulting in a stable, balanced or unchanging system.

Esteem needs: fourth level of Maslow's hierarchy of needs which consists of the need for social and self-esteem.

Ethnocentrism: when an individual judges others' health beliefs in light of their own, which they believe to be superior.

Evaluative: relating to the impact it has on the individual.

Exogenous: illnesses with a cause external to the body.

Exposure-based therapies: facing something that has been avoided because it provokes anxiety.

External (situational) attributions: behaviour that is attributed to external or environmental factors.

Extinction: the reverse of conditioned response where the original stimuli is paired without the conditioned stimuli, which results in the extinction of the previous conditioned response.

Fight or flight: animals react to threats with a general discharge of the sympathetic nervous system, priming the animal for fighting or fleeing.

Filtering process: information that is meaningless is filtered out with only meaningful information begin processed in the sensory memory store.

Five-stage hierarchy of needs model: put together by Abraham Maslow (1954), the model comprises seven levels of needs that a patient can have. In order to reach self-actualisation (the highest level), the preceding levels of needs need to be met first.

Five-stage (DABDA) model: a grief work model of Kubler-Ross that consists of five stages: denial, anger, bargaining, depression and acceptance.

Focusing: stage one of Egan's skilled helper model, which encourages the patient to move forward by focusing on aspects so that a problem is more manageable.

Folk definitions: definitions of health and illness that are developed by non-experts with reference to past experience with family and friends.

Folk sector: healers who cure people with an holistic approach but differ with their approach, depending on the communities' prevailing belief of the causation of ill health. The folk sector range from lifting of spells to addressing social problems which have caused ill-health.

Freud, Sigmund: the pioneer of the psychodynamic approach.

Frustration–aggression hypothesis: theory put forward by Dollard *et al.*, which explores the relationship between frustration and aggression.

Fundamental attribution error: when behaviour is attributed to internal rather than external causes which is also referred to as correspondence bias.

Gate-keeper: an individual (usually a primary-care provider) who coordinates patient care and provides referrals to other specialist medical and health care services.

General adaptation syndrome (GAS): three-stage, universal response to the stressors. Stage one is alarm, in which the fight or flight response is evoked. Stage two is resistance, in which attempts to cope with persistent stressors are made. Stage three is exhaustion, when the body's resources are eventually depleted and the body is unable to maintain normal function.

Generalisation: conditioned stimulus is paired with a similar stimulus which evokes the same conditioned response when the similar stimulus is experienced.

Genuineness: basic ability to be aware of inner experiences and to allow the quality of that inner experience to be apparent in relationships.

Gerontological nursing: specialist area of nursing that focuses on the elderly patient.

Gestalt psychologist: psychologists who give precedence to our tendency to perceive sensory patterns as well-organised wholes rather than as separate isolated parts.

Good grief: also referred to as healthy grief work where the individual experiences the different stages of grief without problems for later acceptance.

Grief: feeling of sadness and sorrow as a result of a loved one's death or loss which can even be one's own loss.

Grief work: emotional process that the individual will experience which consists of many emotional states. Going through grief work is vital in order to reach acceptance.

Grief work models: framework models that identify the stages involved within grief work, such as the model put forward by Kubler-Ross known as the DABDA model.

Grieving: process that an individual experiences after a loss which is characterised by sorrow and external emotions such as crying.

Growth needs: needs that follow higher from the basic needs; the cognitive, aesthetic and self-actualisation needs levels.

Guided imagery: use of relaxation and mental visualisation to improve mood and/or physical well-being.

Health action process approach: suggests that the adoption, initiation and maintenance of health behaviours must be explicitly conceived as a process that consists of at least a motivation phase and a volition phase.

Health belief model: a psychological model developed in the 1950s for studying and promoting the uptake of services offered by health care professionals. It describes the influences and thoughts behind why patients present, and crucially, why they present at that particular moment in their lives.

Health beliefs: health psychology models which highlight and explain factors that result in health behaviours.

Health locus of control: refers to an individual's generalised expectations concerning where control over their health resides.

Heterogeneous: something, an object or system, consisting of a diverse range of different elements or items.

Heuristic: encouraging a person to learn, discover, understand or solve problems on his or her own, by experimenting, evaluating possible answers or solutions, or by trial and error.

Holistic care: care that incorporates biomedical and psychosocial aspects of health and illness explanations.

Humanistic psychology: a perspective within psychology that aims to understand the individual as fully as possible before treating their symptoms.

Humors: balance of the three elements (*Vata, Pitta and Kapha*) within the body which provide the basic understanding within ayurvedic medicine when treating ill-health.

Hypnosis: a process in which critical thinking faculties of the mind are by-passed and a type of selective thinking and perception is established.

Hypothalamus: the part of the brain that lies below the thalamus. Regulates bodily temperature, certain metabolic processes and other autonomic activities.

Id: the primitive part of the personality which is in existence as soon as the child is born and contains basic needs and wants.

Illness perception questionnaire: Based on the self-regulatory model, Leventhal compiled a questionnaire that measures cause, identity, timeline and consequence of illness.

Implicit pain theory: one's own view of pain and its management.

Incidence: the number of new cases of a given problem occurring in a specific period.

Incongruence: inner feelings and thoughts do not match what is being expressed outwardly.

Incongruent: where there is a contradiction between the verbal and non-verbal message, the reverse being congruent where there is a match.

Information-seeking theory: information-seeking theory suggests that uncertainty causes conflict and increases arousal, so finding out what is going on reduces uncertainty and therefore reduces arousal.

Informative intervention: second intervention Heron proposes within his six categories of counselling intervention model which falls within the authoritative category. This intervention requires the practitioner to impart with knowledge, information and meaning to the patient.

Innervate: to stimulate to action.

Instrumental care: care that encompasses providing information, clarification on information and physical as well as routine tasks.

Instrumental passivity hypothesis: unintentional reinforcement of dependency behaviours.

Intentional non-adherence: individual who decides that it is in their best interest not to follow advice or a drug regimen.

Interceding: come between others to mediate where necessary when acting as an advocate.

Internal (dispositional) attributions: behaviour that is attributed to internal factors.

Interview: a guided conversation, in which facts or statements are elicited from another.

Introspective: looking within or from one's own personal experiences.

Inverse care law: the principle that the availability of good medical or social care tends to vary inversely with the need of the population served.

Inverted-U relationship: a relationship between two variables, which when plotted, results in an upside down U-shaped line graph. Increasing values of variable 1 result in increasing values of variable 2 in the lower range of the variable 1 values. In the median range of variable 1 values, changes in variable 1 result in little or no change in values of variable 2. In the upper range of variable 1 values, increasing values of variable 1 result in decreasing values of variable 2.

Johari window: a self-awareness tool put together by Luft.

Labelling: title or label that is given to an individual which then results in the label being seen before the person's individual's qualities.

Last offices: A process that involves the nurse preparing the body of the deceased for viewing or ready to be taken away.

Lay referral system: consulting people with little or no formal knowledge of medicine or health for advice on the matter, such as family or friends.

Levels of processing: the levels, either shallow or deep, at which information is encoded in long-term memory.

Leverage: Egan refers to this as a payoff whereby the completion of one small task contributes to the management of several other related problems/tasks more successfully.

Life events: significant events that occur during a lifespan that may influence an individual's stress levels.

Linear association: relationship between two variables that is illustrated by a straight line.

Linear model: The linear model suggests that pain is a consequence of a linear nerve transmission – from injury through to the brain to observable response.

Locus of control: degree to which a person ascribes the cause, origin or ability to control events to internal or external factors, e.g. own behaviour or actions vs. luck, circumstances or other people.

Long-term memory: the third memory store within Atkinson and Shiffrin's (1968) multi-store memory model which stores information spanning from recently processed information to that of a lifetime.

Low literacy skills: reading and writing skills in any language which are below average and result in the individual finding it difficult to understand written information.

Magical number seven plus or minus two: Miller's (1956) phrase that is used to explain the capacity of short-term memory.

Malnutrition: individual is deficient in essential vitamins and minerals and is losing weight.

Masking: information that is replaced almost immediately with new information within the sensory store.

Medical jargon: terms and abbreviations which health professionals and allied health professions are familiar with.

Medication beliefs: individual's perception and beliefs of the medication stemming from three overarching groups: a negative, a positive and a dual view of medication.

Memory: cognitive systems for storing and retrieving information; the ability to remember the things that we have experienced imagined and learned.

Mental Health Act 1983: an Act of the UK Parliament. It covers the reception, care and treatment of mentally disordered persons, the management of their property and other related matters. In particular, it provides the legislation by which people suffering from a mental disorder can be detained in hospital and have their disorder assessed or treated against their wishes, unofficially known as 'sectioning'.

Mental schema: a mental structure that represents some aspect of the world.

Message framing: how information is portrayed/communicated, e.g. gain health frame or loss health frame.

Meta-analysis: In statistics, combines the result of several studies that address a set of related research hypotheses.

Mirroring: counselling skill which involves reflecting on feelings and thoughts which are reiterated back to the patient. The analogy used is that of holding up a mirror.

Mnemonic device: techniques that make material easier to remember.

Morbidity: The rate of incidence of a disease or illness.

Mortality: death rate; the quality or condition of being mortal.

Motivational interviewing: a counselling approach initially developed by clinical psychologists William R. Miller and Stephen Rollnick. It attempts to increase clients' awareness of the potential problems caused, consequences experienced and risks faced as a result of the behaviour in question in order to increase motivation to change that behaviour.

Mourning: process gone through by the bereaved while adapting to a loss.

Mucositis: painful inflammation and ulceration of the mucous membranes lining the digestive tract.

Multi-modal methods: different modes of treatment used together.

Multi-modal models: models comprised of different modes or psychological concepts.

Myocardial infarction: more commonly known as a heart attack, is a disease state that occurs when the blood supply to a part of the heart is interrupted. The resulting ischemia or oxygen shortage causes damage and potential death of heart tissue.

National Service Framework: Working targets in a definitive document that have been set up by the Department of Health which tackle issues around the elderly when receiving care within the NHS.

Naturalistic systems: an explanation of illness in impersonal, systemic terms from natural forces or conditions.

Negative affect: for example, to respond to a patient appropriately, so encouraging behaviour that results in independence, rather than dependence on the health professional where possible.

Negative punisher: behaviour that is ignored.

Negative reinforcement: the removal, delay or decrease in intensity of an unpleasant stimulus which results in the response becoming stronger or more likely to occur.

Neglect: paying little or no regard to specific areas of the visual field.

Neural mechanisms: mechanisms made up of nerve cells and/or neurons.

Neuroendocrine: interactions between the nervous and endocrine systems, especially in relation to hormones.

Neuroticism: a fundamental personality trait in the study of psychology. It can be defined as an enduring tendency to experience negative emotional states.

Neurotransmitters: a chemical substance, such as acetylcholine or dopamine, that transmit nerve impulses across a synapse.

Nominal: level of measurement at which numbers, if used, are mere labels for discrete categories.

Non-compliance: not following health advice or instructions that have been provided by the nurse.

Non-verbal communication: all behaviour that helps us to understand a message without the use of a verbal language which is expressed consciously or unconsciously every time people interact.

Norms: standards, what is expected.

Nursing culture: rules, regulation and training that nurses are influenced within.

Object permanence: a developmental term that refers to a child's ability to understand that objects still exist after they are no longer in sight.

Objective self-awareness: a feeling where an individual is carrying out a particular behaviour while being aware of others observing or assessing them.

Observational learning: learning that takes place solely through observation where the learner is passive. It forms the main premise of the social learning theory strand of behaviourism.

One-way communication: sender providing a message that the receiver will listen to and not provide any feedback in the form of answering questions or clear up and misunderstanding.

Open questioning: questions that begin with the words such as why, what, when, how and where, which are useful to use when probing a patient to facilitate disclosure of information.

Operant conditioning: strand of behaviourism that explores how likely a response becomes, depending on the consequences of behaviour.

Operants: a response that occurs spontaneously and is identified by its reinforcing or inhibiting effects.

Opioid: analgesics, also known as narcotic analgesics, are pain relievers that act on the central nervous system. Like all narcotics, they may become habit-forming if used over long periods.

Organisational culture: rules and regulations that are both implicit and explicit which are outlined by an organisation to which individuals adhere when in that organisation.

Paralinguistic messages: what is verbally expressed other than words, e.g. tone of voice, speed that words are paced. Also known as para-verbal.

Paraphrasing: reiterating information back to the patient.

Passiveness: where an individual will ignore his or her own rights during an interaction.

Pathology: the scientific study of the nature of disease and its causes, process, development and consequences.

Patient-centred: care that centres around the patient's needs.

Patient culture: health beliefs and previous health care experience of the individual.

Patient satisfaction: how satisfied a patient has been or is with the cognitive, affective and behavioural aspects of the consultation in question.

Peer modelling: the modelling or demonstrating of a behaviour by a peer.

Perception: the brain's interpretation of sensory information so as to give it meaning; the process through which we select, organise and interpret input from our sensory receptors.

Perceptual organisation: process by which we structure the input from our sensory receptors.

Person-centred: from the work of Carl Rogers (1902–1987), who promoted the patient-centred approach on the basis that the patient/client knows what is best for them and knows what is important.

Person-focused approach: originating from person-centred approach (Rogers), which focuses on the person/patient from which care, consultation and treatment is tailored around.

Personalistic systems: belief system which includes supernatural forces.

Persuasive communication: is at the heart of attitude change which is dependent on factors associated with the source of communication, the message itself, the recipient of communication and the channel of communication.

Phantom limb: the illusion that a limb still exists after it has been amputated.

Phobia: an irrational or very powerful fear and dislike of something such as spiders or confined spaces.

Physiological needs: first level of Maslow's hierarchy of needs, which consists of oxygen, sleep, water and other biological needs that are necessary for survival.

Pleasure principle: the id is based in the pleasure principle which largely contains wants and needs that require immediate gratification.

Popular sector: consists of the media, social support networks and the Internet, which influence the health beliefs of individuals.

Population: set of individuals, items or data from which a statistical sample is taken.

Positive punisher: behaviour that gets punished.

Positive reinforcement: reinforcer that is provided after a behaviour which strengthens the association between the stimuli and the response.

Post-traumatic stress disorder: certain severe psychological consequences of exposure to, or confrontation with, stressful events that the person experiences as highly traumatic.

Preconscious: second level or part of the mind which contains experiences, feelings and thoughts from the past which can be readily bought up into the conscious awareness without a problem.

Preparatory-response theory: proposes that in Pavlovian conditioning, the conditioned response is one that prepares the organism for the upcoming unconditioned stimulus.

Prescriptive intervention: Direct the behaviour of the patient which usually is the behaviour outside the nurse–patient relationship. This is the first intervention with the authoritative group of interventions that Heron proposes within his six categories of counselling intervention model.

Pre-therapy: therapy that involves counselling, person centredness and reflections.

Prevalence: total number of cases of a disease or illness in a given population at a specific time.

Primacy effect: the first bit of information that is presented.

Primary memory: also known as short-term memory.

Proactive interference: information already in memory that interferes with new information.

Probing: encouraging patients to disclose information with the use of open questioning, and other counselling skills.

Problem drinking: where an individual drinks heavily, even though they have caused harm, or are causing harm or problems to themselves, their family or society. Many problem drinkers are not dependent on alcohol, but for one reason or another, they continue to drink heavily.

Problem-focused coping: involves dealing with a problem that is the source of stress.

Professional medicine sector: also referred to as the professional sector, based on the biomedical viewpoint when treating and managing ill-health.

Professional self-esteem: the self-evaluative beliefs that nurses hold about themselves.

Progressive muscle relaxation: a technique of stress management developed by American physician Edmund Jacobson in the early 1920s. Individuals undergoing therapy are trained to voluntarily relax certain muscles in their body in order to reduce anxiety symptoms.

Projection: a defence mechanism where the individual attributes one's own unacceptable thoughts, feelings and impulses onto another person.

Prospectively: the individuals are identified and then followed forward in time.

Psychiatric disability: when mental illness significantly interferes with the performance of major life activities, such as learning, thinking, communicating and sleeping.

Psychic determinism: the predominant belief within the psychodynamic approach that all behaviour originates from previous experience which originates within the unconscious part of the mind.

Psychoanalysis: the therapy that stems out of the psychodynamic approach. Also known as psychotherapy.

Psychodynamic: an approach within psychology which aims to explore how the mind (human psyche) especially the unconscious part of the mind is responsible for everyday behaviour.

Psychologically noxious: harmful, hurtful, unpleasant or in any other way aversive to a person psychologically rather than physically.

Psychoneuroimmunology: studying the relationship between the mind, neural activity and immune function.

Psychosocial: involving aspects of both social and psychological behaviour.

Quality of life: your standard of living, including not only money and access to goods and services, but freedom, happiness, culture, environmental health and intellectual stimulation, among others.

Race: a biological construct. Researchers now appreciate that race can be viewed as a social category that varies across societies and cultures, to which the term *ethnicity* is applied.

Radiotherapy: the medical use of ionising radiation as part of cancer treatment to control malignant cells. Also known as radiation therapy.

Ramadan: Muslims practice *sawm*, or fasting, for the entire month of Ramadan. This means that they may eat or drink nothing, including water, while the sun shines.

Rational emotive therapy (RET): is a psychotherapeutic approach which proposes that unrealistic and irrational beliefs cause many emotional problems.

Rationalisation: a defence mechanism where an individual justifies their own behaviour or excuses shortcomings by providing excuses, thereby avoiding criticism, condemnation or disappointment by others.

Reaction formation: a defence mechanism where the individual may conceal his or her true feelings by behaving in the opposite way.

Recency effect: the tendency for items at the end of a list to be remembered better than items in the middle.

Reflecting feeling: listener concentrates on what the speaker expressed in terms of emotional words and feelings, which are paraphrased back to the speaker.

Reflection: where an individual goes beyond merely describing an event or incident and instead learns from the incident or experience that the individual has either been through or observed.

Reflective framework model: enables the process of reflection to be carried out in an effective manner as it allows the individual to ask appropriate questions within an existing framework model.

Regression: a defence mechanism where the individual during times of stress and anxiety will regress back to an earlier childhood state which is comforting.

Reinforcement: the process by which a stimulus or event strengthens or increases the probability of the response that it follows.

Reinforcer: the consequence of behaviour, which further strengthens future behaviour.

Relativism: there are no absolute truths, i.e. truth is always relative to some particular frame of reference, such as a language or a culture.

Repressed: the umbrella defence mechanism which refers to the end result to the process of thoughts, feelings and emotions that are pushed into the unconscious part of the mind by the ego.

Repression: a defence mechanism where unacceptable feelings, thoughts and emotions are pushed into the unconscious.

Retrieval: information that is needed that is taken from memory storage.

Retroactive interference: new material interferes with information already in the long-term memory.

Role clarity: clarifying the roles that each team member has to ensure effective teamwork.

Rote rehearsal: retaining information in memory simply by repeating it over and over.

Royal road into the unconscious: refers to the exploration of the unconscious mind by bringing appropriate thoughts, feelings, memories and emotions into the conscious awareness.

Safety and security needs: second level of Maslow's hierarchy of needs, which consists of protection, security and freedom from anxiety needs.

Safety-signal theory: psychological problems are a result of an individual seeking or desiring safety.

Schemata: set of beliefs or expectations about something that is based on past experience.

Schizophrenia: psychiatric diagnosis that describes a mental illness characterised by impairments in the perception or expression of reality, most commonly manifesting as auditory hallucinations, paranoid or bizarre delusions or disorganised speech and thinking in the context of significant social or occupational dysfunction.

Self: identity and evaluation of oneself.

Self-actualisation: realising personal potential, self-fulfilment, seeking personal growth and peak experiences.

Self-awareness: a state in which one is aware of oneself as an object, much as one might be aware of a tree or another person.

Self-discrepancy theory: theory that describes an individual's self-schema as being split into three categories: actual self (how we currently are), ideal self (how we would like to be) and ought self (how we think we should be).

Self-efficacy: the conviction that one can successfully execute behaviour to produce a specified outcome which is one of the central features that distinguishes one person from another.

Self-esteem: feeling and evaluation about oneself.

Self-fulfilling prophecy: when an individual begins to behave/act or think in the way that they have been treated or expected to behave/act think by another.

Self-growth: ability of a patient to move forward/on.

Self-regulatory model: examines how an individual makes common sense of their present ill-health state.

Self-report questionnaire: a questionnaire completed by oneself.

Semantic: the meaning of words and sentences.

Sensory: relating to sensation, to the perception of a stimulus.

Sensory impairment: functioning on a daily basis without the full function of one or more senses.

Sensory information: information received through the senses, such as sight and sound.

Sensory memory store: the first memory store in Atkinson and Shiffrin's (1968) multi-store memory model which processes information through different sensory modalities, i.e. visual and auditory.

Sensory registers: entry points for raw information from the senses.

Shock: bodily immediate reaction where no emotion is shown.

Silence: a counselling tool used by the nurse to encourage the patient to disclose information and emotions.

Six categories of counselling intervention model: proposed by John Heron, which highlights six types of intervention that can be used when helping a patient. These interventions can be divided into authoritative (practitioner having more power in the relationship) and facilitative (equal weighting of power between the practitioner and the patient, where the patient is encourage to take more responsibility).

Skilled helper model: a framework of basic skills that are involved when helping a patient, which consists of three stages: present, future and getting there (from Egan, 1990).

Social anthropological: the branch of anthropology that studies how currently living human beings behave in social groups. A social anthropological view of phenomena focuses on social and cultural factors.

Social cognition: an understanding of how individuals make sense of the social situation around them.

Social cognition models: models refined to include a role for the social context of the behaviour not just the individual's cognitions or attitudes.

Social comparison: process of comparing one's behaviour and opinions with those of others in order to establish the correct or socially approved way of thinking of being.

Social facilitation: improvement in performance resulting from the presence of individuals or a passive audience.

Social identity: identifying with individuals who are in the same group.

Social inhibition: deterioration of behaviour resulting from the presence of others.

Social learning theory: third strand within behaviourism as pioneered by Bandura, which emphasises learning that requires the learner to be active for learning to occur.

Social perception: how individuals think others perceive them.

Social psychology: the scientific investigation of how the human thoughts, feelings and behaviour of individuals are influenced by the actual, imagined or implied presence of others.

Social reinforcers: non-verbal communication which acts as positive reinforcement to strengthen behaviour or response.

Social role: rights and duties of a person in a given situation (e.g. mother, manager, teacher). The social role is connected to expectations, norms and behaviour a person has to face.

Social stratification: the existence of structured inequalities on life chances between groups in society.

Social support: support around an individual that almost acts as a resource for the individual, of which there are many types, ranging from emotional support to informational support.

Society: a society is a grouping of individuals which is characterised by common interests and may have distinctive culture and institutions. Members of a society may be from different ethnic groups.

Socio-cultural vacuum: stressing the importance of the socio-cultural environment in which the individual operates.

SOLER: acronym provided by Egan, which exemplifies the micro-skills that a helper can use when attending to a patient: Sit squarely, Open posture, Lean forward, Eye contact and Relax.

Specificity theory: developed by Von Frey, who assumed that there were specific sensory receptors responsible for the transmission of sensation, warmth and pain.

Stages of change model: model put together by Prochaska and DiClemente, which emphasises that any proposed change should not be based on the here and now alone. Instead, previous as well as predictive future factors that influence the motivation to change need to be taken into account. This has been reflected with the stages of pre-contemplation, contemplation, preparation, action, maintenance, termination and relapse stages.

State-dependent learning: occurs when aspects of our physical states serve as retrieval cues for information stored in long-term memory.

Stereotypes: characteristics that are applied to a group as sharing all the same characteristics.

Stereotyping: qualities perceived to be associated with particular groups of categories of people.

Storage: information that is attended to and then processed through the different stores of memory.

Strategies: identifying and choosing realistic causes of action for achieving goals, which forms part of the getting there stage in Egan's Skilled Helper Model.

Stress: the disruption of homeostasis through physical or psychological stimuli.

Stress inoculation training (SIT) method: uses a cognitive behavioural framework to help people to be more aware and better interpret perceptions, reduce stress through relaxation and better problem-solving, and apply the learning to real-life situations. The aim is to change emotional responses and behavioural reactions to stressors.

Stress management: encompasses techniques intended to equip a person with effective coping mechanisms for dealing with stress.

Stressors: an event or context that elevates adrenaline and triggers the stress response because it throws the body out of balance and forces it to respond.

Substantia gelatinosa: a narrow, dense, vertical band of gelatinous grey matter forming part of the spinal cord and serving to integrate the sensory stimuli that give rise to the sensations of heat and pain.

Summarising: helper summing up what has been discussed at the end of the interaction.

Superego: component of personality which contains morals and rules within society.

Supernatural health belief model: model based on explanations of health which stem from originating causes such as evil spells.

Supportive intervention: the final intervention within the facilitative category of Heron's six categories of counselling intervention model. This intervention requires the practitioner to affirm the worth and value of the patient's personal qualities, attitudes or actions.

Surgery: the branch of medicine that deals with the diagnosis and treatment of injury, deformity and disease by manual and instrumental means.

Sympathy: an expression of the caregiver's own sorrow at another's (patient's) plight.

Sympathy versus empathy debate: sympathy to comfort, as opposed to empathy where the individual attempts to understand how the individual perceives the world around them.

Systolic blood pressure: the peak pressure in the arteries, which occurs near the beginning of the cardiac cycle.

Tension reduction theory: posits that alcohol is consumed to achieve tension reduction.

Tests of conservation: tests designed to assess whether a child understands that certain properties of a substance remain unchanged even when there are external changes, for example, to shape or arrangement.

Theory of planned behaviour: posits that the intention to perform a behaviour is determined by attitudes towards that behaviour, subjective norms regarding the desirability of the behaviour and perceived control over performing the behaviour. Intention to perform a behaviour impacts upon actual behaviour.

Theory of reasoned action: states that a person's behaviour is determined by their attitude towards the outcome of that behaviour and by the opinions of their social environment.

Third force: the humanistic psychology perspective is referred to as the third force in psychology. Behaviourism is the first and psychodynamic being the second force in psychology.

Three core conditions: Carl Rogers (1902–1987) highlighted the three core conditions, empathy, unconditional positive regard and congruence, as being essential for person-centred counselling and care.

Three-stage memory store model: also referred to as the multi-store memory model put forward by Atkinson and Shiffrin to exemplify the process of memory through the three distinct stages: sensory stores, short-term store and long-term store.

Token economy system: a behaviour modification method based on the principles within operant conditioning where desired behaviours are reinforced with a token that can be exchanged for material goods or other privileges.

Tolerance: the capacity of the body to endure or become less responsive to a substance (as a drug) or a physiological insult, especially with repeated use or exposure.

Top-down process: object being perceived as a whole at once, with the analysis of effect of expectation and prior learning on sensory experience.

Toxic support system: a social environment that exacerbates the condition of a patient.

Traits: distinguishing features of a person's character.

Transactional model: a framework for evaluating the processes of coping with stressful events. Stressful experiences are construed as person-environment transactions.

Transcranial Doppler (TCD) test: a test that measures the velocity of blood flow through the brain's blood vessels.

Transcultural nursing: area of nursing research and practice that explores factors that relate to culture, religion and diversity within care.

Translator(s): one who translates; esp., one who renders into another language; one who expresses the sense of words in one language by equivalent words in another.

Transtheoretical model: Proposes that individuals move through a series of five stages (pre-contemplation, contemplation, preparation, action, maintenance) in the adoption of healthy behaviours or cessation of unhealthy ones.

Two-way communication: an opportunity for the receiver of a message to clarify, pose a question or elaborate on the message back to the sender.

Unconditional positive regard: label given to the nurse's attitude towards the client which values individuality and the patient's thoughts and feelings do not bias this value in any way, which promotes warmth and acceptance for the patient.

Unconditional response: response that is reflexive to an unconditional stimulus which does not require any learning.

Unconditional stimulus: environmental cue or stimulus that evokes an unconditional response that is reflexive or natural.

Unconscious: the third level or largest part of the mind which contains thoughts, feelings, memories and emotions which the individual is not consciously aware of but at the same time motivates the day-to-day behaviour of an individual.

Unpopular patient: label given to patients by nurses resulting from their perception of the patient being difficult, which impacts on the care provided. Coined by Felicity Stockwell (Stockwell, 1972).

Validation therapy: validate and respect the person's feelings in whatever context is real to that person at that time.

Valuing: providing expert care while maintaining individualisation and humanity of the patient, which is a principle of advocacy.

Vicarious learning: learning through observing a model and then practising the skills.

Vipassana: Buddhist meditation.

Visual analogue scale: a simple assessment tool consisting of (usually) a 10 cm line with 0 at one end, representing nothing (e.g., no pain), and 10 at the other, representing the other extreme (e.g. the worst pain ever experienced).

Waiting list controls: a group of individuals currently on a waiting list to receive treatment who are used as a comparison group for individuals receiving an intervention of some kind in order to assess the intervention's effectiveness compared to no treatment.

Wernicke-Korsakoff syndrome: a manifestation of thiamine deficiency, or beri-beri, usually secondary to alcohol abuse.

WHO: the World Health Organization, a specialised agency of the United Nations that acts as a coordinating authority on international public health.

Working memory: short-term memory is referred to as working memory as information that is successfully transferred onto long-term memory tends to be worked with so that it is meaningful or stored away effectively.

References

Aapro, M.S., Molassiotis, A. and Olver, I. (2005) Anticipatory nausea and vomiting. *Support Care Cancer*, **13**, 117–121.

Abas, M., Vanderpyl, J., Prou, T.L., Kydd, R., Emery, B. and Foliaki, S.A. (2003) Psychiatric hospitalisation: reasons for admission and alternatives to admission in South Auckland, New Zealand. *Australian and New Zealand Journal of Psychiatry*, **37** (5), 620–625.

Abraham, C., Sheeran, P., Spears, R. and Abrams, D. (1992) Health beliefs and promotion of HIV – preventive intentions among teenagers – a Scottish perspective. *Health Psychology*, **11** (6), 363–370.

Action on Elder Abuse (1995) Action on Elder Abuse's definition of elder abuse. *Action on Elder Abuse Bulletin*, **2** (http://www.elderabuse.org.uk/What%20is%20abuse/what_is_abuse%20define.htm).

Action on Elder Abuse (2004) *Hidden Voices*. London: Age Concern.

Adegboye, A.A., Roy, P.K. and Emeka, C. (1997) Glove utilization and reasons for poor compliance by health care workers in a Nigerian teaching hospital. *Tropical Doctor*, **27** (2), 93–97.

Ader, R. (1981) *Psychoneuroimmunology*. New York: Academic Press.

Ader, R., Felten, D.L. and Cohen, N. (eds) (2001) *Psychoneuroimmunology*, 3rd edn, Vol. 2. San Diego, CA: Academic Press.

Adler, N.E. and Snibbe, A.C. (2003) The role of psychosocial processes in explaining the gradient between socioeconomic status and health. *Current Directions in Psychological Science*, **12** (4), 119–123.

Aertgeerts, B., Buntinx, F., Ansoms, S. and Fevery, J. (2001) Screening properties of questionnaires and laboratory tests for the detection of alcohol abuse or dependence in a general practice population. *British Journal of General Practice*, **51** (464), 206–217.

Age Concern (2006a) Older people in the United Kingdom: key facts and statistics 2006 (www.ageconcern.org.uk).

Age Concern (2006b) *Hungry to be Heard: The Scandal of Malnourished Older People in Hospital*. London: Age Concern England.

Ajzen, I. (1985) From intentions to actions: a theory of planned behavior. In Kuhl, J. and Beckmann, J. (eds) *Action Control: From Cognition to Behavior*, 11–39. New York: Springer Verlag.

Ajzen, I. (1988) *Attitudes, Personality, and Behaviour*. Homewood, IL: Dorsey Press.

Ajzen, I. and Fishbein, M. (1970) The prediction of behavior from attitudinal and normative variables. *Journal of Experimental Social Psychology*, **6** (4), 466–487.

Akers, R.L. (1977) *Deviant Behaviour: A Social Learning Approach*. Belmont, CA: Wadsworth.

Akhtar, S.G. (2002) Nursing with dignity. Part 8: Islam. *Nursing Times* **98** (16).

Albano, A.M. and Detweiler, M.F. (2001) The development and clinical impact of social anxiety and social phobia in children and adolescents. In Hofmann, S.G. and DiBartolo, P.M. (eds), *From Social Anxiety to Social Phobia: Multiple Perspectives*. Needham Heights, MA: Allyn & Bacon, 162–178.

Alberts, M.S., Lyons, J.S., Moretti, R.J. and Erickson, J.C. III (1989) Psychological interventions in the pre-surgical period. *International Journal of Psychiatry in Medicine*, **19** (1), 91–106.

Aldwin, C.M. and Park, C.L. (2004) Coping and physical health outcomes: an overview. *Psychology and Health*, **19** (3), 277–281.

Alford, P. *et al.* (1995) Should nurses wear uniforms? *Nursing Standard*, **9** (40), 52–53.

Allan, K.D. and Strokes, T.F. (1989) Paediatric behavioural dentistry. In Hensen, M., Eisler, R. and Miller, P. (eds), *Progress of Behaviour Modification*. Newbury Park, CA: Sage Publications, Vol. 24, 60–90.

Allport, F.H. (1920) The influence of group upon association and thought. *Journal of Experimental Psychology*, **3**, 159–182.

Allport, G.W. (1935) Attitudes. In Murchison, C.M. (ed.), *Handbook of Social Psychology*. Worcester, MA: Clark University Press, 789–844.

Alzheimer's Society (2004) *Policy Positions: Demography* (www.alzheimer.org.uk/News_and_campaigns/Policy_Watch/demography.htm).

Alzheimer's Society (2006) http://www.alzheimers.org.uk/site/index.php

Amir, M. and Ramati, A. (2002) Post-traumatic symptoms, emotional distress and quality of life in long-term survivors of breast cancer: a preliminary research. *Journal of Anxiety Disorders*, **16** (2), 191–206.

Amnesty International (1973) *Report on Torture.* London: Duckworth.

An Bord Altranais (2000) *Review of Scope of Practice for Nursing and Midwifery Final Report.* An Bord Altranais, Dublin.

Andersen, B.L., Farrar, W.B., Golden-Kreutz, D.M., Glaser, R., Emery, C.F., Crespin, T.R., Shapiro, C.L. and Carson, W.E. III (2004) Psychological, behavioural and immune changes after a psychological intervention: a clinical trial. *Journal of Clinical Oncology,* **22**, 3570–3580.

Andersen, C., Adamsen, L., Moeller, T., Midtgaard, J., Quist, M., Tveteraas, A. and Rorth, M. (2006) The effect of a multidimensional exercise programme on symptoms and side-effects in cancer patients undergoing chemotherapy – the use of semi-structured diaries. *European Journal of Oncology Nursing,* **10** (4), 247–262.

Anderson, K.O., Dowds, B.N., Pelletz, R.E., Edwards, T. and Peeters-Asdourian, C. (1995) Development and initial validation of a scale to measure self-efficacy beliefs in patients with chronic pain. *Pain,* **63** (1), 77–83.

Anderson, R.M., Fitzgerald, J.T. and, Oh, M.S. (1993) The relationship of diabetes-related attitudes and patients self-reported adherence. *Diabetes Education,* **19**, 287–292.

Andrew, M.M. and Boyle, J.S. (1995) *Transcultural Concepts in Nursing Care,* 2nd edn. Philadelphia: JB Lippincott Co.

Andrews, B., Brewin, C.R., Ochera, J., Morton, J., Bekerian, D.A., Davies, G.M. and Mollon, P. (2000) The timing, triggers and qualities of recovered memories in therapy. *British Journal of Clinical Psychology,* **39**, 11–26.

Antai-Obong, D. (2007) *Nurse–Client Communication: A Lifespan Approach.* Velmans Integrated Support Network. Boston, MA: Jones and Bartlett Publishers.

Antoni, M.H., Cruess, D.G. Cruess, S., Lutgendorf, S., Kumar, M., Ironson, G., Klimas, N., Fletcher, M.A. and Schneiderman, N. (2000) Cognitive-behavioral stress management intervention effects on anxiety, 24-hr urinary norepinephrine output, and T-cytotoxic/suppressor cells over time among symptomatic HIV-infected gay men. *Journal of Consulting and Clinical Psychology,* **68** (1), 31–45.

Antoni, M.H., Cruess, D.G., Klimas, N., Maher, K., Cruess, S., Kumar, M., Lutgendorf, S., Ironson, G., Schneiderman, N. and Fletcher, M.A. (2002) Stress management and immune system reconstitution in symptomatic HIV-infected gay men over time: effects on transitional naive T cells (CD4(+)CD(45)RA(+)CD29(+)). *American Journal of Psychiatry,* **159** (1), 143–145.

Antonovsky, A. (1987) *Unraveling the Mystery of Health: How People Manage Stress and Stay Well.* San Francisco, CA: Jossey-Bass.

Anxiety Care (2007) *Overcoming Medical Phobias.* Essex (http://www.anxietycare.org.uk/docs/medical.asp, accessed 14 June 2007).

Arakawa, S. (1997) Relaxation to reduce nausea, vomiting and anxiety induced by chemotherapy in Japanese patients. *Cancer Nursing,* **20**, 342–349.

Arantzamendi, M. and Kearney, N. (2004) The psychological needs of patients receiving chemotherapy: an exploration of nurse perceptions. *European Journal of Cancer Care,* **13** (1), 23–31.

Archibald, C. (2003) *People with Dementia in Acute Hospital Settings: A Practical Guide for Registered Nurses.* Stirling: The Dementia Services Development Centre.

Argyle, M. (1994) *The Psychology of Interpersonal Behaviour,* 5th edn. London: Penguin.

Armitage, C.J. and Conner, M. (2002) *The Social Psychology of Food.* Philadelphia: Open University Press.

Armstrong-Esther, C.A. and Browne, K.D. (1986) The influence of elderly patients' mental impairment on nurse–patient interaction. *J. Adv. Nurs.* **11** (4), 379–387.

Armstrong-Esther, C.A., Sandilands, M.L. and Miller, D. (1989) Attitudes and behaviours of nurses towards the elderly in an acute care setting. *Journal of Advanced Nursing,* **14**, 34–41.

Arnett, J.J. (2000) Optimistic bias in adolescent and adult smokers and nonsmokers. *Addictive Behaviors,* **25** (4), 625–632.

Arnetz, B.B., Wasserman, J., Petrini, B., Brenner, S.O., Levi, L., Eneroth, P., Salovaara, H., Hjelm, R., Salovaara, L., Theorell, T. and Petterson, I.L. (1987) Immune function in unemployed women. *Psychosomatic Medicine,* **49** (1), 3–12.

Arons, B. (2005) A Review of the Cocktail Party Effect (http://www.media.mit.edu/speech/papers/1992/arons_AVI OSJ92_cocktail_party_effect.pdf, accessed 23 May 2007).

Asch, S.E. (1951) Effects on group pressure upon the modification and distortion of judgements. In Guetzkow, H. (ed.), *Groups, Leadership and Men.* Pittsburgh: Carnegie Press, 177–190.

Asch, S.E. (1952) *Social Psychology.* Englewood Cliffs, NJ: Prentice Hall.

Asch, S.E. (1956) Studies of independence and conformity: a minority of one against a unanimous majority. *Psychological Monographs: General and Applied,* **70** (416), 1–70.

Aseltine, R.H., Gore, S. and Colten, M.E. (1994) Depression and the social developmental context of adolescence. *Journal of Personality and Social Psychology,* **67** (2), 252–263.

ASH (2007) *ASH Facts at a Glance: 01 Smoking Statistics.* London: ASH.

Ashmore, R.D. and Del Boca, F.K. (1981) Conceptual approaches to stereotypes and stereotyping. In Hamilton, D. (ed.), *Cognitive Processes in Stereotyping and Intergroup Behavior,* 37–81. Hillsdale, NJ: Erlbaum Publishers.

Asim, A.J., Stewart, A. and Tavel, L. (2007) *Medication Adherence and Patient Education.* Chapter 7. http://www.faetc.org/PDF/Primary_Care_Guide/Chapter_07-Medication_Adherence.pdf.

Atkins, L. and Fallowfield, L. (2006) Intentional and non-intentional non-adherence to medication amongst breast cancer patients. *European Journal of Cancer,* **42** (14), 2271–2276.

Atkinson, R.C. and Shiffrin, R.M. (1968) Human memory: a proposed system and its control processes. In Spence, K.W. and Spence, J.T. (eds), *The Psychology of Learning and Motivation: Advances in Research and Theory.* New York: Academic Press, 89–195.

Audit Commission (1993) *What Seems to be the Matter: Communication between Hospital and Patients.* National Health Service Report No. 12, London: HMSO.

Auerbach, S.M. (1973) Trait-state anxiety and adjustment of surgery. *Journal of Consulting and Clinical Psychology,* **40** (2), 264–271.

Avis, N.E., Crawford, S. and Manuel, J. (2005) Quality of life among younger women with breast cancer. *Journal of Clinical Oncology,* **23** (15), 3322–3330.

Ayer, S. (1997) Cultural diversity: issues of race and ethnicity in learning disability. In Gates, B. and Beacock, C. (eds), *Dimensions of Learning Disability.* London: Bailliere Tindall, 181–202.

Babor, T.F. and Grant, M. (1992) *WHO Collaborating Investigators Project on Identification and Management of Alcohol Related Problems. Combined analyses of outcome data: the cross national generalizability of brief interventions. Report on phase II: A randomized clinical trial of brief interventions in primary health care.* Copenhagen: WHO.

Bachiocco, V., Rucci, P. and Carli, G. (1996) Request of analgesics in post-surgical pain. Relationships to psychological factors and pain-related variables. *Pain Clinic,* **9** (2), 169–179.

Baddeley, A.D. (1986) *Working Memory.* Oxford: Clarendon.

Baddeley, A.D. and Hitch, G.J. (1974) Working memory. In Bower, G.H. (ed.), *The Psychology of Learning and Motivation: Advances in Research and Theory,* Vol. 8. New York: Academic Press.

Baile, W., Buckman, R., Lenzie, R., Glober, G., Beale, E. and Kundelka, A. (2000) SPIKES – a six-step protocol for delivering bad news: application to the patient with cancer. *The Oncologist,* **5** (4), 302–311.

Bajekal, M., Primatesta, P. and Prior, G. (2003) *Health Survey for England, 2001.* London: Stationery Office.

Baker, A.H. and Wardle, J. (2003) Sex differences in fruit and vegetable intake in older adults. *Appetite,* **40** (3), 269–275.

Baker, D.W., Parker, R.M., Williams, M.V., Coates, W.C. and Pitkin, K. (1996) Use and effectiveness of interpreters in an emergency department. *Journal of the American Medical Association,* **275**, 783–788.

Balint, M., Joyce, D., Marinker, M. and Woodcock, J. (1970) *Treatment or diagnosis: a study of repeat prescriptions in general practice.* London: Tavistock Publications.

Balling, K. and McCubbin, M. (2001) Hospitalized children with chronic illness: parental caregiving needs and valuing parental expertise. *Journal of Pediatric Nursing,* **16**, 110–119.

Baltes, M.M. and Skinner, E.A. (1983) Cognitive performance deficits and hospitalisation: learned helplessness, instrumental passivity, or what? Comment on Raps, Peterson, Jonas and Seligman. *Journal of Personality and Social Psychology,* **45** (5), 1013–1016.

Bandura, A. (1965) Influence of model's reinforcement contingencies on the acquisition of imitative response. *Journal of Personality and Social Psychology,* **1** (6), 589–595.

Bandura, A. (1977) *Social Learning Theory.* Englewood Cliffs, NJ: Prentice Hall.

Bandura, A. (1986) The social learning perspective: mechanisms of aggression. In Toch, H. (ed.), *Psychology of Crime and Criminal Justice.* Prospect Heights, IL: Waveland Press, **xiv**, 198–236; 487.

Bandura, A. (1991) Social cognitive theory of self–regulation [Special issue: Theories of cognitive self regulation]. *Organizational Behaviour and Human Decision Process,* **50** (20), 248–287.

Banks, J., Marmot, M., Oldfield, Z. and Smith, J.P. (2006) Disease and disadvantage in the United States and in England. *Journal of the American Medical Association,* **295** (17), 2037–2045.

Barber, J. (1998) The mysterious persistence of hypnotic analgesia. *International Journal of Clinical and Experimental Hypnosis,* **46** (1), 28–43.

Bardwell, W.A., Natarajan, L., Dimsdale, J.E., Rock, C.E., Mortimer, J.E., Hollenbach, K. and Pierce, J.P. (2006) Objective cancer-related variables are not associated with depressive symptoms in women treated for early-stage breast cancer. *Journal of Clinical Oncology,* **24** (16), 2420–2427.

Barker, P., Manos, E., Novak, V. and Reynolds, B. (1998) The wounded healer and the myth of well-being: ethical issues concerning the mental health status of psychiatric needs. In Barker, P. and Davidson, B. (eds), *Psychiatric Nursing: Ethical Strife.* London: Arnold.

Barnes, K.E. (1990) An examination of nurses' feelings about patients with specific feeding needs. *Journal of Advanced Nursing,* **15**, 703–711.

Baron, R.A. (2001) *Psychology,* 5th edn. Boston, MA: Allyn and Bacon.

Baron, R.A. and Byrne, D. (2000) *Social Psychology* (8th edn). Toronto, ON: Allyn & Bacon.

Barre, T. and Evans, R. (2002) Nursing observations in the acute inpatient setting: a contribution to the debate. *Mental Health Practice,* **5** (10), 10–14.

Bartlett, E.E., Grayson, M., Barker, R., Levine, D.M., Golden, A. and Libber, S. (1984) The effects of physician communications skills on patient satisfaction; recall and adherence. *Journal of Chronic Diseases,* **37** (9/10), 755–764.

Bastable, S. (1997) *Nurse as Educator. Principles of Teaching and Learning.* London: Jones and Bartlett.

Bauman, K.E., Foshee, V.A., Linzer, M.A. and Koch, G.G. (1990) Effect of parental smoking classification on the association between parental and adolescent smoking. *Addictive Behaviors,* **15** (5), 413–422.

Baxter, C. (2002) Nursing with dignity Part 5: Rastafarianism. *Nursing Times,* **98** (13) (www.nursingtimes.net).

Beck, A.T. (1976) *Cognitive Therapy and the Emotional Disorders.* New York: New American Library.

Becker, M.H. (1974) Health belief model and sick role behaviour. *Health Education Monographs,* **2** (4), 409–419.

Becker, M.H. and Rosenstock, I.M. (1987) Comparing social learning theory and the health belief model. In Ward, W.B. (ed.) *Advances in health education and promotion,* Volume 2, 245–249. Greenwich, CT: JAI Press.

Beech, B. and Bowyer, D. (2004) Management of aggression and violence in mental health settings. *Mental Health Practice,* **7** (7), 31–37.

Beecher, H.K. (1959) Generalization from pain of various types and diverse origins. *Science*, 130, 267–268.

Begley, C.M. and White, P. (2003) Irish nursing students' changing self-esteem and fear of negative evaluation during their pre-registration programme. *Journal of Advanced Nursing*, 42 (4), 390–401.

Belloc, N.B. and Breslow, L. (1972) Relationship of physical health status and health practices. *Preventative Medicine*, 1 (3), 409–421.

Bender, B.G. (2002) Overcoming barriers to nonadherence in asthma treatment. *Journal of Allergy and Clinical Immunology*, 109 (6 Supplement), S554–S559.

Bensing, J.M., Kerssens, J.J. and van der Pasch, M. (1995) Patient-directed gaze as a tool for discovering and handling psychosocial problems in general practice. *Journal of Nonverbal Behaviour*, 19 (4), 223–243.

Bentley, J. (2002) *The Experiences of Children Attending Accident and Emergency with Minor Injuries*. Unpublished doctoral thesis. University of West England, Bristol.

Bentley, J. (2004) Distress in children attending A&E. *Emergency Nurse*, 12 (4), 20–26.

Benton, D. (1999) Assertiveness, power and influence. *Nursing Standard*, 13 (52), 48–52.

Bentzen, N., Christiansen, T. and Pedersen, K.M. (1989) Self-care within a model for demand for medical care. *Social Science & Medicine Special Issue: Health Self-care*, 29 (2), 185–193.

Benzeval, M., Judge, K. and Smaje, C. (1995) Beyond class, race, and ethnicity – deprivation and health in Britain. *Health Services Research*, 30 (1), 163–177.

Ben-Zur, H., Gilbar, O. and Lev, S. (2001) Coping with breast cancer: patient, spouse, and dyad models. *Psychosomatic Medicine*, 63 (1), 32–39.

Bergman, A.B. and Werner, R.J. (1963) Failure of children to receive penicillin by mouth. *New England Journal of Medicine*, 268, 1334–1338.

Berichte über die Verhandlungen der Koniglich Sächsischen Gesellshaft der Wissenschaften, 46, 283–297.

Berkman, L.F. and Syme, S.L. (1979) Social networks, host-resistance, and mortality – 9-year follow-up study of Alameda County residents. *American Journal of Epidemiology*, 109(2), 186–204.

Berkman, L.F., Leosummers, L. and Horwitz, R.I. (1992) Emotional support and survival after myocardial-infarction – a prospective, population-based study of the elderly. *Annals of Internal Medicine*, 117 (12), 1003–1009.

Berkman, L.F., Glass, T., Brissette, I. and Seeman, T.E. (2000) From social integration to health: Durkheim in the new millennium. *Social Science and Medicine*, 51 (6), 843–857.

Berlowitz, D.R., Ash, A.S., Hickey, E.C., Friedman, R.H., Glickman, M., Kader, B. and Moskowitz, M.A. (1998) Inadequate management of blood pressure in a hypertensive population. *New England Journal of Medicine*, 339 (27), 1957–1963.

Berlyne, D.E. (1960) *Conflict, Arousal, and Curiosity*. New York: McGraw-Hill.

Bertakis, K.D. (1977) The communication of information from physician to patient: a method for increasing patient retention and satisfaction. *Journal of Family Practice*, 5, 217–222.

Bibace, R. and Walsh, M.E. (1980) Development of children's concept of illness. *Paediatrics*, 66 (6), 912–917.

Biddle, L., Gunnell, D. and Sharp, D. (2004) Factors influencing help seeking in mentally distressed young adults: a cross-sectional survey. *British Journal of General Practice*, 54 (501), 248–253.

Biddle, S.J.H. and Nigg, C.R. (2000) Theories of exercise behaviour. *International Journal of Sport Psychology Special Issue: Exercise Psychology*, 31 (2), 290–304.

Bishop, S. (2000) *Developing Your Assertiveness*, 2nd edn. London: Kogan Page.

Blakely, T.A., Collings, S.C. and Atkinson, J. (2003) Unemployment and suicide. Evidence for a causal association? *Journal of Epidemiology & Community Health*, 57 (8), 594–600.

Blatt, S.J. (2004) *Experiences of Depression. Theoretical, Clinical and Research Perspectives*. Washington, DC: American Psychological Association.

Blaxter, M. (1976) *The Meaning of Disability: A Sociological Study of Impairment*. Cambridge: Heinemann.

Blaxter, M. (1983) Inequalities in health – The Black Report – Townsend, P., Davidson, N. *Journal of Social Policy*, 12, 284–285.

Blaxter, M. (1990) *Health and Lifestyles*. London: Tavistock/Routledge.

Blaxter, M. (1995) What is health? In Davey, B., Gray, A. and Seale, C. (eds), *Health and Disease*. Buckingham: Open University Press.

Block, G., Patterson, B. and Subar, A. (1992) Fruit, vegetables, and cancer prevention: a review of the epidemiological evidence. *Nutrition and Cancer*, 18, 1–29.

Bloom, J.R. (1986) Social support and adjustment to breast cancer. In Andersen, B.L. (ed.), *Women with Cancer: Psychological Perspectives*. New York: Springer, 204–229.

Bloom, J.R. and Spiegel, D. (1984) The relationship of 2 dimensions of social support to the psychological well-being and social functioning of women with advanced breast-cancer. *Social Science and Medicine*, 19 (8), 831–837.

Bloom, J.R., Stewart, S.L., Johnston, M. and Banks, P. (1998) Intrusiveness of illness and quality of life in young women with breast cancer. *Psycho-Oncology*, 7 (2), 89–100.

Blount, R.L., Bachanas, P.J., Powers, S.W., Cotter, M., Franklin, A., Chaplin, W., Mayfield, J., Henderson, M. and Blount, S. (1992) Training children to cope and parents to coach them during routine immunizations: effects on child, parent, and staff behaviours. *Behaviour Therapy*, 23 (4), 689–705.

Bolus, R. and Pitts, J. (1999) Patient satisfaction: the indispensable outcome [online] *Rand Research Paper* (http://www.managedcaremag.com/archives/9904/9904.patsatis.html~#Increasing, accessed 23 January 2004).

Bonow, R.O., Smaha, L.A., Smith, S.C., Mensah, G.A. and Lenfant, C. (2002) World Heart Day 2002 – The international burden of cardiovascular disease: Responding to the emerging global epidemic. *Circulation*, 106 (13), 1602–1605.

Booth, K., Maguire, P.M., Butterworth, T. and Hillier, V. (1996) Perceived professional support and the use of blocking behaviours by hospice nurses. *Journal of Advanced Nursing*, **24** (3), 522–527.

Boscarino, J.A., Adams, R.E. and Galea, S. (2006) Alcohol use in New York after the terrorist attacks: a study of the effects of psychological trauma on drinking behaviour. *Addictive Behaviors*, **31** (4), 606–621.

Bosma, H., Peter, R., Siegrist, J. and Marmot, M. (1998) Two alternative job stress models and the risk of coronary heart disease. *American Journal of Public Health*, **88** (1), 68–74.

Bosscher, R. and Smit, J. (1998) Confirmatory factor analysis of the General Self-efficacy Scale. *Behaviour Research and Therapy*, **36** (3), 339–343.

Bottorff, J.L. and Morse, J.M. (1994) Identifying types of attending patterns of nurses work. *Journal of Nursing Scholarship*, **26** (1), 53–60.

Bottorff, J.L., Johnson, J.L., Irwin, L.G. and Ratner, P.A. (2000) Narratives of smoking relapse: the stories of postpartum women. *Research in Nursing and Health*, **23** (2), 126–134.

Bovbjerg, D.H., Reed, W.H. and Jacobsen, P.B. (1992) An experimental analysis of classically conditioned nausea during cancer chemotherapy. *Psychosomatic Medicine*, **54** (6), 623–637.

Bowers, L. (2005) Reasons for admission and their implications for the nature of acute inpatient psychiatric nursing. *Journal of Psychiatric and Mental Health Nursing*, **12**, 231–236.

Bowlby, J. (1969) *Attachment and Loss*. New York: Basic Books.

Bowling, A. (2004) *Measuring Health: A Review of Quality of Life Measurement Scales*. Buckingham: Open University Press.

Bowling, A. and Gabriel, Z. (2004) An integrational model of quality of life in older age: results from the ESRC/MRC HSRC Quality of Life Survey in Britain. *Social Indicators Research*, **69** (1), 1–36.

Bowling, A., See-Tai, S., Ebrahim, S., Gabriel, Z. and Solanki, P. (2005) Attributes of age-identity. *Aging and Society*, **25**, 479–500.

Bradley, J.C. and Edinberg, M.A. (1990) *Communication in the Nursing Context*, 3rd edn. Connecticut: Appleton and Lange.

Brandon, T.H. and Brandon, K.O. (2005) Brother, can you spare a smoke? Sibling transmission of tobacco use. *Addiction*, **100** (4), 439–440.

Braslis, K.G., Santa-Cruz, C., Brickman, A.L. and Solloway, M.S. (1994) Quality of life 12 months after radical prostatectomy. *British Journal of Urology*, **75** (1), 48–53.

Brennan, A. (1994) Caring for children during procedures. A review of the literature. *Pediatric Nursing*. 20(5), 451–458.

Brewer, S., Gleditsch, S.L., Syblik, D., Tietjens, M.E. and Vacik, H.W. (2006) Paediatric anxiety: child life intervention in day surgery. *Journal of Paediatric Nursing*, **21** (1), 13–22.

Bricker, J.B., Leroux, B.G., Andersen, M.R. *et al.* (2005a) Parental smoking cessation and children's smoking: mediation by antismoking actions. *Nicotine and Tobacco Research*, **7** (4), 501–509.

Bricker, J.B., Peterson, A.V., Rajan, K.B. *et al.* (2005b) Role of close friends' vs. parents' and older siblings' smoking in children's 12th grade smoking: a prospective study. *Nicotine and Tobacco Research*, **7** (4), 686–687.

Bricker, J.B., Rajan, K.B., Andersen, M.R. *et al.* (2005c) Does parental smoking cessation encourage their young adult children to quit smoking? A prospective study. *Addiction*, **100** (3), 379–386.

Brismar, B. and Bergman, B. (1998) The significance of alcohol for violence and accidents. *Alcoholism – Clinical and Experimental Research*, **22** (7) (Suppl.), 299S–306S.

Bristol and District People First (2003) *We are People First*. (Film) Bristol: People First.

Bristol Royal Infirmary Inquiry Report (2001) http://www.bristol-inquiry.org.uk/final_report/report/.

British Deaf Association (2005) *About British Sign Language (BSL)*. London: BDA.

Britt, T.W., Doherty, K. and Schlenker, B.R. (1997) Self-evaluation as a function of self-esteem, performance feedback and self presentational role. *Journal of Social and Clinical Psychology*, **16** (4), 463–483.

Broadbent, D.E. (1958) *Perception and Communication*. London: Pergamon Press.

Bromley, J. and Emerson, E. (1995) Beliefs and emotional reactions of care staff working with people with challenging behaviour. *Journal of Intellectual Disability*, **39**, 341–352.

Browes, S. (2006) Health psychology and sexual health assessment. *Nursing Standard*, **21** (5), 35–39.

Brown, C., Pirmohamed, M. and Park, B.K. (1997) Nurses' confidence in caring for patients with alcohol-related problems. *Professional Nurse*, **13** (2), 83–86.

Brown, P. (2006) Risk versus need in revising the 1983 mental health act: conflicting claims, muddled policy. *Health, Risk and Society*, **8** (4), 343–358.

Bruera, E., Pituskin, E., Calder, K. *et al.* (1999) The addition of an audiocassette recording of a consultation to written recommendations for patients with advanced cancer. *Cancer*, **86**, 2420–2425.

Brummett, B.H., Barefoot, J.C., Siegler, I.C., Clapp-Channing, N.E., Lytle, B.L., Bosworth, H.B., Williams, R.B. and Mark, D.B. (2001) Characteristics of socially isolated patients with coronary artery disease who are at elevated risk for mortality. *Psychosomatic Medicine*, **63** (2), 267–272.

Bruner, J. (1983) Play, thought, and language, *Peabody Journal of Education*, **60** (3), 60–69.

Brunner, L.S. and Suddarth, D.S. (eds) (1993) *Lippincott Manual of Medical Surgical Nursing*, 2nd edn. London: Chapman and Hall.

Bruster, S., Jarman, B., Bosanquet, N. *et al.* (1994) National survey for hospital patients. *British Medical Journal*, **309** (6968), 1542–1546.

Bryan, A.D., Aiken, L.S. and West, S.G. (1996) Increasing condom use: evaluation of a theory-based intervention to prevent sexually transmitted diseases in young women. *Health Psychology*, **15** (5), 371–382.

Bryan, A.D., Aiken, L.S. and West, S.G. (1997) Young women's condom use: the influence of acceptance of sexuality, control over the sexual encounter, and perceived susceptibility to common STDs. *Health Psychology*, **16** (5), 468–479.

BTS and SIGN (2003) British guideline on the management of asthma. *Thorax*, 58 (Suppl. 1), i1–i94.

Buchanan, P. (2001) Skin cancer. *Nursing Standard*, 15 (45), 45–52.

Buchanan-Barrow, E., Barrett, M. and Bati, M. (2005) Children's understanding of illness: the generalisation of illness according to exemplar, *Journal of Health Psychology*, 8 (6), 659–670.

Budd, T. (1999) *Violence at Work: Findings from the British Crime Survey*. London: Home Office.

Bugental, J.F.T. (1964) The third force in psychology. *Journal of Humanistic Psychology*, **4** (1), 19–25.

Bukovic, D., Fajdic, J., Hrgovic, Z., Kaufmann, M., Hojsak, I. and Stanceric, T. (2005) Sexual dysfunction in breast cancer survivors. *Onkologie*, **28** (1), 29–34.

Bull, P.E. (1987) *Posture and Gesture* (Vol. 16). Oxford: Pergamon Press.

Bulman, C. and Schutz, S. (2004) *Reflective Practice in Nursing*, 3rd edn. Oxford: Blackwell Publishing.

Bulsara, C., Ward, A. and Joske, D. (2004) Haematological cancer patients: achieving a sense of empowerment by use of strategies to control illness. *Journal of Advanced Nursing*, **13**, 251–258.

Bunker, S.J., Colquhoun, D.M., Esler, M.D., Hickie, I.B., Hunt, D., Jelinek, V.M., Oldenburg, B.F., Peach, H.G., Ruth, D., Tennant, C.C. and Tonkin, A.M. (2003) 'Stress' and coronary heart disease: psychosocial risk factors. National Heart Foundation of Australia position statement update. *Medical Journal of Australia*, **178** (6), 272–276.

Bupa (2004) *Improving Assertiveness*. Bupa Health Information Fact Sheet. http://hcd2.bupa.co.uk/fact_sheets/html/improving_assertiveness.html

Burgess, C., Ramirez, A.J., Richards, M.A. and Love, S.B. (1998) Who and what influences delayed presentation in breast cancer? *British Journal of Cancer*, **77** (8), 1343–1348.

Burgess, C., Ramirez, A., Cornelius, V., Love, S. and Graham, J. (2002) Do other stressful life experiences increase the risk of depression in women with breast cancer? *Psycho-Oncology*, **11** (6), 548–548.

Burgess, C., Cornelius, V., Love, S., Graham, J., Richards, M. and Ramirez, A. (2005) Depression and anxiety in women with early breast cancer: five year observational cohort study. *British Medical Journal*, **330**, 702–705.

Burgess, L., Page, S. and Hardman, P. (2006) Changing attitudes in dementia care and the roles of nurses. *Nursing Times*, 99 (18).

Burgoon, J.K., Buller, D.B. and Woodall, W.G. (1989) *Nonverbal communication: The unspoken dialogue*. New York: Harper & Row.

Burnard, P. (2002) *Learning Human Skills: An Experiential Guide for Nurses*. Oxford: Heinemann.

Burnard, P. and Morrison, P. (1998) *Know Yourself: Self-awareness Activities for Nurses and Other Health Professionals*. London: Whurr Publishers.

Burnard, P. and Morrison, P. (1991) *Caring & Communicating ... In Nursing*. London: Macmillan.

Bush, T. (2003) Communicating with patients who have dementia. *Nursing Times*, **99** (42).

Butow, P.N., Hiller, J.E., Price, M.A., Thackway, S.V., Kricker, A. and Tennant, C.C. (2000) Epidemiological evidence for a relationship between life events, coping style, and personality factors in the development of breast cancer. *Journal of Psychosomatic Research*, **49** (3), 169–181.

Butz, A.M. (1995) Social factors associated with behavioural problems in children with asthma. *Clinical Pediatrics*, **34** (11), 581–590.

Byrne, A. and Byrne, D. (1992) *Psychology for Nurses: Theory and Practice*. Basingstoke: Macmillan.

Byrne, R.S. (2005) Magical Dreams, Visions of Reality: Guidelines for Developing a Grief Center for Children; Practical Suggestions: Talking to a Grieving Child: A Guide for Classroom Teachers. In Doka, K.J. (ed.) *Living With Grief: Children, Adolescents, and Loss*. Miami Beach, FL: Hospice Foundation of America.

Calley, P. (1990) Moral learning in nursing education: a discussion of the usefulness of cognitive development and social learning theories. *Journal of Advanced Nursing*, **15** (3), 324–328.

Calnan, M. (1987) *Health and Illness – The Lay Perspective*. London: Tavistock.

Calnan, M., Woodhead, G. and Dieppe, P. (2003) Courtesy entitles. *Health Service Journal*, **113** (5843), 30–31.

Calnan, M., Woolhead, G., Dieppe, P. and Tadd, W. (2005) Views on dignity in providing health care for older people. *Nursing Times*, **101**, 38–41.

Cameron, L.D. and Leventhal, H. (2003) *The Self-regulation of Health and Illness Behaviour*. London: Routledge.

Campbell, I.E., Larrivee, P., Field, P.A., Day, R.A. and Reutter, L. (1994) Learning to nurse in the clinical setting. *Journal of Advanced Nursing*, **20** (6), 1125–1131.

Campbell, J.D. (1990) Self-esteem and clarity of the self-concept. *Journal of Personality and Social Psychology*, **59**, 538–549.

Campbell, K.L. and McTiernan, A. (2007) Exercise and biomarkers for cancer prevention studies. *Journal of Nutrition*, **137** (1 Suppl), 161S–169S.

Cannon, W.B. (1929) *Bodily Changes in Pain. Hunger, Fear, and Rage: Researches into the Function of Emotional Excitement*. New York: Harper and Row.

Cappell, H.D. (1987) Reports From The Research Centers. 4. The Addiction Research Foundation of Ontario. *British Journal Of Addiction*, **82** (10), 1081–1089.

Caress, A.L. (2003) Giving information to patients. *Nursing Standard*, **17** (43), 47–54.

Carey, M.P., Kalra, D.L., Carey, K.B., Halperin, S. and Richards, C.S. (1993) Stress and unaided smoking cessation – a prospective investigation. *Journal of Consulting and Clinical Psychology*, **61** (5), 831–838.

Carey, P. (1985) Manner and meaning in West Sumatra: the social-context of consciousness. *The Times Literary Supplement*, **4305**, 112.

Caris-Verhallen, W.M.C.M., Kerkstra, A. and Bensing, J.M. (1997) The role of communication in nursing care for the elderly: a review of the literature. *Journal of Advanced Nursing*, 25, 915–933.

Caris-Verhallen, W.M.C.M., de Gruijter, I.M., Kerkstra, A. and Bensing, J.M. (1999a) Factors related to nurse communication with elderly people. *Journal of Advanced Nursing*, 30 (5), 1106–1117.

Caris-Verhallen, W.M.C.M., Kerkstra, A. and Bensing, J.M. (1999b) Non-verbal behaviour in nurse–elderly patient communication. *Journal of Advanced Nursing*, 29 (4), 808–818.

Carr, E., Brockbank, K., Allen, S. and Strike, P. (2006) Patterns and frequency of anxiety in women undergoing gynaecological surgery. *Journal of Clinical Nursing*, 15 (3), 341–352.

Carr, E.C.J. (1990) Post-operative pain: patients' expectations and experiences. *Journal of Advanced Nursing*, 15, 89–100.

Carr, E.C.J., Thomas, V.N. and Wilson-Barnet, J. (2005) Patient experiences of anxiety, depression and acute pain after surgery: a longitudinal perspective. *International Journal of Nursing Studies*, 42 (5), 521–530.

Carr, M. and Kurtz, B. (1991) Teachers' perceptions of their students' metacognition, attributions and self-concept. *British Journal of Educational Psychology*, 61, 197–206.

Carroll, D. and Seers, K. (1998) Relaxation for the relief of chronic pain: a systematic review. *Journal of Advanced Nursing*, 27 (3), 466–475.

Carson, D.K., Council, J.R. and Gravley, J.E. (1991) Temperament and family characteristics as predictors of children's reactions to hospitalisation. *Journal of Developmental and Behavioural Paediatrics*, 12 (3), 141–147.

Carthey, J. (2006) Involving and communicating with patients and the public. *Nursing Standard*, 20 (17), 50–53.

Cartwright, M., Wardle, J., Steggles, N., Simon, A.E., Croker, H. and Jarvis, M.J. (2003) Stress and dietary practices in adolescents. *Health Psychology*, 22 (4), 362–369.

Caruso, A., Di Francesco, B., Pugliese, P., Cinanni, V. and Corlito, A. (2000) Information and awareness of diagnosis and progression of cancer in adult and elderly cancer patients. *Tumori*, 86 (3), 199–203.

Carver, C.S., Pozo, C., Harris, S.D., Noriega, V., Scheier, M.F., Robinson, D.S., Ketcham, A.S., Moffat Jr, F.L. and Clark, K.C. (1993) How coping mediates the effect of optimism on distress – a study of women with early-stage breast-cancer. *Journal of Personality and Social Psychology*, 65 (2), 375–390.

Carver, C.S., Pozo-Kaderman, C., Price, A.A., Noriega, V., Harrism, S.D., Derhagopian, R.P., Robinson, D.S. and Moffat Jr, F.L. (1998) Concern about aspects of body image and adjustment to early stage breast cancer. *Psychosomatic Medicine*, 60 (2), 168–174.

Carver, E. and Hughes, J. (1990) The significance of empathy. In MacKay, R., Hughes, J. and Carver, E. (eds), *Empathy in the helping relationship*. New York: Springer Publishing Company.

Castledine, G. (1998) The standard of nursing records should be raised. *British Journal of Nursing*, 7 (3), 172.

Castledine, G. (2002) Nurses must ensure they communicate with clients. *British Journal of Nursing*, 11 (21), 1419.

Castoro, C., Drace, C.A. and Baccaglini, U. (2006) Patient information, assessment and preparation of day cases. In Lemos, P., Jarret, P. and Phillip, B. (eds), *Day Surgery: Development and Practice*. Porto: International Association of Ambulatory Surgery, 157–184.

Caumo, W., Schmidt, A.P., Schneider, C.N., Bergmann, J., Iwamoto, C.W., Bandeira, D. and Ferreira, M.B.C. (2001) Risk factors for postoperative anxiety in adults. *Anaesthesia*, 56 (8), 720–728.

Chambers, C.T., Craig, K.D. and Bennett, S.M. (2002) The impact of maternal behaviour on children's pain experience: an experimental analysis. *Journal of Paediatric Psychology*, 27 (3), 293–301.

Chambers, C.T., Finley, G.A., McGrath, P.J. and Walsh, T.M. (2003) The parents' postoperative pain measure: replication and extension to 2–6-year-old children. *Pain*, 105 (3), 437–443.

Chang, G., McNamara, T.K., Orav, E.J., Koby, D., Lavigne, A., Ludman, B., Vincitorio, V.A. and Wilkins-Haug, L. (2005) Brief intervention for prenatal alcohol use: a randomised trial. *Obstetrics and Gynaecology*, 105, 991–998.

Charters, A. (2000) Role modelling as a teaching method. *Emergency Nurse*, 7 (10), 25–29.

Chassin, L., Curran, P.J., Hussong, A.M. and Colder, C.R. (1996) The relation of parent alcoholism to adolescent substance use: a longitudinal follow-up study. *Journal of Abnormal Psychology*, 105 (1), 70–80.

Chenevert, M. (1996) *Professional Nurse Handbook: Designed for the Nurse Who Wants to Thrive Professionally*, 3rd edn. St Louis: Mosby.

Chernoff, R.G., Ireys, H.T., DeVet, K.A. and Kim, Y. (2002) A randomised, controlled trial of a community-based support program for families of children with chronic illness: paediatric outcomes. *Archives of Paediatrics and Adolescent Medicine*, 156 (6), 533–539.

Cherry, C. (1966) *On Human Communication: A Review, a Survey, and a Criticism*, 2nd edn. Cambridge, MA: MIT Press.

Cheston, R. and Bender, M. (2000) *Understanding dementia: The man with the worried eyes*. London: Jessica Kingsley.

Cheung, Y.L., Molassiotis, A. and Chang, A.M. (2003) The effect of progressive muscle relaxation training on anxiety and quality of life after stoma surgery in colorectal cancer patients. *Psycho-Oncology*, 12 (3), 254–266.

Chevannes, M. (1997) Nursing caring for families – issues in a multiracial society. *Journal of Clinical Nursing*, 6, 161–167.

Chick, J., Lloyd, G. and Crombie, E. (1985) Counselling problem drinkers in medical wards: a controlled study. *British Medical Journal (Clinical Research Edition)*, 30, 965–967.

Child-Clarke, A. (2003) Nursing care: following trauma a cognitive behavioural approach. *Mental Health Nursing Practice*, 7 (3), 34–37.

Chives, J. (2003) Care of older people with visual impairment. *Nursing Older People*, 115 (1), 22–26.

Christmas, M. (2002) Nursing with dignity Part 3: Christianity I. *Nursing Times*, 98 (11), 37–39 (www.nursingtimes.net).

Ciccocioppo, R. and Hyytia, P. (2006) The genetic of alcoholism: learning from 50 years of research. *Addiction Biology*, 11 (3–4), 193–194.

Clark, A. (1999) Changing attitudes through persuasive communication. *Nursing Standard*, 13 (30), 45–47.

Clark, A.M. (2003) 'It's like an explosion in your life...': lay perspectives on stress and myocardial infarction. *Journal of Clinical Nursing*, 12, 544–553.

Clatworthy, S., Simon, K. and Tiedeman, M.E. (1999) Child drawing: hospital – an instrument designed to measure the emotional status of hospitalized school-aged children. *Journal of Paediatric Nursing*, 14 (1), 2–9.

Clay, R.A. (2002) A renaissance for humanistic psychology. The field explores new niches while building on its past. *American Psychological Association Monitor*, 33, (8).

Clearly, B. and Gifford, B. (1990) Supporting the bereaved. *American Journal of Nursing*, 90, 49–54.

Closs, S.J. (1994) Pain in elderly patients: a neglected phenomenon. *Journal of Advanced Nursing*, 19, 1072–1081.

Closs, S.J., Fairlough, H.I., Tierney, A.J. and Currie, C.T. (1993) Pain in elderly orthopedic patients. *Journal of Clinical Nursing*, 2, 41–45.

Cobb, N.K., Graham, A.L., Bock, B.C., Papandonatos, G. and Abrams, D.B. (2005) Initial evaluation of a real-world Internet smoking cessation system. *Nicotine and Tobacco Research*, 7 (2), 207–216.

Cohen, L.L. (2002) Reducing infant immunization distress through distraction, *Health Psychology*, 21 (2), 207–211.

Cohen, L., Savary, C. and de Moor, C. (2000) Stress and social support affect immune function in cancer patients receiving vaccine treatment. *Psychosomatic Medicine*, 62 (1), 1137.

Cohen, L.L., Blount, R.L. and Panopoulos, G. (1997) Nurse coaching and cartoon distraction: an effective and practical intervention to reduce child, parent, and nurse distress during immunizations. *Journal of Paediatric Psychology*, 22 (3), 355–370.

Cohen, L.L., Bernard, R.S., Greco, L.A. and McClellan, C.B. (2002) A child-focused intervention for coping with procedural pain: are parent and nurse coaches necessary? *Journal of Paediatric Psychology*, 27 (8), 749–757.

Cohen, R.Y., Brownell, K.D. and Felix, M.R.J. (1990) Age, and sex-differences in health habits and beliefs of school-children. *Health Psychology*, 9 (2), 208–224.

Cohen, S. (2005) The Pittsburgh common cold studies: psychosocial predictors of susceptibility to respiratory infectious illness. *International Journal of Behavioral Medicine*, 12 (3), 123–131.

Cohen, S. and Wills, T.A. (1985) Stress, social support, and the buffering hypothesis. *Psychological Bulletin*, 2, 310–357.

Cohen, S. and Herbert, T.B. (1996) Health psychology: psychological factors and physical disease from the perspective of human psychoneuroimmunology. *Annual Review of Psychology*, 47, 113–142.

Cohen, S., Tyrrell, D.A.J. and Smith, A.P. (1993) Negative life events, perceived stress, negative affect, and susceptibility to the common cold. *Journal of Personality and Social Psychology*, 64 (1), 131–140.

Cohen, S., Frank, E., Doyle, W.J., Skoner, D.P., Rabin, B.S. and Gwaltney Jr, J.M. (1998) Types of stressors that increase susceptibility to the common cold in healthy adults. *Health Psychology*, 17 (3), 214–223.

Cohen, S., Gottlieb, B. and Underwood, L. (2000) Social relationships and health. In Cohen, S., Underwood, L. and Gottlieb, B. (eds), *Measuring and Intervening in Social Support*. New York: Oxford University Press, 3–25.

Cole, F.L. and Abel, C. (2000) Climate of care and nurses attitudes towards AIDS in the emergency department. *Emergency Nurse*, 8 (4), 18–24.

Collins, A. (2002) Nursing with dignity Part 1: Judaism. *Nursing Times*, 98 (09), 33–35 (www.nursingtimes.net).

Conner, M. and Norman, P. (eds) (1996) *Predicting Health Behaviour*. Buckingham: Open University Press.

Conner, M., Fitter, M. and Fletcher, W. (1999) Stress and snacking: a diary study of daily hassles and between meal snacking. *Psychology and Health*, 14, 51–63.

Conner, M., Norman, P. and Bell, R. (2002) The theory of planned behaviour and healthy eating. *Health Psychology*, 21 (2), 194–201.

Conrad, P. (1985) The meaning of medications: another look at compliance. *Social Science and Medicine*, 20 (1), 29–37.

Contro, N.A., Larson, J., Scofield, S., Sourkes, B. and Cohen, H.J. (2004) Hospital staff and family perspectives regarding quality of pediatric palliative care. *Pediatrics*, 114 (5), 1248–1252.

Cook, S. (1981) *Second Life*. New York: Simon and Schuster.

Cook, S.H. (1999) The self in self-awareness. *Journal of Advanced Nursing*, 29 (6), 1292–1299.

Cook, W.W. and Medley, D.M. (1954) Proposed hostility and pharisaic-virtue scales for MMPI. *Journal of Applied Psychology*, 38, 414–418.

Cooke, M., Chaboyer, W., Schulter, P. and Hiratos, M. (2005a) Issues and innovations in nursing practice. The effect of music on preoperative anxiety in day surgery. *Journal of Advanced Nursing*, 52 (1), 47–55.

Cooke, M., Chaboyer, W., Schluter, P. and Hiratos, M. (2005b) The effect of music on preoperative anxiety in day surgery. *Journal of Advanced Nursing*, 52 (1), 47–55.

Coombs, M. and Ersser, S.J. (2004) Medical hegemony in decision-making – a barrier to interdisciplinary working in intensive care? *Journal of Advanced Nursing* 46 (3), 245–252.

Cooper, J. (2001) *Partnerships for Successful Self-management. The Living with Long-term Illness (LILL) Project Report*. London: The Long-Term Medical Conditions Alliance.

Cooper, S. and Bailey, N.M. (2001) Psychiatric disorders amongst adults with a learning disability – prevalence and relationship to ability. *Irish Journal of Psychological Medicine*, 18 (2), 45–53.

Copp, L. (1986) The nurse as an advocate for vulnerable persons. *Journal of Advanced Nursing*, 11 (3), 255–466.

Corr, C.A. (1992) A task-based approach to coping with dying. *OMEGA*, 24 (2), 81–94.

Costanzo, E.S., Lutgendorf, S.K., Bradley, S.L., Rose, S.L. and Anderson, B. (2005) Cancer attributions, distress, and health practices among gynaecologic cancer survivors. *Psychosomatic Medicine*, **67**, 972–980.

Costanzo, E.S., Lutgendorf, S.K., Rothrock, N.E. and Anderson, B. (2006) Coping and quality of life among women extensively treated for gynaecologic cancer. *Psycho-Oncology*, **15** (2), 132–142.

Costello, J. (1995) Helping relatives cope with the grieving process. *Professional Nurse*, **11** (2), 81–94.

Counter Fraud and Security Management Service Division (2003) *New drive to make NHS safe and secure*. Press Release, December 2003. NHS Counter Fraud and Security Management Service. Department of Health. http://www.cfs.nhs.uk/doc/press.release/pr.sms.strat.announcement.pdf

Courtenay, W.H. (2000a) Constructions of masculinity and their influence on men's well-being: a theory of gender and health. *Social Science & Medicine*, **50** (10), 1385–1401.

Courtenay, W.H. (2000b) Behavioural factors associated with disease, injury, and death among men: evidence and implications for prevention. *Journal of Men's Studies*, **9** (1), 81–142.

Courtenay, W.H. (2000c) Engendering health: a social constructionist examination of men's health beliefs and behaviours. *Psychology of Men and Masculinity*, **1**, 4–15.

Courtenay, W.H. (2001) Counselling men in medical settings: the six-point HEALTH plan – *The New Handbook of Psychotherapy and Counselling with Men*.

Courtenay, W.H. (2003) Key determinants of the health and well-being of men and boys. *Men's Studies Press*, **2** (1), 1–30.

Coutts, J.A.P., Gibson, N.A. and Paton, J.Y. (1992) Measuring compliance with inhaled medication in asthma. *Achives of Disease in Childhood*, **67**, 332–333.

Coutts, L. and Hardy, L. (1985) *Teaching For Health*. Edinburgh: Churchill Livingston.

Cowan, N. (1988) Evolving conceptions of memory storage, selective attention, and their mutual constraints within the human information-processing system. *Psychological Bulletin*, **104**, 163–191.

Cox, A., Jenkins, V., Catt, S., Langridge, C. and Fallowfield, L. (2006) Information needs and experiences: an audit of UK cancer patients. *European Journal of Oncology Nursing*, **10** (4), 263–272.

Coyne, J.C. and Anderson, K.K. (1999) Marital status, marital satisfaction, and support processes among women at high risk for breast cancer. *Journal of Family Psychology*, **13** (4), 629–641.

Craik, F.I.M. and Lockhart, R.S. (1972) Levels of processing: a framework for memory research. *Journal of Verbal Learning and Verbal Behaviour*, **11**, 671–684.

Cramer, J.A. and Rosenheck, R. (1998) Compliance with medication regimens for mental and physical disorders. *Psychiatric Services*, **49**, 196–201.

Croghan, E. (2005) An introduction to behaviour change among clients. *Nursing Standard*, **19** (30), 60–62.

Croghan, E. and Johnson, C. (2005) Supporting smoking cessation and dietary change. *Nursing Standard*, **19** (33), 52–54.

Croyle, R.T. and Jemmott, J.B. (1991) Psychological reactions to risk factor testing. In Skelton, J.A. and Croyle, R.T. (eds) *Mental representations in health and illness*, 85–107. New York: Springer-Verlag.

Cummings, K.M. and Hyland, A. (2005) Impact of nicotine replacement therapy on smoking behaviour. *Annual Review of Public Health*, **26**, 583–599.

Cunningham, A. (1999) Nursing stereotypes. *Nursing Standard*, **13** (45), 46–47.

Cunningham, C. (2006) Understanding challenging behaviour in patients with dementia. *Nursing Standard*, **20** (47), 42–45.

Cunningham, C. and Archibald, C. (2006) Supporting people with dementia in acute hospital settings. *Nursing Standard*, **20** (43), 51–55.

Curran, J., Machin, C. and Gournay, K. (2006) Cognitive behavioural therapy for patients with anxiety and depression. *Nursing Standard*, **21** (7), 44–52.

Curtis, A.J. (2000) *Health Psychology*. Routledge Modular Psychology Series, London: Taylor and Francis Group.

Curtis, J., Patrick, D., Shannon, S., Treece, P., Engleberg, R. and Rubenfeld, G. (2001) The Family Conference as a focus to improve communication about end of life in the intensive care unit: opportunities for improvement. *Critical Care Medicine*, **29**, 26–33.

Cutcliffe, J.R. and Barker, P. (2002) Considering the care of the suicidal client and the case for 'engagement and inspiring hope' or 'observations'. *Journal of Psychiatric and Mental Health Nursing*, **9** (5), 611–621.

Dahlquist, L.M., Pendley, J.S., Landthrip, D.S., Jones, C.L. and Steuber, C.P. (2002) Distraction intervention for preschoolers undergoing intramuscular injections and subcutaneous port access. *Health Psychology*, **21** (1), 94–99.

Daniels, K. (2006) Rethinking job characteristics in work stress research. *Human Relations*, **59** (3), 267–290.

Davey, P., Pagliari, C. and Hayes, A. (2002) The patient's role in the spread and control of bacterial resistance to antibiotics. *European Society of Clinical Microbiology and Infectious Diseases*, CMI, **8** (Suppl. 2), 43–68.

Davey-Smith, G., Carroll, D. and Rankin, S. (1992) Socio-economic differentials in mortality: evidence from Glasgow graveyards. *British Medical Journal*, **305**, 1554–1557.

Davey-Smith, G., Blane, D. and Bartley, M. (1994) Explanations for socioeconomic differentials in mortality: evidence from Britain and elsewhere. *European Journal of Public Health*, (4), 131–144.

Davidhizar, R. and Newman Giger, J. (1998) Patients' use of denial: coping with the unacceptable. *Nursing Standard*, **15** (12), 44–46.

Davies, E. (1993) Clinical role modelling: uncovering hidden knowledge. *Journal of Advanced Nursing*, **18** (4), 627–636.

Davies, S.M. (1992) Consequences of division of nursing labour for elderly patients in a continuing care setting. *Journal of Advanced Nursing*, **17**, 582–589.

Dawber, T.R., Moore, F.E. and Mann, G.V. (1957) Measuring the risk of coronary heart disease in the Framingham study. *American Journal of Public Health: Nations Health*, **47**, 4–24.

De Bruin, J.T., Schaefer, M.K., Krohne, H.W. *et al.* (2001) Preoperative anxiety, coping, and intraoperative adjustment: are there mediating effects of stress-induced analgesia? *Psychology & Health*, **16** (3), 253–271.

de Meyrick, J. and Yusuf, F. (2006) The application of household expenditure data in the development of anti-smoking campaigns. *Health Education*, **106** (3), 227–237.

De Santis, L. (1994) Making anthropology clinically relevant to nursing care. *Journal of Advanced Nursing*, **20**, 705–715.

Deakin, N. (1970) *Colour Citizenship and British Society*. London: Cox and Wyman Ltd.

Dean, C. and Surtees, P.G. (1989) Do psychological factors predict survival in breast cancer? *Journal of Psychosomatic Research*, **33** (5), 561–569.

De Araujo. M.M.T., da Silva, M.J.P. and Francisco, M.C.P.B. (2004) Nursing the dying: essential elements in the care of terminally ill patients. *International Nursing Review*, **51** (3), 149–158.

Del Mastro, L., Constantini, M., Morasso, G., Bonci, F., Bergaglio, M., Banducci, S. Viterbori, P., Conte, P., Rosso, R. and Venturini, M. (2002) Impact of two different dose-intensity chemotherapy regimens on psychological distress in early breast cancer patients. *European Journal of Cancer*, **38** (3), 359–366.

Delaney, K.R. (2006) Inpatient psychiatric treatment: should we revive a shrinking system? *Archive of Psychiatric Nursing*, **20** (5), 242–244.

Delp, C. and Jones, J. (1996) Communicating information to patients: the use of cartoon illustrations to improve comprehension of instructions. *Acad Emerg Med*, **3**, 264–270.

Department of Health (1998) *Our Healthier Nation – A Contract for Health. A Consultation Paper*. Command Paper Cm3852. London: Stationery Office.

Department of Health (1999) *Making a Difference: strengthening the nursing, midwifery and health visiting contribution to health and healthcare*. London: HMSO.

Department of Health (2001a) *The Expert Patient*. London: Department of Health.

Department of Health (2001b) *The National Service Framework for Older People. Modern Standards and Service Models*. London: Department of Health.

Department of Health (2001c) *Valuing People: A New Strategy for Learning Disability for the 21st Century*. London: The Stationery Office.

Department of Health (2005a) *Creating a Patient led NHS, Delivering the NHS improvement plan*. London: HMSO.

Department of Health (2005b) *Everybody's Business: Integrated Mental Health Services for Older Adults*. Care Services Improvement Partnership, Department of Health.

Department of Health (2006) *Community Care Statistics 2004–2005 Referrals, Assessments and Packages of Care, for Adults*, table P2s.1 (Estimated number of clients on the books to receive community based services). Cited in Age Concern.

Descartes, R. (1644) *Principles of Philosophy (Principia philosophiae)*.

Detweiler, J.B., Bedell, B.T., Salovey, P., Pronin, E. and Rothman, A.J. (2007) Message framing and sunscreen use: gain-framed messages motivate beach-goers. *Health Psychology*, **18** (2), 189–196.

Dewar, A., Craig, K., Muir, J. and Cole, C. (2003) Testing the effectiveness of a nursing intervention in relieving pain following day surgery. *Ambulatory Surgery*, **10** (2), 81–88.

Dewing, J. and Blackburn, S. (1999) Dementia Part 4: Risk management. *Professional Nurse*, **14**, 803–805; 585–588.

DHSS (1980) *Black Report: Department of Health and Social Security. Inequalities in Health: Report of a Working Group*. London: DHSS.

Diabetes Insight (2006) http://www.diabetes-insight.info/newbies/whats_diabetes/DI_control.asp, accessed 2 October 2007.

Diamond, A.W. and Coniam, S.W. (1991) *The Management of Chronic Pain*. Oxford: Oxford University Press.

Dibble, S.L., Chapman, J., Mack, K.A. and Shih, A.S. (2000) Acupressure for nausea: results of a pilot study. *Oncology Nursing Forum*, **27** (1), 41–47.

DiClemente, C.C. and Prochaska, J.O. (1982) Self-change and therapy change of smoking-behavior – a comparison of processes of change in cessation and maintenance. *Addictive Behaviors*, **7** (2), 133–142.

Dikken, C. and Sitzia, J. (1998) Patients' experiences of chemotherapy: side-effects associated with 5-fluorouracil plus folinic acid in the treatment of colorectal cancer. *Journal of Clinical Nursing*, **7** (4), 371–379.

DiMatteo, M. (1994) Enhancing patient adherence to medical recommendations. *Journal of the American Medical Association*, **271**, 79–83.

DiMatteo, M.R. (2003) Assessing and promoting patient adherence: some lessons from five decades of research. *Journal of Psychosomatic Research*, **55** (2), 137.

DiMatteo, M.R. (2004) Social support and patient adherence to medical treatment: a meta-analysis. *Health Psychology*, **23** (2), 207–218.

DiMatteo, R. (2000) Adherence to treatment in medical conditions. *Contemporary Psychology – APA Review of Books*, **45** (3), 302–304.

Do, C. (2004) Applying the social learning theory to children with dental anxiety. *The Journal of Contemporary Dental Practice*, **5** (1), 126–135.

Dodds, F. (1993) Access to the coping strategies: managing anxiety in elective surgical patients. *Professional Nurse*, **9** (1), 45–52.

Doering, S., Katzlberger, F., Rumpold, G., Roessler, S. Hofstoetter, B., Schatz, D.S., Behensky, H., Krismer, M., Luz, G., Innerhofer, P., Benzer, H., Saria, A. and Schuessler, G. (2000) Videotape preparation of patients before hip replacement surgery reduces stress. *Psychosomatic Medicine*, **62** (3), 365–373.

Dohrenwend, B.P. (1990) Socioeconomic-status (SES) and psychiatric-disorders – are the issues still compelling? *Social Psychiatry and Psychiatric Epidemiology*, **25** (1), 41–47.

Doka, K.J. (2000) Editorial: Challenging our understandings of grief and dying. *OMEGA*, **41** (1), 3–4.

Dolan, B. and Holt, L. (2000) *Accident and Emergency: Theory into Practice*. London: Bailliere Tindall.

Doll, R. and Hill, A.B. (1952) A study of the aetiology of carcinoma of the lung. *British Medical Journal*, **13** (2), 1271–1286.

Dollard, J., Doob, L.W., Miller, N.E., Mowrer, O.H. and Sears, R.R. (1939) *Frustration and Aggression*. New Haven, CT: Yale University Press.

Donovan, J.L. and Blake, D.R. (1992) Patient compliance. Deviance or reasoned decision-making? *Social Science and Medicine*, **34**, 507–513.

Dorset, R. and Marsh, A. (1998) *The Health Trap: Smoking and Lone Parenthood*. London: Policy Studies Institute.

Dosani, S. (2003) Practising medicine in a multi-cultural society. *BMJ*, **326**, s3. http://careerfocus.bmj.com/cgi/content/full/326/7379/S3.

Dowling, M. (2006) The sociology of intimacy in the nurse–patient relationship. *Nursing Standard*, **20** (23), 48–54.

Driggers, D., Nussbaum, J. and Haddock, K. (1993) Role modelling: an educational strategy to promote effective cancer pain management. *Oncology Nursing Forum*, **20** (6), 959–962.

Drotar, D. (1997) Relating parent and family functioning to the psychological adjustment of children with chronic health conditions: what have we learnt? What do we need to know? *Journal of Paediatric Psychology*, **22** (2), 149–165.

Drury, T. (1997) Recognizing the potential for violence in the ICU. *Dimensions of Critical Care Nursing*, **16** (6), 314–323.

Dubois, L. and Girard, M. (2006) Early determinants of overweight at 4.5 years in a population-based longitudinal study. *International Journal of Obesity*, **30**, 610–617.

Dubos, R. (1959) *Mirage of Health, Utopias, Progress and Biological Change*. New York: Harper and Brothers Pub.

Duff, A.J.A. (2003) Incorporating psychological approaches into routine paediatric venepuncture. *Archive of Disorders of Childhood*, **88**, 931–937.

Duijts, S.F.A., Zeegers, M.P.A. and Van der Borne, B. (2003) The association between stressful life events and breast cancer risk: a meta-analysis. *International Journal of Cancer*, **107** (6), 1023–1029.

Dunbar-Jacob, J., Burke, L.E. and Pyczynski, S. (1995) Clinical assessment and management of adherence to medical regimens. In Nicassio, M. and Smith, T. (eds), *Managing Chronic Illness: A Biopsychosocial Perspective*. Washington, DC: American Psychological Association.

Dunne, K. (2005) Effective communication in palliative care. *Nursing Standard*, **20** (13), 57–64.

Dusenbury, L., Kerner, J.F., Baker, E., Botvin, G., James-Ortiz, S. and Zauber, A. (1992) Predictors of smoking prevalence among New York Latino youth. *American Journal of Public Health*, **82**, 55–58.

Duval, S. and Wicklund, R.A. (1972) *A Theory of Objective Self-awareness*. New York: Academic Press.

Dyer, I. (1995) Preventing the ITCU syndrome or how not to torture an ITU patient! Part 1. *Intensive and Critical Care Nursing*, **11** (1), 130–139.

Dysvik, E., Vinsnes, A.G. and Eikeland, O-J. (2004) The effectiveness of a multidisciplinary pain management programme managing chronic pain. *International Journal of Nursing Practice*, **10** (5), 224–234.

Eccleston, C., Morley, S., Williams, A., York, L. and Mastroyannopoulou, K. (2002) Systematic review of randomised controlled trials of psychological therapy for chronic pain in children and adolescents, with a subset meta-analysis of pain relief. *Pain*, **99** (1–2), 157–165.

Edwards, B. and Brilhart, J. (1981) *Communication in Nursing Practice*. St Louis: Mosby.

Egan, G. (1990) *The Skilled Helper*, 4th edn. Pacific Grove, CA: Brooks/Cole.

Egan, G. (1994) *The Skilled Helper: A Problem Management Approach to Helping*, 5th edn. Pacific Grove, CA: Brooks/Cole.

Egan, G. (2000) *The Skilled Helper: A Problem Management Approach to Helping*, Monterey, CA: Brooks/Cole.

Egan, G. (2002) *The Skilled Helper: A Problem-Management and Opportunity-Development Approach to Helping*, 7th edn. Pacific Grove, CA: Brooks/Cole.

Egan, K.J., Ready, L.B., Nessly, M. and Greer, B.E. (1992) Self-administration of Midazlam for postoperative anxiety – a double blinded study. *Pain*, **49** (1), 3–8.

Egbert, L.D., Battit, G.E., Welch, C.E. and Bartlett, M.K. (1964) Reduction of postoperative pain by encouragement and instruction of patients – A study of doctor–patient rapport. *New England Journal of Medicine*, **270**, 825–827.

Eggleston, J., Gallagher, J., Gallagher, M., Hares, T., Murray, E., Naroz, N., Owen, M.B., Owen, T., Price, P., Pym, L., Reed, L. and Robinson, K. (1995) Who should give life-style advice in general-practice and what factors influence attendance at health promotion clinics – survey of patients' views. *British Journal of General Practice*, **45** (401), 669–671.

Eibl-Eibesfeldt, I. (1971) *Liefde En Haat: Over de Biologische Achtergronden Van Elementaire Gedragspatronen [Love and hate: biological backgrounds of elementary behaviour patterns]*. Amsterdam: Uitgeverij Ploegsma.

Eibl-Eibesfeldt, I. (1972) Similarities and differences between cultures in expressive movements. In Hinde, R.A. (ed.), *Nonverbal Communication*. London: Cambridge University Press.

Eiser, J.R. (1990) Environmental threats – perception, analysis and management, *Journal of Environmental Psychology*, **10** (1), 85–87.

Eiser, J.R. (1997) Addiction as a dynamic process. *Addiction Research*, **5** (5), 361–365.

Ekman, P., Friesen, W.V. and Ellsorth, P. (1972) *Emotion in the Human Face: Guidelines for Research and an Integration of Findings*. New York: Pergamon Press.

Elderkin-Thompson, V., Silver, R.C. and Waitzkin, H. (2001) When nurses double as interpreters: a study of Spanish-speaking patients in a US primary care setting. *Social Science and Medicine*. **52** (9), 1343–1358.

Elkins, I.J., King, S.M., McGue, M. and Iacono, M. (2006) Personality traits and the development of nicotine, alcohol, and illicit drug disorders: prospective links from adolescence to young adulthood. *Journal of Abnormal Psychology*, **115** (1), 26–39.

Ellis, A. (1977) *Anger – How to Live With and Without It.* New York: Carol Publishing Group.

Ellis, A. (1994) *Reason and Emotion in Psychotherapy: Revised and Updated.* New York: Birch Lane.

Ellis, R.B., Gates, R.J. and Kenworthy, N. (2001) *Interpersonal Communication in Nursing: Theory and Practice.* Edinburgh: Churchill Livingstone.

Emslie, C., Hunt, K. and MacIntyre, S. (2002) How similar are the smoking and drinking habits of men and women in non-manual jobs? *European Journal of Public Health,* **12** (1), 22–28.

Eng, P.M., Rimm, E.B., Fitzmaurice, G. and Kawachi, I. (2002) Social ties and change in social ties in relation to subsequent total and cause-specific mortality and coronary heart disease incidence in men. *American Journal of Epidemiology,* **155** (8), 700–709.

Engel, G.L. (1977) The need for a new medical model: a challenge for biomedicine. *Science,* **196** (4286), 129–136.

Engel, G.L. (1980) The clinical application of the biopsychosocial model. *American Journal of Psychiatry,* **137** (5), 535–544.

Engel, G.L. (1988) How much longer must medicine's science be bound by a seventeenth century world view? In *The Task of Medicine, Dialogue at Wickenburg.* Menlo Park, CA: The Henry J. Kaiser Family Foundation, 113–136.

Erens, B. and Primatesta, P. (1999) *Health Survey for England 1998. SCPR/UCL for the Department of Health.* London: HMSO.

Erikson, E.H. (1959) *Identity and the Life Cycle.* New York: International Universities Press.

Eriksson, U.F. (2007) Fetal ethanol exposure during pregnancy – how big is the problem and how do we fix it? *Acta Paediatrica* **96** (11), 1557–1559.

Ernst, E. and Köder, K. (1997) An overview of reflexology. *European Journal of General Practice,* **3** (2), 52.

Esselstyn, C.B. (1999) Updating a 12-year experience with arrest and reversal therapy for coronary heart disease (an overdue requiem for palliative cardiology). *American Journal of Cardiology,* **84** (3), 339–341.

Etter, J.F. (2005) Combining psychological theory and new information technology to disseminate smoking-cessation interventions at population level. *Nicotine and Tobacco Research,* **7** (4), 663.

European Nutrition for Health Alliance (2005) *Malnutrition within an Ageing Population: A Call to Action.* Report on the Inaugural Conference of the European Nutrition for Health Alliance, London, 14 September 2005. www.european-nutrition.org.

Evans, D. (2004) Behind the headlines: sexual health implications for nursing ethics and practice. *Primary Health Care,* **14** (8), 40–49.

Evans, D.L., Leserman, J., Perkins, D.O., Stern, R.A., Murphy, C., Zheng, B., Gettes, D., Longmate, J.A., Silva, S.G., van der Horst, C.M., Hall, C.D., Folds, J.D., Golden, R.N. and Petitto, J.M. (1997) Severe life stress as a predictor of early disease progression in HIV infection. *American Journal of Psychiatry,* **154** (5), 630–634.

Evers, K.E., Prochaska, J.O., Johnson, J.L., Mauriello, L.M., Padula, J.A. and Prochaska, J.M. (2006) A randomised clinical trial of a population and transtheoretical model based stress management interventions. *Health Psychology,* **25** (4), 521–529.

Everson-Rose, S.A. and Lewis, T.T. (2005) Psychosocial factors of cardiovascular diseases. *Annual Review: Public Health,* **26**, 469–500.

Eysenck, H. (2002) *Simply Psychology,* 2nd edn. Hove and New York: Psychology Press, Taylor and Francis Group.

Ewing, J.A. (1984) Detecting alcoholism – the cage questionnaire. *Journal of the American Medical Association,* **252** (14), 1905–1907.

Facione, N.C., Miaskowski, C., Dodd, M.J. and Paul, S.M. (2002) The self-reported likelihood of patient delay in breast cancer: new thoughts for early detection. *Preventive Medicine,* **34** (4), 397–407.

Faith, M.S., Berman, N., Heo, M.S., Pietrobelli, A., Gallagher, D., Epstein, L.H., Eiden, M.T. and Allison, D.B. (2001) Effects of contingent television on physical activity and television viewing in obese children. *Paediatrics,* **107** (5), 1043–1048.

Faller, H., Bülzebruck, H., Drings, P. and Lang, H. (1999) Coping, distress, and survival among patients with lung cancer. *Archives of General Psychiatry,* **56**, 756–762.

Faller, H., Bülzebruck, H., Schilling, S., Drings, P. and Lang, H. (1997) Do psychological factors influence survival in cancer patients? 2. Findings of an empirical study with lung cancer patients. *Psychotherapie Psychosomatik Medizinische Psychologie,* **47** (6), 206–218.

Fallowfield, L. (1990) *The Quality of Life: The Missing Measurement in Health Care.* London: Souvenir Press.

Fallsberg, M. (1991) Reflections on medicines and medication: a qualitative analysis among people on long-term drug regimens. Linkoping Studies in Education. Dissertation no. 32. Linkoping University, Sweden.

Falvo, D., Woehlke, P. and Deichmann, T. (1980) Relation of physician behaviour vs patient compliance. *Patient Counselling and Health Education,* **2**, 185–188.

Fan, A. (2002) Psychological and psychosocial effects of prostate cancer. *Nursing Standard,* **17** (13), 33–37.

Farrell, M. (1992) A process of mutual support. Establishing a support network for nurses caring for dying patients. *Professional Nurse,* **8** (1), 10–14.

Farrell, W. (1994) *The Myth of Male Power: Why Men Are the Disposable Sex.* Berkley Pub Group.

Faulkner, G.E.J. and Taylor, A.H. (2006) *Exercise, Health and Mental Health.* London: Routledge.

Faulkner, M. (2002) Instrumental passivity: a behavioural theory of dependence. *Nursing Older People,* **14** (2), 20–21.

Feil, N. (1992) Validation therapy with late-onset dementia patients. In P. Woodrow (1998) Interventions for confusion and dementia 4: alternative approaches. *British Journal of Nursing,* **7** (20), 1247–1250.

Feldman, P.J., Dunkkel-Schetter, C., Snadmand, C.A. and Wadhwa, P.D. (2000) Maternal social support predicts birth weight and fetal growth in human pregnancy. *Psychosomatic Medicine,* **62**, 715–725.

Fennell, P. (1996) *Treatment Without Consent. Law, Psychiatry and the Treatment of Mentally Disordered People Since 1945.* London: Routledge.

Ferguson, S.G. and Miller, O.T. (2001) Environmental influences on craving and the physiological and cognitive effects of cigarette smoking. *New Zealand Journal of Psychology*, 30 (2), 44–52.

Fernandez, E. (1986) A classification system of cognitive coping strategies for pain. *Pain*, 26 (2), 141–151.

Fernando, S. (2002) *Mental Health, Race and Culture*. Palgrave Macmillan.

Ferns, T. (2006) Violence, aggression and physical assault in healthcare settings. *Nursing Standard*, 21 (13), 42–46.

Ferns, T. (2007) Factors that influence aggressive behaviour in acute care settings. *Nursing Standard*, 21 (33), 41–45.

Ferrell, B.A. (1991) Pain management in elderly people. *Journal of the American Geriatrics Society*, 39 (1), 64–73.

Festinger, L. (1957) *A Theory of Cognitive Dissonance*. Stanford, CA: Stanford University Press.

Field, D. and Payne, S. (2003) Social aspects of bereavement. *Cancer Nursing Practice*, 2 (8), 21–25.

Finlay, L. (2005) Difficult encounters. *Nursing Management*, 12 (1), 33–37.

Finlay, L. and Dallimore, D. (1991) Your child is dead. *British Medical Journal*, 302, 1524–1525.

Fiscella, K. and Franks, S.P. (1997) Does psychological distress contribute to racial and socioeconomic disparities in mortality? *Social Science and Medicine*, 45, 1805–1809.

Fishbein, M. (1967) *Attitude and the Prediction of Behavior. Readings in Attitude Theory and Measurement*. New York: Wiley, 477–492.

Fishbein, M. and Ajzen, I. (1975) *Belief Attitude Intention and Behavior: An Introduction to Theory and Research*. Reading, MA: Addison-Wesley.

Fitzgerald, R.G. and Parkes, C.M. (1998) Blindness and loss of other sensory and cognitive functions. *British Medical Journal*, 316, 1160–1163.

Flannigan, C.B., Glover, G.R., Wing, J.K., Bebbington, P.E. and Lewis, S.W. (1994) Inner London collaborative audit of admissions in two health districts: introduction, methods and preliminary findings. *British Journal of Psychiatry*, 165, 734–759.

Fleming, G., McKenna, M., Murchison, V., Wood, Y., Nixon, J., Rogers, T. and Hutcheson, F. (2003) Using self-efficacy as a client-centred outcome measure. *Nursing Standard*, 17 (34), 33–36.

Fleming, M.F., Barry, K.L., Manwell, L.B., Johnson, K. and London, R. (1997) Brief physician advice for problem alcohol drinkers – a randomized controlled trial in community-based primary care practices. *Journal of the American Medical Association*, 277 (13), 1039–1045.

Fletcher, M. (1997) Ethnicity: equal health services for all. *Journal Community Nurse*, 11 (7), 20–24.

Foden, P. and Preston, E. (2001) Teamwork: it's the way forward. *Nursing Times*, 96 (44), 39.

Folkman, S. and Lazarus, R.S. (1988) Coping as a mediator of emotion. *Journal of Personality and Social Psychology*, 54 (3), 466–475.

Fordyce, W.E., Lansky, D., Calsyn, D.A., Shelton, J.L., Stolov, W.C. and Roch, D.L. (1984) Pain measurement and pain behaviour. *Pain*, 18 (1), 53–69.

Forgarty, L., Roter, D., Larson, S., Burke, J., Gillespie, J. and Levy, R. (2002) Patient adherence to HIV medication regimens: a review of published and abstract reports. *Patient Education and Counselling*, 46, 93–108.

Forsen, A. (1991) Psychosocial stress as a risk for breast-cancer. *Psychotherapy and Psychosomatics*, 55, 176–185.

Foss, S., Schmidt, J.R., Andersen, T., Rasmuss, J.J., Damsgaard, J., Schaefer, K. and Munck, L.K. (2004) Congruence on medication between patients and physicians involved in patient course. *European Journal Clinical Pharmacology*, 59, 841–847.

France, E.K., Glasgow, R.E. and Marcus, A.C. (2001) Smoking cessation interventions among hospitalized patients: what have we learned? *Preventive Medicine*, 32 (4), 376–388.

Francis, V., Korsch, B.M. and Morris, M.J. (1969) Gaps in doctor–patient communication. Patients' response to medical advice. *New England Journal of Medicine*, 280, 535–540.

Frank, A.J.M., Moll, J.M.H. and Hort, J.F. (1982) A comparison of three ways of measuring pain. *Rheumatology*, 21, 211–217.

Frank, J.M. (1985) The effects of music therapy and guided visual imagery on chemotherapy induced nausea and vomiting. *Oncology Nursing Forum*, 12, 47–52.

Frasure-Smith, N., Lespérance, F., Gravel, G., Masson, A., Juneau, M., Talajic, M. and Bourassa, M.G. (2000) Social support, depression, and mortality during the first year after myocardial infarction. *Circulation*, 101 (16), 1919–1924.

Fredrickson, B.L., Maynard, K.E., Helms, M.J., Haney, T.L., Siegler, I.C. and Barefoot, J.C. (2000) Hostility predicts magnitude and duration of blood pressure response to anger. *Journal of Behavioral Medicine*, 23 (3), 229–243.

Freemantle, N., Gill, P., Godfrey, C., Long, A., Richards, C., Sheldon, T.A., Song, F. and Webb, J. (1993) Brief interventions and alcohol use. *Quality and Safety in Health Care*, 2 (4), 267–273.

French, S.E., Lenton, R., Walters, V. and Eyles, J. (2000) An empirical evaluation of an expanded nursing stress scale. *Journal of Nursing Measurement*, 8, 161–178.

Freud, S. (1961) *The Ego and the Id*. Standard Edition of the Complete Psychological Works of Freud, Volume XIX. London: Hogarth Press.

Fridfinnsdottir, E.B. (1997) Icelandic women's identifications of stressors and social support during the diagnostic phase of breast cancer. *Journal of Advanced Nursing*, 25, 526–531.

Friedman, M. and Rosenman, R.H. (1959) Association of specific overt behaviour pattern with blood and cardiovascular findings. *Journal of the American Medical Association*, 169, 1286–1296.

Friedman, M. and Rosenman, R.H. (1974) *Type A Behavior and Your Heart*. New York: Alfred A. Knopf.

Friedman, M., Thoresen, C.E., Gill, J.J., Ulmer, D., Powell, L.H., Price, V.A., Brown, B., Thompson, L., Rabin, D.D., Breall, W.S., Bourg, E., Levy, R. and Dixon, T. (1986) Alteration of type-a behavior and its effect on cardiac recurrences in post myocardial-infarction patients – summary results of the recurrent coronary prevention project. *American Heart Journal*, 112 (4), 653–665.

Froggatt, W. (2001) *CBT: A Brief Introduction to REBT* (http://www.rational.org.nz, accessed 10 May 2007).

Fryers, T., Melzer, D. and Jenkins, R. (2003) Social inequalities and the common mental disorders – a systematic review of the evidence. *Social Psychiatry and Psychiatric Epidemiology*, 38 (5), 229–237.

Fryers, T., Melzer, D., Jenkins, R. and Brugha, T. (2005) The distribution of the common mental disorders: social inequalities in Europe. *Clinical Practice and Epidemiology in Mental Health*, September 5, 1–14.

Furler, J.S., Harris, E., Chondros, P., Davies, P.G.P., Harris, M.F. and Young, D.Y.L. (2002) The inverse care law revisited: impact of disadvantaged location on accessing longer GP consultation times. *Medical Journal of Australia*, 177 (2), 80–83.

Fyfe, A. (1999) Anxiety and the pre-operative patient. *British Journal of Theatre Nursing*, 9 (10), 452–454.

Gabel, W. and Piezcker, A. (1985) One-year outcome of schizophrenic patients: the interaction of chronic and neuroleptic treatment. *Psychopharmacology*, 18, 235–239.

Gaberson, K.B. (1995) The effect of humorous and musical distraction on preoperative anxiety. *AORN Journal*, 62 (5), 784–788, 790–791.

Gafney, A. and Dunne, E.A. (1986) Developmental aspects of children's definitions of pain. *Pain*, 26 (1), 105–117.

Galban, C., Montejo, J.C., Mesejo, A., Marco, P., Celaya, S., Sanchez-Segura, J.M., Farre, M. and Bryg, D.J. (2000) An immune-enhancing enteral diet reduces mortality rate and episodes of bacteremia in septic intensive care unit patients. *Critical Care Medicine*, 28 (3), 643–648.

Galdas, P.M., Cheater, F. and Marshall, P. (2005) Men and health help-seeking behaviour: literature review. *Journal of Advanced Nursing*, 49 (6), 616–623.

Gallo, L.C. and Matthews, K.A. (2003) Understanding the association between socioeconomic status and physical health: do negative emotions play a role? *Psychological Bulletin*, 129 (1), 10–51.

Ganz, P.A., Rowland, J.H., Desmond, K., Meyerowitz, B.E. and Wyatt, G.E. (1998) Life after breast cancer: understanding women's health-related quality of life and sexual functioning. *Journal of Clinical Oncology*, 16 (2), 501–514.

García de Lucio, L., García López, F.J., Marín López, M.T., Mas Hesse, B. and Caamaño Vaz, M.D. (2000) Training programme in techniques of self-control and communication skills to improve nurses' relationships with relatives of seriously ill patients: a randomized controlled study, *Journal of Advanced Nursing* 32 (2), 425–431.

Garrison, M.M., Christakis, D.A., Ebal, B.E., Wiehe, S.E. and Rivara, F.P. (2003) A systematic review of smoking cessation interventions for adolescents, *Paediatric Research*, 53 (4), 3206.

Garson, J.Z. (1984) Cancer – a stress disease? *Journal of the Royal College of General Practitioners*, March, 34 (260), 179.

Garssen, B. (2004) Psychological factors and cancer development: evidence after 30 years of research. *Clinical Psychology Review*, 24 (3), 315–338.

Gaston, C.M. and Mitchell, G. (2005) Information giving and decision-making in patients with advanced cancer: a systematic review. *Social Science and Medicine*, 61 (10), 2252–2264.

Gatrad, R. and Sheikh, A. (2002) Palliative care for Muslims and issues after death. *International Journal of Palliative Nursing*, 8 (12), 594–597.

Geersten, H.R., Gray, R.M. and Ward, J.R. (1973) Patient non-compliance within the context of seeking medical care for arthritis. *Journal of Chronic Diseases*, 26, 689–698.

General Household Survey (2001) *Living in Britain, Results from the 2001 General Household Survey*. The Office for National Statistics (ONS), London: TSO.

General Household Survey (2002) *Living in Britain, General Household Survey*, 2002. The Office for National Statistics (ONS), London: TSO.

General Household Survey (2004) *General Household Survey, 2004*. The Office for National Statistics (ONS), London: TSO.

Gerace, L.M., Hughes, T.L. and Spunt, J. (1995) Improving nurses responses toward substance-misusing patients – a clinical-evaluation project. *Archives of Psychiatric Nursing*, 9 (5), 286–294.

Gerrish, K. (1997) Preparation of nurses to meet the needs of an ethnically diverse society: educational implications. *Nurse Education Today*, 17, 359–365.

Gerrish, K. and Papadopoulos, I. (1999) Transcultural competence: the challenge for nurse education. *British Journal of Nursing* 8 (21), 1453–1457.

Gerrish, K., Husband, C. and Mackenzie, J. (1996) *Nursing for a Multiethnic Society*. Buckingham: Open University Press.

Gerson, S. (2006) *The National Institute of Ayurvedic Medicine, USA* (http://niam.com/corp-web/index.htm, accessed 15 August 2006).

Gervais, M.C. and Jovchelovitch, S. (1998) *The Health Beliefs of the Chinese Community in England: A Qualitative Research Study*. London: Health Education Authority.

Gibb, H. and O'Brien, B. (1990) Jokes and reassurance are not enough: ways in which nurses relate through conversation with elderly clients. *Journal of Advanced Nursing*, 15, 1389–1401.

Gibbs, G. (1988) *Learning by Doing: A Guide to Teaching and Learning Methods*. Oxford: Oxford Further Education Unit.

Gibson, P., Powell, H., Coughlan, J., Wilson, A.J., Abramson, M., Haywood, P., Bauman, A., Hensley, M.J. and Walters, E.H. (2002) Self-management education and regular practitioner review for adults with asthma. *Cochrane Database of Systematic Reviews*, Issue 3.

Gidding, S.S., Dennison, B.A., Birch, L.L., Daniels, S.R. Gilman, M.W., Lichtenstein, A.H., Rattay, K.T., Steinberger, J., Stettler, N. and Van Horn, L. (2005) Dietary recommendations for children and adolescents: a guide for practitioners: consensus statement from the American Heart Association. *Circulation*, 112 (13), 2061–2075.

Gidron, Y., Davidson, K. and Bata, I. (1999) The short-term effects of a hostility-reduction intervention on male coronary heart disease patients. *Health Psychology*, 18 (4), 416–420.

Gilbert, D.T. and Malone, P.S. (1995) The correspondence bias. *Psychological Bulletin*, 117, 21–38.

Gill, B.K. (2002) Nursing with dignity – Sikhism. *Nursing Times*, 98 (14).

Gillies, M.A.M. and Baldwin, F.J. (2001) Do patient information booklets increase perioperative anxiety? *European Journal of Anaesthesiology*, 18 (9), 620–622.

Givens, D.B. (2005) *Centre for Nonverbal Studies* (http://members.aol.com/nonverbal2/flashbul.htm).

Glaser, R. and Kiecolt-Glaser, J.K. (2005) Science and society – stress-induced immune dysfunction: implications for health. *Nature Reviews Immunology*, 5 (3), 243–251.

Glasgow, R.E., McCaul, K.D. and Schafer, L.C. (1987) Self-care behaviours and glycaemia control in type 1 diabetes. *Journal Chronic Disease*, 40, 399–412.

Glasgow, R.E., Toobert, D.J., Riddle, M., Donnelly, J., Mitchell, D.L. and Calder, D. (1989) Diabetes-specific social learning variables and self-care behaviors among persons with Type II diabetes. *Health Psychology*, 8 (3), 285-303.

Glintborg, B., Anderson, S.E. and Dalhoff, K. (2007) Insufficient communication about medication use at the interface between hospital and primary care trust. *Qual Saf Health Care*, 16, 34–39.

Godin, G., Valois, P., Lepage, L. and Descharnais, R. (1992) Predictors of smoking behaviour: an application of Ajzen's theory of planned behaviour. *British Journal of Addiction*, 87 (9), 1335–1343.

Godsell, M. and Scarborough, K. (2006) Improving communication for people with learning disabilities. *Nursing Standard*, 20 (30), 58–65.

Godtfredsen, N.S., Vestbo, J., Osler, M. and Prescott, E. (2002) Risk of hospital admission for COPD following smoking cessation and reduction: a Danish population study. *Thorax*, 57 (11), 967–972.

Goffman, E. (1961) *Asylums: Essays on the Social Situations of Mental Patients and Other Inmates*. Oxford: Doubleday.

Goffman, E. (1963) In Finlay (2005) Difficult encounters. *Nursing Management*, 12 (1), 33–37.

Golden, J. (2005) *Message in a Bottle: The Making of Fetal Alcohol Syndrome*. Cambridge, MA: Harvard University Press.

Goldman, D., Oroszi, G. and Ducci, F. (2005) The genetics of addictions: uncovering the genes. *Nature Reviews Genetics*, 6, 521–532.

Gordis, L. (1979) Conceptual and methodological problems in measuring patient compliance. In Haynes, R.B., Taylor, D.W. and Sackett, D.L., *Compliance in Heath Care*. Baltimore: Johns Hopkins University Press, 23–45.

Gordon, D.B., Dahl, J.L., Miaskowski, C., McCarberg, B., Todd, K.H., Paice, J.A., Lipman, A.G., Bookbinder, M., Sanders, S.H., Turk, D.C. and Carr, D.B. (2005) American pain society recommendations for improving the quality of acute and cancer pain management – American Pain Society Quality of Care Task Force. *Archives of Internal Medicine*, 165 (14), 1574–1580.

Gortmaker, S.L., Walker, D.K., Weitzman, M. and Sobol, A.M. (1990) Chronic conditions, socio-economic risks, and behavioural-problems in children and adolescents, *Paediatrics*, 85 (3), 267–276.

Gow, J. and Gilhooly, M. (2003) *Risk Factors for Dementia and Cognitive Failure in Old Age*. Glasgow: NHS Health.

Graham, H. (1987) Women's smoking and family health. *Social Science and Medicine*, 25 (1), 47–56.

Gray, R., Wykes, T. and Gournay, K. (2002) From compliance to concordance: a review of the literature on interventions to enhance compliance with antipsychotic medication. *Journal of Psychiatric and Mental Health Nursing*, 9, 277–284.

Gray-Toft, P. and Anderson, J.G. (1981) The Nursing Stress Scale: development of an instrument. *Journal of Behavioral Assessment*, 3 (1), 11–23.

Green, B., Krupnick, J.L., Rowland, J.H., Epstein, S.A., Stockton, P., Spertus, I. and Stern, N. (2000) Trauma history as a predictor of psychologic symptoms in women with breast cancer. *Journal of Clinical Oncology*, 18 (5), 1084–1093.

Green, C.R., Anderson, K.O., Baker, T.A., Campbell, L.C., Decker, S., Fillingim, R.B., Kaloukalani, D.A., Lasch, K.E., Myers, C., Tait, R.C., Todd, K.H. and Vallerand, A.H. (2003) The unequal burden of pain: confronting racial and ethnic disparities in pain. *Pain Medicine*, 4 (3), 277–294.

Greene, M.G., Adelman, R.D., Friedmann, E. and Charon, R. (1994) Older patient satisfaction with communication during an initial medical encounter. *Social Science and Medicine*, 38, 1279–1288.

Greene, R.L. (1987) Effects of maintenance rehearsal on human memory. *Psychological Bulletin*, 102, 403–413.

Greenfield, S., Kaplan, S. and Ware, J.E. (1985) Expanding patient involvement in care. Effects on patient outcomes. *Ann Intern Med.*, 102, 520–528.

Greeno, C.G. and Wing, R.R. (1994) Stress-induced eating. *Psychological Bulletin*, 115 (3), 444–464.

Greenstreet, W. (2005) Loss, grief and bereavement in inter-professional education, an example of process: anecdotes and accounts. *Nurse Education in Practice*, 5, 281–288.

Greer, S., Morris, T. and Pettingale, K.W. (1979) Psychological response to breast cancer: effect on outcome. *Lancet*, 2 (8146), 785–787.

Greer, S., Morris, T., Pettingale, K.W. and Haybittle, J.L. (1990) Psychological response to breast-cancer and 15-year outcome. *Lancet*, 335 (8680), 49–50.

Griffith, L.S., Field, B.J. and Lustman, P.J. (1990) Life stress and social support in diabetes: association with glycaemia control. *International Journal of Psychiatric Medicine*, 20, 365–372.

Griva, K., Myers, L.B. and Newman, S. (2000) Illness perceptions and self-efficacy beliefs in adolescents and young adults with insulin dependent diabetes mellitus. *Psychology and Health*, 15, 733–750.

Gross, D. (1990) Communication and the elderly. *Physical and Occupational Therapy in Geriatrics*, 9 (1), 49–64.

Gump, B.B., Matthews, K.A. and Raikkonen, K. (1999) Modeling relationships among socioeconomic status, hostility, cardiovascular reactivity, and left ventricular mass in African American and White children. *Health Psychology*, 18(2), 140–150.

Gutschoven, K. and Van den Bulck, J. (2005) Television viewing and age at smoking initiation: does a relationship exist between higher levels of television viewing and earlier onset of smoking? *Nicotine and Tobacco Research*, 7 (3), 381–385.

Hagger, M.S., Chatzisarantis, N., Biddle, S.T.J.H. and Orbell, S. (2001) Antecedents of children's physical activity intentions and behaviour: predictive validity and longitudinal effects. *Psychology & Health*, **16** (4), 391–407.

Hall, G. (1988) Care of the patient with Alzheimer's disease at home. *Nursing Clinics of North America*, **23**, 31–46.

Hall, G. (1994) Chronic dementia: challenges in feeding a patient. *Journal of Gerontological Nursing*, **20**, 21–30.

Hall, J.A. and Doran, M.C. (1990) Patient socio-demographic characteristics as predictors of satisfaction with medical care: a meta-analysis. In Edelmann, R.J. (2000) *Psychosocial Aspects of the Health Care Process*. Harlow: Pearson Education.

Hall, N.R.S. and O'Grady, M. (1991) Psychosocial interventions and immune functioning. In Ader, R., Felton, D.L. and Cohen, N. (eds), *Psychoneuroimmunology*, 2nd edn, 1067–1079. Boston: Academic Press.

Han, W.T., Collie, K., Koopman, C., Azarow, J., Classen, C., Morrow, G.R., Michel, B., Brennan-O'Neill, E. and Spiegel, D. (2005) Breast cancer and problems with medical interactions: relationships with traumatic stress, emotional self-efficacy, and social support. *Psycho-Oncology*, **14** (4), 318–330.

Hand, H. (2006) Promoting effective teaching and learning in the clinical setting. *Nursing Standard*, **20** (39), 55–63.

Hannay, D.R. (1977) Missing patients on a health-center file. *Community Heath*, 8 (4), 210–216.

Harbeck, C. and Peterson, L. (1992) Elephants dancing in my head – a developmental-approach to children's concept of specific pain. *Child Development*, **63** (1), 138–149.

Harbourne, A. and Solly, A. (1996) Challenging behaviours in older people: nurses' attitudes. *Nursing Standard*, **11** (12), 39–43.

Harlow, H.F. (1959) Love in infant monkeys. *Scientific American*, **200** (6), 64–74.

Harlow, H.F. and Zimmermann, R.R. (1959) Affectional responses in the infant monkey; orphaned baby monkeys develop a strong and persistent attachment to inanimate surrogate mothers. *Science*, **130** (3373), 421–432.

Harrington, T. (1998) Perception and physiology psychology in design for older people. Paper presented at the 14th Nordle Geodetic Commission, Trundheim.

Hart, K.E. (1997) A moratorium on research using the Jenkins activity survey for Type A behavior? *Journal of Clinical Psychology*, **53** (8), 905–907.

Haskins, B. (2000) Serving and assessing deaf patients: implications for psychiatry. *Psychiatric Times*, **XVII** (12). www.psychiatrictimes.com/p001229.html (last accessed: 3 January 2006).

Haustein, K.O. (2006) Smoking and poverty. *European Journal of Cardiovascular Prevention and Rehabilitation*, **13** (3), 312–318.

Hawton, K., Salkovskis, P.M., Kirk, J. and Clark, D.M. (eds) (1989) *Cognitive Behaviour Therapy for Psychiatric Problems: A Practical Guide*. Oxford: Oxford University Press.

Haynes, R.B., Taylor, D.W. and Sackett, D.L. (1979) *Compliance in healthcare*. Baltimore, MD: Johns Hopkins University Press.

Haythornwaite, J.A., Lawrence, J.W. and Fauerbach, J.A. (2001) Brief cognitive interventions for burn pain. *Annals of Behavioural Medicine*, **23** (1), 42–49.

Health and Age (2006) The importance of empathy when nursing patients. *Health and Age*, 27 November.

Health and Safety Executive (2007) Workplace violence (http://www.hse.gov.uk/healthservices/violence/index.htm).

Healthcare Commission (2005a) *Day Surgery*. London: Healthcare Commission.

Healthcare Commission (2005b) *Emergency Department: Key Findings. Patient Survey Programme 2004/2005*. London: Commission for Healthcare Audit and Inspection.

Heather, N. (1996) Waiting for a match: the future of psychosocial treatment for alcohol problems. *Addiction*, **91** (4), 469–472.

Heather, N. (2001) Motivational interviewing: effectiveness and cost-effectiveness. *Addiction*, **96** (12), 1772–1773.

Heather, N. (2002) Effectiveness of brief interventions proved beyond reasonable doubt. *Addiction*, **97**, 293–294.

Hedelin, B. and Strandmark, M. (2001) The meaning of mental health from elderly women's perspectives: a basis for health promotion. *Perspectives in Psychiatric Care*, **37** (1), 7–14.

Heffner, K.L., Kiecolt-Glaser, J.K., Loving, T.J., Glaser, R. and Malarkey, W.B. (2004) Spousal support satisfaction as a modifier of physiological responses to marital conflict in younger and older couples. *Journal of Behavioral Medicine*, **27** (3), 233–254.

Heider, F. (1958) *The Psychology of Interpersonal Relations*. New York: Wiley.

Heim, E., Valach, L. and Schaffner, L. (1997) Coping and psychosocial adaptation: longitudinal effects over time and stages in breast cancer. *Psychosomatic Medicine*, **59** (4), 408–418.

Heintzman, M., Leathers, D.G., Parrott, R.L. and Cairns III, A.B. (1993) Nonverbal rapport-building behaviours' effect on perception of a supervisor. *Management Communication Quarterly*, **7** (2), 181–208.

Helgason, L. (1990) Twenty-year follow-up of first psychiatric presentation for schizophrenia: what would have been prevented? *Acta Psychiatrica Scandinavica*, **81**, 231–235.

Hellbom, M., Brandberg, Y., Kurland, J., Arving, C., Thalén-Lindström, A., Glimelius B. and Sjödén P.O. (2001) Assessment and treatment of psychosocial problems in cancer patients: an exploratory study of a course for nurses. *Patient Education and Counselling*, **45** (2), 101–106.

Hellmann, N. (2001) *Higher Prevalence of Drug-resistant HIV Identified in the US*. In Program of the 41st Interscience Conference on Antimicrobial Agents and Chemotherapy, Chicago, IL.

Hellzen, O., Kristiansen, L. and Norberg, K.G. (2003) Nurses' attitudes towards older residents with long-term schizophrenia. *Journal of Advanced Nursing Practice*, **43** (6), 616–622.

Helman, C. (1994) *Culture, Health and Illness*, 3rd edn. Oxford: Butterworth-Heinmann.

Helman, C.G. (2001) *Culture, Health and Illness*, 4th edn. Arnold: Oxford University Press.

Henderson, A. and Zernike, W. (2001) A study of the impact of discharge information for surgical patients. *Journal of Advanced Nursing*, 35 (3), 435–441.

Henley, A. (1983) *Asians in Britain: Caring for Hindus and Their Families*. Cambridge: National Extension College.

Henley, A. and Schott, J. (1999) *Culture, Religion and Patient Care in a Multi-ethnic Society. A Handbook for Professionals*. London: Age Concern Books.

Henson, H.K. (2002) Breast cancer and sexuality. *Sexuality and Disability*, 20 (4), 261–275.

Herlitz, J., Wiklund, I., Caidahl, K., Hartford, M., Haglid, M., Karlsson, B.W., Sjoland, H. and Karlsson, T. (1998) The feeling of loneliness prior to coronary artery bypass grafting might be a predictor of short- and long-term postoperative mortality. *European Journal of Vascular and Endovascular Surgery*, 16 (2), 120–125.

Heron, J. (1975, 2001) *Helping the Client: A Creative Practical Guide*, 1st and 5th edns. London: Sage Publications.

Herzlich, C. (1973) *Health and Illness: A Social Psychological Analysis*. Oxford: Academic Press.

Hesketh, K.L., Duncan, S.M., Estabrooks, C.A., Reimer, M., Giovannetti, P., Hyndman, K. and Acorn, S. (2003) Workplace violence in Alberta and British Columbia hospitals. *Health Policy*, 63 (3), 311–321.

Heslop, P., Smith, G.D., Carroll, D., Macleod, J., Hyland, F. and Hart, C. (2001) Perceived stress and coronary heart disease risk factors: the contribution of socioeconomic position. *British Journal of Health Psychology*, 6 (2), 167–178.

Hester, R.K. and Miller, W.R. (eds) (1995) *Handbook of alcoholism treatment approaches: Effective alternatives*, 2nd edn. Boston, MA: Allyn & Bacon.

Hibbard, J.H. and Pope, C.R. (1993) The quality of social roles as predictors of morbidity and mortality. *Social Science and Medicine*, 36 (3), 217–225.

Higgins, E.T. (1987) Self-discrepancy: a theory relating self and affect. *Psychological Review*, 94, 319–340.

Higginson, I. J. and Carr, A. J. (2001) Measuring quality of life: using quality of life measures in the clinical setting. *British Medical Journal*, 322 (7297), 1297–1300.

Hilakivi-Clarke, L. (1997) Estrogen-regulated non-reproductive behaviors and breast cancer risk: animal models and human studies. *Breast Cancer Research and Treatment*, 46 (2–3), 143–159.

Hilliard, C. (2006) Using structured reflection on a critical incident to develop a professional portfolio. *Nursing Standard*, 21 (2), 35–40.

Hinchliff, S. (2004) *The Practitioner as Teacher*, 3rd edn. London: Elsevier.

Hines, J. (2000) Communication problems of hearing-impaired patients. *Nursing Standard*, 14 (19), 33–37.

Hislop, T.G., Waxler, N.E., Coldman, A.J., Elwood, J.M. and Kan, L. (1987) The prognostic-significance of psychosocial factors in women with breast-cancer. *Journal of Chronic Diseases*, 40(7), 729–735.

Hobfoll, S.E. (1989) Conservation of resources: a new attempt at conceptualising stress. *American Psychologist*, 44, 513–524.

Hockey, L. (1976) *Women in Nursing*. London: Hodder and Stoughton.

Hodnett, E.D. (2002) Caregiver support for women during childbirth. *Cochrane Database of Systematic Reviews* (1): CD000199.

Hogg, M.A. and Vaughan, G.M. (2002) *Social Psychology*, 3rd edn. Harlow: Pearson, Prentice Hall.

Holden-Lund, C. (1988) Effects of relaxation with guided imagery on surgical stress and wound healing. *Research in Nursing & Health*, 11 (4), 235–244.

Holland, K. and Hogg, C. (2001) *Cultural Awareness in Nursing and Health Care: An Introductory Text*. Arnold: London: Hodder Headline Group.

Hollaus, P.H., Pucher, I., Wilfing, G., Wurnig, P.N. and Pridun, N.S. (2003) Pre-operative attitudes, fears and expectations of nonsmall cell lung cancer patients. *Interactive Cardiovascular and Thoracic Surgery*, 2, 206–209.

Hollinger, L.M. (1986) Communicating with the elderly. *Journal of Geronotological Nursing*, 12 (3), 9–13.

Holm, C.J., Frank, D.I. and Curtin, J. (1999) Health beliefs, health locus of control, and women's mammography behavior. *Cancer Nursing*, 22 (2), 149–156.

Holmbeck, G.N. and Shapera, W.E. (1999) *Handbook of Research Methods in Clinical Psychology*. New York: Wiley.

Holmberg, S.K., Scott, L.L., Alexy, W. and Fife, B.L. (2001) Relationship issues of women with breast cancer. *Cancer Nursing*, 24 (1), 53–60.

Holmes, T.H. and Rahe, R.H. (1967) The social readjustment rating scale. *Journal of Psychosomatic Research*, 11, 213–218.

Holyoake, D. (1999) Favourite patients: exploring labelling in inpatient culture. *Nursing Standard*, 13 (16), 44–47.

Holzman, A.D. (1986) *Pain Management: A Handbook of Psychological Treatment Approaches*. Pergamon/Allyn & Bacon.

Holzman, A.D., Turk, D.C. and Kerns, R.D. (1986) The cognitive-behavioral approach to the management of chronic pain. In Holzman, A.D. and Turk, D.C. (eds), *Pain Management: A Handbook of Psychological Treatment Approaches*. Elmsford, NY: Pergamon Press, xi, 31–50, 287

Home, A.M. (1994) Attributing responsibility and assessing gravity in wife abuse situations: a comparative study of police and social workers. *Journal of Social Service Research*, 19 (1–2), 67–84.

Hong, C.S. and Kale, S. (2003) Multiculturalism: a melting pot? *Nursing and Residential Care*, 5 (7).

Hooper, L., Bartlett, C., Davey Smith, G. and Ebrahim, S. (2002) Systematic review of long term effects of advice to reduce dietary salt in adults. *British Medical Journal*, 325 (7365), 628–632.

Horne, D.J. de L., Vatmanidis, P. and Careri, A. (1994) Preparing patients for invasive medical and surgical procedures: I. Adding behavioural and cognitive interventions. *Behavioural Medicine*, 20 (1), 5–13.

Horne, P.J., Tapper, K., Lowe, C.F., Hardman, C.A., Jackson, M.C. and Woolner, J. (2004) Increasing children's fruit and vegetable consumption: a peer-modelling and rewards-based intervention. *European Journal of Clinical Nutrition*, 58 (12), 1649–1660.

Horne, R. (1997) Representations of medication and treatment: advances in theory and measurement. In Petrie, K.J. and Weinman, J. (eds), *Perceptions of Health and Illness: Current Research and Application*, 155–188. London: Harwood Academic.

Horne, R. and Weinman, J. (1999) Patients' beliefs about prescribed medicines and their role in adherence to treatment in chronic physical illnesses. *Journal of Psychosomatic Research*, 47, 555–567.

Horne, R., Weinman, J. and Hankins, M. (1999) The beliefs about your medicines questionnaire: the development of a new method for assessing the cognitive representation of medication. *Psychology and Health*, 14, 1–24.

Horne, R., Frost, S., Hankins, M. and Wright, S. (2001) 'In the eye of the beholder': pharmacy students have more positive perceptions of medicines than students of other disciplines. In Cameron, L.D. and Leventhal, H. (eds) (2003), *The Self Regulation of Health and Illness Behaviour*. London: Routledge.

Hornesten, A., Lundman, B., Selstam, E.K. and Sandstrom, H. (2005) Patient satisfaction with diabetes care. *Journal of Advanced Nursing*, 51 (6), 609–617.

Horwitz, R.I., Viscoli, C.M., Berkman, L., Donaldson, R.M., Horwitz, S.M., Murray, C.J., Ransohoff, D.F. and Sindelar, J. (1990) Treatment adherence and risk of death after a myocardial infarction. *Lancet*, 336 (8714), 542–545.

Hough, M. (2002) *A Practical Approach to Counselling*. Harlow: Pearson Education.

Houldin, A.D. (2000) *Patients with Cancer: Understanding Psychological Pain*. Philadelphia: Lippincott Williams and Wilkins.

Houlding, C. and Davidson, R. (2003) Beliefs as predictors of condom use by injecting drug users in treatment. *Health Education Research*, 18 (2), 145–155.

Houlihan, G.D. (2005) The powers and duties of psychiatric nurses under the Mental Health Act 1983: a review of the statutory provisions in England and Wales. *Journal of Psychiatric and Mental Health Nursing*, 12, 317–324.

Houts, A., Berman, J. and Abramson, H. (1994) Effectiveness of psychological and pharmacological treatments for nocturnal enuresis. *Journal of Counselling and Clinical Psychology*, 62, 737–745.

Houts, P.S., Doak, C.C., Doak, L.G. and Loscaizo, M.J. (2005) The role of pictures in improving health communication: a review of research on attention, comprehension, recall and adherence. *Patient Education and Counselling*, 61 (2), 173–190.

Hovland, C.I., Janis, I.L. and Kelley, H.H. (1953) *Communication and Persuasion*. Newhaven, CT: Yale University Press.

Howells, G. (1997) A general practice perspective. In O'Hara, J. and Sperlinger, A. (eds) *Adults with Learning Disabilities: A Practical Approach for Health Professionals*, 61–79. Chichester: John Wiley and Sons.

HSE (2005) Psychosocial Working Conditions in Great Britain in 2005. Health and Safety Executive (http://www.hse.gov.uk/statistics/causdis/pwc2005.pdf).

HSE (2006) Stress-related and Psychological Disorders. Health and Safety Executive (http://www.hse.gov.uk/statistics/causdis/stress.htm).

http://www.alcoholconcern. org.uk

http://www.mind.org.uk/NR/rdonlyres/907BB333-FC78-4DD7-98C2-38F2592A41B1/0/MHAoutline guide2006.pdf

Huberman, W. and O'Brien, R.M. (1999) Improving therapist and patient performance in chronic psychiatric group homes through goal setting, feedback and positive reinforcement. *Journal of Organisational Behaviour Management*, 19 (1), 13–36.

Hudson, B. (1992) Ensuring an abuse free environment: a learning program for nursing home staff. *Journal of Elder Abuse and Neglect*, 4 (4), 25–36.

Hudson, G.R. (1993) Empathy and technology in the coronary care unit. *Intensive and Critical Care Nursing*, 9, 55–61.

Hughes, S. (2002) The effects of giving patients pre-operative information. *Nursing Standard*, 16 (28), 33–37.

Hughes, S.A. (2004) Promoting self-management and patient independence. *Nursing Standard*, 19 (10), 47–52.

Hunt, P. (1995) Dietary counselling: theory into practice. *Journal of the Institute of Health Education*, 33 (1), 4–8.

Hunt, P. and Hillsdon, M. (1996) *Changing Eating and Exercise Behaviour: A Handbook for Professionals*. London: Blackwell Scientific Publications.

Hunt, P. and Pearson, D. (2001) Motivating change. *Nursing Standard*, 16 (2), 45–52.

Hunter, M.S., Grunfeld, E.A. and Ramirez, A.J. (2003) Help-seeking intentions for breast-cancer symptoms: a comparison of the self-regulation model and the theory of planned behaviour. *British Journal of Health Psychology*, 8, 319–333.

Huver, R.M.E., Engels, R.C.M.E. and de Vries, H. (2006) Are anti-smoking parenting practices related to adolescent smoking cognitions and behavior? *Health Education Research*, 21 (1), 66–77.

HVA (1996) *Integrated Nursing Team – Initial information*, Professional Briefing No. 1. London: Health Visitors' Association.

Hwu, Y.J., Coates, V.E., Boore, J.R.P. *et al.* (2002) The concept of health scale: developed for Chinese people with chronic illness. *Nursing Research*, 51 (5), 292–301.

Hyde, A., Treacy, M.M., Scott, A.P., MacNeela, P., Butler, M., Drennan, J., Kate, I. and Bryne, A. (2006) Social regulation, medicalisation and the nurse's role: Insights from an analysis of nursing documentation. *International Journal of Nursing Studies*, 43 (6), 735–744.

IASP (1979) Pain terms: a list with definitions and notes on usage. Recommended by the IASP Subcommittee on Taxonomy. *Pain*, 6 (3), 249.

IASP (1992) *Classification of Chronic Pain*, 2nd edn. Seattle: International Assocation for the Study of Pain, IASP.

Iconomou, G., Viha, A., Koutras, A., Vagenakis, A.G. and Kalofonos, H.P. (2002) Information needs and awareness of diagnosis in patients with cancer receiving chemotherapy: a report from Greece. *Palliative Medicine*, 16 (4), 315–321.

liffe, S. and Drennan, V. (2001) *Primary Care and Dementia: Good Practical Guides*. London: Jessica Kingsley Publishers.

mmelt, S. (2006) Psychological adjustment in young children with chronic medical conditions. *Journal of Paediatric Nursing*, 21 (5), 362–377.

reys, H.T., Chernoff, R., DeVet, K.A. and Kim, Y. (2001) Maternal outcomes of a randomized controlled trial of a community-based support program for families of children with chronic illnesses. *Archives of Pediatrics & Adolescent Medicine*, 155 (7), 771–777.

rwin, L.G., Johnson, J.L. and Bottorff, J.L. (2005) Mothers who smoke: confessions and justifications. *Health Care for Women International*, 26 (7), 577–590.

srael, Y., Hollander, O., SanchezCraig, M., Booker, S., Miller, V., Gingrich, R. and Rankin, J.G. (1996) Screening for problem drinking and counseling by the primary care physician–nurse team. *Alcoholism – Clinical and Experimental Research*, 20 (8), 1443–1450.

ackson, L.E. (1993) Understanding, eliciting and understanding client's multicultural health beliefs. *Nurse Practitioner*, 18, 30–43.

acobsen, P.B., Meade, C.D., Stein, K.D., Chirikos, T.N., Small, B.J. and Ruckdeschel, J.C. (2002) Efficacy and costs of two forms of stress management training for cancer patients undergoing chemotherapy. *Journal of Clinical Oncology*, 20 (12), 2851–2862.

akobsson, L., Hallberg, I.R. and Lovén, L. (1997) Experiences of daily life and life quality in men with prostate cancer: an explorative study. Part 1. *European Journal of Cancer Care*, 6 (2), 108–116.

ames, D.V., Fineberg, N.A., Shah, A.K. and Priest, R.G. (1990) An increase in violence on an acute psychiatric ward: a study of associated factors. *British Journal of Psychiatry*, 156, 846–852.

ames, W. (1890) *The Principles of Psychology*. New York: Holt.

anis, I.L. (1958) *Psychological Stress: Psychoanalytic and Behavioural Studies of Surgical Patients*. New York: Wiley.

ansma, A., Breteler, M.H., Schippers, G.M., de Jong, C.A. and Van Der Staak, C.F. (2000) No effect of negative mood on the alcohol cue reactivity of in-patient alcoholics. *Addictive Behaviour*, 25 (4), 619–624.

anssen, P., Harris, S., Soolsma, J., Seymour, L. and Klein, M. (2000) Single room maternity care and client satisfaction. *Birth*, 27 (4), 235–243.

Janz, N.K. and Becker, M.H. (1984) The health belief model: a decade later. *Health Education Quarterly*, 11, 1–47.

Jarvis, M.J. (1998) Epidemiology of tobacco dependence. Paper presented at First International Conference of the Society for Research on Nicotine and Tobacco, Copenhagen.

Jay, S.M. (1988) Invasive medical procedures: psychological intervention and assessment. In Routh, D.K. (ed.), *Handbook of Pediatric Psychology*. New York: Guilford Press, 401–425.

Jeffrey, R. (1979) Normal rubbish: deviant patients in casualty department. *Sociology of Health and Illness*, 1 (1), 90–108.

Jellinek, M.S. (1999) Changes in the practice of child and adolescent psychiatry: are our patients better served? *Journal of the American Academy of Child & Adolescent Psychiatry*, 38 (2), 115–117.

Jemmott, J.B. and Jemmott, L.S. (2000) HIV behavioral interventions for adolescents in community settings. In Peterson, J.L. and DiClemente, R.J. (eds), *Handbook of HIV Prevention*. Dordrecht, Netherlands: Kluwer Academic Publishers.

Jenkins, C.D., Zyzanski, S.J. and Rosenman, R.H. (1971) Progress toward validation of a computer-scored test for type-a coronary-prone behavior pattern. *Psychosomatic Medicine*, 33 (3), 193–202.

Jiong, L., Dorthe, H.P., Preben, B.M. and Jørn, O. (2003) Mortality in parents after death of a child in Denmark: a nationwide follow-up study. *Lancet*, 361, 363–367.

Jirojwong, S. and MacLennan, R. (2003) Health beliefs, perceived self-efficacy, and breast self-examination among Thai migrants in Brisbane. *Journal of Advanced Nursing*, 41 (3), 241–249.

Jocobsen, E. (1938) *Progressive Relaxation*. Chicago: University of Chicago Press.

John, J.H., Yudkin, P.L., Neil, H.A.W. and Ziebland, S. (2003) Does stage of change predict outcome in a primary-care intervention to encourage an increase in fruit and vegetable consumption? *Health Education Research*, 18 (4), 429–438.

Johns, C. (1995) Achieving effective work as a professional activity. In O'Callaghan, N (2005) The use of expert practice to explore reflection. *Nursing Standard*, 19 (39), 41–47.

Johnson, D.W. and Johnson, F.P. (1987) *Joining Together: Group Theory and Group Skills*, 3rd edn. Englewood Cliffs, NJ: Prentice Hall.

Johnson, E.H., Jackson, L.A., Hinkle, Y., Gilbert, D., Hoopwood, T., Lollis, C.M., Willis, C. and Gant, L. (1994) What is the significance of black-white differences in risky sexual behavior? *Journal of the National Medical Association*, 86 (10), 745–759.

Johnson, J. (1999) 'Living with radiotherapy': the experiences of women with breast cancer. *Journal of Radiotherapy in Practice*, 1, 17–25.

Johnson, M.E. and Delaney, K.R. (2006) Keeping the unit safe: a grounded theory study. *Journal of the American Psychiatric Nurses Association*, 12 (1), 13–21.

Johnson, M.R. (1992) Transplant coronary disease – nonimmunologic risk factors. *Journal of Heart and Lung Transplantation*, 11 (3), S124–S132 (Part 2 Suppl.).

Johnston, M. (1988) Impending surgery. In Fisher, S. and Reason, J. (eds), *Handbook of life stress, cognition and health*, 79–100. New York: Wiley.

Johnston, M. and Vögele, C. (1993) Benefits of psychological preparation for surgery: a meta-analysis. *Annals of Behavioral Medicine*, 15 (4), 245–256.

Jones, J.M. (1997) In Schneider, D.J. (2004) *The Psychology of Stereotyping*. New York: Guilford Publications.

Jones, D.R. and Goldblatt, P.O. (1986) Cancer mortality following widow(er)hood: Some further results from the office-of-population-censuses and surveys longitudinal-study. *Stress Medicine*, **2** (2), 129–140.

Jones, F. and Bright, J. (2001) *Stress: Myth, Theory and Research*. London: Pearson Education.

Jones, J.R., Huxtable, C.S. and Hodgson, J.T. (2006) *Self-reported Work-related Illness in 2004/05: Results from the Labour Force Survey*. Caerphilly: Health and Safety Executive.

Jones, L.J. (1994) *The Social Context of Health and Health Work*. Basingstoke: Macmillan Press Ltd.

Jootun, D. (2002) Nursing with dignity. Part 7: Hinduism. *Nursing Times*, **98** (15).

Joyce, P. (2005) A framework for portfolio development in postgraduate nursing practice. *Journal of Advanced Nursing*, **14** (4), 456–234.

Kaati, G., Bygren, L.O., Vester, M., Karlsson, A.B. and Sjostrom, M. (2006) Outcomes of comprehensive lifestyle modification in inpatient setting. *Patient Education and Counselling*, **62**, 95–103.

Kain, Z.N., Sevarino, F., Alexander, G.M., Pincus, S. and Mayes, L.C. (2000) Preoperative anxiety and postoperative pain in women undergoing hysterectomy: a repeated-measure design. *Journal of Psychosomatic Research*, **49** (6), 417–422.

Kalman, M. (1967) *Psychiatric Nursing*. New York: McGraw Hill.

Kane, W. (1999) Sight specific. *Nursing Times*, **95** (32), 54–55.

Kanner, A., Coyne, J., Schaefer, C. and Lazarus, R. (1981) Comparison of two modes of stress measurement: daily hassles and uplifts versus major life events. *Journal of Behavioral Medicine*, **4**, 1–39.

Kanner, R. (1986) Pain management. *Journal of the American Medical Association*, **256** (15), 2112–2114.

Kanto, J. (1996) Preoperative anxiety: assessment and treatment, *CNS Drugs*, **6** (4), 270–279.

Kaplan, G.A., Salonen, J.T., Cohen, R.D., Brand, R.J., Syme, S.L. and Puska, P. (1988) Social connections and mortality from all causes and from cardiovascular disease: prospective evidence from Eastern Finland. *Journal of Epidemiology*, **128**, 370–380.

Kaplan, S.H., Greenfield, S. and Ware, J.E. (1989) Assessing the effects of physician-patient interactions on the outcomes of chronic disease. *Med Care*, **27** (3 Suppl.), S110–S127.

Kaprio, J., Koskenvuo, M. and Rita, H. (1987) Mortality after bereavement – a prospective-study of 95,647 widowed persons. *American Journal of Public Health*, **77** (3), 283–287.

Karling, M., Renstrom, M. and Ljungman, G. (2002) Acute and postoperative pain in children. *Acta Paediatrica*, **91** (6), 660–666.

Kashdan, T.B., Vetter, C.J. and Collins, R.L. (2005) Substance use in young adults: associations with personality and gender. *Addictive Behaviours*, **30** (2), 259–269.

Kasl, S.V. (1983) Pursuing the link between stressful life experiences and disease: a time for re-appraisal. In Cooper, C.L. (ed.), *Stress Research: Issues for the Eighties*. Chichester: Wiley.

Kasl, S.V. and Cobb, S. (1966) Health behavior, illness behavior, and sick role behavior. I. Health and illness behavior. *Archives of Environmental Health*, **12** (2), 246–266.

Kater, K.J., Rohwer, J. and Londre, K. (2002) Evaluation of an upper elementary school program to prevent body image, eating, and weight concerns, *Journal of School Health*, **72** (5), 199–204.

Kawachi, I., Kennedy, B.P. and Glass, R. (1999) Social capital and self-rated health: a contextual analysis. *American Journal of Public Health*, **89**, 1187–1193.

Keefe, F.J. (1982) Behavioral assessment and treatment of chronic pain: current status and future directions. *Journal of Consulting and Clinical Psychology*, **50** (6), 896–911.

Keely, B.R. (2002) Recognition and prevention of hospital violence. *Dimensions of Critical Care Nursing*, **21** (6), 236–241.

Kelley, H.H. (1967) Attribution theory in social psychology. In Levine, D. (ed.), *Nebraska Symposium on Motivation*. Lincoln, NE: University of Nebraska Press, 192–238.

Kelley, H.H. (1973) The process of casual attribution. *American Psychologist*, **28**, 107–128.

Kelly, P. and May, D. (1982) Good and bad patients: a review of the literature and a theoretical critique. *Journal of Advanced Nursing*, **7**, 147–156.

Kelly, M., Roberts, J.E. and Bottonari, K.A. (2007) Non-treatment-related sudden gains in depression: the role of self-evaluation. *Behaviour Research and Therapy*, **45**, 737–747.

Kelly, Y.J. and Watt, R.G. (2006) Breast-feeding initiation and exclusive duration at 6 months by social class – results from the Millennium Cohort Study. *Public Health Nutrition*, **8**, 417–421.

Kemeny, M.E. (2003) The psychology of stress. *Current Directions in Psychological Science*, **12** (4), 124–129.

Kendon, A. (1967) Some functions of gaze-direction in social interaction. *Acta Psychologica*, **26**, 22–63.

Kenny, D.T. (1995) Determinants of patient satisfaction with the medical consultation. *Psychology and Health*, **10**, 427–437.

Kenworthy, N.K., Snowley, G. and Gilling, C. (1992) *Common Foundation Studies in Nursing*. Edinburgh: Churchill Livingston.

Kerr, D. (1997) *Down's Syndrome and Dementia: Practitioner's Guide*. Birmingham: Venture Press.

Kerrell, H. (2001) Service evaluation of an autism diagnostic clinic for children. *Nursing Standard*, **15** (38), 33–37.

Kerrigan, D.D., Thevasagayam, S., Woods, T.O., McWelch, I., Thomas, W.E., Shorthouse, A.J. and Dennison, A.R. (1993) Who's afraid of informed consent. *British Medical Journal*, **306** (6873), 298–300.

Key, T.J., Schatzkin, A., Willett, W.C., Allen, N.E., Spencer, E.A. and Travis, R.A. (2007) Diet, nutrition and the prevention of cancer. *Public Health Nutrition*, **7**, 187–200.

Khadilkar, A., Milne, S., Brosseau, L., Robinson, V., Saginur, M., Shea, B., Tugwell, P. and Wells, G. (2005) Transcutaneous electrical nerve stimulation (TENS) for chronic low-back pain. *Cochrane Database of Systematic Reviews*, 2: CD003008.

Kiecolt-Glaser, J.K. and Glaser, R. (1992) Psychoneuro-immunology: can psychological interventions modulate immunity. *Journal of Consulting and Clinical Psychology*, 60 (4), 569–575.

Kiecolt-Glaser, J.K., Glaser, R., Williger, D., Stout, J., Messick, G., Sheppard, S., Ricker, D., Romisher, S.C., Briner, W., Bonnell, G. and Donnerberg, R. (1985) Psychosocial enhancement of immunocompetence in a geriatric population. *Health Psychology*, 4, 25–41.

Kiecolt-Glaser, J.K., Fisher, L.D., Ogrocki, P., Stout, J.C., Speicher, C.E. and Glaser, R. (1987) Marital quality, marital disruption, and immune function. *Psychosomatic Medicine*, 49 (1), 13–34.

Kiecolt-Glaser, J.K., Page, G.G., Marucha, P.T., MacCallum, R.C. and Glaser, R. (1998) Psychological influences on surgical recovery: perspectives from psychoneuroimmunology. *American Psychologist*, 53 (11), 1209–1218.

Kiecolt-Glaser, J.K., Preacher, K.J., MacCallum, R.C., Atkinson, C., Malarkey, W.B. and Glaser, R. (2003) Chronic stress and age related increase in the pro flammatory cytokine IL-6 Proc. *Proceedings of the National Academy of Sciences of the United States of America*, 100, 9090–9095.

Kiecolt-Glaser, J.K., Loving, T.J., Stowell, J.R., Malarkey, W.B., Lemeshow, S., Dickinson, S.L. and Glaser, R. (2005) Hostile marital interactions, proinflammatory cytokine production, and wound healing. *Archives of General Psychiatry*, 62, 1377–1384.

Kincey, J. (1995) Surgery. In Broome, A. and Llewelyn, S. (eds), *Health Psychology – Processes and Applications*, 2nd edn. London: Chapman & Hall.

Kindler, C.H., Harms, C., Amsler, F., Ihde-Scholl, T. and Scheidegger, D. (2000) The visual analog scale allows effective measurement of preoperative anxiety and detection of patients' anesthetic concerns. *Anesthesia and Analgesia*, 90 (3), 706–712.

King, C.R. (1997) Nonpharmacologic management of chemotherapy-induced nausea and vomiting. *Oncology Nursing Forum*, 24 (7), 41–48.

Kingma, M. (2001) Workplace violence in the health sector: a problem of epidemic proportion. *International Nursing Review*, 48 (3), 129–130.

Kirk, S. and Glendinning, C. (2002) Supporting 'expert' parents – professional support and families caring for a child with complex healthcare needs in the community. *International Journal of Nursing Studies*, 39 (6), 625–635.

Kitwood, T. (1997) *Dementia reconsidered: the person comes first*. Buckingham: Open University Press.

Kjelsberg, M.O., Cutler, J.A. and Dolecek, T.A. (1997) Brief description of the multiple risk factor intervention trial. *American Journal of Clinical Nutrition*, 65 (suppl.), 1915–1955.

Kleiber, C., Craft-Rosenberg, M. and Harper, D.C. (2001) Parents as distraction coaches during IV insertion: a randomised control study. *Journal of Pain and Symptoms Management*, 22 (4), 851–861.

Kleinman, A. (1980) *Patients and Their Healers in the Context of Culture*. Berkeley, CA: University of California Press, 49–70.

Knapp, M.L. (1978) *Nonverbal Communication in Human Interaction*, 2nd edn. New York: Holt, Rinehart and Winston.

Knowler, W.C., Barrett-Connor, E., Fowler, S.E., Hamman, R.F., Lachin, J.M., Walker, E.A., Nathan, D.M.; Diabetes Prevention Program Research Group (2002) Reduction in the incidence of type 2 diabetes with lifestyle intervention or metformin. *The New England Journal of Medicine*, 346 (6), 393–403.

Knox, K.A. (1998) Applying psychological theory to visual impairment: something to consider. *Ophthalmic Nursing*, 2 (3), 14–18.

Kobasa, S.C. (1979) Stressful life events, personality, and health: inquiry into hardiness. *Journal of Personality and Social Psychology*, 37 (1), 1–11.

Kohl, H.W. II (200I) Physical activity and cardiovascular disease: evidence for a dose response. *Medicine & Science in Sports & Exercise*, 33 (6), supplement, S472–S483.

Kohnke, M.F. (1982) *Advocacy: Risk and Reality*. St. Louis MO: Mosby.

Kools, M. (2006) A focus on the usability of health education material. *Patient Education and Counselling*, 65 (3), 275–276.

Kownacki, R.J. and Shadish, W.R. (1999) Does Alcoholics Anonymous work? The results from a meta-analysis of controlled experiments. *Substance Use and Misuse*, 34 (13), 1897–1916.

Kralik, D., Koch, T. and Wotten, K. (1997) Engagement and detachment: understanding patients' experiences with nurses. *Journal of Advanced Nursing*, 26 (2), 399–407.

Kramer, K. and Kerkstra, A. (1991) *Eenzaamheid Van Bewoners in Een Verzorgingstehuis (Loneliness of Residents in an Elderly Home)*. Utrecht: NIVEL.

Kreek, M.J., Nielsen, D.A., Butelman, E.R. and LaForge, K.S. (2005) Genetic influences on impulsivity, risk-taking, stress responsivity and vulnerability to drug abuse and addiction. *Nature Neuroscience*, 8, 1450–1457.

Kreitler, S. (1999) Denial in cancer patients. *Cancer Invest*, 17, 514–534.

Kristenson, H., Ohlin, H., Hultén-Nosslin, M.B., Trell, E. and Hood, B. (1983) Identification and intervention of heavy drinking in middle-aged men: results and follow-up of 24–60 months of long-term study with randomized controls. *Alcoholism: Clinical and Experimental Research*, 7 (2), 203–209.

Kruger, J., Yore, M.M. and Kohl, H.W. (2007) Leisure-time physical activity patterns by weight control status: 1999–2002 NHANES. *Medicine & Science in Sports & Exercise*, 39 (5), 788–795.

Krumholz, H.M., Butler, J., Miller, J., Vaccarino, V., Williams, C.S., de Leon, C.F.M., Seeman, T.E., Kasl, S.V. and Berkman, L.F. (1998) Prognostic importance of emotional support for elderly patients hospitalized with heart failure. *Circulation*, 97 (10), 958–964.

Kruse, A. and Schmitt, E. (2006) A multidimensional scale for the measurement of agreement with age stereotypes and the salience of age in social interaction. *Aging and Society*, **26**, 393–411.

Kubler-Ross, E. (1969) *On Death and Dying*. New York: Macmillan.

Kubler-Ross, E. (2001) *Living with Death and Dying*. Huma Horizons Series. New York: Touchstone Books; Simon and Schuster.

Kuhn, D., Langer, J., Kohlberg, L. *et al.* (1977) Development of formal operations in logical and moral judgement. *Genetic Psychology Monographs*, **95** (1), 97–188.

Kuhn, S., Cooke, K., Collins, M., Jones, J.M. and Mucklow, J.C. (1990) Perceptions of pain after surgery. *British Medical Journal*, **300**, 1687–1690.

Kulik, J.A., Moore, P.J. and Mahler, H.I. (1993) Stress and affiliation: hospital roommate effects on preoperative anxiety and social interaction. *Health Psychology*, **12** (2), 118–124.

Kulik, J.A., Mahler, H.I. and Moore, P.J. (1996) Social comparison and affiliation under threat: effects on recovery from major surgery. *Journal of Personality and Social Psychology*, **71** (5), 967–979.

Kunyk, D. and Olson, J.K. (2001) Clarification of conceptualizations of empathy. *Journal of Advanced Nursing*, **35** (3), 317–325.

Kuper, H. and Marmot, M. (2003) Job strain, job demands, decision latitude, and risk of coronary heart disease within the Whitehall II study. *Journal of Epidemiology and Community Health*, **57** (2), 147–153.

Kur Gill, B. (2002) Nursing with Dignity – Sikhism. *Nursing Times*, **98** (14).

Kurtz, S.M.S. (1990) Adherence to diabetes regimens: empirical status and clinical applications. *Diabetics Education*, **16**, 50–56.

Labonte, R. (1994) Health promotion and empowerment: reflections on professional practice. *Health Education Quarterly*, **21**, 253–268.

Lachman, M.E. and Weaver, S.L. (1998) The sense of control as a moderator of social class differences in health and well-being. *Journal of Personality and Social Psychology*, **74** (3), 763–773.

Lal, M.K., McClelland, J., Phillips, J. *et al.* (2001) Comparison of EMLA cream versus placebo in children relieving distraction therapy for venepuncture. *Acta Paediatrica*, **90** (2), 154–159.

Lang, E.V., Benotsch, E.G., Fick, L.J., Lutgendorf, S., Berbaun, M., Berbaum, K., Logan, H. and Spiegel, D. (2000) Adjunctive non-pharmacological analgesia for invasive medical procedure: a randomised trial, *Lancet*, **355** (9214), 1486–1490.

Langley, P., Fonseca, J. and Iphofen, R. (2006) Psychoneuroimmunology and health from a nursing perspective. *British Journal of Nursing*, **15** (20), 1126–1129.

Larner, S. (2005) Common psychological challenges for patients with newly acquired disability. *Nursing Standard*, **19** (28), 33–39.

Latham, J. (1988) *Pain Control*. London: Austin Cornish Publishers, in association with the Lisa Sainsbury Foundation.

Latimer, E. (1998) Ethical care at the end of life. *Canadian Medical Association Journal*, **158** (13), 1741–1747.

Launder, W., Davidson, G., Anderson, I. and Barclay, A. (2005) Self-neglect: the role of judgments and applied ethics. *Nursing Standard*, **19** (18), 45–51.

Lawton, S. and Stewart, F. (2007) Assertiveness: making yourself heard in district nursing. *British Journal of Community Nursing*, **10** (6), 281–283.

Lazarus, A.A. (1973) Multimodal behavior therapy: treating the 'basic id'. *Journal of Nervous and Mental Diseases*, **156** (6), 404–411.

Lazarus, R.S. (1966) *Psychological Stress and the Coping Process*. New York: McGraw-Hill.

Lazarus, R.S. and Folkman, S. (1984) *Stress, Appraisal, and Coping*. New York: Springer.

Lazarus, R.S. and Folkman, S. (1987) Transactional theory and research on emotions and coping. *European Journal of Personality*, **1**, 141–170.

Lazarus, R.S. and Gal, R. (1975) The role of activity in anticipating and confronting stressful situations. *Journal of Human Stress*, **1** (4), 4–20.

Le May, A. (2004) Building a rapport through non-verbal communication. *Nursing and Residential Care*, **6** (10), 488–491.

Le May, A.C. and Redfern, S.J. (1987) A study of non-verbal communication between nurses and the elderly patients. In Fielding, P. (ed.), *Research in the Nursing Care of Elderly People*. Chichester: John Wiley and Sons Ltd, 171–189.

Le Var, R.M.H. (1998) Improving educational preparation for transcultural health care. *Nurse Education Today*, **18**, 519–533.

Leach, E. (1982) *Social Anthropology*. London: Fontana.

Lee, F. (2001) Violence in A&E: the role of training and self-efficacy. *Nursing Standard*, **15** (46), 33–38.

Lee, M. and Rotheram-Borus, M.J. (2001) Challenges associated with increased survival among parents living with HIV. *American Journal of Public Health*, **91** (8), 1303–1309.

Lee, S., Colditz, G.A., Berkman, L.F. and Kawachi, I. (2003a) Caregiving and risk of coronary heart disease in US women – a prospective study. *American Journal of Preventive Medicine*, **24** (2), 113–119.

Lee, S., Colditz, G., Berkman, L. and Kawachi, I. (2003b) Caregiving to children and grandchildren and risk of coronary heart disease in women. *American Journal of Public Health*, **93** (11), 1939–1944.

Leininger, M. (1995) *Transcultural Nursing: Concepts, Theories and Practices*. Maidenhead: McGraw Hill.

Leininger, M. (1997) Transcultural nursing research to nursing education and practice: 40 years. *Image J Nurs Sch*, **29** (4), 341–347.

Lennard-Jones, J.E. (1992) *A Positive Approach to Nutrition as Treatment*. Report of a Working Party on the role of enteral and parenteral feeding in hospital and at home. London: Kings Fund.

Lepore, S.J. and Coyne, J.C. (2006) Psychological interventions for distress in cancer patients: a review of reviews. *Annals of Behavioral Medicine*, **32** (2), 85–92.

Lerman, C., Rimer, B., Blumberg, B., Cristinzio, S., Engstrom, P.F., MacElwee, N., O'Connor, K. and Seay, J.

(1990) Effects of coping style and relaxation on cancer-chemotherapy side-effects and emotional responses. *Cancer Nursing*, **13** (5), 308–315.

Lerner, R.M., Villarruel, F.A. and Castellino, D.R. (1999) *Adolescence: Developmental Issues in the Clinical Treatment of Children*. Boston, MA: Allyn & Bacon, 125–136.

Leserman, J. (2003) HIV disease progression: depression, stress and possible mechanisms. *Biological Psychiatry*, **54** (3), 295–306.

LeShan, L. (1994) *Cancer as a turning point. A handbook for people with cancer, their families and health professionals*, revised edn. New York: Plume.

Leventhal, H. (1993) Theories of compliance, and turning necessities into preferences: application to adolescent health action. In Krasnegor, N.A., Epstein, L., Johnson, S.B. and Yaffe, S.S. (eds), *Development Aspects of Health Behaviour*. New Jersey: Lawrence Erlbaum Associates.

Leventhal, H. (ed.) (2003) *The Self-Regulation of Health and Illness Behaviour*. London: Routledge.

Leventhal, H. and Cameron, L. (1987) Behavioural theories and the problem of compliance. *Patient Education and Counselling*, **10**, 117–138.

Leventhal, H., Meyer, D. and Nerenz, D.R. (1980) The common sense representation of illness danger. In Cameron, L.D. and Leventhal, H. (eds) (2003), *The Self-Regulation of Health and Illness Behaviour*. London: Routledge.

Leventhal, H., Nerenz, D.R. and Steele, D.J. (1984) Illness representations and coping with health threats. In Baum, A., Taylor, S.E. and Singer, J.E. (eds), *Handbook of Psychology and Health, Volume IV: Social Psychological Aspects of Health*. Hillsdale, NJ: Erlbaum, 219–252.

Leventhal, H., Prohaska, T.R. and Hirschman, R.S. (1985) Preventive health behavior across the life span. In Rosen, J.C. and Solomon, L.J. (eds) *Prevention in health psychology*, volume 8, 190–235. Hanover, NH: University Press of New England.

Levine, W.H. (1987) Research on pictures: a guide to the literature. In Willows, D.M. (ed.), *The Psychology of Illustration*, Vol. 1. New York: HA Houghton, 2–50.

Levinson, W., Roter, D.L., Mullooly, J.P., Dull, V.T. and Frankel, R.M. (1997) Physician–patient communication. The relationship with malpractice claims among primary care physicians and surgeons. *Journal of the American Medical Association*, **277**, 553–559.

Lewis, C. and Allen, D. (2003) Nurse prescribing. general prescribing principles, teamwork. *Nursing Standard*, **17** (4).

Ley, P. (1981) Professional non-compliance: a neglected problem. *British Journal of Clinical Psychology*, **20**, 151–154.

Ley, P. (1988) *Communicating with Patients*. London: Croom Helm.

Ley, P. (1989) Improving patients' understanding, recall, satisfaction and compliance. In Broome, A. (ed.), *Health Psychology*. London: Chapman and Hall.

Ley, P. (1990) *Communicating with Patients: Improving Communication Satisfaction and Compliance*. Psychology and Health Series 4. London: Chapman and Hall.

Ley, P., Whitworth, M.A., Skilbeck, C.E., Woodward, R., Pinsent, R.J.F.H., Pike, L.A., Clarkson, M.E. and Clark,

P.B. (1976) Improving doctor–patient communication. In Ley, P. (1990) *Communicating with Patients: Improving Communication Satisfaction and Compliance*. Psychology and Health Series 4. London: Chapman and Hall.

Li, J. *et al.* (2002) Cancer incidence in parents who lost a child. *Cancer*, **95**, 2237–2242.

Liddell, C., Rae, G., Brown, T.R.M., Johnston, D., Coates, V. and Mallett, J. (2004) Giving patients an audiotape of their GP consultation: a randomised controlled trial. *British Journal of General Practice*, **54**, 667–672.

Like, R. and Zyzanski, S.J. (1986) Patient requests in family practice. A focal point for clinical negotiations. *Family Practice*, **3**, 216–228.

Like, R. and Zyzanski, S.J. (1987) Patient satisfaction with the clinical encounter: social psychological determinants. *Soc Sci Med*. **24**, 351–357.

Lillberg, K., Verkasalo, P.K., Kaprio, J., Teppo, L., Helenius, H. and Koskenvuo, M. (2003) Stressful life events and risk of breast cancer in 10,808 women: a cohort study. *American Journal of Epidemiology*, **157**, 415–423.

Lin, M.F., Chiou, J.H., Chou, M.H. and Hsu, M.C. (2006) Significant experience of token therapy from the perspective of psychotic patients. *Journal of Nursing Research*, **14** (4), 315–323.

Lindholm, L., Rehnsfeldt, A., Arman, M. and Hamrin, E. (2002) Significant others' experience of suffering when living with women with breast cancer. *Scandinavian Journal of Caring Sciences*, **16** (3), 248–255.

Lindsey, E. (1996) Health within illness: experiences of chronically ill/disabled people. *Journal of Advanced Nursing*, **24** (3), 465–472.

Linn, B.S., Linn, M.W. and Jensen, J. (1983) Surgical stress in the healthy elderly. *Journal of the American Geriatrics Society*, **31** (9), 544–548.

Lippman, W. (1922) *Public Opinion*. New York: Harcourt Brace.

Lipton, R.B., Losey, L.M., Giachello, A., Mendez, J. and Girotti, M.H. (1998) Attitudes and issues in treating Lation patients with type 2 diabetes: views of health care providers. *Diabetes Educ.*, **24** (1), 67–71.

Litt, M.D., Cooney, N.L., Kadden, R.M. and Gaupp, L. (1990) Reactivity to alcohol cues and induced moods in alcoholics. *Addictive Behaviour*, **15** (2), 137–146.

Litt, M.D., Nye, C.Y. and Shafer, D. (1995) Preparation for oral surgery: evaluating elements of coping. *Journal of Behavioural Medicine*, **18** (5), 435–459.

Little, P., Everitt, H., Williamson, I., Warner, G., Moore, M., Gould, C., Ferrier, K. and Payne, S. (2001) Observational study of effect of patient centredness and positive approach to outcomes of general practice consultations. *British Medical Journal*, **323**, 908–911.

Lobb, M.L., Shannon, M.C., Recer, S.L. and Allen, J.B. (1984) A behavioral technique for recovery from the psychological trauma of hysterectomy. *Perceptual and Motor Skills*, **59** (2), 677–678.

Lock, C.A. (2004) Screening and brief alcohol interventions: what, why, who, where and when? A review of the literature. *Journal of Substance Use*, **9** (2), 91–101.

Lock, C.A., Kaner, E., Lamont, S. and Bond, S. (2002) A qualitative study of nurses' attitudes and practices regarding brief alcohol intervention in primary health care. *Journal of Advanced Nursing*, **39** (4), 333–342.

Locke, E.A. and Latham, G.P. (1984) *Goal Setting: A Motivational Technique That Works*. Englewood Cliffs, NJ: Prentice-Hall.

Lockwood, P. and Kunda, Z. (1999) Increasing the salience of ones best selves can undermine inspiration by outstanding role models. *Journal of Personality and Social Psychology*, **76** (2), 214–228.

Logan, C. (1985) Praise: the powerhouse of self-esteem. *Nursing Management*, **16** (6), 35–38.

Long, A. and Reid, W. (1996) An exploration of the nursing care of the suicidal patient in an acute psychiatric ward. *Journal of Psychiatric and Mental Health Nursing*, **3**, 29–37.

Lorber, J. (1975) Good patients and problem patients: conformity and deviance in a general hospital. *Journal of Health and Social Behaviour*, **16** (2), 213–225.

Lowe, C.F., Horne, P.J., Tapper, K., Bowdery, M. and Egerton, C. (2004) Effects of a peer modelling and rewards-based intervention to increase fruit and vegetable consumption in children. *European Journal of Clinical Nutrition*, **58** (3), 510–522.

Lowe, T. (2000) Aggressive incidents on a psychiatric intensive care unit. *Nursing Standard*, **14** (35), 33–36.

Lowery, K., Buri, H. and Ballard, C. (2000) What is the prevalence of environmental hazards in the home of dementia sufferers and are they associated with falls? *International Journal of Geriatric Psychiatry*, **15** (10), 883–886.

Ludwick-Rosenthal, R. and Neufeld, R.W. (1993) Preparation for undergoing an invasive medical procedure: interacting effects of information and coping style. *Journal of Consulting and Clinical Psychology*, **61** (1), 156–164.

Luft, J. (1969) *On Human Interaction*. Palo Alto, CA: National Press.

Lundberg, U. (2006) Stress, subjective and objective health. *International Journal of Social Welfare*, **15** (1) (suppl.), s41–s48.

Lutgendorf, S.K., Sood, A.K., Anderson, B., McGinn, S., Maiseri, H., Dao, M., Sorosky, J.L., De Geest, K., Ritchie, J. and Lubaroff, D.M. (2005) Social support, psychological distress, and natural killer cell activity in ovarian cancer. *Journal of Clinical Oncology*, **23** (28), 7105–7113.

Lyneham, J. (2000) Violence in New South Wales emergency departments. *Australian Journal of Advanced Nursing*, **18**, 2, 8–17.

Lyonfields, J.D. (1993) In Brewin, C. and Bernice, A. (2000) Psychological defence mechanisms: the example of repression. *The Psychologist*, **13** (12), 615–617.

MacIntyre, S. (1986) The patterning of health by social position in contemporary Britain: directions for sociological research. *Social Science & Medicine*, **23** (4), 393–415.

Mack, D.R.A. (1999) *From Babylon to Rastafari: Origin and History of the Rastafarian Movement*. Chicago, IL: Front Line Distribution International. Available at Amazon.com.

MacKay, R., Hughes, J. and Carver, E. (1990) *Empathy in the Helping Relationship*. New York: Springer Publishing Company.

Mackenbach, J.P. (2005) Genetics and health inequalities: hypotheses and controversies. *Journal of Epidemiology and Community Health*, **59** (4), 268–273.

Macleod, J., Smith, G.D., Heslop, P.F., Metcalf, C., Carroll, D., Hart, C. and Lynch, J. (2002) Psychological stress and cardiovascular disease: empirical demonstration of bias in a prospective observational study of Scottish men. *British Medical Journal*, **324** (7348), 1247–1251.

Macleod Clark, J. (1982) Nurse–patient communication – an analysis of conversations from surgical wards. In Wilson-Barnet, J. (ed.), *Nursing Research Studies in Patient Care*, 25–55. Chichester: John Wiley and Sons.

Maguire, P. and Pitceathly, C. (2002) Key communication skills and how to acquire them. *British Medical Journal*, **325**, 697–700.

Major, S. (2002) Dysfunctional teams: a health and resource warning. *Nursing Management*, **9** (2), 25–28.

Manheimer, E., White, A., Berman, K. and Forys, K. (2005) Meta analysis: accupuncture for low back pain. *Annals of International Medicine*, **142** (19), 651–663.

Manimala, R., Blount, R.L. and Cohen, L.L. (2000) Easier said than done: what parents say they do and what they do during children's immunization. *Children's Health Care*, **29** (2), 79–86.

Mann, T., Sherman, D. and Updegraff, J. (2007) Dispositional motivations and message framing: a test of the congruency hypothesis in college students. *Health Psychology*, **23** (3), 330–334.

Manne, S.L., Sabbioni, M., Bovbjerg, D.H., Jocobsen, P.B., Taylor, K.L. and Redd, W.H. (1994) Coping with chemotherapy for breast-cancer. *Journal of Behavioral Medicine*, **17** (1), 41–55.

Manne, S.L., Taylor, K.L., Dougherty, J. and Kemeny, N. (1997) Supportive and negative responses in the partner relationship: their association with psychological adjustment among individuals with cancer. *Journal of Behavioral Medicine*, **20** (2), 101–125.

Manne, S., Sherman, M., Ross, S., Ostroff, J., Heyman, R.E. and Fox, K. (2004a) Couples' support-related communication, psychological distress, and relationship satisfaction among women with early stage breast cancer. *Journal of Consulting and Clinical Psychology*, **72** (4), 660–670.

Manne, S.L., Ostroff, J.S., Winkel, G., Fox, K., Grana, G., Miller, E., Ross, S. and Frazier, T. (2005) Couple-focused group intervention for women with early stage breast cancer. *Journal of Consulting and Clinical Psychology*, **73** (4), 634–646.

Manne, S.L., Ostroff, J.S., Norton, T.R., Fox, K., Goldstein, L. and Grana, G. (2006) Cancer-related relationship communication in couples coping with early stage breast cancer. *Psycho-Oncology*, **15** (3), 234–247.

Manthorpe, J. and Iliffe, S. (2006) Anxiety and depression. *Nursing Older People*, **18** (1), 24–29.

Maranets, I. and Kain, Z.N. (1999) Preoperative anxiety and intraoperative anesthetic requirements. *Anesthesia and Analgesia*, **89** (6), 1346–1351.

Marazziti, D., Ambrogi, F., Abelli, M., Nasso, E.D., Catena, M., Massimetti, G., Carlini, M. and Dell'Osso, L. (2007) Lymphocyte subsets, cardiovascular measures and anxiety state before and after a professional examination. *Stress*, **10** (1), 93–99.

Marchevsky, D., Leach, C., White, D., Sims, R. and Cottrell, D. (2000) Hospital anxiety and depression scale for use with adolescents – Authors' reply. *British Journal of Psychiatry*, **177**, 89.

Mares, P., Henley, A. and Baxter, C. (1985) *Healthcare Care in Multiracial Britain*. London: Health Education Council.

Marks, D.F. (2005) *Health Psychology: Theory, Research and Practice*. Sage Publications.

Marks, I.M. (1987) *Fears, Phobias and Rituals. Panic, Anxiety and Their Disorders*. New York: Oxford University Press.

Marks, I.M. (1997) *Living With Fear: Understanding and Coping with Anxiety*. Maidenhead: McGraw Hill.

Marks, R.M. and Sachar, E.J. (1973) Under treatment of medical inpatients with narcotic analgesics. *Annals of Internal Medicine*, **78**, 173–181.

Marsh, A. and McKay, S. (1994) *Poor Smokers*. London: Policy Studies Institute.

Marshall, M. (ed.) (2005) *Perspectives on Rehabilitation and Dementia*. London: Jessica Kingsley.

Martell, C.R., Jacobson, N.S. and Addis, M.E. (2001) *Depression in Context: Strategies for Guided Action*. New York: W.W. Norton and Co.

Martikainen, P. and Valkonen, T. (1996) Mortality after the death of a spouse: rates and causes of death in a large Finnish cohort. *American Journal of Public Health*, **86** (8), 1087–1093.

Martin, M.J., Vila, J. and Capellas, R. (2000) A study of nursing students' personality. *Revista Rol de Enfermeria*, **23**, 643–646.

Maslow, A.H. (1943) A theory of human motivation. *Psychological Review*, **50**, 370–396.

Massé, R. (2000) Qualitative and quantitative analyses of psychological distress: methodological complementarity and ontological incommensurability. *Qualitative Health Research*, **10** (3), 411–423.

Mathews, A. and Ridgeway, V. (1984) Psychological preparation for surgery. In Steptoe, A. and Mathews, A. (eds), *Health Care and Human Behaviour*. London: Academic Press.

Matthews, K.A. and Gump, B.B. (2002) Chronic work stress and marital dissolution increase risk of posttrial mortality in men from the multiple risk factor intervention trial. *Archives of Internal Medicine*, **162** (3), 309–315.

Maunsell, E., Brisson, J. and Deschenes, L. (1995) Social support and survival among women with breast cancer. *Cancer*, **76** (4), 631–637.

Maunsell, E., Drolet, M., Brisson, J., Robert, J. and Deschenes, L. (2002) Dietary change after breast cancer: extent, predictors, and relation with psychological distress. *Journal of Clinical Oncology*, **20** (4), 1017–1025.

May, V. (2001) Attitudes to patients who present suicidal behaviour. *Emergency Nurse*, **9** (4), 26–32.

McAleer, M. (2006) Communicating effectively with deaf patients. *Nursing Standard*, **20** (19), 51–54.

McAllister-Williams, R.H., (2006) Relapse prevention in bipolar disorders: A critical review of current guidelines. *Journal of Psychopharmacology*, **20** (2), Supplement (2006), 12–16.

McCaffey, M. (1983) *Nursing Patients in Pain*. London: Harper and Row.

McCallie, M.S., Blum, C.M. and Hood, C.J. (2006) Progressive muscle relaxation. *Journal of Human Behavior in the Social Environment*, **13** (3), 51–66.

McCann, K. and McKenna, H.P. (1993) An examination of touch between nurses and elderly patients in a continuing care setting in Northern Ireland. *Journal of Advanced Nursing*, **18**, 838–846.

McCarthy, A.M. and Kleiber, C. (2006) A conceptual model of factors influencing children's responses to a painful procedure when parents are distraction coaches. *Journal of Paediatric Nursing*, **21** (2), 88–98.

McCarthy, M.C., Ruiz, E., Gale, B.J., Karam, C. and Moore, N. (2004) The meaning of health: perspectives of Anglo and Latino older women. *Health Care for Women International*, **25**, 950–969.

McCormack, B. (2001) Autonomy and the relationship between nurses and older people. *Ageing and Society*, **21**, 417–446.

McDonald, H.P., Garg, A.X. and Haynes, R.B. (2002) Interventions to enhance patient adherence to medication prescriptions. *Journal of the American Medical Association*, **288** (22), 2868–2879.

McDonald, S. *et al*. (2004) Pre-operative education for hip or knee replacement. *The Cochrane Library*, Vol. 1.

McEwen, B. and Lasley, E.N. (2002) *The End of Stress as We Know It*. Washington, DC: Joseph Henry Press.

McGarry, J. and Simpson, C. (2007) Nursing students and elder abuse: developing a learning resource. *Nursing Older People*, **19** (2), 27–30.

McGregor, B.A., Antoni, M.H., Boyers, A., Alferi, S.M., Blomberg, B.B. and Carver, C.S. (2004) Cognitive-behavioral stress management increases benefit finding and immune function among women with early-stage breast cancer. *Journal of Psychosomatic Research*, **56** (1), 1–8.

McHale, S. (1999) From insult to injury. *Nursing Times*, **95** (49), 30.

McKenna, H., Slater, P., McCance, T., Bunting, B., Spiers, A. and McElwee, G. (2001) Qualified nurses' smoking prevalence: their reasons for smoking and desire to quit. *Journal of Advanced Nursing*, **35** (5), 769–775.

McKenzie, K. *et al*. (2004) The impact of nurse education on staff attributions in relation to challenging behaviour. *Learning Disability Practice*, **7** (5), 16–21.

McMullan, M., Endacott, R., Gray, M.A. *et al*. (2003) Portfolios and assessment of competence: a review of the literature. *Journal of Advanced Nursing*, **41** (3), 283–294.

McMullen O'Brien, S. (1998) Health promotion and schizophrenia: the year 2000 and beyond. *Holistic Nursing Practice*, **12** (2), 38–43.

McVicar, A. (2003) Workplace stress in nursing: a literature review. *Journal of Advanced Nursing*, **44** (6), 633–642.

Mearns, D. and Thorne, B. (2005) *Person-centred Counselling in Action*, 2nd edn. Sage Counselling in Action, London: Sage Publications.

Mechanic, D. (1962) The concept of illness behaviour. *Journal of Chronic Diseases*, **15**, 189–194.

Mechanic, D. (1978) Effects of psychological distress on perceptions of physical health and use of medical and psychiatric facilities. *Journal of Human Stress*, **4** (4), 26–32.

Meeting of the Healthcare Commission (2005) Report Head of complaints. Health care Commission. Agenda item 12, CM/05/65. 23 June 2005. http://www.healthcare commission.org.uk/_db/_documents/Chairman_report.pdf.

Mehrabian, A. (1971) *Silent Messages*. Belmont, CA: Wadsworth.

Meichenbaum, D. and Cameron, R. (1983) Stress inoculation training: toward a general paradigm for training coping skills. In Meichenbaum, D. and Jaremko, M.E. (eds), *Stress Reduction and Prevention*. New York: Plenum, 115–154.

Melia, K. (1987) *Learning and Working: The Occupational Socialisation of Nurses*. London: Tavistock.

Meltzer, H., Gill, B., Petticrew, M. and Hinds, K. (1995) *OPCS Surveys of Psychiatric Morbidity in Great Britain: Report 1 The Prevalence of Psychiatric Morbidity Among Adults Living in Private Households*. London: HMSO.

Melzack, R. (1975) The McGill pain questionnaire: major properties and scoring methods. *Pain*, **1**, 277–299.

Melzack, R. and Wall, P.D. (1965) Pain mechanisms: a new theory. *Science*, **150**, 971–979.

Melzack, R. and Wall, P.D. (1973) *The Challenge of Pain*. New York: Basic Books.

Melzack, R., Abbott, F.V., Zackon, W., Mulder, D. and Davies, M.W.L. (1987) Pain on a surgical ward: a survey of the duration and intensity of pain and the effectiveness of medication. *Pain*, **29**, 67–72.

Mendes de Leon, C.F., Powell, L.H. and Kaplan, B.H. (1991) Change in coronary-prone behaviours in the recurrent coronary prevention project. *Psychosomatic Medicine*, **53** (4), 407–419.

Meyer, D., Leventhal, H. and Gutmann, M. (1985) Self-regulation. In Cameron, L.D. and Leventhal, H. (eds) (2003), *The Self Regulation of Health and Illness Behaviour*. London: Routledge.

Meyerowitz, B.E. and Chaiken, S. (1987) The effects of message framing on breast care self examination attitudes, intentions and behaviour. *Journal of Personality and Social Psychology*, **52**, 500–510.

Michael, M. and Tannock, I.F. (1998) Measuring health-related quality of life in clinical trials that evaluate the role of chemotherapy in cancer treatment. *Canadian Medical Association Journal*, **158** (13), 1727–1734.

Michaud, C., Kahn, J.P., Musse, N., Burtlet, C., Nicolas, J.P. and Mejean, L. (1990) Relationships between a critical life event and eating behavior in high-school-students. *Stress Medicine*, **6** (1), 57–64.

Michell, J. (2000) Normal science, pathological science and psychometrics. *Theory & Psychology*, **10** (5), 639–667.

Middlesex University (2001) *Cultural Competence and Awareness Project*. Research Centre for Transcultural Studies in Health, Middlesex University.

Midtgaard, J., Rorth, M., Stelter, R. and Adamsen, L. (2006) The group matters: an explorative study of group cohesion and quality of life in cancer patients participating in physical exercise intervention during treatment. *European Journal of Cancer Care*, **15** (1), 25–33.

Miles, D.R. and Carey, G. (1997) Genetic and environmental architecture of human aggression. *Journal of Personality and Social Psychology*, **72**, 207–217.

Miller, G.A. (1956) The magical number seven plus or minus two: some limits on our capacity for processing information. *Psychological Review*, **63**, 81–97.

Miller, L. (2002) Effective communication with older people. *Nursing Standard*, **17** (9), 45–50.

Miller, S.M. (1980) When is a little information a dangerous thing? Coping with stressful life events by monitoring v blunting. In Levine, S. and Ursin, H. (eds), *Coping and Health*, 54–65. New York: Plenum Press.

Miller, S.M. (1987) Monitoring and blunting: validation of a questionnaire to assess styles of information seeking under threat. *Journal of Personality and Social Psychology*, **52** (2), 345–353.

Miller, S.M. and Mangan, C.E. (1983) Interacting effects of information and coping style in adapting to gynecologic stress: should the doctor tell all? *Journal of Personality and Social Psychology*, **45** (1), 223–236.

Miller, T.Q., Smith, T.W., Turner, C.W., Guijarro, M.L. and Hallet, A.J. (1996) A meta-analytic review of research on hostility and physical health. *Psychological Bulletin*, **119** (2), 322–348.

Miller, W. and Rollnick, S. (1991) *Motivational Interviewing: Preparing to Change Addictive Behaviour*. London and New York: The Guilford Press.

Miller, W.R. and Rollnick, S. (2002) *Motivational Interviewing: Preparing People for Change*, 2nd edn. New York: Guilford Press.

Mills, P. (2005) Establishing a biofeedback (behavioural therapy) service. *Gastrointestinal Nursing*, **3** (3), 35–39.

Mind (2002) *Mental Health Statistics 6: The Social Context of Mental Distress*. London: Mind.

Mitchell, M.J. (2000a) Psychological preparation for patients undergoing day surgery. *Ambulatory Surgery*, **8** (1), 19–29.

Mitchell, M.J. (2000b) Anxiety management: a district nursing role in day surgery. *Ambulatory Surgery*, **8** (3), 119–127.

Mitchell, M. (2005) *Anxiety Management in Adult Day Surgery: A Nursing Perspective*. London: Whurr.

Mitchell, M. (2007) Psychological care of patients undergoing elective surgery. *Nursing Standard*, **21** (30), 48–55.

Mock, V., Dow, K.H., Meares, C.J., Grimm, P.M., Dienemann, J.A., Haisfield-Wolfe, M.E., Quitasol, W., Mitchell, S., Chakravarthy, A. and Gage, I. (1997) Effects of exercise on fatigue, physical functioning, and emotional distress during radiation therapy for breast cancer. *Oncology Nursing Forum*, **24** (6), 991–1000.

Mohamed, I.E., Williams, K.S., Tamburrino, M.B., Wryobeck, J.M. and Carter, S. (2005) Understanding locally advanced breast cancer: What influences a woman's decision to delay treatment? *Preventive Medicine*, 41 (2), 399–405.

Mokdad, A.H., Marks, J.S., Stroup, D.F. and Gerberding, J.L. (2004) Actual causes of death in the United States, 2000. *Journal of the American Medical Association*, 291 (10), 1238–1245.

Molassiotis, A., Yung, H.H.P., Yam, B.M.C. and Mok, T.S.K. (2006) The clinical management of chemotherapy-induced nausea and vomiting with adjuvant progressive muscle relaxation training and imagery techniques in breast cancer patients. *Hong Kong Medical Journal*, 12 (2), S25–27.

Moore, J.R. and Gilbert, D.A. (1995) Elderly residents: perceptions of nurses' comforting touch. *Journal of Gerontological Nursing*, 21 (1), 6–13.

Moore, K. and Estey, A. (1999) The early post-operative concerns of men after radical prostatectomy. *Journal of Advanced Nursing*, 29 (5), 1121–1129.

Moos, R.H. and Billings, A.G. (1982) Conceptualizing and measuring coping resources and processes. In Goldberger, L. and Breznits, S. (eds), *Handbook of Stress: Theoretical and Clinical Aspects*. New York: Macmillan.

Moos, R.H. and Moos, B.S. (2006) Participation in treatment and alcoholics anonymous: a 16-year follow-up of initially untreated individuals. *Journal of Clinical Psychology*, 62 (6), 735–750.

Moos, R.H. and Schaefer, J.A. (1986) Life transitions and crises: a conceptual overview. In Moos, R.H. (ed.), *Coping with Life Crises: An Integrated Approach*. London: Kluwer Academic/Plenum Publishers, 3–29.

Morgan, M. and Watkins, C.J. (1988) Managing hypertension: beliefs and responses to medication among cultural groups. *Sociology of Health and Illness*, 10 (4), 561–578.

Morgan, M.Y. and Ritson, B. (eds) (1998) *Alcohol and Health: Medical Student's Handbook*. London: Medical Council on Alcohol.

Morley, S., Eccleston, C. and Williams, A. (1999) Systematic review and meta-analysis of randomized controlled trials of cognitive behaviour therapy and behaviour therapy for chronic pain in adults, excluding headache. *Pain*, 80 (1–2), 1–13.

Morris, D.C., Silver, B., Mitsias, P., Lewandowski, C., Patel, S., Daley, S., Zhang, Z.G. and Lu, M. (2003) Treatment of acute stroke with recombinant tissue plasminogen activator and abciximab. *Academic Emergency Medicine*, 10 (12), 1396–1399.

Morris, C.G. and Maisto, A.A. (2002) *Psychology: An Introduction*. Englewood Cliffs, NJ: Prentice Hall.

Morris, K. and Ward, K. (2003) Perioperative nursing. In Brooker, C. and Nicol, M. (eds), *Nursing Adults: The Practice of Caring*, 879–922. Edinburgh: Mosby.

Morris, R. (2004) Speak out or shut up? Accountability and the student nurse. *Paediatric Nursing*, 16 (6), 20–22.

Morrow, G.R., Roscoe, J.A., Kirshner, J.J., Hynes, H.E. and Rosenbluth, R.J. (1998) Anticipatory nausea and vomiting in the era of 5-HT3 antiemetics. *Support Care Cancer*, 6, 244–247.

Morse, J.M., Bottorff, J., Anderson, G., O'Brien, B., Solberg. S. and McIlevan, K.H. (1992) Exploring empathy: a conceptual fit for nursing practice? *Image: Journal of Nursing Scholarship*, 24, 273–280.

Morse, J.M., Bottorff, J., Anderson, G., O'Brien, B. and Solberg, S. (2006) Beyond empathy: expanding expressions of caring. *Journal of Advanced Nursing*, 53 (1), 75–90.

Morton, I. (1999) *Person-centred approaches to dementia care*. Bicester: Winslow.

Moyer, A. and Salovey, P. (1996) Psychosocial sequelae of breast cancer and its treatment. *Annals of Behavioral Medicine*, 18 (2), 110–125.

Moynihan, C., Bliss, J.M., Davidson, J., Burchell, L. and Horwich, A. (1998) Evaluation of adjuvant psychological therapy in patients with testicular cancer: randomised controlled trial. *British Medical Journal*, 316, 429–435.

Mumford, A.D., Warr, K.V., Owen, S.J. and Fraser, A.G. (1999) Delays by patients in seeking treatment for acute chest pain: implications for achieving earlier thrombolysis. *Postgrad. Med J*, 75, 90–94.

Munafo, M., Rigotti, N., Lancaster, T., Stead, L. and Murphy, M. (2001) Interventions for smoking cessation in hospitalised patients: a systematic review. *Thorax*, 56 (8), 656–663.

Murphy, J. (2006) Perceptions of communication between people with communication disability and general practice staff. *Health Expectations*, 9, 49–59.

Murray, M. and Jarrett, L. (1985) Young people's perception of health, illness and smoking. *Health Education Journal*, 44 (1), 18–22.

Mutrie, N. and Choi, P.Y.L. (2000) Is 'fit' a feminist issue? Dilemmas for exercise psychology. *Feminism & Psychology*, 10 (4), 544–551.

Mutrie, N., Campbell, A.M., Whyte, F., McConnachie, A., Emslie, C., Lee, L., Kearney, N., Walker, A. and Ritchie, D. (2007) Benefits of supervised group exercise programme for women being treated for early stage breast cancer: pragmatic randomised controlled trial. *British Medical Journal*, 334, 517–520.

Myant, K.A. and Williams, J.M. (2005) Children's concept of health and illness: Understanding of contagious illnesses, non-contagious illness and injuries. *Journal of Health Psychology*, 10 (6), 805–819.

Nagle, A., Schofield, M. and Redman, S. (1999) Australian nurses' smoking behaviour, knowledge and attitude towards providing smoking cessation care to their patients. *Health Promotion International*, 14 (2), 133–144.

Naish, J. (2004) The evolving nurse. *Nursing Standard*, 13, 19 (5), 13.

Narayanasamy, A. (1998) The ACCESS model for transcultural mental health care. University of Nottingham (unpublished).

Narayanasamy, A. (1999) Transcultural mental health nursing 2: race, ethnicity and culture. *British Journal of Nursing*, 8 (12), 741–744.

Narayanasamy, A. (2002) The ACCESS model: a transcultural nursing practice framework. *British Journal of Nursing*, 11 (9), 643–650.

Narayanasamy, A. (2003) Transcultural nursing: how do nurses respond to cultural needs? *British Journal of Nursing*, **12** (3), 185–194.

National Assembly for Wales (2001) *Digest of Welsh Statistics*. Cardiff: National Assembly for Wales.

National Asthma Council (2003) *Asthma Adherence: A Guide For Health Professionals*. Australia [Online] (http://www.nationalasthma.org.au/publications).

National Audit Office (2003) A Safer Place to Work – Protecting the NHS Hospital and Ambulance Staff from Violence and Aggression.

National Cancer Institute (2005) http://www.cancer.gov/cancertopics/pdq/supportivecare/bereavement/patient/allpages, US National Institute of Health.

National Statistics Press Release (2005) Projected increase of 7.2m in UK population by 2031. National Statistics Press Release, 20 October 2005, National Statistics and Government Actuaries Department, table C (Projected population by age United Kingdom 2004–2031).

Navas-Nacher, E.L., Colangelo, L., Beam, C. and Greenland, P. (2001) Risk factors for coronary heart disease in men 18 to 39 years of age. *Annals of Internal Medicine*, **134** (6), 433–439.

Nazroo, J. and King, M. (2002) Psychosis – symptoms and estimated rates. In Sproston, K. and Nazroo, J. (eds), *Ethnic Minority Psychiatric Illness Rates in the Community*, National Centre for Social Research, London: TSO.

Neisser, U. (1967) *Cognitive Psychology*. New York: Appleton-Century-Crofts.

Ness, A.R. and Powles, J.W. (1997) Fruit and vegetables, and cardiovascular disease: a review. *International Journal of Epidemiology*, **26** (1), 1–13.

Ness, A.R., Hughes, J., Elwood, P.C., Whitley, E., Smith, G.D. and Burr, M.L. (2002) The long-term effect of dietary advice in men with coronary disease: follow-up of the Diet and Reinfarction Trial (DART). *European Journal of Clinical Nutrition*, **56**, 512–518.

Nestel, D. and Kidd, J. (2006) Nurses' perceptions and experiences of communication in the operating theatre: a focused group interview. *BMC Nursing*, **5**, 1 (http://www.biomedicalcentral.com/1427-6955/5/1).

Neuberger, J. (1994a) *Caring for Dying People of Different Faiths*, 2nd edn. London: Mosby.

Neuberger, J. (1994b) Cultural issues in palliative care. In Doyle *et al.* (eds), *The Oxford Textbook of Palliative Medicine*. Oxford: Oxford University Press.

NHS (2007) http://www.flyingstart.scot.nhs.uk/Interpersonal Skills.htm.

NICE (2004) *Depression: Management of Depression in Primary and Secondary Care*. Clinical Guidelines no. 23. London: National Institute for Clinical Excellence.

Nickel, C., Lahmann, C., Muehlbacher, M., Pedrosa Gil, F., Kaplan, P., Buschmann, W., Tritt, K., Kettler, C., Bachler, E., Egger, C., Anvar, J., Fartacek, R., Loew, T., Rother, W. and Nickel, M. (2006) Pregnant women with bronchial asthma benefit from progressive muscle relaxation: a randomized, prospective, controlled trial. *Psychotherapy and Psychosomatics*, **75** (4), 237–243.

Nickiln, J. (2002) Improving the quality of written information for patients. *Nursing Standard*, **16** (4), 39–44.

Nolan, P., Soares, J., Dallender, J., Thomsen, S. and Arentz, B. (2001) A comparative study of the experiences of violence of English and Swedish mental health nurses. *International Journal of Nursing Studies*, **38** (4), 419–426.

Norman, P. and Bennett, P. (1996) Health locus of control. In Conner, M. and Norman, P. (eds), *Predicting Health Behaviour: Research and Practice with Social Cognition Models*. Buckingham: Open University Press.

Norman, P., Conner, M. and Bell, R. (1999) The theory of planned behavior and smoking cessation. *Health Psychology*, **18** (1), 89–94.

Northcott, N. (2002) Nursing with dignity Part 2: Buddhism. *Nursing Times*, **98** (10), 36–38.

Northouse, L.L., Templin, T., Mood, D. and Oberst, M. (1998) Couples' adjustment to breast cancer and benign breast disease: A longitudinal analysis. *Psycho-Oncology*, **7** (1), 37–48.

Norton, C. and Chelvanayagam, S. (2004) Conservative management of faecal incontinence in adults. In Norton, C. and Chelvanayagam, S. (eds), *Bowel Continence Nursing*. Beaconsfield: Beaconsfield Publishers.

Nosarti, C., Roberts, J.V., Crayford, T., McKenzie, K. and David, A.S. (2002) Early psychological adjustment in breast cancer patients – a prospective study. *Journal of Psychosomatic Research*, **53** (6), 1123–1130.

NTA (2003) *Black and Minority Ethnic Communities in England: A Review of the Literature on Drug Use and Related Service Provision*. National Treatment Agency for Substance Misuse and the Centre for Ethnicity and Health. University of Central Lancashire.

Nursing and Midwifery Council (2004) *The NMC Code of Professional Conduct, Performance and Ethics. Standards 07.04* (www.nmc-uk.org).

Nyatanga, B. (2005) Cultural issues in palliative care. *International Journal of Pallative Nursing*, **3** (4), 203–208.

O'Brein, A.J. (2001) The therapeutic relationship: historical development and contemporary significance. *Journal of Psychiatric and Mental Health Nursing*, **18** (2), 129–137.

O'Rourke, M. (1993) Nurse-aid management of psychological emergencies: 3. *British Journal of Nursing*, **2** (22), 1133–1136.

Ockene, J.K., Wheeler, E.V., Adams, A., Hurley, T.G. and Hebert, J. (1997) Provider training for patient-centered alcohol counseling in a primary care setting. *Archives of Internal Medicine*, **157** (20), 2334–2341.

Ockene, J.K., Adams, A., Hurley, T.G., Wheeler, E.V. and Hebert, R. (1999) Brief physician- and nurse practitioner-delivered counseling for high-risk drinkers – does it work? *Archives of Internal Medicine*, **159** (18), 2198–2205.

Odell, J. and Holbrook, J. (2006) Improving the hospital experience for older people. *Nursing Times*, **102** (23), 23–24.

Office for National Statistics (1991) *Census*, April 1991, Office for National Statistics. http://www.statistics.gov.uk/CCI/nugget.asap?id=273

Office for National Statistics (2001) *Census*, April 2001, Office for National Statistics. http://www.statistics.gov.uk/CCI/SearchRes.asp?term=ethnicity

Office for National Statistics (2004) *Mortality statistics*. London: Office for National Statistics.

Ogden, J. (2004) *Health Psychology: A Textbook*, 3rd edn. Buckingham: Open University Press.

Ogden, J., Baig, S., Earnshaw, G., Elkington, H., Henderson, E., Lindsay, J. and Nandy, S. (2001) What is health? Where GPs' and patients' worlds collide. *Patient Education and Counseling*, 45 (4), 265–269.

O'Halloran, C.M. and Altmaier, E.M. (1995) The efficacy of preparation for surgery and invasive medical procedures. *Patient Education and Counselling*, 25 (1), 9–16.

Oldham, A. (2007) Changing behaviour: cognitive behavioural therapy: linking thoughts and actions. *Journal of Primary Care Nursing*, 4 (1), 26–29.

Oliver, S. and Ryan, S. (2004) Effective pain management for patients with arthritis. *Nursing Standard*, 18 (50), 43–52.

Ong, L.M.L., Visser, M.R.M., Lammes, F.B., van der Velden, J., Kuenen, B.C. and de Haes, J.C. (2000) Effect of providing cancer patients with the audiotaped initial consultation on satisfaction, recall and quality of life: a randomised double blind technique. *Journal of Clinical Oncology*, 18, 3052–3060.

ONS (1973) *General Household Survey*. London: Office for National Statistics.

ONS (1998) *General Household Survey*. London: Office for National Statistics.

ONS (2001a) Census, Mid-year population estimates, death registrations, ONS Longitudinal Study. London: Office for National Statistics.

ONS (2001b) *General Household Survey*. London: Office for National Statistics.

ONS (2004) *General Household Survey*. London: Office for National Statistics.

ONS (2006) *General Household Survey*. London: Office for National Statistics.

Orem, D.E. (1980) *Nursing: Concepts of Practice*, 2nd edn. New York: McGraw-Hill Book Company.

Orth-Gomer, K., Horsten, M., Wamala, S.P., Mittleman, M.A., Kirkeeide, R., Svane, B., Ryden, L. and Schenck-Gustafsson, K. (1998) Social relations and extent and severity of coronary artery disease: the Stockholm Female Coronary Risk Study. *European Heart Journal*, 19 (11), 1648–1656.

Orth-Gomer, K., Wamala, S.P., Horsten, M., Schenck-Gustafsson, K., Schneiderman, N. and Mittleman, M.A. (2000) Marital stress worsens prognosis in women with coronary heart disease – The Stockholm Female Coronary Risk Study. *Journal of the American Medical Association*, 284 (23), 3008–3014.

Osborn, T.M. and Sandler, N.A. (2004) The effects of preoperative anxiety on intravenous sedation. *Anesthesia Progress*, 51 (2), 46–51.

Osborne, C., Ostir, G.V., Du, X.L., Peek, M.K. and Goodwin, J.S. (2005) The influence of marital status on the stage at diagnosis, treatment, and survival of older women with breast cancer. *Breast Cancer Research and Treatment*, 93 (1), 41–47.

Ost, L.G. and Hugdahl, K. (1985) Acquisition of blood and dental phobia and anxiety response patterns in clinical patients. *Behaviour Research and Theory*, 23 (1), 27–34.

Owens, L., Gilmore, I.T. and Pirmohamed, M. (2000) General practice nurses' knowledge of alcohol use and misuse: a questionnaire survey. *Alcohol and Alcoholism*, 35 (3), 259–262.

Papadopoulos, I. and Lees, I. (2002) Developing culturally competent research. *Journal of Advanced Nursing*, 37 (3), 258–263.

Papadopoulos, I., Tilki, M. and Taylor, G. (1998) *Transcultural Care: A Guide for Healthcare Professionals*. Dinton: Quay Books.

Parent, N. and Fotin, F. (2000) A randomised, controlled trial of vicarious experience through peer support for male first-time cardiac surgery patients: impact on anxiety, self-efficacy expectation, and self reported activity. *Heart and Lung,* 29 (6), 389–400.

Parkes, C.M. (1972) *Bereavement, Studies of Grief in Adult Life*. Harmondsworth: Penguin.

Parkes, C.M. (1986) *Bereavement Studies of Grief in Adult Life*. London: Tavistock.

Parsons, T. (1951a) Illness and the role of the physician: a sociological perspective. *American Journal of Orthopsychiatry*, 21, 452–460.

Parsons, T. (1951b) *The Social System*. London: Routledge & Kegan Paul.

Partridge, C. and Johnston, M. (1989) Perceived control of recovery from physical disability: measurement and prediction. *British Journal of Clinical Psychology*, 28 (1), 53–59.

Partridge, M.R. and Hill, S.R., on behalf of the 1998 World Asthma Meeting Education and Delivery of Care Working Group (2000) Enhancing care for people with asthma: the role of communication, education, training and self-management. *European Respiratory Journal*, 16 (2), 334–349.

Pasacreta, J.V. (1997) Depressive phenomena, physical symptom distress, and functional status among women with breast cancer. *Nursing Research*, 46 (4), 214–221.

Pate, R.R. *et al.* (1995) Physical activity and public health – a recommendation from the Centers for Disease Control and Prevention and the American College of Sports Medicine. *Journal of the American Medical Association*, 273, 402–407.

Paterson, D., Swindells, S., Mohr, J., Brester, M., Vergis, E., Squier, C., Wagener, M. and Singh, N. (1999) How much adherence is enough? A perspective study of adherence to protease inhibitor therapy using MEMSCaps [abstract]. *6th Conference on Retrovirus and Opportunistic Infections*, 31 January to 4 February, Chicago, IL (www.thebody.com/confs/retro99/sessions15.html).

Paterson, R. (2000) *The assertiveness workbook: how to express your ideas and stand up for yourself at work and in relationships*. Oakland: New Harbinger.

Paton, A. (1994) *ABC of Alcohol*, 3rd edn. London: BMJ Publishing Group.

Pavis, S., Cunningham-Burley, S. and Amos, A. (1998) Health related behavioural change in context: young people in transition. *Social Science & Medicine*, 47 (10), 1407–1418.

Payne, T., Etscheidt, M. and Corrigan, S. (1990) Conditioning arbitrary stimuli to cigarette smoke intake: a preliminary study. *Journal of Substance Abuse*, **2**, 113–119.

Peberdy, A. (1997) Communicating across cultural boundaries. In Siddle, M., Jones, L., Katz, J. and Perberdy, A. (eds), *Debates and Dilemmas in Promoting Health: A Reader*. Buckingham: Open University, 99–107.

Pederson, C. (1995) Effect of imagery on children's pain and anxiety during cardiac catheterization. *Journal of Pediatric Nursing*, **10** (6), 365–374.

Pender, M.P. (1996) Recent advances in the understanding, diagnosis and management of multiple sclerosis. *Australian and New Zealand Journal of Medicine*, **26** (2): 157–161.

Penedo, F.J., Molton, I., Dahn, J.R., Shen, B.J., Kinsinger, D., Traeger, L., Siegel, S., Schneiderman, N. and Antoni, M. (2006) A randomized clinical trial of group-based cognitive-behavioral stress management in localized prostate cancer: development of stress management skills improves quality of life and benefit finding. *Annals of Behavioral Medicine*, **31** (3), 261–270.

Perkins, C.C. (1968) An analysis of the concept of reinforcement. *Psychological Review*, **75** (2), 155–172.

Persson, J. and Magnusson, P.H. (1989) Early intervention in patients with excessive consumption of alcohol – a controlled-study. *Alcohol*, **6** (5), 403–408.

Peters, J. (1999a) Eczema. *Nursing Standard*, **14** (16), 49–55.

Peters, J. (1999b) Combining nursing roles in dermatology. *Professional Nurse*, **15** (2), 91–94.

Peters, K.F., Horne, R., Kong, F., Francomano, C.A. and Biesecker, B.B. (2001) Living with Marfan Syndrome II. Medication adherence and physical activity modification. *Clinical Genetics*, **60** (4), 283–292.

Peters-Golden, H. (1982) Breast-cancer – varied perceptions of social support in the illness experience. *Social Science and Medicine*, **16** (4), 483–491.

Petridou, E., Trichopoulos, D., Sotiriou, A., Athanasselis, S., Kouri, N., Dessypris, N., Dounis, E. and Koutselinis, A. (1998) Relative and population attributable risk of traffic injuries in relation to blood-alcohol levels in a Mediterranean country. *Alcohol and Alcoholism*, **33** (5), 502–508.

Petrie, K.J., Cameron, L.D., Ellis, C.J., Buick, D. and Weinman, J. (2002) Changing illness perceptions after myocardial infarction: an early intervention randomized controlled trial. *Psychosomatic Medicine*, **64**, 580–586.

Petro-Nustas, W.I. (2001) Factors associated with mammography utilization among Jordanian women. *Journal of Transcultural Nursing*, **12** (4), 284–291.

Phelan, M. and Parkman, S. (1995) How to work with an interpreter. *British Medical Journal*, **311** (7004), 555–557.

Piaget, J. (1972) Intellectual evolution from adolescence to adulthood. *Human Development*, **15** (1), 1–8.

Piehota, P.W., Pizarro, J., Schnedier, T.R., Mowad, L. and Salovey, P. (2005) Matching health messages to monitor-blunter coping styles to motivate screening mammography. *Health Psychology*, **24** (1), 58–67.

Pillsbury, B.L.K. (1984) 'Doing the month' confinement and convalescence of Chinese women after birth. In Black, N., Boswell, D. and Gray, A. (eds) *Health and Disease*, 17–24. Buckingham: Open University Press.

Pirmohamed, M., Brown, C., Owens, L., Luke, C., Gilmore, I.T., Breckenridge, A.M. and Park, B.K. (2000) The burden of alcohol misuse on an inner-city general hospital. *Qjm – An International Journal of Medicine*, **93** (5), 291–295.

Pistrang, N. and Barker, C. (1995) The partner relationship in psychological response to breast-cancer. *Social Science and Medicine*, **40** (6), 789–797.

Playle, J.F. and Keeley, P. (1998) Non-compliance and professional power. *Journal of Advanced Nursing*, **27**, 304–311.

Pollock, R. (2003) *Designing Interiors for People with Dementia*. Stirling: Dementia Service Development.

Poppa, A., Davidson, O., Deutsch, J., Godfrey, D., Fisher, M., Head, S., Horne, R. and Sherr, L. (2003) *British Association for Sexual Health and HIV (BASHH) Guidelines on Provision of Adherence Support to Individuals Receiving Antiretroviral Therapy*. London: British HIV Association (www.bhiva.org/guidelines/2004/adherence/index.html).

Population Trends (2000) (PP2) 98/1. Official National Statistics. Annual Abstract for Statistics. *Economics of Health Care. The Aging UK Population*. (http://www.oheschools.org/ohech6pg3.html, accessed 5 September 2006).

Population Trends (2005) (PT 122) 122, Winter 2005, National Statistics. Crown Copyright 2005, table 1.4 (Population: age and sex).

Post-White, J. (2002) Clinical indication for use of imagery in oncology practice. In Edwards, D.M. (ed.), *Voice Massage, Scripts for Guided Imagery*. Pittsburgh, PA: Oncology Nursing Society.

Potter, P.A. and Perry, A. (2006) *Basic Nursing Essentials for Practice*, 6th edn. Mobsy, MO: Elsevier.

Power, M.J. and Brewin, C.R. (eds) (1997) *The Transformation of Meaning in Psychological Therapies: Intergrating Theory and Practice*. Chichester: Wiley.

Pradel, F.G., Hartzema, A.G. and Bush, P.J. (2001) Asthma self-management: the perspective of children. *Patient Education and Counselling*, **45** (3), 199–209.

Preti, A. (2003) Unemployment and suicide. *Journal of Epidemiology and Community Health*, **57** (8), 557–558.

Price, B. (2003) Understanding the origins of practice problems. *Nursing Standard*, **17** (50), 47–53.

Price, B. (2006) Exploring person-centred care. *Nursing Standard*, **20** (50), 49–56.

Priest, H.M. (1999) Novice and expert perceptions of psychological care and the development of psychological caregiving abilities. *Nurse Education Today*, **19** (7), 556–563.

Prime Minister's Strategy Unit (2003) *Alcohol misuse: how much does it cost?* London: Cabinet Office.

Pritchard, C. (1995) Unemployment, age, gender and regional suicide in England and Wales 1974–90: a harbinger of increased suicide for the 1990s? *British Journal of Social Work*, **25** (6), 767–790.

Prochaska, J.O. and DiClemente, C.C. (1982) Transtheoretical therapy: Toward a more integrative model of change. *Psychotherapy: Theory, Research and Practice*, **19** (3), 276–288.

Prochaska, J. and DiClemente, C. (1986) Towards a comprehensive model of change. In Miller, W. and Heather, N. (eds), *Treating Addictive Behaviours: Processes of Change*. New York: Plenum.

Prochaska, J.O., Velicer, W.F., Rossi, J.S., Goldstein, M.G., Marcus, B.H., Rakowski, W., Fiore, C., Harlow, L.L., Redding, C.A., Rosenbloom, D. and Rossi, S.R. (1994) Stages of change and decisional balance for 12 problem behaviors. *Health Psychology*, **13**, 39–46.

Pronzato, P., Bertelli, G., Losardo, P. and Landucci, M. (1994) What do advanced cancer-patients know of their disease – a report from Italy. *Supportive Care in Cancer*, **2** (4), 242–244.

Prouty, G. (1990) Pre Therapy: A theoretical evolution in the person centered/experiential psychotherapy of schizophrenia and retardation. In Lietaer, G., Rombauts, J. and Van Balen, R. (eds), *Client Centered and Experiential Psychotherapy in the Nineties*, 645–648. Leuven, Belgium: Leuven University Press.

Prus, S.G. (2007) Age, SES, and health: a population level analysis of health inequalities over the lifecourse. *Sociology of Health & Illness*, **29** (2), 275–296.

Purnell, L.D. and Paulanka, B.J. (1998) *Transcultural Health Care*. Philadelphia, PA: F.A. Davis Co.

Quadrel, M.J. and Lau, R.R. (1989) Health promotion, health locus of control, and health behavior: two field experiments. *Journal of Applied Social Psychology*, **19** (18, Pt 2), 1497–1521.

Quinn, F.M. (2001) *Principles and Practice of Nurse Education*, 4th edn. Cheltenham: Nelson Thornes.

Quist-Paulsen, P. and Gallefoss, F. (2003) A nurse led smoking cessation intervention increased cessation rates after hospital admissions for coronary heart disease. *British Medical Journal*, **327**, 1254–1257.

Quitkin, F., Riftkin, A., Kane, J.M., Ramos-Lorenzi, J.R. and Klein, D.F. (1978) Long action versus injectable antipsychotic drugs in schizophrenics. A 1-year double-blind comparison in multiple episode schizophrenics. *Archives of General Psychiatry*, **35**, 889–892.

Radhakrishnan, S. (1968) *The Principal Upanishads*. London: Allen and Unwin.

Rakos, R. (1997) In Hargie, O. (1997) *The Handbook of Communication Skills*, 2nd edn. London: Routledge.

Ramirez, A.J., Westcombe, A.M., Burgess, C.C., Sutton, S., Littlejohns, P. and Richards, M.A. (1999) Factors predicting delayed presentation of symptomatic breast cancer: a systematic review. *Lancet*, **353** (9159), 1127–1131.

Ramsay, M., Baker, P., Goulden, C., Sharp, C. and Sondhi, A. (2001) *Home Office Research Study 224: Drug Misuse Declared in 2000: Results from the British Crime Survey*. London: Home Office Research, Development and Statistics Directorate.

Rand, C.A. (1997) Comprehensive review of the history, content, issues and measurement of adherence. In *Asthma Adherence Workshop Report*, Melbourne. Victoria: National Asthma Campaign, 12–15.

Rand, C.S. (2002) Adherence to asthma therapy in the preschool child. *Allergy*, **57** (74), 48–57.

Randle, J. (2003) Bullying in the nursing profession. *Journal of Advanced Nursing*, **43** (4), 395–401.

Ransom, S., Jacobsen, P.B., Schmidt, J.E. and Andrykowski, M.A. (2005) Relationship of problem-focused coping strategies to changes in quality of life following treatment for early stage breast cancer. *Journal of Pain and Symptom Management*, **30** (3), 243–253.

Rantz, M. and McShane, R. (1995) Nursing interventions for chronically confused home residents. *Geriatric Nursing*, **16**, 22–27.

Ranzijn, R., Keeves, J., Luszcz, M. and Feather, N.T. (1998) The role of self-perceived usefulness and competence in the self-esteem of elderly adults: confirmatory factor analysis of the Bachman Revision of Rosenberg's self-esteem scale. *Journal of Gerontology Series B: Psychological Sciences, Social Sciences*, **53**, 96–104.

Rao, J.K., Weinberg, M. and Kroenk, K. (2000) Visit-specific expectations and patient-centered outcomes: a literature review. *Archives Family Medicine*, **9**, 1148–1155.

Rapoff, M.A. (1999) *Adherence to Paediatric Medical Regimens*. New York: Kluwer Academic/Plenum Publishers.

Rappaport, J. (1984) Studies in empowerment: introduction to the issue. *Prevention in Human Sciences*, **3**, 1–7.

Rasberry, R.W. and Lemoine, L.F. (1986) *Effective Managerial Communications*. Massachusetts: Kent Publishing.

Rassool, G.H. (1993) Nursing and substance misuse – responding to the challenge. *Journal of Advanced Nursing*, **18** (9), 1401–1407.

Rassool, G.H. (2006) Substance abuse in black and minority ethnic communities in the United Kingdom: a neglected problem? *Journal of Addictions Nursing*, **17**, 59–63.

Raudonis, B.M. (1993) The meaning and impact of empathetic relationships in hospice nursing. *Cancer Nursing*, **16**, 304–309.

Rayner, M. and Scarborough, P. (2005) The burden of food related ill health in the UK. *Journal of Epidemiology and Community Health*, **59** (12), 1054–1057.

RCN (1994) Black and ethnic minority clients: meeting needs. *RCN Nursing Update*, **7**, 3–13.

RCN (1995) *Advocacy and the Nurse. Issues in Nursing and Health*, No. 22. London: Royal College of Nursing.

RCN (2006) *Clinical Teams Programme: Developing Effective Teams, Delivering Effective Services, Executive Summary*. London: Royal College of Nursing.

RCN (2007) *Role of the rehabilitation nurse. RCN Guidance* (Hawkey, B. and Williams, J.) London: Royal College of Nursing.

Read, S. (1998) Feedback – Re: Conference report – Clinical Nurse Specialism Conference organised by Professional Nurse, November 1996, reported in *Journal of Advanced Nursing* 1997, **25**, 867–870. *Journal of Advanced Nursing*, **27** (1), 230.

Redd, W.H., Montgomery, G.H. and DuHamel, K.N. (2001) Behavioral intervention for cancer treatment side effects. *Journal of the National Cancer Institute*, **93** (11), 810–823.

Reece, M. and Whitman, R. (1962) Expressive movements, warmth and verbal reinforcement. *Journal of Abnormal Social Psychology*, **64**, 234–236.

Rees, D. (1997) *Death and Bereavement: The Psychological Religious and Cultural Interfaces*. London: Whurr Publishers.

Reid-Galloway, C. (1998) *African Caribbean Community in Britain*. London: Mind Factsheet.

Resnick, B. and Jenkins, L. (2000) Testing the reliability and validity of the self-efficacy for exercise scale. *Nursing Research*, 49 (3), 154–159.

Reynolds, P., Boyd, P.T., Blacklow, R.S., Jackson, J.S., Greenberg, R.S., Austin, D.F., Chen, V.W. and Edwards, B.K. (1994) The relationship between social ties and survival among black and white breast cancer patients. *Cancer Epidemiology Biomarkers and Prevention*, 3 (3), 253–259.

Reynolds, P., Hurley, S., Torres, M., Jackson, J., Boyd, P. and Chen, V.W. (2000) Use of coping strategies and breast cancer survival: results from the black/white cancer survival study. *American Journal of Epidemiology*, 152 (10), 940–949.

Reynolds, W. and Scott, B. (1999) Empathy: a crucial component of the helping relationship. *Journal of Psychiatric and Mental Health Nursing*, 6, 363–370.

Reynolds, W.J. and Scott, B. (2000) Do nurses and other professional helpers normally display much empathy? *Journal of Advanced Nursing*, 31 (1), 226–234.

Rhee, H. (2005) Racial/ethnic differences in adolescents' physical symptoms. *Journal of Pediatric Nursing*, 20 (3), 153–162

Rhodes, V.A. and McDaniel, R.W. (2001) Nausea, vomiting and retching: complex problems in palliative care. *CA Cancer Journal for Clinicians*, 51, 232–248.

Richards, K.C., Gibson, R. and Overton-McCoy, A.L. (2000) Effects of massage in acute and critical care. *AACN Clinical Issues*, 11 (1), 77–96.

Richards, M.A., Westcombe, A.M., Lowe, S.B., Littlejohns, P. and Ramirez, A.J. (1999) The influence of delay on survival in patients with breast cancer: a systematic review. *Lancet*, 353, 1119–1126.

Riekert, K.A. and Drotar, D. (2000) Adherence to medical treatment in pediatric chronic illness: critical issues and answered questions. In Drotar, D. (ed). *Promoting Adherence to Medical Treatment in Chronic Childhood Illness: Concepts, Methods and Interventions*, 9–32. Hillsdale, NJ: Lawrence Earlbaum Associates.

Riley, M.W. and Riley, J.W. Jr (1994) Age integration and the lives of older people. *Gerontologist*, 34, 110–115.

Risk estimation and the prevention of cardiovascular disease. A national clinical guideline. (2007) (http://www.sign.ac.uk/pdf/sign97.pdf).

RNID (2004a) *A Simple Cure*. March. London: Royal National Institute for Deaf People.

Roach, J.A., Tremblay, L.M. and Bowers, D.L. (1995) A pre-operative assessment and education program: implementation and outcomes. *Patient Education and Counseling*, 25 (1), 83–88.

Rock, C.L. and Demark-Wahnefried, W. (2002) Can lifestyle modification increase survival in women diagnosed with breast cancer? *Journal of Nutrition*, 132 (11 Suppl.), 3504S–3507S.

Roelofs, J., Peters, M.L., De Jong, J.R. and Vlaeyen, J.W.S. (2002) Psychological treatments for chronic low back pain: past, present and beyond. *Pain Reviews*, 9 (1), 29–40.

Roffe, L., Schmidt, K. and Ernst, E. (2005) A systematic review of guided imagery as an adjuvant cancer therapy. *Psycho-Oncology*, 14 (8), 607–617.

Rogers, C.R. (1961) *On Becoming a Person*. Boston, MA: Houghton Mifflin.

Rogers, J. (1998) Nocturnal enuresis should not be ignored. *Nursing Standard*, 13 (9), 35–38.

Rogers, J. (2002) Managing daytime and night-time enuresis. *Nursing Standard*, 16 (32), 45–52.

Rogers, P., Curran, J. and Gournay, K. (2002) Depression: nature, assessment and treatment using behavioural activation (Part I). *Mental Health Practice*, 5 (10), 32–37.

Rogers, R.W. (1975) A protection motivation theory of fear appeals and attitude change. *Journal of Psychology*, 91, 93–114.

Rogers, R.W. (1983) Cognitive and physiological processes in fear appeals and attitude change: a revised theory of protection motivation. In Cacioppi, T. and Petty, R.E. (eds), *Social Psychology*. New York: Guilford, 153–176.

Rogers, R.W. (1985) Attitude change and information integration in fear appeals. *Psychological Reports*, 56, 183–188.

Rondahl, G., Innala, S. and Carlsson, M. (2004) Nurses' attitudes towards lesbians and gay men. *Journal of Advanced Nursing*, 47 (4), 386–392.

Rooda, L.A., Clements, R. and Jordon, M. (1999) Nurses' attitudes toward death and caring for dying patients. *Oncology Nursing Forum*, 26 (10), 1683–1687.

Room, R., Babor, T. and Rehm, J. (2005) Alcohol and public health. *Lancet*, 365 (9458), 519–530.

Roper, N. *et al.* (eds) (1983) Edinburgh: Churchill Livingstone.

Rose, N.B. (1995) *Essential Psychiatry*, 2nd edn. Oxford: Blackwell Science.

Rose, R.J., Kaprio, J., Williams, C.J., Viken, R. and Obremski, K. (1990) Social contact and sibling similarity: facts, issues, and red herrings. *Behav Genet*. 20 (6), 763–778.

Rosenberg, H. (1993) Prediction of controlled drinking by alcoholics and problem drinkers. *Psychological Bulletin*, 113 (1), 129–139.

Rosenfeld, H.M. (1978) Conversational control functions of non-verbal behaviour. In Siegman, A.W. and Feldstein, S. (eds), *Nonverbal Behaviour and Communication*. New York: Wiley, 291–328.

Rosenman, R.H., Brand, R.J., Jenkins, C.D., Friedman, M., Straus, R. and Wurm, M. (1975) Coronary heart-disease in western collaborative group study – final follow-up experience of $8\frac{1}{2}$ years. *Journal of the American Medical Association*, 233 (8), 872–877.

Rosenstock, I.M. (1974) Historical origins of the health belief model. *Health Education Monographs*, 2 (4), 328–335.

Rosenthal, T. and Zimmerman, B. (1987) *Social Learning and Cognition*. New York: Academic Press.

Ross, L. (1977) The intuitive psychologist and his short-comings. In Berkowitz, L. (ed.), *Advances in Experimental Social Psychology*, Vol. 10. New York: Academic Press, 174–220.

Roter, D.L. and Hall, J.A. (1992) *Doctors Talking to Patients/Patients Talking with Doctors: Improving Communication in Medical Visits*. Westport, CT: Auburn House.

Rotter, J.B. (1966) Generalized expectancies for internal versus external control of reinforcement. *Psychological Monographs: General & Applied*, 80 (1), 1–28.

Rowe, J.L., Montgomery, G.H., Duberstein, P.R. and Boybjern, D.H. (2005) Health locus of control and perceived risk for breast cancer in healthy women. *Behavioral Medicine*, 31 (1), 33–40.

Rowland, N. and Maynard, A.K. (1989) Alcohol education for patients: some nurses need persuading. *Nurse Education Today*, 9 (2), 100–104.

RNIB (2002) www.rnib.org.uk, accessed 12 May 2007.

Royal College of Nursing (1994) Black and ethnic minority clients: meeting needs. *RCN Nursing Update*, 7, 3–13.

Royal Pharmaceutical Society of Great Britain (1997) From compliance to concordance: achieving shared goals in medication taking. London: RPS.

Ruble, D.N. (1977) Premenstrual symptoms – reinterpretation. *Science*, 197, 291–292.

Rudolph, K.D., Dennig, M.D. and Weisz, J.R. (1995) Determinants and consequences of children's coping in the medical setting – conceptualisation, review, and critique. *Psychological Bulletin*, 118 (3), 328–357.

Rummans, T.A., Clark, M.M., Sloan, J.A., Frost, M.H., Bostwick, J.M., Atherton, P.J., Johnson, M.E., Gamble, G., Richardson, J., Brown, P., Martensen, J., Miller, J., Piderman, K., Huschka, M., Girardi, J. and Hanson, J. (2006) Impacting quality of life for patients with advanced cancer with a structured multidisciplinary intervention: a randomized controlled trial. *Journal of Clinical Oncology*, 24 (4), 635–642.

Russell, S., Daly, J., Hughes, E. and Hogg, C.O. (2003) Nurses and 'difficult' patients: negotiating non-compliance. *Journal of Advanced Nursing*, 43 (3), 281–287.

Rutter, D. and Calnuan, M. (1987) Do health beliefs predict health behaviour?: A further analysis of breast self–examination. In Dent, H. (ed.), *Clinical Psychology: Research and Developments*. New York: Croom Helm, 35–41.

Rutter, D.R. (2000) Attendance and reattendance for breast cancer screening: a prospective 3-year test of the Theory of Planned Behaviour. *British Journal of Health Psychology*, 5 (Part 1), 1–13.

Rutter, M. (1980a) The long-term effects of early experience. *Developmental Medicine and Child Neurology*, 22 (6), 800–815.

Rutter, M. (1980b) Youth in society. 4. Disorders in adolescence. *New Society*, 52 (918), 296–299.

Rutter, M. (1980c) Youth in society. 5. Psychosocial adolescence. *New Society*, 52 (917), 225–226.

Ryan, T., Reid, D. and Enderby, P. (2000) *A Strategic Review of Services for Carers of People with Dementia*, unpublished report, Institute of General Practice and Primary Care, University of Sheffield.

Sachie, K.W. and Willis, S.L. (1996) *Adult Development and Aging*, 4th end. Harper Collins College Publishers. Harper Collins Publishers Inc.

Sadur, C.N., Moline, N., Costa, M., Michalik, D., Mendlowitz, D., Roller, S., Watson, R., Swain, B.E., Selby, J.V. and Javorski, W.C. (1999) Diabetes management in a health maintenance organization. Efficacy of care management using cluster visits. *Diabetes Care*, 22 (12), 2011–2017.

Sahinler, B.E. (2002) A review of pediatric pain management in acute and chronic setting. *Pain Practice*, 2 (2), 137–150.

Saines, J.C. (1999) Violence and aggression in A&E: recommendations for action. *Accident and Emergency Nursing*, 7 (1), 8–20.

Salber, E.J., Welsh, B. and Taylor, S.V. (1963) Reasons for smoking given by secondary school children. *Journal of Health and Human Behavior*, 4 (2), 118–129.

Salmon, P. (1993) Interactions of nurses with elderly patients: relationship to nurses' attitudes and to formal activity periods. *Journal of Advanced Nursing*, 18, 14–19.

Salmon, P. and Hall, G.M. (1997) A theory of postoperative fatigue: an interaction of biological, psychological, and social processes. *Pharmacology, Biochemistry and Behaviour*, 56 (4), 623–628.

Sander Wint, S., Eshelman, D., Steele, J. and Guzzetta, C.E. (2002) Effects of distraction using virtual reality glasses during lumbar punctures in adolescents with cancer. *Oncology Nursing Forum*, 29 (1), E8–E15.

Sanders, D. and Wills, F. (2003) *Counselling for Anxiety Problems*, 2nd edn. Counselling in Practice, London: Sage Publications.

Sandman, P., Adolfsson, R., Nygren, C., Hallmans, G. and Winblad, B. (1987) Nutritional status and dietary intake in institutionalised patients with Alzheimer's disease and multi-infarct dementia. *Journal of the American Geriatrics Society*, 35, 31–38.

Sangster, D., Shiner, M., Patel, K. and Sheikh, N. (2001) *Delivering Drug Services to Black and Minority Ethnic Communities*. DPAS 16; London: HMSO.

Saracci, R. (1997) The World Health Organisation needs to reconsider its definition of health. *British Medical Journal*, 314 (7091), 1409–1410.

Sarafino, E.P. (2005) *Research Methods: Using Processes and Procedures of Science to Understand Behaviour*. Upper Saddle River, NJ: Pearson/Prentice Hall.

Sarafino, E.P. and Ewing, M. (1999) The hassle assessment scale for students in college: measuring the frequency and unpleasantness of and dwelling on stress events. *Journal of American College Health*, 48 (2), 75–83.

Sarafino, E.P. and Goehring, P. (2000) Age comparisons in acquiring biofeedback control and success in reducing headache pain. *Annals of Behavioral Medicine*, 22 (1), 10–16.

Sarason, I.G., Levine, H.M., Basham, R.B. and Sarason, B.R. (1983) Assessing social support – the social support questionnaire. *Journal of Personality and Social Psychology*, 44 (1), 127–139.

Sarna, L., Bialous, S.A., Wewers, M.E., Froelicher, E.S. and Danao, L. (2005) Nurses, smoking, and the workplace. *Research in Nursing and Health*, 28 (1), 79–90.

Scambler, A., Scambler, S. and Craig, D. (1981) Kinship and friendship networks and women's demand for primary care. *The Journal of the Royal College of General Practitioners*, 31 (233), 746–750.

Scanlon, P.D., Connett, J.E., Waller, L.A., Altose, M.D., Bailey, W.C., Buist, A.S. and Tashkin, D.P. (2000) Smoking cessation and lung function in mild-to-moderate chronic obstructive pulmonary disease – The Lung Health Study. *American Journal of Respiratory and Critical Care Medicine*, 161 (2), 381–390.

Schabracq, M.J. (1987) Bekrokkenheid En Onderlinge Gelijkheid in Sociale Interacties (Involvement and equality in social interactions). PhD Thesis, Leuven: Katholieke.

Schachter, S. (1977) Nicotine regulation in heavy and light smokers. *Journal of Experimental Psychology*, 106, 5–12.

Schaie, K.W. and Willis, S.L. (1996) *Adult Development and Aging*, 4th edn. New York: Harper Collins Publishers Inc.

Schapira, M.M., Meade, C. and Nattinger, A.B. (1997) Enhanced decision-making: the use of videotape decision-aid for patients with prostate cancer. *Patient Education Counselling*, 30, 119–127.

Schapiro, I.R., Ross-Petersen, L., Saelan, H., Garde, K., Olsen, J.H. and Johansen, C. (2001) Extroversion and neuroticism and the associated risk of cancer: a Danish cohort study. *American Journal of Epidemiology*, 153 (8), 757–763.

Scheier, M.F., Matthews, K.A., Owens, J.F., Magovern, G.J. Sr, Lefebure, R.C., Abbot, R.A. and Carver, C.S. (1989) Dispositional optimism and recovery from coronary artery bypass surgery: the beneficial effects on physical and psychological well-being. *Journal of Personality and Social Psychology*, 57 (6), 1024–1040.

Schermerhorn, J., Hunt, J.G. and Osborn, R.N. (2004) *Organisational Behaviour*. New York: John Wiley and Sons.

Schmieding, N. (1999) Reflective inquiry framework for nurse administrators. *Journal of Advanced Nursing*, 30 (3), 631–639.

Schneider, D.G. (2004) *The psychology of stereotyping*. New York: Guilford Press.

Schnittker, J. (2004) Education and the changing shape of the income gradient in health. *Journal of Health and Social Behavior*, 45 (3), 286–305.

Schoenberg, N.E., Amey, C.H., Stoller, E.P. and Muldoon, S.B. (2003) Lay referral patterns involved in cardiac treatment decision making among middle-aged and older adults. *Gerontologist*, 43 (4), 493–502.

Schott, J. (1999) Lessons from the Lawrence Inquiry. *British Journal of Midwifery*, 7 (4), 208–210.

Schott, J. and Henley, A. (1996) *Culture, Religion and Childbearing in a Multiracial Society*. Oxford: Butterworth-Heinmann.

Schuckit, M.A., Smith, T.L., Pierson, J., Danko, G.P. and Beltran, I.A. (2006) Relationships among the level of response to alcohol and the number of alcoholic relatives in predicting alcohol-related outcomes. *Alcoholism: Clinical and Experimental Research*, 30 (8), 1308–1314.

Schuckit, M. (2006) *Drug and Alcohol Abuse: A Clinical Guide to Diagnosis and Treatment*, 6th edn. Springer.

Schwarzer, R. (1992) Self-efficacy in the adoption and maintenance of health behaviors: theoretical approaches and a new model. In Schwarzer, R. (ed.), *Self-efficacy: Thought Control of Action*. Washington, DC: Hemisphere Publishing Corp.

Scott, D.W., Donahue, D.C., Mastrovito, R.C. and Hakes, T.B. (1986) Comparative trial of clinical relaxation and an antiemetic drug regimen in reducing chemotherapy-related nausea and vomiting. *Cancer Nursing*, 9, 178–187.

Scott, H.K., Irvine, J. and Mann, R.E. (2005) Can psychological interventions reduce mortality rates in patients with coronary heart disease and cancer? A review of randomized trials. *International Journal of Mental Health and Addiction*, 2 (2), 13–24.

Scott, J., Harmsen, M., Prictor, M.J., Entwistle, V.A., Snowden, A.J. and Watt, I. (2006) Recordings or summaries of consultations for people with cancer (Cochrane Review). *The Cochrane Library*, Issue 3. Oxford: Update Software/Chichester: John Wiley.

Scott, J.L., Halford, W.K. and Ward, B.G. (2004) United we stand? The effects of a couple-coping intervention on adjustment to early stage breast or gynecological cancer. *Journal of Consulting and Clinical Psychology*, 72 (6), 1122–1135.

Seaton, R. (2005) *HRSACAREACTION: Providing HIV/AIDS Care in a Changing Environment*. May. US Department of Health and Human Services (http://hab.hrsa.gov/publications/may2005/).

Sederer, L.I. and Summergrad, P. (1993) Criteria for hospital admission. *Hospital & Community Psychiatry*, 44 (2), 116–118.

Seedhouse, D. (1986) *Health: The Foundations for Achievement*. Chichester: Wiley.

Seers, C.J. (1987) Pain, anxiety and recovery in patients undergoing surgery. Unpublished PhD thesis, Department of Nursing Studies, University of London, London.

Segal, R., Evans, W., Johnson, D., Smith, J., Colletta, S., Gayton, J., Woodward, S., Wells, S., Wells, G. and Reid, R. (2001) Structured exercise improves physical functioning in women with stages I and II breast cancer: results of a randomized controlled trial. *Journal of Clinical Oncology*, 19 (3), 657–665.

Seigal, C. (1972) Changes in play therapy behaviours over-time, on a function of different levels of therapists offered conditions. *Journal of Clinical Psychology*, 28, 235.

Seligman, M.E.P. (1971) Phobias and preparedness. *Journal of Behavior Therapy*, 2, 307–320.

Selye, H. (1956) What is stress? *Metabolism*, 5 (5), 525–530.

Sepúlveda, C. (1990) Palliative Care: The World Health Organization's Global Perspective. *Journal of Pain and Symptom Management*, 24 (2), 91–96.

Serrant Green, L. (2001) Transcultural nursing education: a view from within. *Nurse Education Today*, 21 (8), 670–678.

Seymour-Smith, S., Wetherell, M. and Phoenix, A. (2002) 'My wife ordered me to come!': A discursive analysis of doctors' and nurses' accounts of men's use of general practitioners. *Journal of Health Psychology*, 7 (3), 253–267.

Shannon, C. and Weaver, W. (1949) *The Mathematical Theory of Communication*. Urbana: University of Illinois Press.

Sharma, S. (1996) *Applied Multivariate Techniques*. New York: John Wiley and Sons.

Shaw, C., Mccoll, E. and Bond, S. (2003) The relationship of perceived control to outcomes in older women undergoing surgery for fractured neck of femur. *Journal of Clinical Nursing*, 12 (1), 117–123.

Shaw, M. and Dorling, D. (2004) Who cares in England and Wales? The positive care law: cross-sectional study. *British Journal of General Practice*, 54 (509), 899–903.

Shaw, M., Smith, G.D. and Dorling, D. (2005) Health inequalities and New Labour: how the promises compare with real progress. *British Medical Journal*, 330 (7498), 1016–1021.

Sheikh, A. and Gatrad, A.R. (2000) *Caring for Muslim Patients*, Abingdon: Radcliffe Medical Press.

Sherbourne, C.D., Hays, R.D., Ordway, L., DiMatteo, M.R. and Kravitz, R.L. (1992) Antecedents of adherence to medical recommendations: results from the Medical Outcomes Study. *Journal of Behavioral Medicine*, 15 (5), 447–469.

Sherman, D.K., Mann, T. and Updegraff, J. (2006) Approach/avoidance motivation, message framing and health behaviour: understanding the congruency effect. *Motivation and Emotion*, 30, 165–169.

Shi, L.Y. (1998) Sociodemographic characteristics and individual health behaviors. *Southern Medical Journal*, 91 (10), 933–941.

Shipley, R.H. (1981) Maintenance of smoking cessation: effect of follow-up letters, smoking motivation, muscle tension, and health locus of control. *Journal of Consulting and Clinical Psychology*, 49 (6), 982–984.

Shneidman, E.S. (1989) The Indian summer of life: a preliminary study of septuagenarians. *American Psychologist*, 44, 684–694.

Shrier, L.A., Harris, S.K., Sternberg, M. and Beardslee, W.R. (2001) Associations of depression, self-esteem, and substance use with sexual risk among adolescents. *Preventive Medicine: An International Journal Devoted to Practice and Theory*, 33 (3), 179–189.

Siahpush, M. and Carlin, J.B. (2006) Financial stress, smoking cessation and relapse: results from a prospective study of an Australian national sample. *Addiction*, 101 (1), 121–127.

Sidley, G. and Renton, J. (1996) General nurses' attitudes to patients who self-harm. *Nursing Standard*, 10 (30), 32–36.

Siegel, L.J. and Conte, P. (2001) Hospitalization and medical care of children. In Walker, C.E. and Roberts, M.C. (eds), *Handbook of Clinical Child Psychology* (3rd edn), 895–909. New York: Wiley Inc.

SIGN (2007) Risk estimation and the prevention of cardiovascular disease. A national clinical guideline. At http://www.sign.ac.uk/pdf/sign97.pdf. Edinburgh: Scottish Intercollegiate Guidelines Network.

Simmons, S.J. (1989) Health: a concept analysis. *International Journal of Nursing Studies*, 26 (2), 155–161.

Simon, A.B., Feinleib, M. and Thompson, H.K. (1972) Components of delay in the pre-hospital phase of acute myocardial infarction. *American Journal of Cardiology*, 30, 476–482.

Simoni, J.M., Frick, P., Pantalone, D. and Turner, B.J. (2003) Antiretroviral adherence interventions: a review of current literature and ongoing studies. *Topic HIV Med*, 11, 185–198.

Simons, J., Franck, L. and Roberson, E. (2001) Parent involvement in children's pain care: views of parents and nurses. *Journal of Advanced Nursing*, 36 (4), 591–599.

Simpson, J. (2002) Nursing with dignity. Part 9: Jehovah's Witnesses. *Nursing Times*, 98 (17), 36–37.

Simpson, M., Buckman, R., Stewart, M. and Maguire, P. (1991) Doctor–patient communication: the Toronto consensus statement. *British Medical Journal*, 303, 1385–1387.

Sivanandan, A. (1991) *Deadly Silence: Black Death in Custody*. London: Institution of Race Relations (IRR).

Skinner, B.F. (1956) A case history in scientific method. *American Psychologist*, 11, 221–233.

Slangen, K., Kleemann, P.P. and Krohne, H.W. (1993?) Coping with surgical stress. In Krohne, H.W. (ed.), *Attention and Avoidance: Strategies in Coping with Aversiveness*. Ashland, OH: Hogrefe & Huber Publishers, xiv, 321–346, 363.

Slater, R. (1995) *The Psychology of Growing Old: Looking Forward. Rethinking Ageing*. Buckingham: Open University Press.

Slovic, P. (2000) What does it mean to know a cumulative risk? Adolescents' perceptions of short-term and long-term consequences of smoking. *Journal of Behavioral Decision Making*, 13 (2), 259–266.

Smith, D. (1979) A decade of patient advocacy. *Heart and Lung*, 8 (5), 926–928.

Smith, M. (1975) *When I Say No, I Feel Guilty*. New York: Bantam.

Smith, M. (1998) Who should run intensive care units? *Care of the Critically Ill*, 14, 113–115.

Smith, N.A., Seale, J.P., Ley, P., Shaw, J. and Bracs, P.U. (1986) Effects of intervention on medication compliance in children with asthma. *Med. Journal of Australia*, 144, 119–122.

Smith, P. (1992) *The Emotional Labour of Nursing*. London: MacMillan.

Snelgrove, S. (2006) Factors contributing to poor concordance in health care. *Nursing Times*, 102 (2).

Sosa, R., Kennell, J., Klaus, M., Robertson, S. and Urrutia, J. (1980) The effect of a supportive companion on perinatal problems, length of labor, and mother–infant interaction. *New England Journal of Medicine*, 303 (11), 597–600.

Spanos, N.P. and Katsanis, J. (1989) Effects of instructional set on attributions of nonvolition during hypnotic and nonhypnotic analgesia. *Journal of Personality and Social Psychology*, 56 (2), 182–188.

Spector, R. (1996) *Cultural Diversity in Health and Illness*. Stamford, CT: Appleton and Lange.

Spencer, S.M., Lehman, J.M., Wynings, C., Arena, P., Carver, C.S., Antoni, M.H., Derhagopian, R.P., Ironson, G. and Love, N. (1999) Concerns about breast cancer and relations to psychosocial well-being in a multiethnic sample of early-stage patients. *Health Psychology*, 18 (2), 159–168.

Sperling, G. (1960) The information available in brief visual presentations, *Psychological Monographs*, **74** (11).

Spielberger, C., Gorsuch, R. and Lushene, R. (1977) *STAI Manual for the State-Trait Anxiety Inventory*. Palo Alto, CA: California Consulting Psychologists Press.

Spíndola, T. and Macedo, M. (1994) A morte no hospital e seu significado para os profissionais; The significance of the patients' death in the eyes of health professionals. *Revista Brasileira de Enfermagem*, **47** (2), 108–117.

Spinks, C. (2003) Can written and verbal consultation reduce non-attendance for colonoscopy procedures? *Gastrointestinal Nursing*, **1** (9), 33–39.

Sprague, B.L., Trentham-Dietz, A., Newcomb, P.A., Titus-Ernstoff, L., Hampton, J.M. and Egan, K.M. (2007) Lifetime recreational and occupational physical activity and risk of *in situ* and invasive breast cancer. *Cancer Epidemiology Biomarkers and Prevention*, **16** (2), 236–243.

Sprah, L. and Sostaric, M. (2004) Psychosocial coping strategies in cancer patients. *Radiological Oncology*, **38** (1), 35–42.

Sriwatanakul, K., Weis, O.F., Alloza, J.L., Kelvie, W., Weintraub, M. and Lasagna, L. (1983) Analysis of narcotic usage in the treatment of postoperative pain. *Journal of the American Medical Association*, **250**, 926–929.

Stanton, A.L. (2006) Psychosocial concerns and interventions for cancer survivors. *Journal of Clinical Oncology*, **24**, 5132–5137.

Stanton, N. (1990) *Communication*. London: Macmillan Press Ltd.

Stavraky, K.M., Donner, A.P., Kincade, J.E. and Stewart, M.A. (1988) The effect of psychosocial factors on lung-cancer mortality at one year. *Journal of Clinical Epidemiology*, **41** (1), 75–82.

Stegen, K., Van Diest, I., Van de Woestijne, K.P. and Van den Bergh, O. (2000) Negative affectivity and bodily sensations induced by 5.5% CO_2-enriched air inhalation: is there a bias to interpret bodily sensations negatively in persons with negative affect? *Psychology and Health*, **15**, 513–525.

Stiegelis, H.E., Ranchor, A.V. and Sanderman, R. (2004) Psychological functioning in cancer patients treated with radiotherapy. *Patient Education and Counselling*, **52**, 131–141.

Stirling, L. (2006) Reduction and management of perioperative anxiety. *British Journal of Nursing*, **15** (7), 359–361.

Stockhorst, U., Spennes-Saleh, S., Korholz, D., Gobel, U., Schneider, M.E., Steingruber, H.J. and Klosterhalfen, S. (2000) Anticipatory symptoms and anticipatory immune responses in paediatric cancer patients receiving chemotherapy: features of a classically conditioned response? *Brain Behaviour and Immunity*, **14**, 198–218.

Stockwell, F. (1972) *The Unpopular Patient*. Beckenham: Croom Helm.

Stoddard, J.A., White, K.S., Covino, N.A. and Strauss, L. (2005) Impact of a brief intervention on patient anxiety prior to day surgery. *Journal of Clinical Psychology in Medical Settings*, **12** (2), 99–110.

Stokes, C. (2000) *Challenging Behaviour in Dementia: A Person-centred Approach*. Oxfordshire: Winslow Press.

Stoller, N. (2003) Space, place and movement as aspects of health care in three women's prisons. *Social Science and Medicine*, **56** (11), 2263–2275.

Stone, A.A. and Brownell, K.D. (1994) The stress-eating paradox – multiple daily measurements in adult males and females. *Psychology and Health*, **9** (6), 425–436.

Straker, N. (1998) Psychodynamic psychotherapy for cancer patients. *Journal of Psychotherapy Practice and Research*, **7** (1), 1–9.

Strober, M. (2000) Controlled family study of anorexia nervosa and bulimia nervosa: evidence of shared liability and transmission of partial syndromes. *American Journal of Psychiatry*, **157** (3), 393–401.

Stroebe, M.S. (1998) New directions in bereavement research: exploration of gender differences. *Palliative Medicine*, **12**, 5–12.

Stroebe, W. (2000) *Social Psychology and Health*, 2nd edn. Buckingham: Open University Press.

Strong, P.M. (1979) Sociological imperialism and the profession of medicine – critical-examination of the thesis of medical imperialism. *Social Science & Medicine Part A – Medical Sociology*, **13** (2A), 199–215.

Strydom, A. and Hall, I. (2001) Randomized trial of psychotropic medication information leaflets for people with intellectual disability. *Journal of Intellectual Disability Res*, **45** (pt 2), 146–151.

Stürmer, T., Hasselbach, P. and Amelang, M. (2006) Personality, lifestyle, and risk of cardiovascular disease and cancer: follow-up of population based cohort, *British Medical Journal*, **332** (7554), 1359.

Sue, D.W. (1990) Culture-specific strategies in counselling: a conceptual framework. *Professional Psychology: Research and Practice*, **21** (6), 424–433.

Suls, J. and Wan, C.K. (1989) Effects of sensory and procedural information on coping with stressful medical procedures and pain – a meta analysis. *Journal of Consulting and Clinical Psychology*, **57** (3), 372–379.

Sutherland, J.A. (1993) The nature and evolution of phenomenological empathy in nursing: an historical treatment. *Archive of Psychiatric Nursing*, **7** (6), 369–376.

Sutton, S. (2002) Influencing optimism in smokers by giving information about the average smoker, *Risk, Decision & Policy*, **7** (2), 165–174.

Suzman, R. and Riley, M.W. (1985) Introducing the 'oldest old'. *Milbank Memorial Fund Quarterly: Health and Society*, **63**, 177–185.

Svedberg, P., Jormfeldt, H., Fridlund, B. and Arvidsson, B. (2004) Perceptions of the concept of health among patients in mental health nursing. *Issues in Mental Health Nursing*, **25** (7), 723–736.

Swenson, S.L., Buell, S., Zettler, P., White, M., Ruston, D.C. and Lo, B. (2004) Patient-centered communication: do patients really prefer it? *Journal of General Internal Medicine*, **19** (11), 1069–1079.

Tadd, W., Dieppe, P. and Bayer, T. (2002) Dignity in health care: reality or rhetoric. *Reviews in Clinical Gerontology*, **12**, 1–4.

Tan, G., Waldman, K. and Bostick, R. (2002) Psychosocial issues, sexuality, and cancer. *Sexuality and Disability*, **20** (4), 297–318.

Tanghe, A., Paridaens, R., Evers, G., Vantongelen, K., Aerts, R., Lejeune, M. and Vermeiren, P. (1996) Case study of quality assurance in the administration of chemotherapy. *Cancer Nursing*, **19** (6), 447–454.

Tapper, K., Horne, P.J. and Lowe, C.F. (2003) The Food Dudes to the rescue! *The Psychologist*, **16** (1), 18–21.

Taylor, B.J. (2000) *Reflective Practice: A Guide for Nurses and Midwives*. Buckingham: Open University Press.

Taylor, C. (1997) Problem solving in clinical nursing practice. *Journal of Advanced Nursing*, **26** (2), 329–336.

Thatcher, D.L. and Clark, D.B. (2006) Adolescent alcohol abuse and dependence: development, diagnosis, treatment and outcomes. *Current Psychiatry Reviews*, **2** (1), 159–177.

The Adult Dental Health Survey of 1988. Adult Dental Health Survey: Oral Health in the United Kingdom 1998. Norwich: The Office for National Statistics, TSO.

Thomas, R., Daly, M., Perryman, B. and Stockton, D. (2000) Forewarned is forearmed – benefits of preparatory information on video cassette for patients receiving chemotherapy or radiotherapy – a randomised control trial. *European Journal of Cancer*, **356**, 1536–1543.

Thomas, V., Heath, M., Rose, D. and Flory, P. (1995) Psychological characteristics and the effectiveness of patient-controlled analgesia. *British Journal of Anesthesia*, **74** (3), 271–276.

Thomson, R. and McKenzie, K. (2005) What people with a learning disability understand and feel about having a learning disability. *Learning Disability*, **8** (6), 29–32.

Thorndike, E.L. (1898) Animal intelligence: an experimental study of the associative processes in animals. *Psychological Review Monograph Supplement*, **2** (8).

Tierney, A.J. (1996) Undernutrition and elderly hospital patients: a review. *Journal of Advanced Nursing*, **23**, 228–236.

Timberlake, N., Klinger, K., Smith, P., Venn, G., Treasure, T., Harrison, M. and Newman, S.P. (1997) Incidence and patterns of depression following coronary artery bypass graft surgery. *Journal of Psychosomatic Research*, **43** (2), 197–207.

Timmins, F. and McCabe, C. (2005) How assertive are nurses in the workplace? A preliminary pilot study. *Journal of Nursing Management*, **13** (1), 61–67.

Timms, P. (2001) *Mental Health Information: Older People, Memory and Dementia*. London: Royal College of Psychiatrists.

Tod, A.M., Read, C., Lacey, A. and Abbott, J. (2001) Barriers to uptake of services for coronary heart disease: qualitative study. *British Medical Journal*, **323**, 214–217.

Tosevski, D.L. and Milovancevic, M.P. (2006) Stressful life events and physical health. *Current Opinion in Psychiatry*, **19** (2), 184–189.

Townsend, P. and Davidson, N. (1982) *Inequalities in Health: The Black Report*. London: Penguin.

Trinh, K.V., Phillips, S.D., Ho, E. *et al.* (2004) Acupuncture for the alleviation of lateral epicondyle pain: a systematic review. *Rheumatology*, **43** (9), 1085–1090.

Triplett, N. (1898) The dynamogenic factors in pace making and competition. *American Journal of Psychology*, **9**, 507–533.

Troesch, L.M., Rodehaver, C.B., Delaney, E.A. and Yanes, B. (1993) The influence of guided imagery on chemotherapy-related nausea and vomiting. *Oncology Nursing Forum*, **20** (8), 1179–1185.

Trost, S.G., Sallies, J.F., Pate, R.R., Freedson, P.S., Talor, W.C. and Dowda, M. (2003) Evaluating a model of parental influence on youth physical activity. *American Journal of Preventative Medicine*, **25** (4), 277–282.

Tschuschke, V., Hertenstein, B., Arnold, R., Bunjes, D., Denzinger, R. and Kaechele, H. (2001) Associations between coping and survival time of adult leukemia patients receiving allogeneic bone marrow transplantation: results of a prospective study. *Journal of Psychosomatic Research*, **50** (5), 277–285.

Tuckman, B.W. (1965) Developmental sequences in small groups. *Psychological Bulletin*, **63** (6), 384–399.

Tudor-Hart, J. (1971) The inverse care law. *Lancet*, **1**, 405–412.

Turk, D. (1997) Psychological aspects of pain. In Norris, J. (ed.), *Springhouse Guide to Expert Pain Management*, 124–178. Pennsylvania: Springhouse Corporation.

Turner, P. (1993) Activity nursing and the changes in the quality of life of elderly patients: a semi-quantitative study. *Journal of Advanced Nursing*, **18**, 1727–1733.

Tylor, E. (1920) [1871] *Primitive Culture*. New York: J.P. Putnam's Sons.

Uchino, B.N. (2004) *Social Support and Physical Health: Understanding the Health Consequences of Relationships*. New Haven, CT: Yale University Press.

UKCC (1996) *Guidelines for Professional Practice*. London: United Kingdom Central Council for Nursing, Midwifery and Health Visiting.

UKCC (1999) *Practitioner–Client Relationships and the Prevention of Abuse*. London: UKCC.

UKCC (2002) *The Recognition, Prevention and Therapeutic Management of Violence in Mental Health Care*. Report prepared for the UKCC by the Health Services Research Department, Institute of Psychiatry. London: UKCC.

Ulrich, R.S. (1984) View through a window may help recovery from surgery. *Science*, **224** (4647), 420–421.

UN (1999) United Nations Development Program, Human Development Report 1999. New York: Oxford University Press.

Underman Boggs, K. (2003) In Arnold, E. and Underman Boggs, K., *Interpersonal Relationships. Professional Communication Skills for Nurses*, 4th edn. Missouri: Saunders.

Urberg, K.A., Shyu, S.J. and Liang, J. (1990) Peer influence in adolescent cigarette-smoking. *Addictive Behaviors*, **15** (3), 247–255.

Vaillant, G.E. (1983) *The Natural History of Alcoholism*. Cambridge, MA: Harvard University Press.

Valente, T.W., Unger, J.B. and Johnson, C.A. (2005) Do popular students smoke? The association between popularity and smoking among middle school students. *The Journal of Adolescent Health*, **37** (4), 323–329.

Van Cott, M.L. (1993) Communicative competence during nursing admission interviews of elderly patients in acute care settings. *Qualitative Health Research*, **3** (2), 184–208.

Van den Bosch, J.E., Moons, K., Bonsel, G.J. and Kalkman, C.J. (2005) Does measurement of preoperative anxiety have added value for predicting postoperative nausea and vomiting? *Anesthesia and Analgesia*, **100** (5), 1525–1532.

Van der Smagt-Duijnstee, M., Hamers, J.P. and Abu-Saad, H.H. (2000). Relatives of stroke patients: Their needs and experiences in hospital. *Scandinavian Journal of Caring Sciences*, **14**, 44–51.

Van Hout, H.P.J., Beekman, A.T.F., De Beurs, E., Comijs, H., Van Marwijk, H., De Haan, M., Van Tilburg, W. and Deeg, D.J.H. (2004) Anxiety and the risk of depression in older men and women. *British Journal of Psychiatry*, **185**, 399–404.

van Rossum, C.T.M., Shipley, M.J., van de Mheen, H., Grobbee, D.E. and Marmot, M.G. (2000) Employment grade differences in cause specific mortality. A 25 year follow up of civil servants from the first Whitehall study. *Journal of Epidemiology and Community Health*, **54** (3), 178–184.

Van Werde, D. and Morton, I. (1999) The Relevance of Prouty's Pre-Therapy to Dementia Care. In Morton, I. *Person-Centred Approaches to Dementia Care*, 139–166. Bicester, Oxon: Winslow Press.

Van Zuuren, F.J., de Groot, KL., Mulder, N.L. and Muris, P. (1996) Coping with medical threat: an evaluation of the medical threatening situations inventory (TMSI). *Personality and Individual Differences*, **21** (1), 21–31.

Vargas, P.A. and Rand, C. (1999) A pilot study of electronic adherence monitoring in low-income, minority children with asthma. *American Journal of Respiratory Critical Care Medicine*, **159**, A260.

Varni, J.W., Seid, M. and Kurtin, P.S. (2001) The PedsQL™ 4.0: Reliability and Validity of the Pediatric Quality of Life Inventory™ Version 4.0 Generic Core Scales in healthy and patient populations. *Medical Care*, **39**, 800–812.

Vasudeva, S., Claggett, A.L., Tietjen, G.E. and McGrady, A.V. (2003) Biofeedback-assisted relaxation in migraine headache: relationship to cerebral blood flow velocity in the middle cerebral artery. *Headache: The Journal of Head and Face*, **43** (3), 245–250.

Velicer, W.F., Prochaska, J.O., Bellis, J.M., DiClemente, C.C., Rossi, J.S., Fava, J.L. and Steiger, J.H. (1993) An expert system intervention for smoking cessation. *Addictive Behaviors*, **18** (3), 269–290.

Ventura, S.J., Mathews, T.J. and Curtin, S.C. (1999) Declines in teenage birth rates, 1991–1998: update of national and state trends, *National Vital Statistics Reports*, **47** (26).

Verbrugge, L.M. (1980) Health Diaries. *Medical Care*, **18**, 73–95

Victor, C.R., Healy, J., Thomas, A. and Seargent, J. (2000) Older patients and delayed discharge from hospital. *Health and Social Care in the Community*, 8 (6), 443–452.

Vivar, C.G. and McQueen, A. (2005) Informational and emotional needs of long-term survivors of breast cancer. *Journal of Advanced Nursing*, **51** (5), 520–528.

Volicer, B.J., Isenberg, M.A. and Burns, M.W. (1977) Medical-surgical differences in hospital stress factors. *Journal of Human Stress*, 3 (2), 3–13.

Volicer, L., Seltzer, B., Rheaume, Y. *et al.* (1987) Progression of Alzheimer-type dementia in institutionalised patients: a cross sectional study. *The Journal of Applied Gerontology*, **6**, 183–194.

Von Cranach, M. (1971) The role of orientating behaviour in human interaction. In Esser, A.H. (ed.), *Behaviour and Environment*. New York: Plenum Press.

Von Frey, M. (1894) Beiträge zur Physiologie des Schmerzsinns (2. Mitteilung). *Berichte über die Verhandlungen der Königlich Sächsischen Gesellshaft der Wissenschaften*, **46**, 283–297.

Voogt, E., van Leeuwen, A.F., Visser, A.P., Heide, A. and Maas, P.J. (2005) Information needs of patients with incurable cancer. *Supportive Care in Cancer*, **13** (11), 943–948.

Vygotsky, L.S. (1978) *Mind and Society: The Development of Higher Mental Processes*. Cambridge, MA: Harvard University Press.

Wade, C. and Tavris, C. (2003) *Psychology*, 7th edn. Upper Saddle River, NJ: Pearson Education Inc., Prentice Hall.

Wagner, C.D., Bigatti, S.M. and Storniolo, A.M. (2006) Quality of life of husbands of women with breast cancer. *Psycho-Oncology*, **15** (2), 109–120.

Wai Ming, V.M. (2002) Psychological predictors of marital adjustment in breast cancer patients. *Psychology, Health and Medicine*, **7** (1), 37–51.

Waitzkin, H. (1989) A critical theory of medical discourse. *Journal of Health and Social Behaviour*, **30**, 220–239.

Waldron, I. and Johnson, S. (1976) Why do women live longer than men? *Journal of Human Stress*, 2 (2), 19–30.

Walker, J. (2001) *Control and the Psychology of Health*. Buckingham: Open University Press.

Walker, J. (2002) Caring for patients with a diagnosis of cancer and spinal metastasis disease. *Nursing Standard*, **16** (42), 41–44.

Wallston, B.S., Wallston, K.A., Kaplan, G.D. and Maides, S.A. (1976) Development and validation of the Health Locus of Control (HLC) Scale. *Journal of Consulting and Clinical Psychology*, **44** (4), 580–585.

Wallston, K.A. and Wallston, B.S. (1982) Who is responsible for your health: the construct of health locus of control. In Sanders, G. and Suls, J. (eds), *Social Psychology of Health and Illness*, 65–98. Hillsdale, NJ: Lawrence Erlbaum & Associates.

Wallston, K.A., Wallston, B.S. and DeVellis, R. (1978) Development of the Multidimensional Health Locus of Control (MHLC) scales. *Health Education Monographs*, **6** (2), 160–170.

Walsgrove, H. (1999) A sanctuary from anxiety. *Nursing Standard*, **14** (8), 61.

Walsh, K. (2006) Reason, commonsense and imagination in the service of our shared humanity. *Contemporary Nurse*, **21** (1).

Walsh, K. and Kowanko, I. (2002) Nurses' and patients' perceptions of dignity. *International Journal of Nursing Practice*, **8**, 143–151.

Walsh, M. (1995) The health belief model and use of accident and emergency services by the general public. *Journal of Advanced Nursing*, **22** (4), 694–699.

Walsh, S.R., Manual, J.C. and Avis, N.E. (2005) The impact of breast cancer on younger women's relationships with their partner and children. *Families, Systems, & Health*, **23**, 80–93.

Wardle, J. and Steptoe, A. (2003) Socioeconomic differences in attitudes and beliefs about healthy lifestyles. *Journal of Epidemiology and Community Health*, 57, 440–443.

Wartman, S.A., Morlock, L.L., Malitz, F.E. and Palm, E.A. (1983) Patients' understanding and satisfaction as predictors of compliances. *Medical Care*, **21**, 886–891.

Watkinson, S. and Scott, E. (2004) Managing the care of patients who have visual impairment. *Nursing Times*, 1, 40–42.

Watson, H.E. (1999) Minimal interventions for problem drinkers: a review of the literature. *Journal of Advanced Nursing*, 30 (2), 513–519.

Watson, M., Homewood, J., Haviland, J. and Bliss, J.M. (2005) Influence of psychological response on breast cancer survival: 10-year follow-up of a population-based cohort. *European Journal of Cancer*, **41** (12), 1710–1714.

Watson, P.W.B. and Myers, L.B. (2001) Which cognitive factors predict clinical glove use amongst nurses? *Psychology, Health and Medicine*, 6 (4), 399–409.

Watson, R. (1994) Measuring feeding difficulty in patients with dementia: replication and validation of the EdFED Scale#1. *Journal of Advanced Nursing*, 19, 850–855.

Watson, R. and Deary, I.J. (1997) Feeding difficulty in elderly patients with dementia: confirmatory factor analysis. *International Journal of Nursing Studies*, 34, 405–414.

Waugh, N. and Norman, D.A. (1960) Primary memory. *Psychological Review*, 72, 89–104.

Webb, C. and Hope, K. (1995) What kind of nurses do patients want? *Journal of Clinical Nursing*, 4 (2), 101–108.

Webb-Johnson, A. (1992) *A Cry for Change – An Asian Perspective on Developing Quality Mental Health Care.* London: Confederation of Indian Organisations.

Webster, J. (2002) Teamwork: understanding multi-professional working. *Nursing Older People*, 14 (3), 14–19.

Webster, M.E. (1981) Communication with dying patients. *Nursing Times*, 4, 999–1002.

Weekes, N., Lewis, R., Patel, F., Garrison-Jakel, J., Berger, D.E. and Lupien, S.J. (2006). Examination stress as an ecological inducer of cortisol and psychological responses to stress in undergraduate students. *Stress*, 9 (4), 199–206.

Weinman, J. and Johnston, M. (1988) Stressful medical procedures: an analysis of the effects of psychological interventions and of the stressfulness of the procedures. In Maes, S. *et al.* (eds), *Topics in Health Psychology*. London: John Wiley, 205–217.

Weinstein, N.D. (1983) Reducing unrealistic optimism about illness susceptibility. *Health Psychology*, 2 (1), 11–20.

Weinstein, N.D. (1984) Why it won't happen to me: perceptions of risk factors and susceptibility. *Health Psychology*, 3 (5), 431–457.

Weinstein, N.D. (1987) Unrealistic optimism about susceptibility to health problems: conclusions from a community-wide sample, *Journal of Behavioral Medicine*, 10 (5), 481–500.

Weinstein, N.D., Slovic, P. and Gibson, G. (2004) Accuracy and optimism in smokers' beliefs about quitting. *Nicotine & Tobacco Research*, 6 (Suppl 3), 375–380.

Weinstein, N.D., Slovic, P. and Gibson, G. (2005) Accuracy and optimism in smokers' beliefs about quitting: erratum. *Nicotine & Tobacco Research*, 7 (2), 307.

Weisenberg, M. (1977) Pain and pain control. *Psychological Bulletin*, **84** (5), 1008–1044.

Weiss, M. and Britten, N. (2003) What is concordance? *The Pharmaceutical Journal*, **271**, 493.

Weitoft, G.R. and Rosen, M. (2005) Is perceived nervousness and anxiety a predictor of premature mortality and severe morbidity? A longitudinal follow up of the Swedish survey of living conditions. *Journal of Epidemiological and Community Health*, 59 (9), 1768–1774.

Wellings, K., Field, J., Johnson, A., Wadworth, J. with Bradshaw, S. (1994) *Sexual Behaviour in Britain.* London: Penguin.

Wells, J. and Bowers, L. (2002) How prevalent is violence towards nurses working in general hospitals in the UK? *Journal of Advanced Nursing*, 39 (3), 230–240.

Wells, J.K., Howard, G.S., Nowlin, W.F. and Vargas, M.J. (1986) Presurgical anxiety and postsurgical pain and adjustment – effects of a stress inoculation procedure. *Journal of Consulting and Clinical Psychology*, 54 (6), 831–835.

Wendell Moller, D. (1996) *Confronting Death: Values, Institutions, and Human Mortality.* New York: Oxford University Press.

Werch, C.E., Anzalone, D.M., Brokiewicz, L.M., Felker, J., Carlson, J.M. and Castellon-Vogel, E.A. (1996) An intervention for preventing alcohol use among inner-city middle school students. *Archives of Family Medicine*, 5 (3), 146–152.

Werch, C.E., Pappas, D.M., Carlson, J.M. and DiClemente, C.C. (1999) Six-month outcomes of an alcohol prevention program for inner-city youth. *American Journal of Health Promotion*, 13 (4), 237–240.

Werch, C.E., Owen, D.M., Carlson, J.M., DiClemente, C.C., Edgemon, P. and Moore, M. (2003) One-year follow-up results of the STARS for Families alcohol prevention program. *Health Education Research*, 18 (1), 74–87.

Wessel, J. and Buscher, U. (2002) Denial of pregnancy: population based study. *British Medical Journal*, 324, 458.

Wheeler, P. (2000) Is advocacy at the heart of professional practice? *Nursing Standard*, 14 (36), 39–41.

Whitehead, M. (1992) The concept and principles of equity and health. *International Journal of Health Services*, 22 (3), 429–445.

Whitely, E., Gunnell, D., Dorling, D. and Davey-Smith, G. (1999) Ecological study of social fragmentation, poverty, and suicide. *British Medical Journal*, 319, 1034–1037.

Whittington, R., Shuttleworth, S. and Hill, L. (1996) Violence to staff in a general hospital setting. *Journal of Advanced Nursing*, 24 (2), 326–333.

WHO (1946) Preamble to the Constitution of the World Health Organization as adopted by the International Health Conference, New York, 19–22 June. *Official Records of the World Health Organization*, 2, 100.

WHO (1990) *Cancer Pain Relief and Palliative Care* (World Health Organisation technical report series 804). Geneva: World Health Organization.

WHO (1993) *The ICD-10. The Classification of Mental and Behavioural Disorders*. Geneva: World Health Organization.

WHO (2000) *Report on Infectious Diseases. Overcoming antimicrobial resistance*. Geneva: World Health Organization (http://www.who.int/infectious-disease-report/2000/index.html).

WHO (2006) Gender. Accessed at: http://www.who.int/topics/gender/en/ on 13 December 2007.

WHO (2007) Health statistics and health information. Accessed at: http://www.who.int/healthinfo/morttables/en/index.html on 13 December 2007.

WHOQOL Group (1993) *WHOQOL Measuring Quality of Life*. http://www.who.int/mental_health/media/68.pdf

Whykes, T. (1994) *Violence and Healthcare Professionals*. London: Chapman and Hall.

Whyte, L. (2007) The Team Wheel. *Nursing Management*, **13** (9), 22–24.

Wicker, P. (1995) Pre-operative visiting: making it work. *British Journal of Theatre Nursing*, **5** (7), 16–19.

Wieland, D. (2000) Abuse of older persons: an overview. *Holistic Nursing Practice*, **14** (4), 40–50.

Wikman, A., Marklund, S. and Alexanderson, K. (2005) Illness, disease, and sickness absence: an empirical test of differences between concepts of ill health. *Journal of Epidemiology and Community Health*, **59** (6), 450–454.

Wilkinson, S. (1991) Factors which influence how nurses communicate with cancer patients. *Journal of Advanced Nursing*, **16**, 677–688.

Wilkinson, S., Locker, J., Whybrow, J., Percival, J. and Owen, L. (2004) The nurse's role in promoting smoking cessation. *Nursing Standard*, **19** (14–16), 45–52.

Wilkinson, S., Roberts, A. and Aldridge, J. (1998) Nurse–patient communication in palliative care: an evaluation of a communication skills programme *Palliative Medicine*, **12** (1), 13–22.

Williams, B., Poulter, N.R., Brown, M.J., Davis, M., McInnes, G.T., Potter, J.F., Sever, P.S. and Thorn, S. McG. (2004) Guidelines for management of hypertension: report of the fourth working party of the British Hypertension Society. *Journal of Human Hypertension*, **2004** (18), 139–185.

Williams, D.R. (1995) Primary care for women – the nurse-midwifery-legacy, *Journal of Nurse-Midwifery*, **40** (2), 57–58.

Williams-Piehota, P., Schneider, T.R., Pizarro, J., Mowad, L. and Salovey, P. (2004) Matching health messages to health locus of control beliefs for promoting mammography utilization. *Psychology & Health,* **19** (4), 407–423.

Wilson, K., Gibson, N., Willan, A. and Cook, D. (2000) Effect of smoking cessation on mortality after myocardial infarction – meta-analysis of cohort studies. *Archives of Internal Medicine*, **160** (7), 939–944.

Wilson, R.W., Taliaferro, L.A. and Jacobsen, P.B. (2006) Pilot study of a self-administered stress management and exercise intervention during chemotherapy for cancer. *Supportive Care in Cancer*, **14** (9), 928–935.

Wilson-Barnett, J. and Batehup, L. (1988) *Patient Problems: A Research Base for Nursing Care*. London: Scutari Press.

Wimberly, S.R., Carver, C.S., Laurenceau, J.P., Harris, S.D. and Antoni, M.H. (2005) Perceived partner reactions to diagnosis and treatment of breast cancer: Impact on psychosocial and psychosexual adjustment. *Journal of Consulting and Clinical Psychology*, **73** (2), 300–311.

Wing, J.K., Marriott, S., Palmer, C. and Thomas, V. (1998) *The Management of Imminent Violence: Clinical Practice Guidelines to Support Mental Health Services*. Occasional Paper OP41. London: Royal College of Psychiatrists.

Wolf, M.H., Putnam, S.M., James, S.A. and Stiles, W.B. (1978) The Medical Interview Satisfaction Scale: development of a scale to measure patient perceptions physician behaviour. *Journal of Behaviour Medicine*, **1**, 391–401.

Wong, D.L., Hockenberry-Eaton, M., Wilson, D., Winkelstein, M.L. and Schwartz, P. (2001) *Wong's Essentials of Pediatric Nursing*, 6th edn, St. Louis: Mosby.

Wood, B. (1999) Deaf patients in the OR: a mile in someone else's shoes. *Today's Surgical Nurse*, **21** (3), 34–36.

Woollard, J., Beilin, L., Lord, T., Puddey, I., MacAdam, D. and Rouse, I. (1995) A controlled trial of nurse counselling on lifestyle change for hypertensives treated in general practice: preliminary results. *Clinical and Experimental Pharmacology and Physiology*, **22** (6–7), 466–468.

Workman, E.A. and La Via, M.F. (1987) T-lymphocyte polyclonal proliferation: effects of stress and stress response style on medical students taking national board examinations. *Clinical Immunology and Immunopathology*, **43** (3), 308–313.

Wu, A. (2001) Report from Buenos Aires: lessons in adherence. *Hopkins HIV Report*, **13** (5), 9–11.

Yang, M.H. and Mcilfatrick, S. (2001) Intensive care nurses' experiences of caring for dying patients: a phenomological study. *International Journal of Palliative Nursing*, **7** (9), 435–441.

Yarbrough, S.S. and Braden, C.J. (2001) Utility of health belief model as a guide for explaining or predicting breast cancer screening behaviours. *Journal of Advanced Nursing*, **33** (5), 677–688.

Yeandle, S. and Macmillan, R. (2003) The role of health in labour market detachment. In Alcock, P., Beatty, C., Fothergill, S., Macmillan, R. and Yeandle, S., *Work to Welfare: How Men Become Detached from the Labour Force*. Cambridge: Cambridge University Press, Ch. 8.

Yeates, S. (1995) The incidence and importance of hearing loss in people with severe learning disabilities: the evolution of a service, *British Journal of Learning Disability*, **23**, 79–84.

Yehuda, R. and McEwen, B. (2004) Biobehavioral stress response – protective and damaging effects – introduction. *Annals of the New York Academy of Sciences*, **1032**, XI–XVI.

Zajonc, R.B. (1965) Social facilitation. *Science,* **149**, 269–274.

Zaza, C. and Baine, N. (2002) Cancer pain and psychosocial factors: a critical review of the literature. *Journal of Pain and Symptom Management*, **24** (5), 526–542.

Zborowski, M. (1952) Cultural components in response to pain. *Journal of Social Issues*, **8** (4), 16–30.

Zimmermann, T., Heinrichs, N. and Baucom, D.H. (2007) Does One Size Fit All? Moderators in Psychosocial Interventions for Breast Cancer Patients: A Meta-Analysis. *Annals of Behavioural Medicine*, **34** (3), 225–239.

Zucker, R.A. and Wong, M.M. (2005) Prevention for children of alcoholics and other high risk groups. *Recent Developments in Alcoholism*, **17**, 299–320.

Zvara, D., Manning, M., Stewart, T., McKinley, A.C. and Cran, W. (1994) Pre-operative anaesthetic concerns: perceptions versus reality in men and women. *Anesthesiology*, **81** (3A).

Index